THE ROUTLEDGE COMPANION TO PAKISTANI ANGLOPHONE WRITING

The Routledge Companion to Pakistani Anglophone Writing forms a theoretical, comprehensive, and critically astute overview of the history and future of Pakistani literature in English. Dealing with key issues for global society today, from terrorism, religious extremism, fundamentalism, corruption, and intolerance, to matters of love, hate, loss, belongingness, and identity conflicts, this *Companion* brings together over thirty essays by leading and emerging scholars, and presents:

- the transformations and continuities in Pakistani anglophone writing since its inauguration in 1947 to today;
- contestations and controversies that have not only informed creative writing but also subverted certain stereotypes in favour of a dynamic representation of Pakistani Muslim experiences;
- a case for a Pakistani canon through a critical perspective on how different writers and their works have, at different times, both consciously and unconsciously, helped to realise and extend a uniquely Pakistani idiom.

Providing a comprehensive yet manageable introduction to cross-cultural relations and to historical, regional, local, and global contexts that are essential to reading Pakistani anglophone literature, *The Routledge Companion to Pakistani Anglophone Writing* is key reading for researchers and academics in Pakistani anglophone literature, history, and culture. It is also relevant to other disciplines such as terror studies, post-9/11 literature, gender studies, postcolonial studies, feminist studies, human rights, diaspora studies, space and mobility studies, religion, and contemporary South Asian literatures and cultures.

Aroosa Kanwal is Assistant Professor in English Literature at International Islamic University, Pakistan. She is an author of *Rethinking Identities in Contemporary Pakistani Fiction: Beyond 9/11* (2015), which was awarded the KLF-Coca-Cola award for the best non-fiction book of the year in 2015.

Saiyma Aslam is Assistant Professor in English Literature at International Islamic University, Pakistan. She is a researcher in postcolonial studies and English literature, with a focus on travelling theory, mobility, globalisation, and Islamic feminism. She is the author of *From Stasis to Mobility: Arab Muslim Feminists and Travelling Theory* (2017).

ROUTLEDGE COMPANIONS TO LITERATURE SERIES

Also available in this series:

The Routledge Companion to Anglophone Caribbean Literature
Also available in paperback

The Routledge Companion to Asian American and Pacific Islander Literature
Also available in paperback

The Routledge Companion to the Environmental Humanities

The Routledge Companion to Experimental Literature
Also available in paperback

The Routledge Companion to Inter-American Studies

The Routledge Companion to International Children's Literature

The Routledge Companion to Latino/a Literature
Also available in paperback

The Routledge Companion to Literature and Human Rights

The Routledge Companion to Literature and Religion

The Routledge Companion to Literature and Science
Also available in paperback

The Routledge Companion to Native American Literature

The Routledge Companion to Picturebooks

The Routledge Companion to Science Fiction
Also available in paperback

The Routledge Companion to Travel Writing

The Routledge Companion to World Literature
Also available in paperback

The Routledge Companion to Pakistani Anglophone Writing

For further information on this series visit: www.routledge.com/literature/series/RC4444

THE ROUTLEDGE COMPANION TO PAKISTANI ANGLOPHONE WRITING

Edited by Aroosa Kanwal and Saiyma Aslam

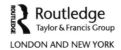

LONDON AND NEW YORK

First published 2019
by Routledge
2 Park Square, Milton Park, Abingdon, Oxon OX14 4RN

and by Routledge
711 Third Avenue, New York, NY 10017

Routledge is an imprint of the Taylor & Francis Group, an informa business

© 2019 selection and editorial matter, Aroosa Kanwal and Saiyma Aslam; individual chapters, the contributors

The right of Aroosa Kanwal and Saiyma Aslam to be identified as the authors of the editorial material, and of the authors for their individual chapters, has been asserted in accordance with sections 77 and 78 of the Copyright, Designs and Patents Act 1988.

All rights reserved. No part of this book may be reprinted or reproduced or utilised in any form or by any electronic, mechanical, or other means, now known or hereafter invented, including photocopying and recording, or in any information storage or retrieval system, without permission in writing from the publishers.

Trademark notice: Product or corporate names may be trademarks or registered trademarks, and are used only for identification and explanation without intent to infringe.

British Library Cataloguing-in-Publication Data
A catalogue record for this book is available from the British Library

Library of Congress Cataloging-in-Publication Data
Names: Kanwal, Aroosa, 1974– editor. | Aslam, Saiyma, editor.
Title: The Routledge companion to Pakistani Anglophone writing /
edited by Aroosa Kanwal and Saiyma Aslam.
Description: London ; New York, NY : Routledge, 2018. |
Series: Routledge companions to literature series |
Includes bibliographical references and index.
Identifiers: LCCN 2018016204 | ISBN 9781138745520 (hardback) |
ISBN 9781315180618 (e-book)
Subjects: LCSH: Pakistani literature (English)–20th century–History and criticism. |
Pakistani literature (English)–21st century–History and criticism. |
Pakistani literature (English)–Great Britain–History and criticism.
Classification: LCC PR9540 .R68 2018 | DDC 820.9/95491–dc23
LC record available at https://lccn.loc.gov/2018016204

ISBN: 978-1-138-74552-0 (hbk)
ISBN: 978-1-315-18061-8 (ebk)

Typeset in Bembo
by Out of House Publishing

CONTENTS

Notes on contributors ix
Acknowledgements xv

    Introduction 1
    Aroosa Kanwal and Saiyma Aslam

PART I
Reimagining history: the legacy of war and partition 11

1 'All these angularities': spatialising non-Muslim Pakistani identities 13
   Cara Cilano

2 1971: reassessing a forgotten national narrative 22
   Muneeza Shamsie

3 History, borders, and identity: dealing with silenced memories of 1971 35
   Daniela Vitolo

PART II
9/11 and beyond: contexts, forms, and perspectives 47

4 Global Pakistan in the wake of 9/11 49
   Ulka Anjaria

5 Pakistani inoutsiders and the dynamics of post-9/11 dissociation in Pakistani anglophone fiction 58
   Claudia Nördinger

Contents

6 The nuclear novel in Pakistan 68
 Michaela M. Henry

7 Uses of humour in post-9/11 Pakistani anglophone fiction:
 H.M. Naqvi's *Home Boy* and Mohammed Hanif's
 A Case of Exploding Mangoes 80
 Ambreen Hai

8 Comic affiliations/comic subversions: the use of humour in
 contemporary British-Pakistani fiction 94
 Sarah Ilott

9 Resistance and redefinition: theatre of the Pakistani diaspora
 in the UK and the US 106
 Suhaan Mehta

10 Historiographic metafiction and renarrating history 116
 Nisreen T. Yousef

PART III
The dialectics of human rights: politics, positionality, controversies 125

11 Pakistani fiction and human rights 127
 Esra Mirze Santesso

12 Divergent discourses: human rights and contemporary Pakistani
 anglophone literature 138
 Shazia Sadaf

13 The taming of the tribal within Pakistani narratives of progress,
 conflict, and romance 151
 Uzma Abid Ansari

14 Phoenix rising: the West's use (and misuse) of anglophone
 memoirs by Pakistani women 162
 Colleen Lutz Clemens

15 Writing back and/as activism: refiguring victimhood and
 remapping the shooting of Malala Yousafzai 172
 Rachel Fox

PART IV
Identities in question: shifting perspectives on gender — 183

16 Doing history right: challenging masculinist postcolonialism in Pakistani anglophone literature — 185
Fawzia Afzal-Khan

17 Love, sex, and desire vs Islam in British Muslim literature — 200
Kavita Bhanot

18 Transgressive desire, everyday life, and the production of 'modernity' in Pakistani anglophone fiction — 213
Mosarrap Hossain Khan

PART V
Spaces of female subjectivity: identity, difference, agency — 223

19 Agency, gender, nationalism, and the romantic imaginary in Pakistan — 225
Abu-Bakar Ali

20 Conjugal homes: marriage culture in contemporary novels of the Pakistani diaspora — 236
Rahul K. Gairola and Elham Fatma

21 British-Pakistani female playwrights: feminist perspectives on sexuality, marriage, and domestic violence — 248
Aqeel Abdulla

PART VI
Shifting contexts: new perspectives on identity, space, and mobility — 259

22 Identifying Islamic spaces of worship in contemporary British-Pakistani Muslim life writing — 261
Georgia Stabler

23 Homes and belonging(s): the interconnectedness of space, movement, and identity in British-Pakistani novels — 274
Éva Pataki

24 Committed and communist: negotiating political allegiances in the diaspora — 285
Miquel Pomar-Amer

PART VII
Unsettling narratives: imagining post-postcolonial perspectives   295

25 Non-human narrative agency: textual sedimentation in Pakistani
    anglophone literature   297
    Asma Mansoor

26 Post-postcolonial experiments with perspectives   307
    Hanji Lee

27 Peripheral modernism and realism in British-Pakistani fiction   318
    Asher Ghaffar

PART VIII
New horizons: Towards a Pakistani idiom   333

28 'Brand Pakistan': global imaginings and national concerns in
    Pakistani anglophone literature   335
    Barirah Nazir, Nicholas Holm, and Kim L. Worthington

29 Competing habitus: national expectations, metropolitan market,
    and Pakistani writing in English (PWE)   348
    Masood Ashraf Raja

30 De/reconstructing identities: critical approaches to contemporary
    Pakistani anglophone fiction   360
    Faisal Nazir

31 On the wings of 'poesy': pakistani diaspora poets and the
    'Pakistani idiom'   370
    Waseem Anwar

32 Brand Pakistan: the case for a Pakistani anglophone literary canon 381
    Aroosa Kanwal and Saiyma Aslam

Index   *394*

CONTRIBUTORS

Aqeel Abdulla is an associate lecturer in drama at the University of Exeter, a visiting lecturer in human geography also at Exeter, and a drama facilitator at acta community theatre company in Bristol. He received his PhD in Drama in 2016 from Exeter. The title of his PhD dissertation was *Representations of Muslim Women in Contemporary British Theatre*. He also received his MA degree from Exeter in 2010, his MA dissertation was titled *Representations of Arabs in Contemporary British Theatre*. He is currently developing a practice-led research project on refugee theatre in the UK. Aqeel is a Syrian national born in Saudi Arabia, and has been living in the UK since 2009.

Fawzia Afzal-Khan is University Distinguished Scholar and Professor of English at Montclair State University, where she was Director of Gender, Sexuality, and Women's Studies for six years. She has published five books, including a memoir about growing up in Pakistan, is a published poet and playwright, as well as a trained vocalist in Indo-Pakistani classical music. She has been the recipient of several awards and fellowships, including the Fulbright-Hays, the National Endowment of the Humanities, the American Institute of Pakistan Studies, The Rotary, and the W.E.B. Dubois fellowship at Harvard University.

Abu-Bakar Ali was awarded a doctorate in September 2012. His thesis, entitled *Agency and its Discontents: Nationalism and Gender in the Work of Pakistani Women Writers*, explored the work produced by Pakistani women writers, from the moment the country was 'created' sixty years ago, to present-day diasporic texts. His research interests lie in the field of postcolonial literature, specifically the work of Pakistani writers. He explores the extent to which contemporary theorisations within postcolonial studies of agency, performativity, and the politics of sexual and particularly gendered identities can be employed to approach such a diverse body of work.

Ulka Anjaria is Associate Professor of English at Brandeis University, Massachusetts. She is the author of *Realism in the Twentieth-Century Indian Novel: Colonial Difference and Literary Form* (Cambridge University Press, 2012) and *Reading India Now: Contemporary Formations in Literature and Popular Culture* (Temple University Press, 2019), and editor of *A History of the Indian Novel in*

English (Cambridge University Press, 2015). She has also published articles on literature in *The Boston Review, Scroll.in* and *Public Books*.

Uzma Abid Ansari is a PhD fellow at the Amsterdam School for Cultural Analysis (ASCA), a research school of the Faculty of Humanities at the University of Amsterdam. Her PhD dissertation is on *Orhan Pamuk's City and the Turkish Republic: An Engagement with the Nation State*. Her areas of interest include the cross-pollination of arts and culture in West and Central Asia, nomadism, postcolonialism, decolonisation, and orientalism among others. She is currently a teaching research associate at the International Islamic University Islamabad.

Waseem Anwar is Professor of English and Former Dean of Humanities and Former Chairperson (English), Forman Christian College (A Chartered University) Lahore, Pakistan; a member of the Executive Committee, SALA (South Asian Literary Association, USA); and has been a President of PUAN (Pak-US Alumni Network) Lahore. He has twice been a Fulbright Fellow (1995 for doctoral and 2007 for postdoctoral research) and a Gale Group *American Scholar*. He received the HEC 'Best Teacher Award – 2003' and the Pakistan Punjab Education Department 'Salam Teacher Award – 2004'. He is the author of *'Black' Women's Dramatic Discourse* (VDM Verlag, 2009) and in 2010 was co-guest editor of *South Asian Review* 31(3) on Pakistani creative writing. He is a member of the advisory and editorial boards of several literary journals and has numerous national and international publications and conference presentations.

Saiyma Aslam is Assistant Professor in English Literature at International Islamic University, Pakistan, where she teaches modern drama, modern fiction, postcolonial literatures, globalisation, and South Asian literature. She is a researcher in postcolonial studies and English literature, with a focus on travelling theory, mobility, globalisation, and Islamic feminism. She is the author of *From Stasis to Mobility: Arab Muslim Feminists and Travelling Theory* (Oxford University Press, 2017). She has published essays within the broader spectrum of feminist ethnography and the intersections of Arab feminism, travelling theory, nation, and self. Her most recent research interests include connections between the Arab world and South Asia in women's writing.

Kavita Bhanot's fiction, non-fiction, and reviews have been published and broadcast widely. She is editor of the anthology *Too Asian, Not Asian Enough* (Tindal Street Press, 2011) and the forthcoming *Book of Birmingham* (Comma Press, 2018), and co-editor of the first *Bare Lit Anthology* (Brain Mill Press, 2017). She has a PhD from Manchester University, is a reader and mentor with The Literary Consultancy, and is an Honorary Fellow at Leicester University.

Cara Cilano is Professor and Chair of the Department of English at Michigan State University in the United States. She has published several monographs and more than a dozen journal articles and chapters on Pakistani anglophone literature.

Colleen Lutz Clemens is Associate Professor of Non-Western literatures and Director of Women's and Gender Studies at Kutztown University. She is a regular contributor to the Teaching Tolerance project and has overseen dozens of author entries for the Contemporary Literary Criticism series. Her work on gender in postcolonial contexts has been published in several peer-reviewed journals. She is the co-host of the feminist podcast Inside254.

Elham Fatma is a PhD candidate in English within the Department of Humanities & Social Sciences at the Indian Institute of Technology Roorkee, India. She focuses on gender and trauma in contemporary Kashmiri novels. She was a Fulbright Scholar at Davis & Elkins College, USA, and holds an MA in English from Aligarh Muslim University (AMU), where she won the Gold Medal for achieving the highest marks in her cohort. She has more than two years of undergraduate teaching at AMU, and also teaches at IIT Roorkee. She has written and published on issues including the Qur'an bride, matriarchy, marriage, diaspora, and rape epidemics. Her areas of interest include trauma literature, South Asian fiction, feminist studies, and Partition literature.

Rachel Fox is an associate lecturer and research student in the Department of English Literature and Creative Writing at Lancaster University. Her research interests include post-9/11 literature, postcolonial feminisms; Muslim women's writing, representations of Western Asia and the Middle East, and the relationship between written text and visual media. Her article 'Capturing Iraq: Optical Focalization in Contemporary War Cinematography' has recently been published in *Interventions*.

Rahul K. Gairola is the Krishna Somers Lecturer in English & Postcolonial Literature, School of Arts, and Fellow of the Asia Research Centre, at Murdoch University, Perth, Australia. He is the author of *Homelandings: Postcolonial Diasporas & Transatlantic Belonging* (Rowman & Littlefield, 2016), and co-editor of *Revisiting India's Partition: New Essays in Memory, Culture, & Politics* (Lexington, 2016). He is an article editor for *Postcolonial Text*, and serves as a manuscript reviewer for a number of reputable journals and presses. His fellowships include a DAAD at Leipzig University; a Macmillan Center fellowship at Yale University; the Pembroke Fellowship at Cambridge University; an SCT fellowship at Cornell University; two writing fellowships at the Simpson Center for the Humanities; a Mellon fellowship at the University of Washington, Bothell; and a graduate fellowship at the University of Washington, Seattle. In addition to teaching at the latter two institutions, he has also taught at Rhode Island College; Cornish College of the Arts; Seattle University; the University of Maryland, Baltimore County; Queens College and York College of The City University of New York; and the Indian Institute of Technology Roorkee, India. He holds a joint PhD in English literature and theory and criticism from the University of Washington, Seattle.

Asher Ghaffar is a PhD candidate in Social and Political Thought at York University. Asher is the editor of the Routledge anthology, *History, Imperialism, Critique: New Essays in World Literature* (2018). His research monograph, *Muslims in World Literature: Political Philosophy and Continental Thought*, is forthcoming with Routledge in 2019. In addition to working as a coordinator of a writing centre, Asher is also completing a second poetry collection.

Ambreen Hai is Professor of English Language and Literature at Smith College, USA, where she teaches anglophone postcolonial literature from South Asia, Africa, and the Caribbean; literature of the British Empire; literary theory; and women's and gender studies. She is the author of *Making Words Matter: The Agency of Colonial and Postcolonial Literature* (Ohio University Press, 2009), and of many scholarly articles and book chapters on postcolonial and transnational writing. She is currently writing a book titled *Postcolonial Servitude: Domestic Servants in Contemporary Transnational and South Asian English Fiction*.

Michaela M. Henry is Assistant Professor of Literary and Cultural Studies at FLAME University, Pune, India. She received her PhD from Brandeis University, Massachusetts in 2017, and her current project in progress, *Narrative's Nuclear Spring: The South Asian Novel* *after the Nuclear Bomb*, explores the twinned South Asian history of nuclear armament and the anglophone novel.

Nicholas Holm is a senior lecturer in the School of English & Media Studies, Massey University, New Zealand. He specialises in cultural studies, in particular the role of humour as an aesthetic category, and the interrelation of aesthetic theory, political economics, and popular culture. He is the author of *Advertising and Consumer Society* (Palgrave, 2017) and *Humour as Politics* (Palgrave, 2017).

Sarah Ilott is a lecturer in literature and film at Manchester Metropolitan University, UK. Her main research and teaching interests are in postcolonial literature and genre fiction. She has published a monograph, *New Postcolonial British Genres: Shifting the Boundaries* (Palgrave, 2015) and an edited collection with Chloe Buckley, *Telling it Slant: Critical Approaches to Helen Oyeyemi* (Sussex Academic Press, 2017). Her publications also include multiple book chapters and journal articles in *The Journal of Commonwealth Literature*, *The Journal of Postcolonial Writing*, and *Postcolonial Text*. She serves on the editorial board of *Postcolonial Text*.

Aroosa Kanwal is Assistant Professor in English Literature at International Islamic University, Pakistan. She is the author of *Rethinking Identities in Contemporary Pakistani Fiction: Beyond 9/11* (Palgrave, 2015), which was awarded the KLF-Coca-Cola award for the best non-fiction book of the year 2015. Her current research interests include post-9/11 constructions of Muslims and Islam in relation to Islamophobic discourse, politics of representation, and questions of migration, identity, and resistance in contemporary Pakistani anglophone fiction. Her chapters on these connections can be found in Claire Chambers and Caroline Herbert (eds.), *Imagining Muslims in South Asia and the Diaspora* (Routledge, 2014) and Daniel Meyer-Dinkgräfe (ed.), *Consciousness, Theatre, Literature and the Arts* (Cambridge Scholars, 2012).

Mosarrap Hossain Khan is Assistant Professor at Lovely Professional University, Punjab, India. He obtained his doctorate from the Department of English, New York University, USA. He is a founding editor at *Café Dissensus* magazine.

Hanji Lee is a PhD candidate at Western University (London, Canada). Her main research interest is metafictional narratives that are self-consciously experimental. Her present dissertation project examines the late Victorian adventure fiction of Robert Louis Stevenson, Rudyard Kipling, and Joseph Conrad as nostalgic rewritings of the adventure tradition. She examines nostalgia in their texts as a form of metafictionality.

Asma Mansoor is an assistant professor in the Department of English at the International Islamic University, Islamabad, Pakistan. She is currently pursuing a PhD degree in English Literature. Her research papers have been published in international journals including *Asiatic*, *New Writing: The International Journal for the Theory and Practice of Creative Writing*, *South Asian Review*, *Curriculum Inquiry*, and *Palgrave Communications*.

Suhaan Mehta was born and raised in Mumbai. He is currently an assistant professor in the English Department at the University of Colorado, Colorado Springs. He works on postcolonial literature and cinema with a particular focus on South Asia. He has published scholarly articles on Indian and Pakistani anglophone novels and comics. He has taught a range of undergraduate courses in composition, literature, and film at Case Western Reserve University, the Ohio State University, and St. Xavier's College, Mumbai.

Notes on Contributors

Barirah Nazir is a lecturer at the University of Sargodha, Punjab, Pakistan and is currently completing her PhD studies at Massey University, New Zealand. Her doctoral research focuses on the global reception of Pakistani anglophone fiction. Her research interests are postcolonial studies, literary commodification, and language preservation/revitalisation.

Faisal Nazir is an assistant professor at the Department of English, University of Karachi, where he teaches courses in literary theory and criticism, postcolonial literature and criticism, and world literature. His research interests are mainly in Pakistani anglophone fiction and its critical reception around the world, but also include the relation between religion, culture, and literature, and generally academic study of literature in the twenty-first century. His doctoral thesis analysed the influence of orientalism on fictional representations of Islam in post-9/11 Pakistani anglophone fiction. He is currently working on the possibility of developing a specifically Pakistani Muslim literary-critical discourse based on Pakistani sources.

Claudia Nördinger currently teaches English as a foreign language and works as a translator in Frankfurt am Main, Germany. She has previously been associated with anglophone studies departments at the universities of Frankfurt, Duisburg-Essen, and Stuttgart where she taught courses on anglophone literature and film. She has contributed to the 'Cities and Cultures' programme at Amsterdam University College, where her classes dealt with the global city and literatures of exclusion. For her study on US-American inoutside perspectives in globalised anglophone literatures, she received a PhD from the University of Duisburg-Essen. Her research interests include globalised anglophone studies, anti-Americanism, transculturality, cosmopolitanism, fundamentalism, literary adaptation, film narratology, literary translation, and EFL didactics.

Éva Pataki is an assistant lecturer at the Institute of Modern Philology at the University of Miskolc, Hungary. She defended her doctoral dissertation – *Space, Movement and Identity in Contemporary British Asian Fiction* – in 2015. Her field of interest includes the literature, film, and culture of the British-Asian diaspora, as well as postcolonial literature, cultural identity studies, and gender studies. She has published two book chapters (in *Cultural Imprints in the Age of Globalization: Writing Region and Nation*, 2012, and *Space, Gender and the Gaze in Literature and Art*, 2017) as well as essays and reviews about British-Asian fiction in *The AnaChronisT* and the *Hungarian Journal of English and American Studies*, among others.

Miquel Pomar-Amer has been an associate lecturer at the University of the Balearic Islands since 2015. He completed his PhD in the University of Manchester with a dissertation that compared a selection of novels and autobiographical works written by British-Pakistani and Catalan-Moroccan authors. His research interests include the representation of identity in literature, especially in postcolonial contexts of migration and diaspora, the ethical and political relations between text and context, and the representation of the encounter between locals and tourists in works set in the Mediterranean. He has given presentations at several conferences on these topics and his research has been published as articles and book chapters. He is currently working on romantic novels set in the Balearic Islands within the research project HER (FFI-2016 75130-P, AEI/FEDER, UE).

Masood Ashraf Raja is an associate professor of English at University of North Texas and the editor of *Pakistaniaat: A Journal of Pakistan Studies*. He is the author of *The Religious Right and the Talibanization of America* (Palgrave, 2016) and *Constructing Pakistan* (Oxford University Press, 2010).

Notes on Contributors

Shazia Sadaf teaches Human Rights and Social Justice in the Institute of Interdisciplinary Studies at Carleton University, Ottawa, Canada. Her research interest lies in the intersectional areas of War on Terror Studies, human rights discourse, and post-9/11 anglophone literature. She has had articles published in *Interventions: International Journal of Postcolonial Studies, South Asian History and Culture, ARIEL: A Review of International English Literature,* and *The European Journal of English Studies*. She is currently working on the manuscript of her book on human rights and Pakistani literature.

Esra Mirze Santesso is Associate Professor in the Department of English at the University of Georgia. Her book *Disorientation: Muslim Identity in Contemporary Anglophone Literature* (Palgrave Macmillan, 2013) investigates displaced Muslim women as they negotiate their identities in their adopted homes in the West. Her co-edited collection *Islam and Postcolonial Literature* (Routledge, 2017) includes essays that examine Islam as a significant and complex component of postcolonial identity. Esra's articles have appeared in numerous edited collections and journals, including *Recherche Littéraire/Literary Research, The Comparatist, Postcolonial Text,* and *Postcolonial Intervention*. An interview she conducted with Orhan Pamuk appeared in *PMLA*.

Muneeza Shamsie's extensive writings on Pakistani anglophone literature include the literary history, *Hybrid Tapestries: The Development of Pakistani Literature in English* (Oxford University Press, 2017). She is Bibliographic Representative (Pakistan) for *The Journal of Commonwealth Literature*, and serves on the International Advisory Board of *The Journal of Postcolonial Writing* and the Advisory Committee of the DSC Prize for South Asian Literature. In 2009–2011 she was the Regional Chairperson (Eurasia) of the Commonwealth Writers' Prize.

Georgia Stabler is a postgraduate researcher specialising in postcolonial texts and theory and literary studies at Nottingham Trent University. Her doctoral work is concerned with the representation of literary texts by black, Asian, minority ethnic (BAME) British writers at UK literature festivals. Her research interests include literary marketplaces, literary cultures, postcolonial and neocolonial contexts, black British writing, life writing, and texts by and from the South Asian and African diaspora. Georgia's PhD is supported by the AHRC-funded Midlands3Cities Doctoral Training Partnership.

Daniela Vitolo holds a PhD from the Department of Literary, Linguistic, and Comparative Studies of the University of Naples 'L'Orientale'. Her research is focused on Pakistani anglophone literature and she is interested in discourses concerning the representation of Pakistani identity both within Pakistani society and among diasporas. She is author of the essay 'Relocating the Memory of the Partition in Bapsi Sidhwa's *Defend Yourself Against Me*'. Other works have appeared in *Transnational Literature, Anglistica,* and *Quaderni della ricerca*.

Kim L. Worthington is a senior lecturer in the School of English and Media Studies, Massey University, New Zealand. Her research interests include contemporary global fiction (notably from South Asia and South Africa), subjectivity, narratology, and narrative ethics. She is the author of *Self as Narrative: Subjectivity and Community in Contemporary Fiction* (Clarendon, 1996) and has published book chapters and journal articles on a wide range of contemporary fiction.

Nisreen T. Yousef is an Assistant Professor at the Department of English at Middle East University, Jordan, where she teaches a variety of courses on English literature. Dr Yousef is currently the Director of Language and Translation Centre at MUE. Her research interest focuses on postcolonial and historical literature. She was awarded her PhD from the University of Leicester, in 2017.

ACKNOWLEDGEMENTS

It is with warm heart and sincere gratitude that we extend our thanks to those who have supported us during this endeavour, and who have made it possible for us to complete this ambitious book. We are immensely grateful to our brilliant contributors whose scholarship and deeply probing chapters introduced us to some new aspects of Pakistani anglophone writing, as they will most likely do for you.

Special thanks are due to Polly Dodson at Routledge for commissioning the Companion and to Zoe Meyer and Elizabeth Cox for their patient assistance at every stage of the project. We would like to make special acknowledgement of the extraordinary assistance provided by the production team, Fiona Hudson and Liz Davey, and in particular our copy-editor Alwyn Harrison.

Claire Chambers, Cara Cilano, and Charles Altieri have been very generous in their advice on the concluding chapter. Our thanks to Sarah Ilott for her suggestions and insights on various occasions.

Our gratitude goes to Professor Mohammad Bashir Khan, Vice President, Academics and Professor Munawar Gondal, Dean Faculty of Languages and Literature, International Islamic University, for their timely support and encouragement throughout this project. We would like to acknowledge the intellectual investment of our mentor Prof. S.M.A. Rauf, which has enormously shaped our writing over the years. He has taught us more than we could ever give him credit for here.

We are grateful to our families for their love and support over the years and we dedicate this book to their long-suffering support.

INTRODUCTION

Aroosa Kanwal and Saiyma Aslam

In 'Poetry, Pakistani Idiom in English, and the Groupies', Alamgir Hashmi reminds us that:

> the proponents of the idea of a Pakistani idiom are not only interested in certain literary techniques but also try to assume an active role in the politics of culture [...] to decide who is a Pakistani writer [...] The matter should thus make one raise questions not only about a Pakistani idiom in English but also about 'Pakistaniness': what constitutes this, that, and the other? And who may best exemplify these?
>
> (1990: 268–271)

In keeping with Hashmi's dynamic way of thinking about the artistic and the political, this Companion aims to conceptually organise representations by and of Pakistani Muslims by focusing on the theories, themes, and methodologies distinctive to the study of Pakistani anglophone literature and related cultural productions since 1947. In so doing, it rehearses the ways in which literary critics and international and multigenerational groups of scholars of Pakistani anglophone writing have scrutinised and analysed shifts in foci over the decades in order to foreground the continuities and transformations within this trajectory of Pakistani anglophone writing since its inauguration in 1947. Literature produced by writers of Pakistani origin, both at home and in the diaspora, is not seen merely as aesthetic objects created in isolation, but as cultural products tremendously influenced and constrained by national and international religious and political grievances and the sociopolitical circumstances of their times, as well as by geographical and environmental factors.

The last two decades have witnessed an extraordinary blossoming of fiction, poetry, drama, and life writings by writers of Pakistani origin who have been prominent not only on bestseller lists but also when prestigious literary awards have been announced such as the Orange Prize, the DSC prize, the Booker Prize, the Windham-Campbell Literature Prize, or the Nobel Prize. And the fact that their works now appear in numerous university syllabi underscores the timeliness of this volume. What makes Pakistani anglophone literature all the more appealing as a subject for serious academic pursuit is its critical and creative engagement with generational, regional, religious, ethnic, class-based, and migratory tensions and frictions that continue to have far-reaching repercussions for Pakistan on both local and global levels. Ranging from Muslim and non-Muslim minority issues, censorship, human rights, terrorism, religious extremism, fundamentalism, corruption, and intolerance to matters of love, hate, loss, sexualities, belonging, and identity conflicts – nothing is outside its ambit. The complexity underlying this flowering outburst is unique, as Daniyal Mueenuddin's astute observation shows: 'We're not lying in sort of a bath of warm water and reflecting upon, you know, our sort of quirky, funny families. There's an edginess to our writing, I believe, which is distinctive' (Tiwari 2009: n.p.). The ever-burgeoning creative literature produced by writers from various backgrounds in Pakistan, and the Pakistani diaspora, demands studies encompassing the rich and kaleidoscopic tapestry of themes in order to ascertain the depth and scope that Pakistani writing in English has attained thus far. Despite the fact that Pakistani anglophone literature has become an established field in institutions of higher learning around the world, very few handbooks and companions have surveyed the critical debates and interpretive orientations influencing this literary trajectory.

Therefore, the fundamental aim of this Companion is to provide a comprehensive yet manageable introduction to cross-cultural relations and to historical, regional, local, and global contexts that are essential to reading Pakistani anglophone literature. As stated earlier, what has made Pakistani anglophone writing and literary criticism such an enthralling and rewarding field is the ways in which these situate contemporary Pakistan on the world map. The chapters in this Companion, focused on the aforementioned themes, map out contestations and controversies that have not only informed creative writing and critical enquiry but have also continued to subvert and ultimately render static certain stereotypes in favour of a dynamic representation of Pakistani Muslim experiences. The contributions in this Companion emphasise that the historical trajectories and forms of Pakistani creativity are quite distinctive and cannot easily be situated within the usual Euro-American theoretical paradigms. We propose instead that, given its evolving aesthetic and generic complexity, its circulatory market potential and increasing translocal viability, Pakistani anglophone literature, as a morphing episteme, is arguably on an epochal itinerary of canon formation. (We take up this debate in the concluding chapter.) Therefore, this Companion uniquely examines in considerable depth a variety of texts and genres created by writers of Pakistani origin. We would like to emphasise here that the Companion pays special attention to authors and texts that have not always received adequate attention in times past. Since any discussion of canon formation focuses not only on texts but also on production, market, readership, and criticism, this Companion hopes to enrich our understanding of the Pakistani anglophone literary tradition, tracing the impact of reception, marketing, and audience on its formation along the way. Most significantly, this is but a small step towards the development of a transnational perspective of canon constitution in Pakistani literature. To this end we have been joined by scholars from Jordan, Syria, Saudi Arabia, Germany, Hungary, Italy, New Zealand, Spain, Britain, Canada, America, India, and, of course, Pakistan. We can safely assume that this is one of the first books academics and scholars will use in what will be a continuing self-education in the Pakistani anglophone literary tradition.

This Companion specifically concentrates on works written against the backdrop of Partitions and civil wars, works deeply enmeshed in the history of the region in a variety of conspicuous, mutated, or vestigial ways. In so doing, we hope to reinforce the 'presentness' of historical contexts and memory and their enormous relevance to what we think of as contemporary Pakistan. In this way, this Companion conveys a sense of the interconnectedness of Pakistani anglophone texts and their historical contexts; the chapters in this Companion aim to ground Pakistani anglophone literature in historical awareness and history's continued impact on contemporary realities. It would not be wrong to say that Pakistani writers are mindful of the literary dimension of the historicity of experience. The eight sections of this Companion offer distinctive if overlapping paradigms and contextualisations for thinking about Pakistani anglophone literature; it is precisely with this intention that individual sections are

Introduction

read contrastively and dialogically, rather than in isolation. The eight sections of the Companion provide historical genealogies for several phenomena, such as migration, otherness, civil wars, military dictatorships, ethnic and sectarian crises, human rights, gender and minority issues, the Islamisation or secularisation of the state in various eras, the Talibanisation of Pakistan, and the historical pathologies of Islamic extremism and contemporary violence. For instance, these contexts and connections cannot be grasped in their entirety without the backdrop of the social and political history of Pakistan during Zia's dictatorial regime (1977–1988); US-led Afghan *jihad* and intra-Muslim sectarian violence, manipulated by the US during the Afghan and the Gulf Wars; the Talibanisation of Pakistan in the '80s; the post-9/11 war against terrorism in the region; and multigenerational ethnic and sectarian rivalries that date back to the 1947 and 1971 Partitions.

Given this complex historical contextualisation, the entries are grouped under sections that correspond to a hugely variegated field of events and activities. Part I, which includes three chapters collected under the heading 'Reimagining history: the legacy of war and partition', focuses on two key defining historical moments in the history of Pakistan and South Asia, the 1947 and 1971 Partitions. Both these conflicts have continued to influence the ways in which South Asians envisage their past, present, and future. In reimagining our history and the legacy of war and Partition, we begin Part I with Cara Cilano's '"All these angularities": Spatialising non-Muslim Pakistani identities'. Cilano argues that Muhammad Ali Jinnah envisaged that these 'angularities' would 'vanish' between majority and minority communities, but different sects within Muslims communities were in fact 'sharpened' in the new nation state. Cilano traces how these 'produce the spatialisation of Islam and [...] shape the lived spaces and mobilities of these [non-Muslim] minorities alongside those of the majority'. These angularities were later seen sharpening among East and West Pakistani Muslims on the basis of ethnicity, leading to the 1971 War. Muneeza Shamsie 'reassesses a forgotten national narrative' of 1971 by tracing the 'angularities' that cleaved East and West Pakistan, peoples, friends, and spouses living on both sides of the divide and thereafter in subsequent years. Providing insights into a valuable body of work on the 1971 War, such as writing by Tariq Rahman, Sorayya Khan, Aamer Hussein, Aquila Ismail, Shahbano Bilgrami, Sara Suleri, Kamila Shamsie, and Roopa Farooqi, among others, Shamsie underscores the need to shatter the national amnesia. She writes that 'These traumatic events have yet to be addressed at a national level, but they are being tackled increasingly in Pakistani anglophone fiction'. Daniela Vitolo's essay broadens our understanding of how this event continued to sharpen 'angularities' in the 'postmemory generation' (i.e. the generation born after the 1971 War, who only know as much as the older generation have divulged about it). Through her deft analysis of Sorayya Khan's *Noor* and Kamila Shamsie's *Kartography*, she proposes that envisioning the unpleasant and long-repressed memories is important in coming to terms with selves ruptured by division in space or time.

Part II of our Companion attests to the enduring pressures of these 'angularities', which are further compounded by Pakistan's role in Afghanistan as a US ally, the 9/11 attacks, the war on terror, and the growing Islamophobia and stereotyping that Muslims and Pakistanis have experienced. This section, '9/11 and beyond: contexts, forms, and perspectives', aims, therefore, to engage with the varied and intersecting pre- and post-9/11 contexts, forms, and perspectives that Pakistani anglophone writers use in dealing with 9/11 and beyond, thereby taking a prospective and retrospective glance at the growing terrorism and intolerance and their aftermaths. In reading about Pakistan outside the dominant discourse of 9/11, Ulka Anjaria's 'Global Pakistan in the wake of 9/11' discusses how literature written since 2001, especially by internationally recognised writers such as Kamila Shamsie, Mohsin Hamid, and Mohammed Hanif, situates Pakistan in a global imaginary where a conglomerate of global, national, regional, and local concerns has added to the challenges facing Pakistan today. The novelists' wider glance at the global power inequities and 'alternative spatial formations' encompass 'truths outside of the current US-sponsored rhetoric of "Islamic Terrorism"'. The US involvement in the Afghan War and Pakistan's role as a go-between led to identity crises not only for Pakistanis in the home country but also in the US. Focusing on 'Pakistani "inoutsiders" and the dynamics of post-9/11 dissociation in Pakistani anglophone fiction', Claudia Nördinger advances the idea of 'inoutsiders' in the US, meaning those who have 'acquired access to a sphere that is not originally [their] own' (such as Mohsin Hamid's Changez) and those who feel alienated despite having birth rights (such as Ayad Akhtar's Amir). She relates the challenges that 'inoutsiders' face to 'the precariousness of identity formation in a modern world of embattled absolutes and shifting boundaries'. She situates this within the troubled relationship between the US and Pakistan and its repercussions for the Pakistani nation, people, and diaspora, in particular the 'inoutsiders' in the US. The matrices of problems that the Pakistani nation has to face on account of its uneasy relation with the US and its troubled relationship with India are further explored in Michaela M. Henry's 'The nuclear novel in Pakistan', which sees Pakistan's nuclearisation as deriving from 'existential fear' due to 'swimming in [a] history of unresolved conflicts', namely, Partitions and subsequent wars with India, growing sectarianism, fundamentalism, US intervention, 9/11, etc. It is also against this backdrop that Henry reads Pakistanis' hope in the 'bomb', especially in a bid to confront the tense relations with Indian and US violations of Pakistani territory in the form of drone attacks.

To correct the unidimensional representation of Muslims in Britain and America, Ambreen Hai and Sarah Ilott explore the potential of humour in questioning the inanity of stereotyping Muslims and Pakistanis in a post-9/11 world. Hai's 'Uses of humour in post-9/11 Pakistani anglophone fiction: H.M. Naqvi's *Home Boy* and Mohammed Hanif's *A Case of Exploding Mangoes*' discusses how writers engage with 'benign humour as a form of resistance and challenge to domination as a sign and reassertion of humanity, resilience, intelligence, and as a way to build community and foster rethinking'. Ilott's 'Comic affiliations/comic subversions: The use of humour in contemporary British-Pakistani fiction' examines how chick lit provides comic engagements with and subversions of patriarchal, political, and Islamophobic attitudes. Particularly detailing Ayisha Malik's works among many others in this genre, Ilott discusses how Malik gleefully engages with and rebuts stereotypes regarding Muslims and Pakistanis, in particular, Muslim ceremonial rituals and veiling. Ilott discusses how the 'gentle mockery' of Sofia (Ayisha Malik's protagonist) resists numerous 'homogenising discourses through Sofia's varied modes of identification (as Muslim, as Pakistani, as a Londoner, as a woman) and an internal othering of certain Asians and Muslims'. Against this backdrop, Sofia Khan's blog, 'Yes I'm Muslim, Please Get Over It', effectively calls for a new community founded on the 'prioritisation of similarity over difference'. Suhaan Mehta's 'Resistance and redefinition: Theatre of the Pakistani diaspora in the UK and the US' focuses on the creative outburst from playwrights of Pakistani origin. In line with the title, the resistance comes from growing racism in the two host lands, as well as from pursuing a life attenuated by pressures from religion, customs, peers, community expectations, and social respectability, all adding to myriad levels of redefinitions in the characters. Nisreen Yousef's 'Historiographic metafiction and renarrating history' examines Tariq Ali's *The Book of Saladin* and Kamran Pasha's *Shadow of the Swords* 'as a means of complicating, refuting or reinforcing established present-day ideas about Islam and the West'.

Part III, 'The dialectics of human rights: Politics, positionality, controversies', takes into its ambit important debates on how human rights became such a contested field in the Pakistani context and an important catch-all in global power politics. As a result of continued local

Introduction

tensions and foreign interventions (as the essays in the previous sections show), human rights debates need to be wary of the operating dialectics: who says what, when, and why, from what side of the power divide, and unleashing what controversies. The essays in this section are sensitive to this Gordian knot. Esra Mirze Santesso's 'Pakistani fiction and human rights' engages precisely with the period of heightened and amorphous human rights: the era in which Zia-ul-Haq adjusted to American needs in Afghanistan and enlisted the support of the local subaltern classes. The way in which these diametrically opposed agendas were harnessed to buttress political Islam and to silence dissenting voices, according to Santesso, has required a breaking away from traditional realism for magic realist ventures, as in Mohammed Hanif's *A Case of Exploding Mangoes* and Kamila Shamsie's *Broken Verses*. The mix of conflicting positions and politics, the characters in Pakistani anglophone fiction shown aiding and abetting, and the controversies these are shown to air, all come layered with meanings as we read Santesso's analyses. Shazia Sadaf's 'Divergent discourses: Human rights, and contemporary Pakistani anglophone literature' provides a comprehensive view of how human rights debates have become ambivalent due to the locational and locutional differences/positionalities of characters/writers and would-be audiences, which again are just as heterogenous and variegated as the debates in these works. Pakistani anglophone writers, Sadaf rightly points out, tread a tightrope: to escape the trap of being pro-Western and yet name local flaws while at the same time not twisting foreign interventions. She observes that 'the future of international human rights can only be meaningful if there is a careful balance between representations of local cultures and the globalised world, and regional political movements are not completely neglected in the face of larger political claims'.

The next three essays in this Part underscore the nuances of local cultures and native/human agency as correctives to neo-orientalised versions of this world. Focusing on three narratives on the tribal areas of Pakistan, Uzma Abid Ansari's 'The taming of the tribal within Pakistani narratives of progress, conflict, and romance' discusses the ways in which tribal cultures are presented in essentially skewed ways, and how tribals 'tamed' as 'potential militants' are shown to possess life trajectories that are 'running against the grain of progressivism and modernity'. Colleen Lutz Clemens' 'Phoenix rising: The West's use (and misuse) of anglophone memoirs by Pakistani women' rebuts the essentialised image of Pakistani women and culture which the West appropriates for its rhetoric of the war on terror. Laying bare the modalities spurring any interest in the rights of Muslim women and the conflationary rhetoric lumping together all Muslim women irrespective of regional differences, Clemens claims that the reception of stories of phoenixes who rose unscathed from the ashes of their miseries, such as Malala and Mukhtar Mai, to find 'liberation' may stir Western concern for the liberation and autonomy of all those dispossessed, but it does not usher in any genuine collaboration. Closely paralleling Clemens' essay, Rachel Fox's 'Writing back and/as activism: Refiguring victimhood and remapping the shooting of Malala Yousafzai' also talks about how Yousafzai's image of a wounded victim was appropriated by the 'neo-imperial project of cosmopolitan interest, sympathy, charity, and "rescue" within the context of the War on Terror'. Nonetheless, Fox moves away from the implications of the paratextual features of this memoir and focuses on its written content to assert that Malala 'refigures – or remaps – the events she narrates in her memoir in ways that allow her to return to her position of advocacy for education'. By shifting the emphasis away from her status of victimhood, Fox calls attention towards an often neglected facet: how the event galvanised Malala's quest to highlight the politics of girls' education.

Closely aligned with, and in fact extending, the debates initiated in the preceding sections, we move towards 'Identities in question: Shifting perspectives on gender' in Part IV. As our sections so far make clear, the 'angularities' facing the new nation state never vanished, rather they have returned with a vengeance and greater complexity at every crucial stage of our social, cultural, political, and religious history. Because of this constant flux, multiple pressures and interests have continued to jostle for dominance over our quite heterogenous, flexible, and ephemeral precepts of identity. As a result, identities, especially the shifting perspectives on gender, naturally become more volatile. Fawzia Afzal-Khan's 'Doing history right: Challenging masculinist postcolonialism in Pakistani anglophone literature' questions the 'erotic' masculinist History that has merely exacerbated the problems of the marginalised. Propelled by a deep realisation that 'When the voices of the marginalised remain trapped in masculinist ideologies, the future remains captive to the past', she urges a materialist conception of history for a better 'feminist futurity'. 'Breaking out of the prison-house of masculinist (self-hating) melancholia' can only provide the apotheosis of this conflict-ridden world of charged binaries, an effort Afzal-Khan partly reads in Tayeb Salih's *Season of Migration to the North*, and more so in Mohsin Hamid's *Exit West*. Nihilist and atavistic urges paralyse characters such as the Amir (Ayad Akhtar's *Disgraced*), Changez (Hamid's *The Reluctant Fundamentalist*), and the nameless narrator of Ali Eteraz's *Native Believer*. Analysing Hanif Kureishi's *The Black Album*, Nadeem Aslam's *Maps for Lost Lovers*, and Sarfraz Manzoor's *Greetings from Bury Park*, Kavita Bhanot's 'Love, sex, and desire vs Islam in British Muslim literature' presents Western liberalism and political Islam as in contention over matters of love, desire, pleasure, and sexuality manifested through 'abstract notions of music, literature, creativity, imagination, beauty, and freedom'. While Bhanot focuses on characters in the diaspora, Mosarrap Hossain Khan's 'Transgressive desire, everyday life, and the production of "modernity" in Pakistani anglophone fiction' focuses on shifting gendered identities due to transgressive desires, deriving primarily from '"modern" Muslim subjectivity' and contests traditional gender norms in Pakistani society.

As its title suggests, Part V, 'Spaces of female subjectivity: Identity, difference, agency' focuses on multiple modalities of gender, nationalism, class, religion, sexuality, and generation. Abu-Bakar Ali's chapter, 'Agency, gender, nationalism, and the romantic imaginary in Pakistan', examines the ways in which the popular romance genre 'can potentially serve as a site on which Pakistani women writers refashion and reconfigure their role in their country's nationalist imaginary'. By focusing on the national and state ideologies within the Pakistani romantic imaginary, Ali's chapter discusses how the Pakistani women novelists Qaisra Shahraz, Shaila Abdullah, and Kamila Shamsie respond to the challenges and subsequent implications of nationalist ideologies for gendered expressions of sexuality and agency. Rahul K. Gairola and Elham Fatma's chapter, 'Conjugal homes: Marriage culture in contemporary novels of the Pakistani diaspora', compares three novels by Pakistani diasporic writers – Bapsi Sidhwa's *An American Brat* (1993), Azhar Abidi's *Twilight* (2008), and Nadeem Aslam's *Maps for Lost Lovers* (2004) – to offer critical insights into conflicting intergenerational familial relationships against a backdrop of sociocultural and religious dynamics. They argue that the first and second generations' conflict of perspectives on matrimonial relations', informed by their respective cultural topographies, not only 'exert[s] influence on the matrimonial spaces of domesticity in the Pakistani diaspora' but also exacerbates feelings of detachment and cultural dissonance in the West. Aqeel Abdulla's chapter, 'British-Pakistani female playwrights: Feminist perspectives on sexuality, marriage, and domestic violence', focuses exclusively on the current wave of new feminist British-Pakistani playwrights – Alia Bano, Nadia Manzoor, and Emteaz Hussain – who engage with issues of marriage, sexuality, and domestic violence to problematise perceived generalisations about Pakistani Muslim men's 'particular fixation with controlling women's sexuality', predominantly constructed and hijacked by 'self-appointed community leaders, radical religious speakers, and the manipulative and sensationalist British media'.

Part VI, 'Shifting contexts: New perspectives on identity, space, and mobility', focuses on the ways in which identity and a sense of belonging are informed by notions of space and mobility. Georgia Stabler draws attention to personal and intergenerational encounters with Islamic spaces of worship and how these impact on writers' construction of the self in their life writings. By juxtaposing domestic and religious spaces as well as social practices, rituals, and religious observance in Sarfraz Manzoor's *Greetings from Bury Park* (2007), Zaiba Malik's *We Are a Muslim, Please* (2010), and Yasmin Hai's *The Making of Mr Hai's Daughter: Becoming British* (2008), Stabler demonstrates the ways in which each writer has a dynamic relationship with Islam, thereby 'complicating the idea of a homogenous British-Pakistani Muslim experience'. Éva Pataki focuses on the construction of mobile subjectivities within urban and suburban diaspora spaces by examining the interrelatedness of divergent forms of belonging with a certain kind of movement such as mapping, nomadic paths, or mental movement. She compares three British-Pakistani novels – Nadeem Aslam's *Maps for Lost Lovers* (2004), Hanif Kureishi's *The Buddha of Suburbia* (1990), and Suhayl Saadi's *Psychoraag* (2004) – to offer insights into complex ways of 'self-identification' and 'imaginary shared belongings'. 'By placing the white English and the Asian as configuring two different social spaces', Miquel Pomar-Amer's essay complicates the notion of politics of difference and the precariousness of Pakistanis through their egalitarian and peaceful coexistence in the diaspora, through assimilation, multiculturalism, or interculturality. Pomar-Amer argues that the characters of Shamas and Mr Hai in *Maps for Lost Lovers* and *The Making of Mr Hai's Daughter*, respectively, 'use their cultural and social capital to cope with the social downgrading that migration often entails', despite their cultural differences, subaltern positions, and disadvantageous situations. Nevertheless, taking on with pride the role of 'organic intellectuals', both characters aim not to 'become rich but to act as mediating agents between their respective diasporic communities and society as a whole'.

Contesting the identities marked by the history of colonisation, Part VII, 'Unsettling narratives: Imagining post-postcolonial perspectives', collects essays that explore the possibilities of emergence of post-postcolonial subjectivities, informed by the pressures of globalisation. With the intention of escaping from the colonial past, Asma Mansoor envisions a post-postcolonial selfhood outside binaristic identity quandaries through negotiation between humans and the material environment. She conceptualises Pakistani Muslims as global citizens with diverse mobile identities informed by historical and cultural archives which continue to slide across time and space, blending into malleable individual and collective human histories. Hanji Lee's chapter focuses on the post-postcolonial generation of writers who fictionalise their conflicting relationships with the nation and the world under the pressures of globalisation. By comparing the narratological perspectives and curiosities within Mohsin Hamid's *The Reluctant Fundamentalist* (2007) and *How to Get Filthy Rich in Rising Asia* (2013), and Bilal Tanweer's *The Scatter Here is Too Great* (2013), Lee proposes that the 'narrative unsteadiness' represented in these novels is reflective of 'the authors' own Pakistani subjectivit[ies] caught in a tension between the local and the global'. Asher Ghaffar's essay focuses on the ways in which Ghose's experimental writing style dissociates him from the politics of postcolonial identities. Taking on an anticolonial dimension through a resistance to the categories of 'local' and 'Western' – which shape the postcolonial field, and which confirm his non-canonical status in postcolonial studies – Ghose's writing opens up the possibilities of 'alternative modernities' through aesthetic mediations of disjuncture between exile and nationalism, centre and periphery, realism and modernism.

The essays in the final Part of this collection, 'New horizons: towards a Pakistani idiom', are primarily focused on the debates surrounding the reception and dissemination of 'brand Pakistan' within the global literary marketplace. Pakistani diasporic writers are often pigeonholed as investigators of exoticism for metropolitan audiences and readers. The essays by Masood Raja and Barirah Nazir, Nicholas Holm, and Kim L. Worthington foreground the complexities and contradictions inherent in self-identification and the critical reception of Pakistani writers at home and within the diaspora, in terms of the marketing strategies adopted by global publishers. The first essay in this section, 'Brand Pakistan': Global imaginings and national concerns in Pakistani anglophone literature', raises important concerns regarding 'who should be counted as an "authentic" Pakistani author in the contemporary cosmopolitan literary market' against the backdrop of the West's fascination with Islamic fundamentalism and Muslim identity after 9/11. In so doing, the authors enumerate the ways in which those writers who are 'branded' as Pakistani respond to allegations such as exoticising and stereotyping Pakistani (Muslim) culture for metropolitan readers. Masood Ashraf Raja, in 'Competing habitus: National expectations, metropolitan market, and Pakistani writing in English (PWE)', draws our attention to the tension between national expectations of PWE and its reception within and beyond the nation. According to him, Pakistani writing in English and 'its critique within Pakistan can be better understood by taking a deeper look at the habitus that determines writing and the habitus that structures the expectations and aspirations of Pakistani readers critical of PWE'. Extending these debates on the critical reception of 'brand' Pakistan within the global market in relation to its identitarian and aesthetic corollaries in the immediate aftermath of 9/11, Faisal Nazir's 'De/reconstructing identities: Critical approaches to contemporary Pakistani anglophone fiction' is the only essay that analyses selected literary criticism on Pakistani anglophone literature. Nazir engages those critical works on contemporary Pakistani anglophone fiction that focus on the theme of the deconstruction of an exclusivist and hegemonic national identity and that tend to propose the reconstruction of this identity within a more inclusive national and/or global cosmopolitan frame. Nazir, however, argues that 'while the critics [such as Cilano, Morey, Clements, and Kanwal] discussed in this chapter do appreciate writers' efforts to emphasise religious, cultural, ethnic, class, and gender diversity in Pakistan, they do not address the essentialism that this strategy [deconstruction/reconstruction] often involves'. Waseem Anwar's essay, 'On the wings of "poesy": Pakistani diaspora poets and the "Pakistani idiom"', is a genuine effort to address the concerns and questions raised by the first three essays in this section: What does it mean to be a true Pakistani? Who should be counted as the authentic voice of Pakistan in the contemporary cosmopolitan literary market? In response to these questions, Anwar's essay unhesitatingly suggests a move 'towards a Pakistani idiom' and *Pakistaniat*, one informed by spatiotemporal frames beyond borders and territories. By extending the debates raised in different ways by contributors to this section, in the concluding essay, Aroosa Kanwal and Saiyma Aslam underscore claims for a move towards the canonisation of Pakistani anglophone literature. By taking into consideration ideas and ideals about any literary canon, they investigate the 'normative' (innovations and experiments in genre and style), 'curatorial' (exemplary attitudes and wisdom), and 'dialogical' (interaction with other literary cultures and textual fields) functions performed by different categories of Pakistani anglophone literature. Taking a synoptic, yet deftly engaged, view of the treasure trove of Pakistani anglophone literature, they show how, 'in dialogue with literary trends of Asian, Muslim, and subcontinental cultures and civilisations, Pakistani literary tradition has morphed into a distinct Pakistani idiom'. Being the last essay in this Companion, this also sits very well with the editors' desire to invite more global and local voices to enter conversations on the canonisation of Pakistani anglophone literature.

The very probing essays in this Companion, by scholars from across the globe, are indeed a step towards this end.

Bibliography

Hashmi, A. (1990) 'Poetry, Pakistani Idiom in English, and the Groupies'. *World Literature Today* 64(2), 268–271.

Tiwari, P. (2009) 'All Eyes on them'. *Deccan Herald* [online]. Available from <www.deccanherald.com/content/19771/all-eyes-them.html> [12 January 2018].

PART I

Reimagining history
The legacy of war and Partition

1
'ALL THESE ANGULARITIES'
Spatialising non-Muslim Pakistani identities

Cara Cilano

The reality of minority status animated the idea of Pakistan, a decolonising movement intent on securing a homeland for India's Muslims. From the moment of the term's coinage, 'Pakistan' already hinted at what has since become a significant challenge: how to spatialise or territorialise a nationalism itself subject to contested views of the role of Islam in the nation's identity. Chaudhary Rahmat Ali's pamphlet, 'Now or Never: Are We to Live or Perish Forever?', first published in January 1933, introduced the term 'Pakistan' into the many anti-colonial discourses gaining purchase in South Asia in the first decades of the twentieth century. In the first clause of his pamphlet, Rahmat Ali coined the term as an acronym for the territories that would, in part, eventually make up West Pakistan: 'PAKISTAN by which we mean the five Northern units of India viz: Punjab, North-West Frontier Province (Afghan Province), Kashmir, Sind, and Baluchistan' (1933: n.p.). The term also means 'land of the pure', a definition that neatly connects space and concept (here, religious identities).[1] Within this neat connection lies an irony: the territories encompassed by Rahmat Ali's term were Muslim majority so while, in the grander context of the British exit from South Asia, Muslims were a minority in relation to Hindus, in the space (partially) identified as Pakistan, the minority-majority ratios swung in a different direction. The minorities were the non-Muslims. And, as the process of decolonisation accelerated after the Second World War, this idea took on increasingly concrete dimensions, culminating in the actual territorialisation of Pakistan into a new nation bisected across the north of the South Asian subcontinent. Consequently, the minority-majority ratios, especially in what became West Pakistan, tilted even more in favour of the Muslim majority.[2] Thus, the physical reality of Pakistan added new dimensions to the reality of minority status, especially in spatial terms.

Muhammad Ali Jinnah's speech to the Constituent Assembly on 11 August 1947 takes on added prescience in this spatially oriented context. Jinnah assures his soon-to-be fellow Pakistanis that they 'are free; you are free to go to your temples, you are free to go to your mosques or to any other place of worship in this State of Pakistan' (Jinnah 1947: n.p.). These lines encapsulate a founding spatial vision for Pakistan not only in terms of the actual physical existence of temples, mosques, churches, etc., but also in terms of mobility. Non-Muslims, in this vision, would be free to move about cities and villages to get to their respective houses of worship. This vision is at once both descriptive, insofar as it captures the everyday lived experience of people currently inhabiting the territories that would shortly become Pakistan, and prescriptive in that Jinnah and members of the Muslim League were highly cognisant of the need to ensure the safety of minorities throughout the decolonising process. Earlier in this address, Jinnah says:

> [I]n the course of time all these angularities of the majority and minority communities, the Hindu community and the Muslim community – because even as regards Muslims you have Pathans, Punjabis, Shias, Sunnis and so on, and among the Hindus you have Brahmins, Vashnavas, Khatris, also Bengalees, Madrasis and so on – will vanish.
>
> (1947: n.p.)

Jinnah adds dimension to the 'angularities' of majority and minority interactions by parsing out differences within each group. This effort to embody abstractions with reference not only to religious groups but also to ethno-regional ones subtly identifies the spaces these abstractions occupy and in which they move. In other words, geometrically, the vanishing of angles suggests an inductive wholeness wherein the edges of difference lose visibility. In predicting that the sharp corners of these 'angularities' will vanish, Jinnah also offers an image of an idealised, cohesive, near-homogenous view of national identity. Significantly, though, when taken alongside the spatial vision I have identified, this homogeneity does not align with the markedly shifted political relations that came about via the demographic homogeneity caused by Partition's migrations (Rahman 2012: 303). Speaking in the abstract on 8 November 1945, nearly two years before Pakistan's creation, Jinnah noted, for instance, that neither Hindus nor 'anyone else' would experience 'social barriers of any kind' in the 'Muslim state' of Pakistan (Jinnah 1945: n.p.). Nonetheless, politics and the power wielded through them did change dramatically upon the establishment of Pakistan due to the ongoing and heightening tensions between a conceptualisation of Muslim nationhood and an Islamic state. The angles sharpened.[3]

Although my focus relies upon Jinnah's spatial vision, my purpose is not to gauge the (in)sincerity of Jinnah's secularism. Rather, the point is to analyse how textual representations of non-Muslim minorities in Pakistan in fictive and non-fictive texts help produce the spatialisation of Islam (as inclusive of but not wholly coterminous with Islamisation) and help shape the lived spaces and mobilities of these minorities alongside those of the majority. With primary reference to three novels, Saad Ashraf's *The Postmaster* (2004), Sorayya Y. Khan's *Five Queen's Road* (2009), and Nadeem Aslam's *Season of the Rainbirds* (1993), I examine the fictive portrayals of non-Muslim characters' abilities to occupy and move through space with specific reference to significant events and dynamics in Pakistani history, namely the 1947 Partition and the slow burn of de-secularisation in Aslam's depiction of Pakistan in the 1980s, to develop in spatial terms Sadia Saeed's arguments regarding how the Pakistani state produces appropriate citizens by producing inappropriate ones – that is, non-Muslims (2007: 133).[4]

By taking a spatial turn – that is, by attending to the territorialisation or spatialisation of Islam in Pakistan – I extend Saeed's analysis of how the Pakistani state inflected and took shape from 'a new definition of the national community by equating the nation with Islam', a move that, in Saeed's view, led to the 'construction of new social imaginaries' (2007: 133). I am interested in how these imaginaries take material form, especially with respect to minority mobility. Jørgen Ole Baerenholdt's term 'governmobility', which he describes as a form of regulation that 'works through bodily, technological and institutional forms of self-government, which are enacted relationally and embedded in systems', highlights the spatial materialisation of such social imaginaries (2013: 29). The concept of governmobility captures how the connectedness of representation and space work along with lived experience. In working with representations to grasp lived spaces, I deliberately turn to both imaginative and government writings, not just to scrutinise textual hierarchies, but also to initiate dynamic analyses that refuse to fix the spatial aspects of representation as unchanging or mimetic. As Doreen Massey argues, the long history of fusing representation to spatialisation, thought of as the antithesis of temporality, encourages a flattening of both in contrast to the dynamism of time rather than productive efforts to grapple with representing space-time (2005: 27–28). Instead, through reading texts of varying provenances together, I consider representation and space as connected 'in a continuous production' – a mutual production, even (Massey 2005: 28). With respect to my goals here, time in the sense of specific historical events, including Partition and the following decades through to the 1980s, thus matters a great deal to how representations and space are mutually constitutive.

Not long after the emergence of the nations of Pakistan and India on 14 and 15 August 1947, respectively, the two new governments realised that the mass migrations accompanying their nations' creation affected property, the lived spaces of everyday lives. According to Joseph Schechtman, in early September 1947, the governments of both nations thought that those who had departed would return, and so agreed upon the 'unconditional and automatic restoration of property to returning refugee-owners' (1951: 407). Yet, before that month was through, the governments of Pakistan and India recognised that return was unlikely (Schechtman 1951: 407). Consequently, policies for distributing evacuee property sprang up. Pakistan was in particular need of such policies for, as Ayesha Jalal points out, it 'ended up with twice as many evacuee properties than Muslim migrants abandoned in India, creating a deep vested interest in the acquisition of evacuee properties by those with political connections' (2014: 44). Rather than focus on returnees, then, Pakistan and India turned their bureaucratic efforts to finding space for their new compatriots. The initial anticipation of return, which readily demonstrates what Kavita Daiya identifies as a fetish in much migrant literature (2005: 185), as well as the deals and entitlements accompanying the distribution of evacuee property, appear again and again in South Asian English-language Partition fiction. The Muslims in Khushwant Singh's *Train to Pakistan* (1956) entrust their possessions to their Sikh neighbours, for instance, while Lenny's family promises to safeguard their non-Muslim neighbours' items in Bapsi Sidhwa's *Cracking India* (1988).

That the house next door to the main family's home in Sidhwa's *Cracking India*, abandoned by non-Muslims departing for India, becomes a rehabilitation centre for abducted women begins to illustrate how literary representations spatialise the presence and absence of non-Muslim minorities in Pakistan. Lenny's Hindu nanny Ayah stays at this ad hoc centre temporarily as Lenny's godmother arranges for her return to her family in what is now India. Notably, Ayah's 'rescue' comes about through the godmother's efforts, though the novel does reveal that Lenny's mother and aunt also manage to locate and return other abducted women apparently outside of the state-sanctioned mechanisms for doing so.[5] And the centre's guard is a stalwart and intimidating Sikh (1988: 288). Through its function as a haven for abducted women – one protected by a non-Muslim male – this space avoids appropriation into any evacuee property disbursement plan, as though it existed, for some short span of time, outside the state's workings (though not the state's patriarchal mandates). The un-narrated mobility which Lenny's mother and aunt possess goes even further, hinting at the possibility of spaces wherein non-Muslim minorities can act purposefully and in resistance to the threatening forces that would otherwise violently impose majority identifications on non-Muslim female characters. That both spaces with their attendant confinement or mobility exist coextensively illustrates how the assertion of a dominant definition of Pakistani identity – one characterised in Sidhwa's novel as masculinist and violent – becomes starkly visible in relation to attempts to occupy and move through the spaces of the new nation while bearing the brunt of the former's force.

Ashraf's novel *The Postmaster* (2014) focuses on the absence of non-Muslims in the distribution of evacuee property to highlight the failings of the state's efforts to consolidate a national identity through spatial allocation. Ashraf's novel effectively fictionalises Jalal's critique of Pakistan's handling of evacuee property:

> A psychology of looting and disregard for the rule of law took hold of the ruling coterie in Pakistan early on. The initial gold mine was the allotment of properties abandoned by Hindus and Sikhs in Punjab and, subsequently, also in Sindh.
>
> (2014: 57–58)[6]

The Pakistan to which Ghulam Rasool, Ashraf's protagonist, migrates reflects this debased approach to spatialising national belonging for the new Pakistanis. After having served with distinction in British India's civil service, Rasool opts to join Pakistan's service and in his new role is responsible for reassigning evacuee properties in Lahore (2004: 293). Believing he has received 'honest answers' from a refugee from India about the place the latter inhabited prior to migrating, Rasool allots the man, referred to as Sheikh Mohammed, 'a bungalow near the university grounds which has recently been abandoned by a Sikh engineer who had migrated to India' (2004: 293). Happening upon the house by chance, Rasool stops to greet the refugee, who has rifled through the previous owner's possessions choosing for himself and his wife the finest clothes, jewellery, and houseware (2004: 294). Without compunction, Sheikh Mohammed tells Rasool:

> It seems that [the Sikh engineer] had a daughter who was to be married soon because we found her jewelry and her trousseau in a large steel trunk. It is a strange coincidence that the clothes fit my wife perfectly and the jewelry too looks good on her, just as if everything was made for her.
>
> (2004: 294)

Rasool understands then that Sheikh Mohammed was 'an uneducated and corrupt individual devoid of sensitivity who felt no qualms about grabbing and using the wealth of others as his own' (2004: 295). The episode leaves Rasool 'wondering how people like the Sheikh and his progeny would build and run the new state of Pakistan' (Ashraf 2004: 296).

Significantly, the refugee's ability to establish his status in Pakistan requires the occupation of the Sikh's space and the donning of his family's possessions. Indeed, in claiming the betrothed daughter's trousseau and jewellery, Sheikh Mohammed's wife metaphorically even wears the identity of the departed daughter. Subtly, then, Ashraf's novel also implicates the gendered aspects of spatial occupation in the sense that the purloined finery which Sheikh Mohammed's wife enjoys marks her as a woman whose honour remains intact through the migration process, in high contrast to the female characters who inhabit the temporary shelter – another abandoned property – in Sidhwa's novel. The disbursement of evacuee property hinged upon connectedness and patronage, as Ashraf's novel and Jalal's historical commentary suggest, as it physically located new Pakistanis. Such locatedness, however, required not only movement across the newly created border but also the incorporation of non-Muslim residential spaces to the point of erasure. Even while the Pakistani government established units such as the Evacuee Trust Property Board, whose aim was to preserve properties left by non-Muslims, the fictional portrayals of the handling of evacuee properties ask readers to recognise the lived experience of the places' reframing within the Pakistani nation.[7]

Khan's *Five Queen's Road* (2009) also attempts to portray minority absence as foundational to the establishment of belonging for those characters deemed appropriately Pakistani. As a minority still resident in Lahore after the creation of Pakistan, the character Dina

Lal gauges both belonging and displacement through the occupation of space. The protagonist purchases a grand home at Five Queen's Road, initially as a direct rebuke to the British. Conceding his own complicity with empire building, for 'He had profited from the railway lines expanding across his village land' (2009: 15), Dina Lal nonetheless has 'had enough' by the time 1947 rolls around; Radcliffe's cartographic 'etchings' spur Dina Lal to 'teach [the British] a lesson. On this side of the lines' in Pakistan (2009: 15). Spatial occupation, for Dina Lal, is an assertion of legitimacy: he is 'Like the country, *land of the pure*, just born' (2009: 25). Anti-colonial resentment translates into national belonging. Dina Lal's invocation of Pakistan as 'land of the pure' is not about religious identity but, instead, appears to refer to the British departure from the subcontinent.

Khan's novel highlights the futility of Dina Lal's anti-colonial sentiments as the violent realities of Partition and its aftermath for Pakistan's minority populations becomes evident. Dina Lal effectively erases himself by converting to Islam. At the same time, he partitions his grand home and invites a Muslim tenant, Amir Shah, thinking that doing so will secure his and his wife's belonging, spatially and nationally. In Dina Lal's mind, these acts constitute 'whatever was necessary to claim [Lahore] back' (2009: 52) even as they signal the dissipation of Dina Lal's sense of having begun a new life in the land of the pure. Within months of Amir Shah's arrival, however, Dina Lal's wife is abducted by unidentified men (2009: 85). That Amir Shah's presence does nothing to deter this act of violence leads Dina Lal to conclude that Amir Shah 'had failed in his obligation to protect him and his wife' (2009: 91), a figurative representation of the vexed majority-minority tensions occurring extra-fictionally. Indeed, Dina Lal's expectation of Amir Shah's obligation to protect and his allegation of his tenant's failure to do so invoke assurances made by Jinnah, cited above, in the years leading to Partition, as well as those reasserted (though with different emphases) by Liaquat Ali Khan and Jawaharlal Nehru in 1950. In a joint agreement, the Prime Ministers declared:

> The Governments of India and Pakistan solemnly agree that each shall ensure, to the minorities throughout its territory, complete equality of citizenship, irrespective of religion, a full sense of security in respect of life, culture, property and personal honour, freedom of movement within each country and freedom of occupation, speech and worship, subject to law and morality.
>
> (Nehru and Khan 1950: 344)

When added to the prevailing gender and communal economy of this historical moment as portrayed in Khan's novel, Liaquat and Nehru's agreement appears inattentive to the lived experiences of the non-Muslim minorities who remained in Pakistan. Dina Lal goes from feeling as though he could claim belonging to Pakistan via ownership of Five Queen's Road to recognising 'The truth was [that] he was left behind' (Khan 2009:96).

The image of Dina Lal's abandonment complicates his spatialised belonging just as much as Amir Shah's attempts to delegitimise it over the course of the two characters' long association. In the novel's first reference to Dina Lal, for instance, readers learn that 'Amir Shah wasted as little energy as he could on a person [Dina Lal] who had made it his mission to rob him of his peace and property alike' (2009: 11). This initial presentation of Dina Lal, made early in the novel but ten years into his and Amir Shah's acquaintance, invites the conclusion that Amir Shah is the proprietor of Five Queen's Road, as it is Dina Lal who seeks 'to rob' his 'peace'. Although the novel makes Dina Lal's ownership of the house clear when it introduces the earlier narrative plane in the next chapter, Amir Shah's claims of ownership in the later plane promote confusion in the reader and demonstrate the imbalanced interdependence of both characters' identities.

The time span traversed by Khan's novel gestures towards the fictionalisation of Pakistan's development beyond Partition and its representation of the effects which a more widely spatialised Islam has had on non-Muslim minorities. The plot of Aslam's *Season of the Rainbirds* (1993), unfolds over the course of a week in 1982, the very week when, extra-fictionally, an attempt was made on General Zia's life. Yet, in its depiction of non-Muslim minorities, especially Ahmadis, the novel draws upon a longer history, one that stretches back to the nation's earliest moments, when anti-Ahmadi rhetoric could already be heard alongside calls for the institutionalisation of a codified Islam. Historically, two major events punctuate this span: the 1953 anti-Ahmadi disturbances in the Punjab and the ratification in 1973 of the Second Amendment to the Constitution, which identified Ahmadis as non-Muslim. In the penultimate chapter of *Season of the Rainbirds*, an enraged anonymous mob breaks down the door of the Deputy Commissioner's house in order to gain access to his mistress, Elizabeth Massih, a Christian woman whom the villagers had earlier taken to be his domestic help. Readers learn indirectly in the next chapter that this mob, inflamed by a *maulana*'s impassioned Friday afternoon sermon in which he condemns the lovers, 'dragged [the woman] through the streets' and tore her clothes off (1993: 187–189). The mob's reaction to the affair and the *maulana*'s condemnation, which manifest much of the village's discontent with the situation, far outshine any reaction to the murder of the village judge, the primary event that opens the novel. The third-person narrator conveys the consensus view that the judge, apparently corrupt to the core, got what he deserved (1993: 75). In one way of thinking, Elizabeth, too, receives just treatment, as the *maulana*'s fixation with what's pure and what isn't suggests. Significantly, given this fixation, the authorities, led by Elizabeth's lover, want to question her father, Benjamin, about the judge's murder. Elizabeth objects, however, on the grounds that her father only 'unblock[s] the gutters and drains in [the] street [where the judge lived]' (1993: 52). The only character who attempts to intervene on Elizabeth's behalf during this attack is Mr Kasmi, the village's retired schoolmaster, who is also an Ahmadi. All the narrator reveals about Mr Kasmi's professional past is that, years ago while he was still working, the school consisted of only one room, and the classroom was actually a walled-in yard (1993: 29). In the novel's present, the school has grown. Rubbish provided by the villagers serves as the concrete-encased foundations for the school's extension, creating a nauseating stench that permeates the entire structure (1993: 30).

These brief sketches of plot and character establish the basis of a preliminary inquiry into how Aslam's novel's representation of non-Muslim minorities troubles the emplacement of Islam in the geographical space of Pakistan. Three primary points emerge from the novel's non-Muslim characters, all of which insist upon the necessity of these characters for the functioning of the majority characters' lives. First, the work of all three characters contributes to the social reproduction of community in the sense that they maintain public and private spaces (Benjamin and Elizabeth) and are responsible for educating the village's children (Mr Kasmi). Second, all three characters' work somehow deals with waste, literally and figuratively. Benjamin, for instance, literally cleans the village's gutters, filthy but necessary work, and his occupation may well stand in for the marginal but crucial role which Christians, as one type of non-Muslim minority, played as a minority in a majority Muslim context. Elizabeth's doubled role is similar, though her 'wasted' work results from the futility of her efforts to maintain a domestic space for herself and her Muslim lover in the face of communal disapprobation. Mr Kasmi's identity as schoolmaster connects him directly to the reproduction of existing structures, a role that implicates him in the oppression and violence he suffers as an Ahmadi. His wasted effort to educate his students otherwise finds its physical manifestation in the garbage-filled foundations of the school itself. Third and relatedly, all three characters' occupation of specific places is crucial to the functioning of the other villagers, either as a collective or as individuals. This third point differs from the first, which speaks to the characters' contributions to the work of social reproduction in that, with respect to this latter, the actual occupation of space is irreducible. Despite prejudices, religious edicts, and laws, these characters are 'there', so to speak, taking up space that no one else can also inhabit at the same time. And, Elizabeth's desire to downplay her father's usefulness to the authorities aside, both she and Mr Kasmi forcefully occupy their spaces, deliberately bucking the social conventions that discriminate against them.

The Muslim community in Aslam's novel denies the three non-Muslim characters any freedom of movement or occupation of space, however. All three characters experience some form of explicit hostility, Elizabeth and Mr Kasmi most of all, as she is dragged through the streets and he is beaten by the same mob as he tries to protect her. Kasmi's assault only deepens the violence he has suffered, as the novel also mentions – though does not fully narrate – how his native village was razed and his family killed in the process, a development he learns about only through 'the two maulana-jis [of the novel's central village] rejoicing on their loudspeakers that the country was being purged' (Aslam 1993: 141). Further, Aslam's narrator makes repeated though subtle references to how the main mosque dominates the village's topography. From the balcony above the butcher's shop, for instance, the 'tips of the two minarets' are visible (1993: 57). Similarly, the narrator describes how, 'Behind the courthouse, above the roofs and the tops of trees, […] the minarets of the two mosques [appeared to be] holding up the drizzly sky' (1993: 78). The images of the mosques' omnipresence make of these structures more than landmarks; they can also be read as structuring the layout of the entire village – their minarets are holding up the sky, after all. This topographical imagining of Islam's dominance in the novel, coupled as it is with the violent restrictions placed upon the non-Muslim minorities – the novel's Christians must go to another village to attend mass – mirrors Manan Ahmed's structural metaphor for the position of non-Muslim Pakistanis in Pakistani politics: 'Pakistan resembles a house designed and built from the inside, piecemeal […]. In the […] basement are the 'minorities' – those deemed capable of sanctuary but incapable of being seen above the surface' (1993: 233). Ahmed's house and basement imagery goes to the foundational yet invisible presence of minorities in relation to majority identities as Aslam's novel represents the relations and their spatial dimensions.

What remains as yet unexamined though crucial to this analysis of space and mobility in relation to non-Muslim minorities in Pakistan are the broader geopolitical dynamics that may have shaped the domestic politics of the nation. Jinnah closes his 1947 address, for instance, with mention of George Marshall's greetings. Marshall, as US Secretary of State in the post-Second World War era was, of course, the architect of the Marshall Plan and thus a prime mover in the US' Cold War ascendancy and its identification of Pakistan as a crucial ally because of its geopolitical location.

Significantly, literary production at the time – namely, Saadat Hasan Manto's 'Letters to Uncle Sam' – presciently encapsulates these internal and external dynamics in ways that, even in present-day scholarship, neither historians nor international relations scholars do. Manto wrote his series of satirical letters at the behest of the US Information Services, at least initially. The USIS approached Manto in 1950/1951 to see if he would use his literary esteem to forward a pro-American agenda in Pakistan. Keen for the money the Americans offered, and yet turned off by the naked interest in propaganda, Manto submitted the first letter, for which he received an advance of 300 rupees, only for the Americans to refuse to publish it. Undeterred, Manto published that first letter and eight more in local Lahori periodicals from 1951 to 1954. The provenance of the 'Letters' makes clear their direct line to Cold War politics. Manto's satire extends this line with a particularly keen eye towards the spatialisation of Islam and its effects on non-Muslim minorities. During the time Manto was writing and subversively serialising his satire (1953), John Foster Dulles was the US Secretary of State (Dulles was serving as the US delegate to the UN in 1947). US Department of State cables passed between Dulles and the American diplomatic staff in Karachi make clear the Secretary's preference for dealing with Pakistan because of its Muslim majority population over India, due to the latter's polytheistic majority. Dulles, a staunch Christian, believed that 'people of the book' bore a natural affinity and aversion to the threat of godless communism, whereas polytheists were less stringent regarding others' belief systems. Thus, Dulles set a religiously tinged tone at a crucial formative moment in US-Pakistan relations.

Of significance, too, is the extra-fictional context which Aslam incorporates into his novel: the attempted assassination of Zia. That specific military dictator was a particular darling of President Ronald Reagan's administration due to the arrangements provided and accommodations made for the US' proxy war against the Soviet Union in Afghanistan. Of course, these arrangements followed the logic established by Dulles' Muslim preference: devoted monotheists were more likely to recognise godless communism as a threat to their way of life. These historical realities add dimensions to – though cannot be said to determine – majority-minority relations in Pakistan, as, no doubt, do the Raj's legacies, including the way the British conception of the liberal subject fed into religious freedom and territorial sovereignty.

Notes

1 See Chapter 7 of my *National Identities in Pakistan* (2011) for a lengthier discussion of Rahmat Ali's engagement from afar with the Pakistan Movement.
2 Tariq Rahman (2012) gives hard figures from census data in the 1940s and 1950s that demonstrates the stunning shifts in religious demographics in what became Pakistan.
3 In *Politics of Desecularization*, Sadia Saeed focuses on the legal status of the Ahmadi community in Pakistan to illustrate the process of 'unsettled desecularization', which 'defines those national cases in which religion has been selectively folded into political life but in ways that are continually contested from various quarters' (2016: 28).
4 Other novels that portray non-Muslim minority characters include Muhammad Hanif's *Our Lady of Alice Bhatti*, Bina Shah's *The Slum Child*, and Omar Shahid Hamid's *The Prisoner*.
5 See my 'Spatial Visions' (2016), where I argue that Lenny's mother and aunt, as non-Muslim female characters, gesture towards an alternative social order in immediate post-Partition Pakistan.
6 Non-Muslims were not alone in being overlooked in the distribution of evacuee property. Unprivileged Muslims experienced a similar marginalisation, as Jalal says: 'Individual citizens with little or no influence had to settle for whatever was left over, which in most cases was very modest' (2014: 58).
7 See Feisal Khan's 'How Not to Control Corruption, Pakistani Style' (2016) and Ilyas Chattha's 'Competition for Resources' (2012) for analyses of how the government's attempts to institutionalise the management of evacuee properties were hobbled by corruption.

Bibliography

Ahmed, M. (2011) *Where the Wild Frontiers Are: Pakistan and the American Imagination*. Charlottesville: Just World Books.
Ali, C.R. (1933) 'Now or Never: Are We to Live or Perish Forever?' *Islam in South Asia: Some Useful Study Materials*. [online]. Available from <www.columbia.edu/itc/mealac/pritchett/00islamlinks/txt_rahmatali_1933.html> [3 June 2017].
Ashraf, S. (2004) *The Postmaster*. New Delhi: Penguin.
Aslam, N. (1993) *Season of the Rainbirds*. London: Faber and Faber.
Baerenholdt, J.O. (2013) 'Governmobility: The Powers of Mobility'. *Mobilities* 8(1), 20–34.
Chatta, I. (2012) 'Competitions for Resources: Partition's Evacuee Property and the Sustenance of Corruption in Pakistan'. *Modern Asian Studies* 46(5), 1182–1211.
Cilano, C. (2016) 'Spatial Visions: Mobility and the Social Order in Pakistani Women's English-Language Partition Fiction'. *Asiatic* 10(1), 113–127.

Cilano, C. (2011) *National Identities in Pakistan: The 1971 War in Contemporary Pakistani Fiction*. London: Routledge.
Jalal, A. (2014) *The Struggle for Pakistan: A Muslim Homeland and Global Politics*. Cambridge, MA: Harvard University Press.
Jinnah, M.A. (1945) 'Interview to a Representative of the Associated Press of America, Clarifying Various Aspects of Pakistan' [online]. Available from <www.oocities.org/sadna_gupta/Extra1C_Jinnahspeeches4345.html> [12 June 2017].
Jinnah, M.A. (1947) 'First Presidential Address to the Constituent Assembly of Pakistan'. [online]. Available from <www.columbia.edu/itc/mealac/pritchett/00islamlinks/txt_jinnah_assembly_1947.html> [3 June 2017].
Khan, F. (2016) 'How Not to Control Corruption, Pakistani Style'. [online]. Available from <http://blogs.lse.ac.uk/southasia/2016/05/31/how-not-to-control-corruption-pakistani-style/> [31 August 2017].
Khan, S.Y. (2009) *Five Queen's Road*. New Delhi: Penguin.
Manto, S.H. (2001) *Letters to Uncle Sam*. Trans. by Hasan, K. Islamabad: Alhamra.
Massey, D. (2005) *For Space*. London: Sage Publications.
Nehru, J. and Khan, L.A. (1950) 'Agreement between India and Pakistan on Minorities'. *Middle East Journal* 4(3), 344–346.
Rahman, T. (2012) 'Pakistan's Policies and Practices towards Religious Minorities'. *South Asian History and Culture* 3(2), 302–315.
Saeed, S. (2007) 'Pakistani Nationalism and the State Marginalisation of the Ahmadiyya Community in Pakistan'. *Studies in Ethnicity and Nationalism* 7(3), 122–152.
Saeed, S. (2016) *Politics of Desecularization: Law and the Minority Question in Pakistan*. New York: Cambridge University Press.
Schechtman, J.B. (1951) 'Evacuee Property in India and Pakistan'. *Pacific Affairs* 24(4), 406–413.
Sidhwa, B. (1998) *Cracking India*. Minneapolis: Milkweed.
Singh, K. (1956) *Train to Pakistan*. New York: Grove.

2
1971

Reassessing a forgotten national narrative

Muneeza Shamsie

In 1947, Pakistan was created as a unique country, on the basis of its Muslim identity as a unifying force, although its two major provinces, East and West Pakistan, were divided by 1,000 miles. The population ratio was 54:46. The larger population was in East Pakistan. The seat of government was in West Pakistan (Karachi, then Islamabad). The fragile, newly independent country faced many problems, including ongoing hostilities with India. Consequently, 'the demands of the military establishment on the state's meagre resources left little for development in the provinces' (Jalal 2014: 146). In December 1970, following political turmoil and martial law, Pakistan saw its first free and fair election. The results revealed a country deeply ethnically divided. The Awami League, led by Sheikh Mujibur Rahman in East Pakistan, won a clear overall majority, but it had no support in West Pakistan. His election campaign was based on 'six points' demanding greater provincial autonomy due to East Pakistan's anger with West Pakistan's domination. But the bureaucratic military elite, dominated by West Pakistanis, considered this tantamount to treason. To complicate this, in West Pakistan, Zulfikar Ali Bhutto's Pakistan People's party won a majority in Punjab and Sindh, the two most populous provinces, but in Baluchistan and North-West Frontier, a majority voted for Wali Khan's National Awami Party, which was willing to join Mujibur Rahman and form a government in Islamabad.

The military government of Yahya Khan refused to hand over power to Mujibur Rahman. The two most senior West Pakistani officials in East Pakistan, the governor, Admiral S.M. Ahsan, and the chief martial law administrator, Lt General Sahabzada Yaqub-Khan, urged a political solution, not a military one (Yaqub-Khan 2005: 280). Their advice was ignored, and they resigned in protest in early March. On the night of 25–26 March 1971, the army embarked on a ruthless military action in Dhaka.

In West Pakistan, there was great outrage at Bengalis' killing of non-Bengalis in East Pakistan. In September 1971, the expatriate Pakistani-American academic Eqbal Ahmed tried to set the record straight by publishing 'Letter to a Pakistani Diplomat' in the *New York Times*. He explained that he originally belonged to Bihar and most of his people had migrated to East Pakistan, where several 'were killed by Bengali zealots during the period immediately preceding the military's intervention' (Ahmed 2006: 416), but he was 'able to find neither a political nor an economic nor a moral justification for the current policy of military intervention'. He added that the white paper published in August 1971 by the Pakistan military authorities exaggerated tenfold the number of people killed by the Bengalis and was 'obviously intended to justify trials and death sentences for opposition leaders' (Ahmed 2006: 419) in East Pakistan.

The conflict culminated in December 1971 with war with India and defeat for the Pakistani army. East Pakistan became independent Bangladesh. Ayesha Jalal writes: 'The army's campaign against Bengali resistance, a tragic mixture of human folly and capacity for brutality, was abruptly cut short by Indian military intervention and the disintegration of Pakistan' (1991: 312–313). Tariq Ali describes the military action of 1971 and its ethnic violence as 'shocking, shameful and one of the worst blots in our history'. He says, 'Jinnah's Pakistan died on March 26, 1971, with East Pakistan drowned in blood' (qtd. in M. Shamsie 1996: 91).

Defeat by the Indian army and the loss of half a country came as a shock to most West Pakistanis, thanks to a censored press and a policy of disinformation. Reports in the foreign media, such as the *Daily Telegraph*'s lead story 'Genocide' by Anthony Mascarenhas, a Pakistani journalist, were condemned as lies and foreign propaganda.[1] In December 1971, a new truncated Pakistan came into being. Zulfikar Ali Bhutto, who now held the majority vote, formed a government. He established the Hamoodur Rahman Commission 'to enquire how the 1971 defeat came about' (Cilano 2011: 2). The Commission's report was submitted in 1974, but suppressed until 2000. Pakistan's literary response to 1971 was also very limited for years. Pakistanis 'simply wanted to be done with the events of 1971 and not be reminded time and again' (Zaman and Farrukhi qtd. in Cilano 2011: 6). The year 1971 passed into official and public amnesia.

In 2002, the then-president of Pakistan, General Pervez Musharraf, 'offered regrets for the war to Bangladeshis' (Cilano 2011: 2) during a visit to Dhaka, but this apology 'raises questions about the meaning of the past'. To this day, in textbooks used 'in a field called "Pakistan studies" Jalal sees the use of "bigoted narrative styles" that are in her opinion "consistent with the state's homogenising agendas of proclaiming a national culture by fiat"' (Cilano 2011: 30). The declassified Hamoodur Rahman Commission's report also revealed contradictions and elisions which gave 'an inadequate account of what happened', creating 'a narrative vacuum at the national level' (2011: 2). Today, Musharraf's 'regret' has slipped from public memory.

In marked contrast, as my literary history *Hybrid Tapestries* (2017) reveals, there has been a growing literary response to 1971 in Pakistani anglophone literature, particularly after 2000, creating a body of work possibly as extensive as post-9/11 Pakistani anglophone fiction, but little known. Cara Cilano's *National Identities in Pakistan: The 1971 War in Contemporary Pakistan Fiction* (2011) remains the only major critical work on the subject. This essay looks at the representation of 1971 in English-language fiction by Pakistanis and discusses the few twentieth-century works alongside those of a younger generation.

In the aftermath of 1971: breaking the silence

Tariq Rahman's courageous story 'Bingo', published in *The Frontier Post* in 1975, was the first response to 1971 in Pakistani anglophone fiction, while Rahman was a serving officer in the Pakistan army. He had opposed the military action in East Pakistan, though he was never posted there and resolved to leave the army, which he did in 1978. Today he is a distinguished academic. The title 'Bingo' refers to the derogatory West Pakistani term for Bengalis in 1970–1971. The narrator, Safeer, and a Bengali cadet, Tajassur, are classmates at the military academy. Tajassur is popular with juniors, but scorned by contemporaries for his easy-going attitude towards drill and discipline and his eccentric interest in books. Safeer recalls that shortly before graduation, 'East Pakistan had started kicking up one hell of a row to get separated from West Pakistan. We called him [Tajassur] "Bingo", and "a traitor" and "Sheikh Mujibur Rehman's ADC"' (Rahman 1997: 313). Safeer and Tajassur are then posted to East Pakistan as second lieutenants. Soon, 'the Mukti Bahini – i.e. rebel Bingo troops – had started to play havoc with our supply lines' (1997: 317). Safeer never uses the words 'parliament', 'election' or 'vote', but sums up Mujibur Rahman's 'six points' with the comment, 'anything coming from a loony like Mujib must have been crap' (1997: 317). In Sorayya Khan's *Noor*, young Pakistani soldiers in East Pakistan dismiss Bengalis as 'dim-wits' (2003: 152).

The influence of obsolete, racist, and colonial textbooks is embodied in a commanding officer's admiration for General Nicholson's role in 1857 – in quelling the uprising – and his dismissive comment on the Vietcong as 'a short statured people' who 'don't seem to be a martial race' (Rahman 1997: 316). Tajassur says, 'I believe there are no martial races [...] People are forced to fight when they are exploited and transgressed against. And bravery is only good if it is used in a just cause' (1997:316). Later Safeer tells Tajassur that 'the Bingos' want to divide the country and are 'Pakistan's enemies' and 'Indian agents' (1997:318). Tajassur answers: 'Listen, Safeer. This is all propaganda' (1997:318). To Safeer's horror, he speaks of army excesses, 'and of exploitation and tyranny' – and Tajassur soon deserts (1997:318).

Safeer's matter-of-fact descriptions of shooting, killings, rapes, and the razing to the ground of entire villages, in which he takes part as a duty against 'the enemy', are truly chilling, as is his inability to distinguish between right and wrong, including the rape of a frightened girl, provided for him by his senior officer to celebrate his twenty-first birthday. Khan's *Noor* (2003) provides a more graphic and shocking description of a young Pakistani soldier being encouraged by his superior to prove his masculinity by violating a Bengali woman (182). Khan's research on 1971 for *Noor* underpins these texts.[2] According to Yasmin Saikia, 'The Pakistanis hoped that the tactics of fear and extreme punishment and humiliation of Bengali honour would prevent further rebel recruitment of the Mukti. But this was not the case. Their ranks swelled' (2011: 49–51). Safeer is captured by the Mukti Bahini and discovers Tajassur is a captain in the unit. He helps Safeer escape, sheltering him with his own family. But Safeer is 'rescued' by Pakistani commandos. They kill Tajassur, violate his sister, and their mother goes mad with grief: Safeer shoots her to put her out of her misery. He knows there will be no one to accuse him. This dénouement is a reminder of 1971's horror, and the complicating, unrecorded narratives of civil war, men in opposite camps who had once served together – as had many Mukti and Pakistani soldiers – often honour that comradeship, despite the bitterness of conflict: a detail reinforced by Khan's research too.

The violence that Rahman captures is exceptional for the Pakistani anglophone literature of that time; and predates the harrowing descriptions of Partition in Bapsi Sidhwa's novels *The Bride* (1982) and *Ice-Candy Man* (1988): the difference is that, in 1971, the wanton killings and crimes were committed by a state institution – the army – in the name of law and order. Rahman's critically acclaimed story did not raise any great public awareness in Pakistan. Interestingly, Aminatta Forna's novel *The Memory of Love* (2010), revolving around the savage civil war in Sierra Leone, portrays a similar national silence, only to reveal, ultimately, equally terrifying stories. Forna's use of a psychiatrist as a main protagonist draws parallels between the silence, memory lapses, and disorientation of individuals suffering from post-traumatic stress with those of an entire nation.

Beyond trauma and amnesia

The need to move beyond trauma and amnesia in order to remember and forgive is central to Khan's remarkable novel *Noor*, the first Pakistani anglophone novel to portray East Pakistan in 1971. The book juxtaposes Islamabad in the 1990s with the unravelling of suppressed memories of East Pakistan in 1971. Khan employs, as a catalyst, the subcontinental superstition that the mentally challenged are endowed with clairvoyant powers: the uncanny drawings of Noor, a special child, 'different' from the others (doctors employs terms such as Asperger's Syndrome, Rhett Syndrome), unleash unexpected images of the past for Ali, her grandfather, and Sajida, her mother.

Sajida believes that she and Noor, her third child, have a special connection. Noor appears to her in a vision, long before she is born. Sajida and her husband Hussein, her erstwhile classmate, live with her foster father, Ali, an estate agent, at Ali's insistence. In 1971, Ali was a serving army officer in East Pakistan. He had rescued Sajida, a Bengali orphan of 'fiveandsix' (Khan 2003: 11). He adopted her and brought her up in Islamabad, with the help of his widowed mother, Nanijan. This appellation – maternal grandmother – represents an absence in Ali's home, embodying 'the narrative vacuum' (Cilano 2011: 2) of Pakistan, since Ali never married and Sajida has never known any mother in Islamabad.

Noor starts to paint from the age of five. The earliest paintings, of fish, remind Sajida that her father was a fisherman; another painting 'brought the cyclone back to Sajida' (Khan 2003: 103) – in which she believes her parents died. Noor unwittingly continues to produce brilliantly coloured images which exhume Ali's and Sajida's buried memories of 1971. Noor's drawings increasingly impel Ali to confront his memories, that he participated in more than military combat in East Pakistan. He recalls rape, the wholesale slaughter of Bengalis, and mass graves to bury them – one such muddy pit, included fresh, recently shot bodies of Bengali passers-by, where a little girl struggled through the dead, crying out 'Mukhtiar'. As Ali's confession unfolds, it transpires that that child was Sajida, and Mukhtiar her baby brother: Ali had killed her family. But Khan moves beyond guilt and recrimination to look at the possibilities of love and atonement, though 'the family is by no means fully consolidated at the novel's close; a shattered mirror cannot be put back together. It does, however, stand a chance of being reconstituted along different lines, with a different narrative to tell its story' (Cilano 2011: 65–66).

Masculinity, war, and violence against women

Khan often refers to gender, which, Cilano suggests,

> hints at a genuine queering of conventional masculinity by having Ali's tour in East Pakistan last for the nine months it would take for a woman to gestate a baby. Ali's paternity then depends on his own corresponding and unnatural maternity.
> (2011: 56)

On Ali's return to Islamabad in 1971, to exorcise his memories, he forces himself into a tub of boiling water, 'enveloped by steam' until 'his genitals were burned and blistered'. De-sexed, Ali's 'paternal body' becomes 'a metaphor for the violence carried out in the nation's name' (Cilano 2011: 56). He recalls the treatment of a young Bengali girl who 'didn't wear a sari blouse, a preference of the officer in charge' and who, having been violated by his superior, is then offered to Ali, who 'felt sick to his stomach', for which he is taunted: 'you are not a soldier' (Khan 2003: 182). The fact that Ali tries to oblige but his attempt to violate the girl ends in failure muddles guilt and masculinity. His attempt to 'blanch his memories' by self-inflicted torture becomes 'an act to stabilize himself for the larger good of his new "ready-made family" in Islamabad' (Cilano 2011: 56).

The discourse on patriarchy, masculinity, war, and violence against women is central to Khan's narrative, and also to Shahbano Bilgrami's *Without Dreams* (2007) Moni Mohsin's *The End of Innocence* (2006) and Kamila Shamsie's *Kartography* (2003). In *Noor*, Ali joined the army against the wishes of his mother, with dreams of making his country proud, although she warned of imminent conflict in 1970–1971 and said: 'war is an animal gone mad' (Khan 2003: 70). The novel shatters another illusion when it transpires that the loving Nanijan, the family matriarch, was a battered wife: her husband would punch her, 'slamming her against the display cabinet, knocking knick knacks from their places' (Khan 2003: 176).

In *Without Dreams*, Bilgrami depicts silence as complicity, drawing parallels between the division of Pakistan in 1971 and Pakistan's divisions of ethnicity, class, and gender. The novel links a family's amnesia with that of Pakistan, when Haroon returns to Pakistan after nineteen years, but cannot remember how his father died. The teenage Haroon had in fact killed him. Haroon had toppled a bookshelf on his father to stop him beating Haroon's beautiful mother, Tahira. Accustomed to hiding her bruises to avert social scandal, Tahira protects her son, too, by allowing Abdul, their Bengali servant boy, to be accused and jailed in his stead. She is unaware that her 'vulnerability to violence prompts Abdul to connect her victimhood to his dreams and memories, allowing him to eventually recall his own mother's vulnerability' (Cilano 2013: 73) in East Pakistan, where she was violated and killed in 1971 by West Pakistani soldiers. In another ironic comment, Abdul had then come to Karachi with other poor Bengali migrants in search of employment.

Patriarchal violence against women is central to Mohsin's *The End of Innocence*, which looks at the 1971 conflict from the distance of rural Punjab, culminating metaphorically with an unexploded bomb which falls in the vicinity during the war. The narrative, presented from the perspective of Laila, a privileged child, links the demise of a united Pakistan with the murder of Rani, an unmarried, pregnant girl – both in the name of 'honour' – and, Cilano argues, also 'links Rani's increasingly desperate situation with the violence and coming war in East Pakistan' (2013: 79). Laila, admires and loves the teenage Rani, the family maidservant's daughter, but cannot understand Rani's romantic dreams, inspired by the Punjabi folk tale of Heer Ranjha. The worthless young man with whom Rani falls in love abandons her; and her stepfather kills her for her crime. Laila cannot forgive herself for her inadvertent, uncomprehending words which betrayed Rani. Laila's liberal, aristocratic, landowning parents are among a minority of people in the area who are shocked by Rani's death, as they also are by the military action in East Pakistan. They voice their concern 'at the atrocities going on in East Pakistan' to Colonel Butt at the nearby cantonment. He replies that 'Civil war is not a polite sanitary affair. It's like within a household. Between husband and wife, if you will!' (Mohsin 2006: 105). Cilano points out that, in traditional Pakistani society, the man of the family is responsible for the family's honour based on due obedience, this metaphor 'effeminizes the East Pakistanis' who need to be disciplined, and justifies the price Rani pays for her 'sin' (2013: 80). Rani is buried on 3 December 1971, the day that India invaded Pakistan, providing one of many 'structural linkages' (Cilano 2013: 80).

Marxism: an interlude

Shahryar Fazli's *Invitation* (2011) takes history back to the 1951 Rawalpindi Conspiracy Case, in which the father of the narrator, Shahbaz, is accused, together with other left-wing officers, activists, writers, and trade unionists, of planning an alleged military coup; the episode enabled the authorities to clamp down on communist activities in Pakistan. Fazli juxtaposes that era with the expatriate Shahbaz's encounter with the all-powerful 1970 military, particularly his father's old friend, the retired Brigadier Imtiaz, who owns a nightclub famous for its cabarets. Shahbaz is looked after by his father's one-time driver, Ghulam Hussain, in Karachi. But Ghulam Hussain is Bengali, and as the country veers into the crisis of 1970–1971, Shahbaz is sucked into corruption and state violence, and betrays Ghulam Hussain, whose very ethnicity renders him suspect to the authorities. Tariq Ali's novel *The Night of the Golden Butterfly* (2010) encapsulates sixty years of Pakistan's history, including the demise of communism and the rise of military power and religious extremism. The narrator lives in exile, unable to forget that in the 1960s his Bengali friend Tipu, a fellow communist activist and student in Lahore, was betrayed and handed over to the military authorities, symbolising the betrayal of East Pakistan. The novel is an intertextual engagement with Ali's non-fiction work *The Duel: Pakistan on the Flight of American Power* (2008), which includes his bond with Maulana Bhashani (1880–1976) and his popular peasant-based movement in East Pakistan (after the 1970 cyclone, Bhashani withdrew from contesting polls).

Confronting the reality

There are few portrayals in Pakistani anglophone literature of Pakistan's immediate reaction to the 1971 surrender. In her creative memoir *Meatless Days* (1989), Sara Suleri writes:

> something in our spirits broke in the war of 1971. It was not so much the country's severing that hurt as the terrible afterimages we had to face: censorship lifted for a flash, flooding us with photographs and stories of what the army actually did in Bangladesh during the months of emergency before the war, 'I am not talking about the two-nation theory,' I wept to my father, 'I am talking about blood.'
>
> (1989: 122)

In a narrative replete with analogies, symbolism, and subtexts, Suleri links family history with that of the nation. Her narrative revolves around her sister, Ifat, and their Welsh-born mother, Mair, both killed in traffic accidents. She writes, too, of Ifat's impetuous marriage in Lahore to Javed, an army officer. After the surrender of 1971, he was one of 93,000 soldiers in East Pakistan taken as prisoners of war in India, but 'the country made quick provisions to forget the war in Bangladesh' (1989: 144). When the soldiers were repatriated after two years, they 'came back to a world that did not really want to hear the kind of stories they had to tell'. At home there came that horrific moment 'when he began to describe what he had felt during his first killing'. Terrified, Suleri wondered, 'How will Ifat do it, how will she make Javed's mind a human home again and take those stories from his head?' (1989: 144).

Amid cyclone, floods, and gunfire

In *Noor*, Sajida is haunted by memories of the cyclone in East Pakistan. The cyclone – one of the worst in recent history – struck shortly before the 1970 election; people died in their hundreds of thousands, millions were left homeless. The government's inability to cope and the criticism of its relief operations ensured Mujibur Rahman's sweeping electoral victory.

Adam Zameenzad's novel *Cyrus Cyrus* (1991) focuses on the lives of the poor and marginalised, albeit across several continents. His narrator, Cyrus, a Choodah (the lowest Hindu caste), a latrine cleaner and Christian convert in India, is falsely accused of murder. He flees with his family to East Pakistan where, overtaken by the tragedies of 1970–1971, only he survives. His agony at loved ones falling prey to natural disasters – snakes, crocodiles, and wild beasts during the cyclone and floods – pales in comparison to mankind's brutality: Cyrus' mother, sister, and brother are tortured and murdered in their *jhuggi* (mud hut). The fact that the assailants' identity and ethnicity remain unknown captures the savagery and hatred of 1971.

Cyrus' comment that he and his family were 'certainly not political […] but we too were quite excited about the excitement, and vociferously and heartily agreed with whoever expressed an opinion' (Zameenzad 1991: 139) made them doubly vulnerable; and this is also a reminder that in countries with huge social disparities, the daily struggles of most people are for food, employment, and survival.

In *Cyrus Cyrus*, Zameenzad criticises politicians, the army, and Indian interference for the sufferings of 1971. He adds that the foreign press 'failed to see […] the massacre of the Biharis and the Urdu-speaking, pro-Pakistan citizens of Bangla Desh by the Bengalis, though it rightly saw and rightly reported the genocidal waves of attacks by the Pakistan Army upon the Bangla-speaking people' (1991: 141). As Saikia says, 'The story of violence committed by the Bengalis is less well known and is poorly represented in the news media, except the Pakistani Urdu press' (2011: 59).

In nowhere land

Zameenzad's suggestion that language, Bangla and Urdu, defined loyalties in East Pakistan during the 1971 conflict conforms to widespread perceptions in Pakistan and Bangladesh that belie a more complex history. In the pre-Partition era, Urdu became a symbol of Muslim unity and was made the language of government in Pakistan, alongside English. The refusal to accept East Pakistan's demand that Bengali should be a national language led to conflict, riots, and the growth of Bengali nationalism. Bengali was accepted as a national language of Pakistan in 1956, rescinded in 1959, and reinstated shortly before the 1970 election. At the same time, a number of Bengalis, albeit an urban minority, were traditionally Urdu-speaking and included leading politicians. In 1971, many Urdu-speaking Bengalis identified with Bengali nationalists, which Bangladeshi novelist Tahmima Anam skilfully captures in her novel *The Golden Age* (2008). However, the Biharis, Urdu-speaking migrants from India to East Pakistan (mostly from the province of Bihar), 'were targeted as "the enemy" of the Bengalis' in 1970/71' (Saikia 2011: 50).

Aamer Hussein's nuanced story 'Karima' in the collection *Mirror to the Sun* (1993) 'draws upon Bihari history, but it does so in order to identify the silences enveloping the displacement that Biharis figuratively represent' (Cilano 2011: 103). This tale of dislocation and loss, takes Karima, a woman of Bihari origin, from Dhaka to Karachi, then London, and is reconstructed by a nameless Urdu-speaking British-Asian narrator. Though Karima was born in Dhaka and 'could speak Bengali like her mother tongue' (Hussein 1993: 63), at home she spoke Urdu. Her literate Bihari husband Badshah, a mechanic, had set up a small business, and so Karima didn't have to work, unlike most of her neighbours. Badshah longed to move to Karachi because 'that's where they speak our language, that's the real Pakistan. These Bengalis, he said, he couldn't really understand them' (Hussein 1993: 35). Karima is alarmed by the 'Punjabi soldiers [who] had come in from across the sea and begun to pillage around the edges of city' in 1971, but Badshah regarded them as friends who would rescue them 'from those marauding Bengalis' (Hussein 1993: 36). Karima's once-friendly neighbours taunt her: 'Dirty Biharis […] go home or we'll come and get you' (Hussein 1993: 36). Four Bengali men enter her home and threaten her. Badshah comes at them with a broken bottle, shouting 'Pakistan Zindabad' [long live Pakistan] (Hussein 1993: 37). They set him on fire.

Karima escapes to Karachi with Shahzeb, her two-year-old son, and Badshah's family. Ironically, despite the national rhetoric of 'belonging' and 'unity', the Biharis find themselves different to Karachi's inhabitants, as is their Urdu and their appearance: the Biharis are smaller and darker and in Karachi they are known as 'Bengali log' [Bengali people] (Hussein 1993: 38). The Biharis are confined in an overcrowded camp, because Pakistan refused to accept

Biharis from East Pakistan after 1971, 'due to instability born of ethno-regional unrest' (Cilano 2011: 84). Karima reluctantly marries Badshah's younger brother, Rahim, in self-protection and has a child by him, but Rahim considers Badshah's son a financial burden. Both husband and wife finally find work, as a driver and an *ayah*, respectively, for a rich family. But when the employers take Karima to London to look after their disadvantaged son and her eldest, Shahzeb, dies, she runs away. She ends up living in London with a Bengali butcher and working as virtual slave labour in his shop: since they are not married, she dares not accompany him on his visits to Bangladesh, in case she is recognised. Her state of limbo embodies that of the Biharis, who find they belong nowhere and have nowhere to go.

Aquila Ismail's loosely autobiographical novel *Of Martyrs and Marigolds* (2012) is perhaps the only Pakistani anglophone novel to portray the perspective of Biharis. Ismail, a Bihari, born and brought up in in Dhaka, speaks Bengali fluently, as does her protagonist, Suri (like Hussein's Karima). In a memoir essay, 'Leaving Bangladesh', Ismail describes being rounded up with other Biharis in Dhaka and incarcerated in a camp. She escaped thanks to 'a family friend in the Bangladeshi army [who] took the risk of literally whisking us away at great peril to himself' (Ismail 2011: 139). Ismail developed this into her novel *Martyrs*.

Suri is in love with Rumi, a Bengali boy. She belongs to a cultured family which identifies with East Pakistan and criticises West Pakistan's policies. But in the political tensions of 1970–1971, they are tarred as 'non-Bengali' and 'West Pakistani sympathisers'; many 'Urdu-speakers' are killed. In the newly created Bangladesh, Suri realises that 'all those whose mother tongue was not Bengali had no place in this land whatsoever' (Ismail 2012: 2). In February 1972, she and her family and Bihari neighbours are herded out of their homes. The men and women are separated. The men are driven away in buses, the women are confined to a house; at night, some women are 'taken away' by the Bangladeshi soldiers. Suri and her women companions are sent by ship to a camp – a former juvenile home. There is no sign of the men. Rumi, now an officer in the Bangladesh army, helps Suri, her mother, and sister escape. His father helps her locate her father, in a jail, but Suri cannot find her brothers. Ultimately, she learns that when the men were taken away, the young were separated and killed by Bangladeshi soldiers bent on revenge. Suri and her surviving family are among the few Biharis to obtain a passage to unknown and alien Karachi.

Dreams of unity

Mehr Nigar Masroor's posthumously published novel *Shadows of Time* (1987) remains the only work in Pakistani anglophone fiction to span over a century, including the divisions of 1947 and 1971. She leads up to the rise of religious extremism during the Zia regime in the 1980s. The novel is also unique because it begins in Bengal in 1883 and provides an important portrayal of Bengal's leading role in the politics of Muslim identity, which becomes a foil to the post-independence derailment of the political process in Pakistan and West Pakistan's exploitation of East Pakistan.

Masroor tells the tale of the friendship in the late nineteenth century between Akbar, a Muslim aristocrat, and three Hindus in Calcutta, the then-imperial capital. She describes Bengal's political awakening, the birth of Indian nationalism, and the Partition of Bengal into Hindu and Muslim majority areas by the British to create schisms between the two communities. The rise of Hindu extremism, the establishment of the Muslim League in Dhaka, Bengal's leading role in the Pakistan movement, and the colonial resolve to create a new imperial capital in Delhi, thus marginalising Bengal, are all built into the narrative, as are enduring love affairs between Hindu and Muslim protagonists. The resulting intertwined bloodlines suggest a syncretic Indo-Muslim society 'in sharp contrast [...] [to] the political, ideological and cultural stances, bent on purity and fundamentalisms' (Cilano 2013: 45).

Masroor's main protagonist, Maheen, grows up in Lahore. She is the daughter of Farhan, a Muslim League activist, whose family includes a Punjabi father, a mother from Delhi, and a much-loved Bengali uncle – Akbar. These interprovincial family bonds assert the ideals of a multi-ethnic, united Muslim Pakistan. This concept finds expression in Zaib-un-Nissa Hamidullah's story collection *The Young Wife* (2008), which includes fiction set in East Pakistan, where she was born, and West Pakistan, where she married. She says: 'Both wings are beloved to me' (Hamidullah 2008: xxi). Masroor wrote her novel while suffering from terminal cancer and may not have had time for further revisions. As Niaz Zaman points out, 'Masroor's reading of the politics of [pre-1947] Bengal and her moulding of it to fit her fictional characters is better than her use of political history in the later section of the book' (2000: 305).

The obstacles to freedom of cultural expression in Pakistan are central to the post-independence section, since Maheen concentrates on fostering the arts and classical dance (as did Masroor). But past 'Muslim ruler[s] had patronized all art forms in India', whereas 'in Pakistan the homeland required for the Muslims of India to live and grow' (Masroor 1987: 386). Maheen 'and other Lahore artists struggled in their respective fields but they received neither patronage nor encouragement' (Masroor 1987: 387). The marginalisation of Maheen's artistic vision embodies that of East Pakistan, including the Bengali language and the songs, music, and dance so intrinsic to Bengali culture.

The reclamation of pre-1971 Pakistan and its loss run through *Bengal Raag* (2006) by Durdana Soomro and Ghazala Hameed, twin daughters of a Punjabi civil servant posted in East Pakistan. Narrated in the third person, the novel is filled with finely observed details which describe the carefree pre-1971 Bengal known and loved by fictional twins Gaity and Diya. Their father's postings take them to Chittagong and Dhaka; they also travel to the Chittagong Hill Tracts, Rangamati, and Cox's Bazaar. Their eldest sister, Aynee, marries a Bengali (as did the co-authors' sister, the Bangladeshi critic, Niaz Zaman). At the time of the military action in Dhaka, the twins are at college in Lahore and their father has been transferred to West Pakistan permanently. Their concerns and fears for their loved ones, particularly Aynee in Dhaka, amid tales of excesses by the army and the Mukti, are built into the plot and lead up to December 1971 – and the loss of the Pakistan they knew. Their account of 1971 has interesting links to Zaman's recollections in *Fault Lines* (2008: xiv–xvii).

In the new millennium: excavating memories of 1971

In the twenty-first century, a growing number of novels about 1971 'enact a specific relationship to history that posits the author as mediator of conflicting memorial legacies' (Kabir 2013: 62). These authors include those born after 1971, such as Bilgrami, Roopa Farooki, Mohsin Hamid, and Shamsie. Hamid's *Moth Smoke* (2000), explores themes of fratricide in a historical, political, and personal context. Symbolically framed by a tale of Mughal rivalry and Aurangzeb's execution of Dara Shikoh, his elder brother and the heir apparent, the plot, set in contemporary Pakistan, tells of the life-and-death rivalry between the corrupt, rich Aurangzeb (Ozi) and the poor, orphaned Dara (Daru). In 1971, Ozi's father, Khurram, had used his influence 'to obtain a cushy job as ADC in Rawalpindi' (Hamid 2000: 73). Daru's father, 'a quiet, courageous man, a soldier's soldier', served in East Pakistan 'and died of gangrene in a prisoner-of-war camp in Chittagong' (2000: 73–74); it later transpires that Daru and Ozi are both Khurram Uncle's sons. Thus, references to 1971 become integral to themes of illusion, rivalry, and twinning which challenge narratives of Otherness. This extends to class, gender, and Indo-Pakistan rivalry resulting in the 1998 nuclear tests.

Confused bloodlines and/or twins run through several South Asian English novels, including Rushdie's *Midnight's Children* (1981), Masroor's *Shadows of Time*, Farooki's *Half Life* (2010), and Shamsie's *Kartography*. Shobhana Bhattacharji writes that 'mirroring and twinning are used to offer alternative perspectives on Partition which left ragged, incomplete histories on both sides of the border' (2017: 389); this applies to 1971, too. The narrator of *Kartography*, Raheen, and her friend, Karim, 'share a crib as babies, know the contentment of sleeping spine to spine, finish each other sentences and eventually fall in love' (Bhattacharji 2017: 364). Their parents are close friends. To Raheen, the Civil War of 71 is a distant event, which occurred at the time when her father, Zafar, and Karim's mother, Maheen, swapped fiancé(e)s.

In 1985, Raheen and Karim's hometown, Karachi, is engulfed by ethnic violence, as was East Pakistan in 1970; similarly, a curfew is declared. Shamsie creates another resonance with the past when Raheen is shocked into the realisation that her parents, Yasmin and Zafar, migrants – *muhajirs* (refugees) (who came to Karachi from India in great numbers in 1947) are regarded in their close group as ethnically 'different'. She overhears Uncle Ali (Karim's father) declare, 'I am not a Muhajir', while discussing the current riots with landowning friends, Uncle Asif and Aunty Laila, who rail against 'those bloody Muhajirs' (Bhattacharji 2017: 38). Laila, belonging to an old Karachi family, goes a step further and expresses her resentment 'at the way Zafar and Yasmin talk about "their Karachi"? […] "Who the hell are these Muhajirs to pretend it is their city?"' (Bhattacharji 2017: 38).

The reverberations of words, the prejudiced narratives they create, and thus complicity with brutality and violence, run through the book. Raheen realises that she had always known that Karim's mother, 'Aunty Maheen […] was Bengali […] because every so often aunts or cousins would arrive from Bangladesh to visit, bearing giftwrapped saris and a reminder that Aunty Maheen grew up in another language' (Bhattacharji 2017: 39).

This insight into Maheen's 'difference' provides a telling comment on the space that Bengalis who remained in Pakistan after 1971 had to negotiate. This is accentuated by Raheen's recollection of an incident at school, when she and Karim were little. Their friend, Zia, is so shocked to hear Karim say that his mother is from Bangladesh and so he is half Bengali that Zia starts to kick him and shout, 'He's not Bengali, he's not. He's my friend. Why is he lying?' (Bhattacharji 2017: 39–40). The consternation that follows among the parents of Karim, Raheen, and Zia culminates with Zia's father shouting at the *ayah*, and Zia trying to say that the *ayah* isn't responsible, whereupon 'his mother yelled at him to be quiet' (2017: 40). The incident highlights the refusal to ask questions and accept responsibility, and the collusion between 1971's verbal violence in West Pakistan and physical violence in East Pakistan.

The story of Zafar and Maheen in 1971 is central to the plot of *Kartography*. Both regarded Karachi as their home and they got engaged while the post-election political crisis was escalating. But Maheen begins to be regarded as 'the enemy' because she is Bengali. She is abused in the street by strangers. She receives obnoxious telephone calls. Ali urges them to leave the country and says that Zafar is regarded as 'treasonous' by many. Ali laments that the 'country has turned rabid' and that drawing-room conversations condone the rape of women in East Pakistan 'to improve their genes' (Bhattacharji 2017: 173). Zafar is taunted as a 'Bingo lover' at the tennis courts and beaten up. His repudiation of Maheen takes place shortly afterwards. He confesses the details to Raheen twenty years later: he comes home to find that his neighbour, Shafiq's brother has been brutally murdered by the Mukti Bahini. Zafar bursts out (and Maheen overhears): 'How can I marry one of them? How can I let one of them bear my children? Think of it as my civic duty, I'll be diluting her Bengali bloodline' (Bhattacharji 2017: 210). His sense of shame and his apology are lost on Raheen. She flees from the house, repulsed. Her anger and trauma embody that of the nation, but unlike Pakistan, she is gradually forced to re-examine the past, confront it, and forgive, with the help of her mother and Maheen – and the letter her father wrote to Maheen long ago:

> What happens when you work so hard to forget a horror that you also forget that you have forgotten it? It doesn't disappear – the canker turns inwards and mutates into something else. In this city, that we both love and claim – even though our families' histories lie elsewhere – what will this canker become?
>
> (Bhattacharji 2017: 179)

My brother, my enemy

Roopa Farooki is unique among the writers discussed here as she is the daughter of a Bangladeshi mother, Nilofer Farooki, and a Pakistani father, Nasir Ahmed Farooki (an early post-independence Pakistani anglophone writer). Her novels *Bitter Sweets* and *The Flying Man* include intermarriages between East and West Pakistanis. Her fourth, *Half Life*, explores the friendship between Anwar, a Punjabi army officer, and Bangladeshi poet Hari Hassan, who 'has been in the thick of the civil war between East and West Pakistan' (2010: 11). They had been at Oxford together. Family relationships, secrets, and the emotional upheavals caused by an absent father are central to the novel. Farooki removes the impediments of visas by placing her protagonists in the South Asian diaspora: Britain, Singapore, and Malaysia. The narrative moves between three people; the dying Hari Hassan, in Malaysia; a Singaporean academic, married to an Englishman, Dr Aroona Ahmed Jones (Roony), who is researching Hari; and Jazz (Ejaz Ahsan), her erstwhile lover in Singapore. Roony and Jazz's relationship collapses when a DNA test reveals they are siblings. The theme of intertwined bloodlines is given an added twist when Hari Hassan turns out to be the pen name of Jazz's estranged father. Unknown to Jazz and Rooney, Hari Hassan has a secret. In pre-Partition Calcutta, during the Second World War, he fell in love with a young woman, who died expecting his child. He has lived with the guilt ever since. Anwar visits Hari in Chittagong, shortly before the outbreak of civil war. He believes he can help Hari atone for the past: Anwar asks Hari to marry Anwar's pregnant cousin, Zaida: the child born to her is Jazz (and no, Anwar is not the father).

In hospital, Hari is visited by Anwar's son, Khalid, after Anwar dies. The exchange of letters between Anwar and Hari, referring to 1971 and Anwar's diaries, captures the shock, despair, and horror of West Pakistanis who did not support the military action and provides an interesting intertextual engagement with E.M. Forster's words, 'If I had to choose between my country or my friends, I hope I would have the guts to betray my country'. Anwar had 'heard of the atrocities third-hand in the direct comfort of senior ranks' and 'now found himself with the blood of multitudes on his hands' (Farooki 2010: 199). He wrote to Hari:

> I have the choice of betraying my country, or betraying all that I hold good. I do not have the strength to betray my country, and so I am betraying my integrity, and my friends. I will always be your brother, but now I am your enemy.
>
> (2010: 199)

Hari never knew if Anwar received his letter, so he published his answer, addressed to a nameless Pakistani:

My brother enemy. There will always be a place for you in my heart, but there is no longer a place for you in my country. The green and pleasant land is red with the blood of brave men, broken women and innocent children, and the calls for vengeance will not and should not be silenced. My brother, my enemy. It is time to stop fighting and go home.

(2010: 11)

Farooki's dual Bengali-Punjabi inheritance adds to the richness of her narrative and to the sensitivity with which she writes of human frailty and family histories amid the bitter divisions of 1947 and 1971. As Shamsie says:

We act as if history can be erased. Of course we want to believe that – the cost of remembering may break our wilted spirits. But if we believe in erasure we tell ourselves it is possible to have acts without consequences. The finger squeezing the trigger becomes a thing apart from the bullet that speeds along the sands, which becomes a thing apart from the child looking down at his blood pumping out of his heart. And that child, that bullet, they become things way, way apart from our lives, here, in rooms where we look upon our own sleeping children.

(2003: 180)

Notes

1 See Muneeza Shamsie's memoir essay 'When We Were Young' (2013).
2 See Soraya Khan (2015), where she describes her research including the unravelling of buried memories by former soldiers.

Bibliography

Ahmed, E. (2006) 'Letter to a Pakistani Diplomat'. In *Selected Writings of Eqbal Ahmed*. Ed. by Bengelsdorf, C., Cerullo, M., and Chandrani, Y. Karachi: Oxford University Press.
Ali, T. (2008) *The Duel: Pakistan on the Flight of American Power*. London: Verso.
Ali, T. (2010) *The Night of the Golden Butterfly*. London: Verso.
Anam, T. (2008) *The Golden Age*. London: John Murray.
Bhattacharji, S. (2017) 'Kamila Shamsie'. In *Hybrid Tapestries: The Development of Pakistani Literature in English*. Ed. by Shamsie, M. Karachi: Oxford University Press, 384–395.
Bilgrami, S. (2007) *Without Dreams*. New Delhi: Harper Collins.
Cilano, C. (2011) *National Identities in Pakistan: The 1971 War in Contemporary Pakistani Fiction*. Abingdon: Routledge.
Cilano, C. (2013) *Contemporary Pakistani Fiction in English: Idea, Nation, State*. Abingdon: Routledge.
Farooki, R. (2007) *Bitter Sweet*. London: Pan Macmillan.
Farooki, R. (2010) *Half Life*. London: Pan Macmillan.
Farooki, R. (2012) *The Flying Man*. London: Headline.
Fazli, S. (2011) *Invitation*. Chennai: Tranquebar.
Forna, A. (2010) *The Memory of Love*. London: Bloomsbury.
Hamid, M. (2000) *Moth Smoke*. New York: Picador.
Hamidullah, Z. (2008) *The Young Wife and Other Stories*. Karachi: Oxford University Press.
Hussein, A. (1993) *Mirror to the Sun*. London: Mantra Publishing.
Ismail, A. (2001) 'Leaving Bangladesh'. In *Leaving Home: Towards a New Millennium: A Collection of English Prose by Pakistani Writers*. Ed. by Shamsie, M. Karachi: Oxford University Press, 135–140.
Ismail, A. (2012) *Of Martyrs and Marigolds*. North Charleston: CreateSpace.
Jalal, A. (1991) *The State of Martial Rule: The Origins of Pakistan's Political Economy of Defence*. Lahore: Vanguard.
Jalal, A. (2014) *The Struggle for Pakistan: A Muslim Homeland and Global Politics*. Cambridge: Belknap Press.

Kabir, A.J. (2013) *Partition's Post Amnesias: 1947, 1971 and Modern South Asia*. New Delhi: Women Unlimited.
Khan, S. (2003) *Noor*. Karachi: Alhamra.
Khan, S. (2015) 'The Silence and Forgetting That Wrote *Noor*'. *The Journal of Narrative Politics* 1(2), 121–132.
Masroor, M.N. (1987) *Shadows of Time*. New Delhi: Chanakya Publications.
Mohsin, M. (2006) *The End of Innocence*. London: Penguin.
Rahman, T. (1997) 'Bingo'. In *A Dragonfly in the Sun: An Anthology of Pakistani Writing in English*. Ed. by Shamsie, M. Karachi: Oxford University Press, 311–324.
Rushdie, S. (1981) *Midnight's Children*. London: Jonathan Cape.
Saikia, Y. (2011) *Women, War and the Making of Bangladesh*. Karachi: Oxford University Press.
Shamsie, K. (2003) *Kartography*. Orlando: Harcourt Books.
Shamsie, M. (1996) 'Controversial Comrade: The Life and Times of Tariq Ali: Interview'. *Newsline*, 89–93.
Shamsie, M. (2013) 'When We Were Young: Karachi 1965–1971'. *Moving Worlds* 13(2), n.p.
Shamsie, M. (2017) *Hybrid Tapestries: The Development of Pakistani Literature in English*. Karachi: Oxford University Press.
Sidhwa, B. (1982) *The Bride*. London: Jonathan Cape.
Sidhwa, B. (1988) *Ice-Candy Man*. London: Heinemann.
Soomro, D. and Hameed, G. (2006) *Bengal Raag*. Dhaka: Writers Ink.
Suleri, S. (1989) *Meatless Days*. Chicago: Chicago University Press.
Yaqub-Khan, S. (2005) *Strategy, Humanity, Diplomacy: The Life and Work of Sahabzada Yaqub-Khan*. San Diego: Intercultural Forum.
Zaman, N. (2000) *A Divided Legacy: The Partition in Selected Novels of India, Pakistan and Bangladesh*. Karachi: Oxford University Press.
Zaman, N. and Farrukhi, A. (eds.) (2008) *Fault Lines: Stories of 1971*. Dhaka: University Press Ltd.
Zameenzad, A. (1991) *Cyrus, Cyrus*, London: Minerva.

3
HISTORY, BORDERS, AND IDENTITY
Dealing with silenced memories of 1971

Daniela Vitolo

Looking at the country through the lens of Benedict Anderson's theory, which states that a nation is an 'imagined community' (1991), Salman Rushdie defined Pakistan as an 'insufficiently imagined community' in his novel *Shame* (1995: 87). Studies by scholars in different fields echo Rushdie's words when they state that Pakistan is a country where the process of national formation has failed (Cohen 2004; Jafferlot 2002; Jalal 1995). The reasons for this failure are found partly in the fact that, in Pakistan, the sense of collective belonging to the nation seems to give way to stronger forms of affiliation, such as to ethnic, regional, or religious groups. For this reason, nationalism has emerged as a possible solution to the problem, as it proposes a clear definition of national identity by stressing the Muslim origins of the state, fostering the idea that a sense of collective belonging lies in the religious belief that unites the citizens of the state. However, not only has nationalism failed to heal the cracks that divide Pakistani society, it also seems to have played a part in deepening the split between the majority of the population and its minorities, principally because proposing the image of a prototypical Pakistani has favoured discrimination against those who do not fit that model. It is not surprising that Pakistani society should experience an identity crisis as a consequence, and that writers feel a need to participate in a debate addressing the issue. While society seems to be looking for a definition of the Pakistani nation and of Pakistani identity, Cara Cilano's study of a corpus of works of Pakistani anglophone literature demonstrates that on reading the texts it is possible to note they do not convey a uniform representation of Pakistani identity. Rather, they 'offer readings that conjure a myriad of possibilities, creating a spectrum that runs from a reinforcement of dominant modes of belonging to a reinvention of the terms of collective attachments' (Cilano 2013: 1). Consequently, Cilano states that because they show that the sense of belonging to a nation can theoretically be conceived in a limitless number of ways, these works of fiction respond both to nationalist narratives that promote a monolithic definition of Pakistani identity, and to the idea that Pakistan has failed in the process of creating an 'imagined community'.

Postmodern thought conceives identity not as something unique and clearly defined but rather as something composed of various fragments. In 'The Question of Cultural Identity', Stuart Hall explains how the understanding of the nature of identity has changed over time, moving from an early phase when it was thought to be a stable entity whose essential core was internal to the subject and remained unchanged throughout the lifetime. Today, identity is believed to be a product of the interaction between the subject and society, on which depends the shaping of personal and collective identities. If, in the past, the individual experienced society as composed of organised blocks creating an ordered picture where elements like class, race, gender, and ethnicity had a determined place and frame, today the internal coherence of those blocks has crumbled, each revealing its complex nature. This transformation has undermined the sense of integrity of the individual who, being unable to relate to a stable pattern, has found himself to be partial, composed of a number of fragments that interact and articulate themselves in different ways according to the circumstances. Therefore, being fragmented and continuously changing, 'the structure of identity remains open' (Hall 1996: 600).

Following Hall's analysis, a question arises as to how the contemporary subject relates to cultural identities and, in particular, how s/he deals with national identity. Hall reminds us that national identity is also fragmented, being composed of different elements: on the one hand, a person can be a member of a nation state and, on the other, feel part of a national culture. Even the latter is not unitary because, as Anderson's theory implies, any nation is a product of the encounter between people of different origins and cultures who become part of one political entity. However, a nation is a 'structure of cultural power', where national culture constitutes 'a *discursive device* which represents difference as unity or identity' (Hall 1996: 61).

If it is true that a nation cannot exist as such if it does not define its concrete limits and exercise a form of control over them, then borders play a part so relevant in Pakistan's life that the country's history can be retraced by recalling several episodes and situations involving the creation or protection of borders. Pakistan was created by drawing lines that partitioned the Indian subcontinent in 1947, forming a state comprising two separate wings. From that moment, the wars that have broken out between Pakistan and India have been major events involving a border constantly in the spotlight. Since the tensions between the two countries have not softened over time, the line separating them stands as a concrete sign of the wound inflicted by Partition – not yet healed in either nation – whilst also standing as a reminder of the 'two nations theory'; it further serves to define Pakistan itself in a negative way with respect to 'the "other nation"' (Jafferlot 2002: 8). In 1971, Pakistan witnessed another reconfiguration of its territory when, at the end of the conflict between the two wings of the country, East Pakistan became an independent state, Bangladesh. Furthermore, the war had been fought between Muslims who, in 1947, had become part of the same state, finding in religion the element that kept them together and distinguished them from Hindu and Sikh communities. Being fought in the name of ethnic diversity and resulting from politics that did not guarantee a fair share of political and economic power, the war prompted reconsideration of what defines Pakistani identity. Moreover, the Kashmir issue and the course of events that, since the 1980s, have unfolded on the troubled border between Pakistan and Afghanistan have had a direct impact on society, serving as further examples of how 'identity' and 'border' are two intertwined concepts that participate in compelling discourses that affect Pakistan's everyday life.

The phrase 'line which separates two countries' is one of the definitions of the term 'border', which also describes a frontier zone, an area of transition where the traits that characterise one region give way to the aspects that define an adjacent region. In this sense, we can think of a border not as a line separating sharply distinct identities but as a space where different elements converge, such as those characterising two national cultures, and where the fixity of identities is questioned. As theorists such as Gloria E. Anzaldúa (1987), Edouard Glissant (1989), and Homi Bhabha (1994) have argued, a deconstruction of identities otherwise supposed to be invariable can take place within a frontier dimension generating potential transformative energy. A liminal space can be thought of as a hybrid terrain of cultural difference where subjects and communities can think in a new and critical way about their identities. Finding themselves in a space where imposed conceptions of identity are contested, individuals and groups can also redefine their idea of the society to which they belong. As Homi Bhabha writes, 'It is in the emergence of the interstices – the overlap and displacement of domains of difference – that the intersubjective and collective experiences of *nationness*, community interest, or cultural value are negotiated' (1994: 2). Within the interstitial space, individuals and groups can thus redefine their relationship with a place, a culture, or a nation.

Sorayya Khan's novel *Noor* (2003), which revolves around the consequences of the war between East and West Pakistan, is part of a consistent production dealing with the role played by memories of traumatic past events, such as the 1947 Partition and the 1971 conflict, in the shaping of identities. For this reason, while proposing a reading of Khan's novel, this essay suggests reading the novel within its literary context. As authors tend to create stories that move between the present and memories of the past, their works seem to convey the idea that certain determining episodes, which have both a public and private nature, are still affecting the lives of individuals and communities. Since recalling and transmitting memories implies creating a narrative version of the past, authors can pay attention to the roles played and the power retained by narratives that participate in shaping how people think about their common past and understand their relationship with the nation. In *Salt and Saffron* (2000), for example, Kamila Shamsie holds that because certain narratives of the past can be partial and distorted, younger generations need to examine events related to Partition in order to develop their understanding of that fundamental moment in history. In addition, several stories approach historical fact from a minor perspective that narrates the event from the point of view of characters that experienced it from a marginal position. The most famous case is Bapsi Sidhwa's *Cracking India* (1991), which chooses as narrator an adult woman who recalls her memories of 1947. The novel narrates Partition as experienced by women through adopting the point of view of a child belonging to a middle-class Parsi family – and therefore a context not touched directly by the clashes between rival groups. Shahbano Bilgrami's *Without Dreams* (2007) makes comparisons between the country's history from 1971 onwards and the life experiences and identity formation of two boys, one from East and one from West Pakistan, introducing two different perspectives on the conflict as well as on Pakistani history and society in the years that followed the war.

Among the most relevant features which emerge from novels and short stories like those cited above is their focus on the relationship between memory, narrative, and identity. The authors point out that recalling and narrating the past are fundamental parts of a process that allows younger generations to understand the country's history as they develop their relationship with the nation and, as a consequence, their national identity. Likewise, such a process participates in the shaping of personal identity. According to the theory of narrative identity, the construction of personal identity happens through the construction of a story. Indeed, in order to understand who they are and what is their relationship with the world around them, individuals need to create a narrative version of their life experience and produce a story that combines the present, as they perceive it, and the past, as they reconstruct it, projecting themselves into an imagined future. Likewise, the studies proposed by Anderson (1991) and Bhabha (1990) move from the idea that, for a national identity to be developed, it is necessary that citizens access the same narrations which disseminate the same stories and ideas about the past and the present of the community that forms the nation, thus creating among the citizens a sense of belonging. Marianne Hirsh coined the phrase 'postmemory generation' (2008: 111) to refer to the generation born after a major dramatic event who develop deep knowledge of events they never witnessed through memories shared with them by older generation. Consequently, they need to confront those memories in order to create their own understanding of past events they have not experienced yet which form part of their identity. The concept proposed by Hirsh becomes particularly relevant in works of fiction about the 1971 conflict because, when writing about younger generations' awareness of that event, authors address the absence of a 'postmemory generation' in Pakistani society.

The war between East and West Pakistan and the victory of the former over the latter were a shock to the population of the then West Pakistan, which was unprepared to face the turn of events that reshaped Pakistan within just a few weeks. Indeed, as military operations took place, the media coverage did not reveal the actual situation on the ground, for which reason news of the defeat was entirely unexpected. Likewise, in the aftermath of the war, the state's approach to the matter was one of promoting a general amnesia about what had actually happened. After the conflict, Pakistani society confronted the need to understand the reasons for a war fought because ethnic diversity had proved stronger than religious unity, during which there had been high numbers of casualties on both sides and in which the West Pakistan army had committed systematic atrocities against the local population.[1] The solution favoured by the authorities was to avoid any public discussion of the subject that, when it was addressed, was mainly presented as a consequence of Indian interference in Pakistan's internal matters, given that East Pakistan had prevailed in the war in part thanks to support from the Indian army.

Recalling the war in *Noor*

The two protagonists of Khan's *Noor* experienced the 1971 war in different ways: Ali, as a soldier, arrived from West Pakistan to fight in East Pakistan, while Sajida was an orphaned Bangladeshi child. They later formed an unusual kind of family, living in Pakistan, when a few months after his arrival in East Pakistan, Ali was discharged, having contracted typhoid, and brought home the little Sajida, whom he found living alone on the streets of Dhaka. Before the war broke out, Sajida had been the sole survivor of a cyclone that killed her family in the village where they lived by the Gulf of Bengal. From the moment she reaches West Pakistan, Sajida thinks of Ali as her father, while Ali's mother, Nanijaan, becomes a maternal figure for the girl. The novel's eponymous character, the youngest child of Sajida and her husband Hussein, has a special gift that gives her insights into the experiences of older members of the family. Realising that Noor knows their past, the principal characters are forced to deal with memories of the war that they had put aside after 1971, thus mirroring the public demeanour adopted by the state. As they recall past traumas, the characters begin a process that helps them to recall what they experienced in East Pakistan. During this process, they also come to realise that before Ali found Sajida in Dhaka, the two had already once met, when Ali and his comrades had opened fire on a group of helpless villagers, killing almost all of them, sparing a child, only by chance – Sajida.

As the story reveals, *Noor* is a novel that addresses the silence that fell on 1971 and which, in the absence of public discussion, prevented citizens from developing an awareness of what had taken place. In an interview given to Cilano, Khan explains that her aim was:

> to address the silence, to pinpoint it as something that is out there, that defines the history of '71 in Pakistan, the way we think about who we are, as a way of not taking responsibility for what's been done. It's in the doing of the writing – that I'm writing 'about' the silence.
>
> (Cilano 2011: 221)

Through a story set in the present yet which could not develop without characters able to recall the past, the author highlights the intertwined nature of both private and public memories of the 1971 war, making it clear by opening with a quote from Agha Shahid Ali: 'your history gets in the way of my memory'. Pierre Nora (1989) has explained the difference between history and memory, stating that while the former is the reconstruction, problematic and incomplete, of a succession of past events, memory is the product of a collective process based on the continuous elaboration of something that happened in the past and which, for this reason, is never complete. Since the official version of history has been manipulated, Khan stresses both the discrepancies between personal memories and official histories and how the public record affects the manner in which people can relate to their experiences. Creating a novel which recalls such a problematic event, and thus participating in the development of a shared narrative, the author develops characters who are directly involved in factual events that happened during the conflict, but who can relate to those facts from marginal perspectives.

In *Noor* the interwoven nature of the processes that produce self and national narrative identities is presented through a story in which unsilencing memories of war means that the characters move from a state of acceptance of an official behaviour towards the 1971 events, to a position of reviewing events as they remember them. This journey parallels the characters' personal progress from a condition in which they try to fit within a normative definition of a Pakistani citizen to a state of acceptance of their composite nature and of their complex relationship with the nation. When Ali returns from the front, bringing Sajida with him, Nanijaan, who had warned him of the risks of leaving for East Pakistan, asks no questions, either about Ali's experiences or about the child, and her curiosity seems to be satisfied when Ali says just a few words about Sajida: 'She says she's fiveandsix. Little girl from East Pakistan. She'll stay with us' (Khan 2003: 52). When, many years later, Sajida asks Nanijaan why she did not enquire about her story and the reasons why she joined their family, the old woman answers: 'Your father told me. He brought you from Dhaka. You told me about the cyclone, when you were pregnant with Noor. Remember?' (2003: 122). Given her choice to remain ignorant about things that happened in East Pakistan, Nanijaan can be regarded as a representative of that part of Pakistani society that did not question the censorship of the war, accepting as exhaustive the partial official accounts. When, many years after the war, Nanijaan asks Ali if he ever killed someone during the conflict and learns that indeed he did, she understands that, 'until then, she hadn't wanted to know, and still didn't want to know, because she had been afraid of the answer' (2003: 136). Although Nanijaan knew that, for her, it would have been difficult to bear the truth about the brutalities committed by soldiers, once she exposes herself to the facts, she is obliged to elaborate her personal understanding of the situation and comes to accept her son's deeds as part of his past. Ali appears as a symbol of that part of society that knew and chose to hide the truth about the war and the atrocities perpetrated by the army against civilians. When he arrives home, he takes a long purifying bath which he performs as a symbolic act that will allow him to put aside memories of the war in order to return to his life: 'He imagined his story, the sum of horrible details, so neatly stored away, he'd done away with any reason to retrieve it. Ever. And that was how Ali had planned to return to life' (2003: 55). Since she was very young when the event happened, Sajida possesses only scattered pieces of memory of her life in Bangladesh. These are fragments of her first years and the cyclone that killed her family – 'My mother was a seamstress' (2003: 10), 'In one swoop. The water […] was as high as the hills. […] The water, it was alive' (2003: 11) – and of the moment Ali found her:

> A man got out of the jeep. She heard him, but she didn't turn to look. She was suddenly exhausted, so overcome that when this man – Ali, Aba, her father – picked her up […] from the side of the road, she let him.
>
> (2003: 108)

In the beginning, it seems that she has no memory of what happened between those two key events, and therefore of the war that began after the cyclone. Unlike Nanijaan and Ali, Sajida does not choose to forget; rather she prefers not to interrogate her past, which tries to come back to her in the form of dreams and flashbacks. This is a sign of her unwitting effort to put aside her Bangladeshi identity and integrate herself into Pakistani society, where she has built her new life, a life where she is a daughter, a happy wife, and a mother. She sees this as a second chance, and thus she lives her life in a positive way, in contrast to her previous existence: 'As much as He took, He gave much more. Love, laughter, children, second chances. Especially second chances. She believed that her big, healthy son was God's way of giving her another chance' (2003: 15).

Noor, a child 'born not of this world, but of another' (2003: 81), whose drawings are 'windows into another world' (2003: 106), embodies both knowledge of the past and a need to deal with it. For this reason, she represents a social group that seems difficult to find in Pakistani society but which might have formed naturally. To address the absence of a 'postmemory generation', Khan gives Noor special gifts, thus introducing to the novel an element of magic realism, and uses her to unmask a trait that also defines other characters. Ali and Sajida share with this special child both a peripheral position within society and personal knowledge of a historical event. However, although the child proves to be aware of her family's past, she also appears as a projection of the adults' need to give space to something that they have repressed. This seems to be suggested in the incipit of the novel – 'Noor was Sajida's secret' (2003: 1) – which literally refers to the fact that, soon after conceiving her, Sajida has a premonition about the fact that her daughter will be different to other children yet chooses to hide this from other members of the family. The moment that Noor begins to name the places in Bangladesh that she illustrates in her drawings, Ali and Sajida, who associate those places with specific memories, understand that they cannot escape their past any longer. Noor's pictures hanging on the walls of their home create a gallery of memories suddenly made public and encourage the protagonists to go back to 1971 and Bangladesh. A definition of *lieux de mémoire*, as first proposed by Pierre Nora, is that of physical sites to which a specific function is attributed, that of recalling and symbolising historical events. Because 'memory attaches itself to sites' and 'takes root in the concrete, in spaces, gestures, images and objects' (Nora, 1989: 22, 9), a *lieu de mémoire* is, according to Nora, a place to which is attributed a specific, symbolic and usually public, meaning that helps to remember a specific event whilst being different from the event itself. A site of memory is something concrete, like a monument or an archive, which creates a public memory preserving and recalling something that a community risks forgetting. Although Bangladesh does not entirely fit Nora's definition in *Noor*, it might be read as a site of memory as long as it is presented as a physical place in which determining events happened and to which the protagonists metaphorically return to face their past. The concreteness of a geographical space which belonged to the Pakistani nation and whose partition left Pakistan severed of a piece of its identity is rendered through detailed descriptions of the places Ali sees: 'East Pakistan was beautiful. Lush and green the way West Pakistan never was, even during the monsoons. Snaking rivers and endless tributaries flowing like life itself through the rich fields' (2003: 84). The vivid pictures of places are echoed by similarly strong images of the violence suffered by West Pakistani soldiers – 'The roads were raised. They were the only elevation in the fucking flat land. [...] We were target practice for them. Dead, we rolled [...] down slopes. Our blood and guts fertilized their fields' (2003: 165) – and of the cruelties enacted by them – 'The mother shaking, begging for the life of her child. The child whimpering. The smell of a mother's milk: sweet. She: wet, cut open, on the desk' (2003: 182). Thus, while 1971 Bangladesh is appointed a symbolic role and becomes a tangible sign of Pakistan's past, the house where the family moves soon after Noor's birth also becomes a symbolic site of memory. Indeed, it hosts Noor and her pictures, each of which has a title and is placed on the walls in alphabetical order, showing a need to organise memories in a clear way. As with her gallery, Noor also characterises the house as a private space of memory that she soon refuses to leave, showing herself to be afraid of borders: 'of walls that marked the property, the doorways she was forced to pass under, the cracks on the brick walkways' (2003: 42). Noor's fear of crossing borders, which helps to characterise the house as a distinct site symbolically related to Bangladesh, might be explained either as a reminder of the violence that the child associates with the scission of the nation or as a mirror of what the characters feel about the possibility of recalling the past.

When the characters begin to help each other to remember – 'You killed someone?' (2003: 133), Nanijaan asks Ali, while Sajida enquires, 'What *was* it like? There?' (2003: 183) – a process starts which allows them to become self-aware, aware of how they place themselves concerning the 1971 events. They thus become conscious of the relationships that bond their unusual family while they reveal the intricacies of the subject's connection with the nation. Ali's war trauma has resulted in his loss of faith in God. This loss of faith means that he distances himself from the founding value of Pakistani society, something that he keeps private but which can be noticed by those living with him, as Sajida makes clear: 'she'd never seen her father pray or hear him utter commonplace, daily phrases like "inshallah," the minute references to God that peppered everyone else's speech in Pakistan' (2003: 146).

His changed relation to God becomes an indicator of the way in which the war modified Ali's connection with the nation. Indeed, for Ali, remembering means admitting to himself that his ideals crumbled as soon as he confronted reality in the field. As a young soldier, he asked to be sent to East Pakistan, where the war was soon to begin, driven by the desire to live an adventure, but also because he was proud to fight for his nation, as he told his mother: 'I'm going [...] I'll fight for my country. You'll be proud' (2003: 49). However, his nationalist ideals soon die after he finds himself in the field: 'It took one day to know he wasn't fighting the war for his country, yet another to realize he wasn't fighting for Nanijaan or, for that matter, any family. On the fourth day he felt like a mercenary' (2003: 167). Years after that moment, Ali expresses his scepticism regarding the politics adopted by the central government based in West Pakistan towards the eastern part of the country: 'Now, he wasn't certain any of the things he'd been told (except the facts about the Indians) had ever rung true to him. That Bengalis, dark and stupid, not *really* Muslims, didn't deserve their own country, their own leaders' (2003: 167). At the same time, this critical position does not exclude his racist attitude towards Bengalis remaining unaltered. Voicing a position common in West Pakistan, Ali recalls 'Those people, we used to call them Bingos' (2003: 120), and on more than one occasion represents them as stupid (2003: 115), dark, and short (2003: 190). Likewise, he entertains Noor with some expressions and commonplaces about Bengalis that were frequently heard at that time:

> Effortlessly, as if he'd learned them yesterday, Ali remembered several similar jokes. *How can you tell a Bengali from a fly? Bengalis smell.* [...] *What does independence mean for a Bengali? Not having to be told to wash his hands after having a shit.*
>
> (2003: 118)

Even Nanijaan demonstrates that she has acquired a stereotyped image of the citizens of East Pakistan when she is surprised to hear Sajida whisper '"alhamdulillah," giving praise to God' (2003: 61). Nanijaan shows that she has unwittingly received an idea common at the time, that Bengalis also differed from Pakistanis because they were not proper Muslims: 'Nanijjan's first thought was, *Where did she learn that?* Before the thought was complete, she was ashamed.

East Pakistanis, Bengalis, were Muslims, too' (2003: 61). Giving space to the issue of the racist representation of Bengalis, Khan highlights one of the aspects of the narrative that supported the war and seems to suggest that between the two wings of the country there was a sort of colonial relation. Unsurprisingly, Sajida is a victim of such racism because her complexion is darker than is common in Pakistan, and so she is recognisably Bengali. For this reason, for example, her classmates call her, '*kohl-ki-larki*' (2003: 9), the girl made of coal.

Notwithstanding their parental love for Sajida, both Ali and Nanijaan have an ambiguous relationship with the girl. Indeed, their actions are the reason why she has abandoned her motherland and lost her original culture. This means that, for Sajida, dealing with her memories also means reconsidering her family relations. Ali's choice to take the girl with him might be the act that saved Sajida, and yet, because the child did not consent, and could not have consented, to follow him, the man's act also looks like an abduction. Read as such, this is the second act of violence against Sajida, the child whom Ali might have shot dead some time before in the village. In addition, as soon as she reaches Ali's house, she begins to undergo a process of redefining her identity, because she soon forgets her mother tongue – 'a different language – Bengali – which she had long since lost' (2003: 74) – in favour of Urdu – 'the first Urdu word she learned [was] *razai*, for the stack of quilts at the foot on Nanijaan's bed' (2003: 110). Likewise, she finds herself unable to remember her brother's name or the name of the village she was from. At the same time, in an effort to make her feel Pakistani, Nanijaan tells her that her dark skin is nothing but a consequence of God's choice to give her more colour (2003: 9). However, Sajida's reaction to her rediscovery of the past means that she becomes conscious of what happened to her without regarding Ali and Nanijaan as culpable of depriving her of her identity, and she is able to rethink her identity and connections with Pakistan and Bangladesh. Thus, the woman, who can remember that as a child she knew that 'Bangladesh, simply translated, meant home for Bengalis' (2003: 175), can herself eventually claim to be Bengali – 'I'm from somewhere else, really. […] I'm not from here. […] I am from somewhere else' (2003: 176) – which also requires her to recognise openly that Ali is not her father. In this way, she also lets the other characters understand that she fully accepts her life in Pakistan and them as her family.

Unveiling a hidden past in *Kartography*

A comparative reading of *Noor* and Kamila Shamsie's *Kartography* (2002), another work that revolves around the consequences of 1971, allows one to notice how both novels engage in similar ways with issues of narrative, identity, and memory. Shamsie's novel follows Karim and Raheen, a boy and a girl who grew up together in Karachi, the children of two couples of long-time friends, Ali and Maheen and Zafar and Yasmin. While the story is set in the 1980s and 1990s, in a violent Karachi that experiences crime as well as ethnic tensions, the two protagonists learn that their existence is inextricably bound to 1971, when there was a fiancée swap between their parents. Learning that behind the reasons that made their parents exchange their partners was Maheen's Bengali identity, leads Karim and Raheen to face the implications of an event of which they had no awareness but that they understand to be fundamental in determining who they are and how they relate to people around them. In the novel, the silence that fell on the conflict and the discomfort generated by it are mirrored in the silence that Karim's and Raheen's parents have imposed on their past, a choice explained by the fact that Zafar, and to some extent Yasmin, betrayed Maheen at a time when, in West Pakistan, she was perceived as the enemy. This explains why the four adults feel ashamed of what happened and find it difficult to explain it to their children and why they remained friends. As the story moves between the present and the adults' memories of the past, the reader discovers with Raheen (the last to learn about the secret) that, in 1971, Zafar was engaged to Maheen, whom he had tried to protect from the social discrimination she faced, himself accepting to be regarded as a traitor. However, one of his accusers had attacked him, saying: 'You're going to marry one of them. You're going to let her have your children. How?' (2002: 231), and he had answered, while Maheen was listening, 'Think of it as a civil duty. I'll be diluting her Bengali blood line' (2002: 232). With this statement, he seems to demonstrate that beneath his claims in favour of Bengali independence lies a racist view that made him share the most common attitude towards East Pakistan. Notwithstanding, he reveals the ambiguity of his position when he admits that he is not sure whether he said those words to prevent his attacker from hurting Maheen or because he believed that it was a way to break off an engagement whose social consequences had become a burden too heavy to bear (2002: 335).

The ambiguous position of this character regarding Bengalis and their war for independence pairs with other episodes where the author points out the persistent racism towards Bengalis. Rather than being pictured as racists, the characters appear complex when faced with the necessity of confronting narratives concerning Bengali identity and the reasons behind the civil war. The difficulty of taking a clear position for or against a certain perspective shows the power of the narratives developed at the time as well as the tensions that crossed Pakistani society. 'There was violence in the air those days, and why should your father have been expected not to get terrified of it?' (2002: 308), explains Maheen to Raheen, who finds it difficult to justify her father's actions. Such a tense atmosphere of violence is cause and consequence of condemnable behaviours which, during those days, involved every single citizen: 'if you hold everyone accountable for what they said and did in '71 hardly anyone escapes whipping' (2002: 278). Being aware of this, the older generation in *Kartography* does not hold Zafar accountable for what he did, and encourages the younger characters to forgive their past faults as a way of dealing with the war and its consequences, opening up to a past-aware future.

In *Kartography* the narrator gives space to consideration of the development of narratives (2002: 4), boundaries (2002: 26), the ways memories are shaped (2002: 58–59) and belonging (2002: 165), thus giving the reader the keys to the main themes of the novel. The 'absence of narrative' (2002: 6) about what happened to the two couples of friends in 1971 becomes an issue when Raheen and Karim begin to try to match the few fragments of information they have and thus understand what happened. Karim learns the story quite early in his life but he is unable to share it with his friend, thus himself becoming a symbol of the difficulty of talking about an event which, if faced, implies unearthing issues affecting personal relationships. Therefore, as Karim suddenly becomes a sort of representative of the 'postmemory generation', he too tries to find ways to communicate to his friend that there is something unsaid in their past, but she is unable to read his silence. Consequently, Raheen, who as a young girl had been curious about her parents' story but had stopped asking questions after a while, learns the story only when Karim chooses to deal openly with knowledge that has tormented his adolescence. Indeed, he sees in Zafar's betrayal the reasons for his mother's suffering, but his anger also seems to be explained by the fact that he sees that Zafar's act as an injustice perpetrated by Pakistani society against Bengalis. When Raheen has to face the knowledge of her father's actions she is obliged to contextualise them within the political moment in which they occurred. And so she realises, for the first time, that her generation does not have awareness of what happened in 1971 because no one has told them anything about the events of that year, besides a few scattered snippets of information insufficient to reconstruct a clear picture.

As that compromising statement means Zafar 'stepping into history' (2002: 238), Shamsie maintains the importance of individuals taking a position on what happened as well as on the contemporary political situation in which they live. This is rendered more clearly in *Kartography* than in *Noor* through discussions between the characters who prove to be aware of the significance of being active citizens and thus not pretending that their private lives are not affected by what happens in the public sphere. For example, Karim also wants Raheen to know about the family secret because she needs to understand the importance of perceiving oneself as part of a social and political reality. After that act which altered the course of events in the characters' lives, Zafar's self-awareness as a Pakistani citizen emerges in discussions about politics and society that he has with his friends. In this context, he defines himself as a Mohajir, thus claiming a specific kind of relationship with Pakistan. Likewise, particularly in the face of ethnic tensions experienced, Raheen reflects on definitions of identity in terms of ethnicity, for example thinking of her friends and herself as Mohajirs, Pathans, Panjabi, Sindhis, while Karim claims his 'Bengaliness' (2002: 176), choosing to identify with his mother's ethnic identity. Thus, while in *Noor* identity issues concern how the characters relate to Pakistan and Bangladesh, here the 1971 war becomes part of a broader discussion that highlights Pakistan's composite nature, as Shamsie seems to suggest that Pakistan's identity lies precisely in its hybridity.

While Karim obliges Zafar to face the past by telling his story to his daughter, *Kartography* also stresses the importance of questioning narratives of the past. Indeed, both protagonists are induced to investigate that past moment, which is only vaguely referred to by their parents. Discovery of what happened poses questions of identity and belonging that are developed through the relationship that Karim and Raheen establish with each other and with the city. Here, the creation and crumbling of borders define the stages of the relationship between the two friends. A divide arises between them when Karim learns about Zafar's betrayal and racism towards his mother and begins to believe that, being Zafar's daughter, Raheen would behave in a similar way. The separation is strengthened by the parting of their ways when Karim moves to England and, some years later, Raheen attends university in the United States. It is her discovery of the secret of 1971 that starts a process that reunites the friends when both are able to process their common past in a way that allows them to look towards the future. Within the story, identity is also looked at through the ways in which the characters relate to Karachi, a city that Karim wants to map, and about which he develops knowledge that associates topography with a chronicle of major events, thus suggesting that the identity of a place lies in its inhabitants and in the events that occur in its streets. Karim's need to create a 'kartography' of Karachi allows the author to propose a reflection on home and belonging that conceives identity as bound to a place and its defining traits. For this reason, besides the different ways in which each character understands personal identity and perceives their relationship with Pakistan, their shared identity lies in their common social and cultural experiences.

Like *Noor*, *Kartography* emanates from the idea that the country needs to enact a process through which memories of what happened in 1971, both on the battlefield and to Pakistani society, must be handed down to younger generations. Thus, the authors highlight that dealing with that event should imply questioning official narratives. This would allow citizens to develop their narratives of a crucial moment whose comprehension participates in private and collective understandings of Pakistani identity. Therefore, the novels produce representations that point out the potentially rhizomatic nature of the relationship that the subject can establish with the nation while developing multiple, non-fixed, and fragmented conceptions of national identity.

Note

1 At the end of the war, the *Report of the Hamoodur Rehman Commission of Inquiry into the 1971 War* (published 2001) proved that acts of violence were committed by the army of West Pakistan.

Bibliography

Anderson, B. (1991) *Imagined Communities: Reflections on the Origin and Spread of Nationalism*. London and New York: Verso.
Anzaldúa, G.E. (1987) *Borderlands/La Frontera. The New Mestiza*. San Francisco: Aunt Lute Books.
Bhabha, H. (ed.) (1990) *Nation and Narration*. London and New York: Routledge.
Bhabha, H. (1994) *The Location of Culture*. London and New York: Routledge.
Bilgrami, S. (2007) *Without Dreams*. New York: Harper Collins.
Cilano, C. (2011) *National Identities in Pakistan: The 1971 War in Contemporary Pakistani Fiction*. London and New York: Routledge.
Cilano, C. (2013) *Contemporary Pakistani Fiction in English: Idea, Nation, State*. London: Routledge.
Cohen, S. (2004) *The Idea of Pakistan*. Washington: Brookings Institution Press.
Glissant, É. (1989) *Caribbean Discourse. Selected Essays*. Charlottesville: University of Virginia Press.
Hall, S. (1996) 'The Question of Cultural Identity'. In *Modernity: An Introduction to Modern Societies*. Ed. by Hall, S., Held, D., Hubert, D., and Thompson, K. Oxford: Wiley-Blackwell, 596–632.
Hamoodur Rehman Commission (2001) *The Report of the Hamoodur Rehman Commission of Inquiry into the 1971 War as Declassified by the Government of Pakistan*. Islamabad: Vanguard.
Hirsh, M. (2008) 'The Generation of Postmemory'. *Poetics Today* 29, 103–128.
Jafferlot, C. (ed.) (2002) *Pakistan. Nationalism without a Nation?* New York: Zed Books.
Jafferlot, C. (ed.) (2004) *A History of Pakistan and its Origins*. London: Anthem.
Jalal, A. (1995) 'Conjuring Pakistan: History as Official Imagining'. *International Journal of Middle East Studies*, 27, 73–89.
Khan, S. (2003) *Noor*. Karachi: Alhamra.
Nora, P. (1989) 'Between Memory and History: *Les Lieux de Mémoire*'. *Representations* 26, 7–24.
Rushdie, S. (1995) *Shame*. London: Vintage.
Shamsie, K. (2000) *Salt and Saffron*. London: Bloomsbury.
Shamsie, K. (2002) *Kartography*. London: Bloomsbury.
Sidhwa, B. (1991) *Cracking India*. Minneapolis: Milkweed.

PART II

9/11 and beyond

Contexts, forms, and perspectives

4
GLOBAL PAKISTAN IN THE WAKE OF 9/11

Ulka Anjaria

The events of 9/11 brought Pakistan once again into a global light, but largely through negative representations. I argue that anglophone Pakistani[1] literature written since 2001 has been the key site of contesting these negative representations by offering a new understanding of Pakistan's place in the global imaginary. The chapter will show how internationally well-known authors Kamila Shamsie, Mohammed Hanif, and Mohsin Hamid are among those involved in rethinking Pakistan's place in the world through their novels and, in this way, in thinking the global novel anew. Their works offer new imaginaries that take into account global power inequalities, but also present alternative spatial formations. In *Burnt Shadows* (2009), Shamsie develops the concept of postcolonial globality to situate Pakistan within a transnational and transhistorical episteme that both celebrates cosmopolitanism and draws attention to its limits in the contemporary, post-2001 world. In *A Case of Exploding Mangoes* (2008), Hanif uses the logic of conspiracy to both underline global complicity in Pakistani politics and to imagine new networks and collectivities as a response to it. And in *The Reluctant Fundamentalist* (2007), *How to Get Filthy Rich in Rising Asia* (2013), and *Exit West* (2017), Hamid questions the relationship between identity and place, first by allegorising cultural misunderstanding, and second by eliminating the specificity of place altogether. Together, these three authors offer new modes of representing global Pakistan outside of the dominant discourse of 9/11.

Postcolonial globality

The postcolonial novel has always been a place of interchange and mixing, as epitomised by the works of Salman Rushdie (Jani 2010) and Amitav Ghosh, in particular his Ibis trilogy (Luo 2013). Origins are presented as mixed and hybrid, power as weak rather than strong, and language as a key site of subject-formation (Bhabha 1994). This is clear in postcolonial theory and has been evinced in the anglophone Indian novel, though perhaps less so in its Pakistani counterpart.[2] But in the wake of 9/11 and the explosion of globally successful Pakistani novels, we see more of a turn to a representation of globality. We might even say that those events are what made the Pakistani novel 'postcolonial'.[3]

Shamsie's *Burnt Shadows* represents this global turn in anglophone Pakistani fiction through the globe-crossing story of Hiroko Tanaka and her transnational group of family and acquaintances from 1945 to 2002. The novel's epic sweep is markedly different from Shamsie's earlier novel *Kartography* (2002), which briefly follows Raheen in her college years abroad, but is intensely located and particular in its discussion of what it means to love the wounded city of Karachi. By contrast, *Burnt Shadows* refuses to be anchored in any one place, moving from Nagasaki to Delhi to Karachi to Afghanistan to New York. Displacement becomes the prerequisite of narrative here, as it is with Rushdie and Ghosh – the idea that it is in travel and movement that stories are born and that, conversely, the huge thing we understand as the globe can only be understood by means of stories. Translation and polyglottism are also tropes in global postcolonial fiction, and we see that in this novel as well, with Hiroko beginning as a German teacher (Shamsie 2009: 12) and then translating for the American army in the wake of the atomic bomb (2009: 63), and Raza as a teenager doing a multilingual crossword puzzle with ease, 'with its Japanese and Urdu clues and German and English solutions' (2009: 131).

But in Shamsie's version, this vision of twentieth-century cosmopolitan fluidity and movement is born in wounds, in this case two wounds occurring almost simultaneously: the atomic bomb dropped on Nagasaki and the Partition of India two years later. While Hiroko retains literal scars from the first, the second causes emotional scars for her husband Sajjad, as he is forced to rediscover home all over again when, after their honeymoon in Istanbul, he is not let back into the country: 'They said I chose to leave [...] They said I'm one of the Muslims who chose to leave India. It can't be unchosen [...] They said I can't go back to Dilli, I can't go back home' (2009: 127). Partition leaves its mark on several generations in Pakistan, and particularly in Karachi, a city fundamentally changed by the division of the subcontinent and the mass migrations that followed. Sajjad's hope for his own son's professional success is thus part of a larger wish across the city that the impact of Partition will finally be overcome: 'Every father in this neighbourhood of migrants, each with stories of all they had lost and all they had started to rebuild after Partition, made a similar speech to his son' (2009:138).

But Shamsie's innovation in *Burnt Shadows* is to take this global imaginary and give it a contemporary gloss by beginning and ending the story in a specific, post-2001 moment and thus registering the consequences of this movement and fluidity in the post-9/11 world. For despite his multilingualism, Raza's relationship to movement and travel is much more uneasy than his parents'. While his parents ultimately adjust to life in Pakistan, despite living there initially against their will, Raza is perennially out of place (Henry 2017: 78–80). Even at a young age, he finds his racial difference from others a source of shame: 'He only spoke Japanese within the privacy of his home [...] Why allow the world to know his mind contained words from a country he'd never visited?' (Shamsie 2009:141). His fluid multilingualism, which on one hand he loves, also has an underside, as when faced with his school exams he sees a 'jumble of words' rather than meaning, 'and nonsensical answers to questions he didn't even understand kept coming to mind in Japanese' (2009: 146). In part this is because although he loves languages, the world around him seems to be getting more provincial and he is increasingly out of place in it:

> [Languages] was a passion that could have no fulfilment, not here. Somewhere in the world perhaps there were institutions where you could dive from vocabulary to vocabulary and make that your life. But not here. 'Polyglot' was not any kind of practical career choice.
>
> (2009: 148)

Transnational movement, which had been so transformative for his parents, becomes for Raza a form of loss. This is until he meets Harry Burton, in whom he finds a fellow polyglot (2009: 154), and, around the same time, Abdullah, the Hazara boy who mistakes him for an

Afghani and introduces him to the world of the *mujahideen*. In the late twentieth century, in the midst of the Cold War, these are the two fates for a shape-shifting hybrid such as Raza: the CIA or the *jihad*.

Following September 11 and the increased culture of paranoia it spawns, Raza's chameleon-like quality and his cultural fluidity end up costing him his freedom, as he is accused of being a spy by an American at the security firm to which he has been so loyal, and even the daughter of his family's long-time friends, Kim Barton, ends up putting him in danger because of her unfounded suspicions of his Hazara friend, Abdullah. Raza's ability to be 'at home' in so many different contexts is in fact a liability in a world increasingly divided between those who 'are either with us or against us', in George W. Bush's infamous words (CNN 2001). This is a somewhat ironic twist on the postcolonial global novel, which has long been considered an antidote to provincialist ways of thinking. Shamsie's novel is certainly that, but is also aware that the nuances of translation and an open, cultural relativity – those bastions of postcolonial thought – might not, in times of war, be the most feasible stances. It is precisely nuance and relativity that the so-called war on terror wanted to exterminate, and thus the fate of the postcolonial imagination is presented as tenuous.

Conspiracy and network

If 9/11 stands as an impasse in Shamsie's vision of a world of global interchange, it – or rather the conspiracy-oriented logic it represented and caused to intensify – is deployed as a primary mode of meaning-making in Hanif's *A Case of Exploding Mangoes*. Here, conspiracy and plot, two key words that emerged out of the events of 11 September 2001, are reframed as novelistic structuring principles. Not only is the story about a series of conspiracies to assassinate the Pakistani president General Zia-ul-Haq, but its structure is itself one of mystery, in which the end is presented at the beginning, the various characters' intentions *vis-à-vis* the general are only gradually revealed, and related stories like that of Ali's father's death are told only towards the end. If a conspiracy is marked by deep levels of interconnectedness between people and/or things that at first do not seem related, then Hanif's novel recreates this logic in fictional form.

Conspiracy theories aside, US intelligence after September 11 noted 'the existence of a vast and complex transnational conspiracy behind the hijackings' (Crenshaw 2001: 425) which spoke of networks of influence and collaboration that went beyond what the world had seen before. Mainstream renderings of the event in the US stopped short of extending this network of transnational influences to America's own actions in the Cold War and beyond, leaving that work up to progressive and alternative media. The most significant of these actions was of course the US involvement in the Afghanistan war, in which Pakistan played the go-between, changing the nature of Pakistani society as much as it had a profound effect on geopolitics. Linking the CIA to the very *mujahideen* and Saudi financiers who backed the attacks on September 11, with the ISI and the Pakistani army as middle men, is part of the work of this novel, which is not so much uncovering a conspiracy as it is giving a full historical account which includes truths outside of the current US-sponsored global rhetoric of 'Islamic terrorism'. (US involvement in Afghanistan is also touched on, for this same reason, in *Burnt Shadows*.) Marieke de Goede argues that the network has become a key metaphor in thinking about 'global connectivity' and 'contemporary social life', including 'transnational danger' (2012: 215) such as 'the dispersed global terrorism threat, [...] the spread of (computer) viruses, [...] the identification of organized crime "hubs"' and 'the depiction of al Qaeda terrorism' (2012: 216). In Hanif's novel, the network is animated with the US as a constitutive part in order to counter dominant narratives of 9/11.

A Case of Exploding Mangoes does this by alternating between the first-person narration of Ali Shigri, an officer in the Pakistani army, and third-person description – much of it satirical – of General Zia-ul-Haq, featuring, at close range, his religiosity, his paranoia, his irrationality, and even his stomach parasites. This fictionalised insider's account of the dictator is supplemented by various additional perspectives, including that of his wife, US ambassador Arnold Raphel and his wife, and General Akhtar. Raphel's own worries about the growing power of the CIA in Pakistan in relation to the US government underlines the sense of intrigue; he describes Islamabad as 'a whirl of conspiracies and dinner parties; there were more CIA subcontractors and cooks per household than meals in a day' (Hanif 2008: 76). Indeed, General Akhtar is shown secretly meeting Bill Casey, the CIA director (2008: 79); General Zia is consorting with businessmen in Lufkin, Texas (2008: 110); and Osama bin Laden (called OBL) 'of Laden and Co. Constructions' (2008: 230), shows up to a US-government party, saying that 'Allah has been very kind. There is no business like the construction business in times of war' (2008: 233). There is an element of farce to these representations as well, in scenes such as that where General Akhtar rehearses for the speech he will give when he wins the Nobel Peace Prize for his role in fighting the Soviets (2008: 200) and a US government Fourth of July party where American guests dress up like tribal Afghans.

But Hanif not only represents these real or fictional networks and conspiracies; we also have conspiracy and network as a fictional device, which presents different parts of the story as seemingly unrelated and then gradually linked together as the novel proceeds. *A Case of Exploding Mangoes* begins at the end, at the moment right before Pak One takes off on the fatal flight. The novel's prologue describes a grainy clip as one might see in footage taken by an amateur on what later became a crime scene, so that 'everything in it is sun-bleached and slightly faded' (2008: 3). This falls into conventions of representing video security footage from crime scenes, where a few seconds of footage get played over and over again on the news following a crime or disaster. The main players in the conspiracy feature in the clip: General Zia, Arnold Raphel, and General Akhtar. This moment, the narrator tells us, marks the end of the war in Afghanistan 'and these men we see in the TV clip are the undisputed victors' (2008: 5). But they are all about to die in a plane crash whose cause will never be found: 'There will be no autopsies, the leads will run dry, investigations will be blocked, [and] there will be cover-ups to cover cover-ups [...] It would be said that this was the biggest cover-up in aviation history since the last biggest cover-up' (2008: 5). The only surviving witness is Ali, our narrator: 'I was the one who got away' (2008: 5).

The rest of the novel tells us not only how Ali got away, but how he got there in the first place, how the various other characters got there – most of them based on real-life individuals – and how they were involved in plotting General Zia's demise. Ali, for his part, wanted to kill General Zia in order to avenge his father's death, likely at the hands of Zia's men. Ali's plan, 'a fucked-up idea, which, like most fucked-up ideas, was conceived at the end of a very hot day in the Academy' (2008: 97), involved injecting General Zia with a drop of krait venom during a silent swordsman exercise performed for the general by a highly skilled squadron of soldiers. The truth behind this 'silent drill conspiracy' (2008: 97) is revealed in a series of flashbacks, in which Ali's seemingly innocent demeanour gradually gives way to a dark side.

Ali goes through with the 'sword manoeuvre' (2008: 180) and poisons General Zia, but he 'gets away' in the end because so many others kill Zia at the same time. Indeed, almost every other character in the novel wants to kill Zia for his or her own reasons, and in his or her own way. General Akhtar wants Zia's power and so he plants air fresheners in Zia's plane loaded with poisonous VX gas. (In one of the many humorous scenes of the novel, General Akhtar tries to get CIA Director Coogan's support for getting rid of Zia, but Coogan is too involved watching a replay of a Redskins-Buccaneers football game to listen. Thus when, with one eye on the television, he shouts, 'Go get him' (2008: 237), Akhtar takes it as a sign that he should proceed with his plan.) The union of mango farmers wants to kill Zia for his anti-union policies and send him the eponymous case of exploding mangoes as a gift. And the blind rape victim Zainab, one of many women adversely affected by Zia's implementation of the Hudood ordinance in 1979 (Imran 2005), casts a curse upon Zia, which is heard by a crow flying overhead, who then flies kamikaze-style into Pak One.

There is certainly a jab here at Zia's paranoia – when Zia repeatedly asks his security officer, 'Who wants to kill me?' (2008: 65), the answer is always, 'Everyone' (2008: 66) – but it is also a product of fiction itself, in which Hanif imagines a network that takes the place of what we might have earlier called 'solidarity' in response to authoritarian governments. The populace is so fragmented and has different aims, most of them petty and self-serving, and so the possibility of real solidarity or a grass-roots movement where all of Zia's enemies might unite as one is largely precluded from the outset. What we have instead is a network or conspiracy of interlocking interests, and one utopic moment in which all the interests coincide, in this case to produce the spectacular event not only of Zia's death, but of his death 'many times over' (2008: 323). The flip side of paranoia is that in fact, Zia *is* killed by everyone, in an inadvertent act of pseudo-collective revolt.

The doubleness of the title, the 'case' being both the mangoes gifted to Zia by the mango farmers' union and the case as an incident to be investigated, offers a play on the idea of conspiracy, a lightness that pervades what could otherwise be a heavy – and even depressing – novel. Hanif registers both the truth about conspiracies – there are more connections than often meet the eye – but also their absurdity and their potential to cause paranoia. This balance between fate and agency appears throughout the novel, in Brigadier TM's comment that 'Life is in Allah's hands […] but I pack my own parachute' (2008: 64) and in Ali's self-referential commentary in the novel as a whole, such as when he asks his lover Obaid about the book he is reading, Gabriel García Márquez's *Chronicle of a Death Foretold*: 'Why keep reading it when you already know that the hero is going to die?' (Hanif 2008: 279). The conspiracy form demands this new structure: action, then retrospective solution.

In this way, by counteracting the real and still-buried connections between the US and the Pakistani state with a conspiracy plot of his own – and one which includes homosexual love and elements of the absurd – Hanif rewrites conspiracy as a fruitful aesthetic space, rather than merely a geopolitical stranglehold on individual action and freedom. The novel offers a space where humour and love can flourish, even amidst the intensive connectivities that offer a spectacular future of state violence, with insidious collaborations between governments like those of America and Pakistan. In doing so, Hanif reclaims the global conspiracy as a thing of the imagination.

The problem of place

If Shamsie and Hanif raise questions about new modes of connectivity in a world that, after 9/11, looks more broken or disconnected than ever, Hamid pushes these questions further through an intense questioning of place. While his first novel, *Moth Smoke*, is intensely located, following Darashikoh as he criss-crosses the streets and byways of Lahore, in the three novels that followed Hamid seems to be approaching the question of Pakistan askance, as it were, progressively emptying out place signifiers while still telling uniquely Pakistani stories – or, more specifically, stories that engage with the problem of what it means to be Pakistani in a post-9/11 world.

There is no doubt that the image of Pakistan in the world changed following 9/11, culminating, perhaps, in the discovery of Osama bin Laden in Abbottabad in 2011. This change was twofold: a suspicion of Pakistan in its role as a US ally and simultaneously a suspicion of all Muslim men as potential terrorists, which manifested in various hate crimes in the United States as well as increased scrutiny at airports and elsewhere. *The Reluctant Fundamentalist* is set in this particular moment when Muslim men, even those who have completely bought into the American capitalist dream, are still suspected of being disloyal. It traces Changez as he gets a high-profile job with the investment banking firm Underwood Samson after graduating from Princeton. Changez does very well at the firm until the events of 9/11 compel him to rethink his place in America. But beyond this narrative of progressive alienation, the novel raises questions about empathy and relatability in the way we read as a whole. The story is structured around an encounter between Changez and an anonymous interlocutor in Lahore. Changez and his interlocutor mistrust one another, not knowing whether the story each is telling is true or whether the other is, respectively, a terrorist and an assassin. The story ends on this mutual mistrust: 'It seems an obvious thing to say, but you should not imagine that we Pakistanis are all potential terrorists, just as we should not imagine that you Americans are all undercover assassins' (Hamid 2007: 183). As the two men part, the American can see nothing but a waiter who 'is rapidly closing in […] [and] waving at me to detain you' and the protagonist hopes that the 'glint of metal' in the interlocutor's jacket is 'the holder of your business cards' (2007: 184) – but the novel ends there, and we are never sure if they are who they say they are. The uncertainty of the encounter becomes the crucial frame of the book, raising questions about cultural misunderstanding and stereotypes: it is likely that while some readers would interpret the protagonist as a terrorist, others might see the American as a CIA agent, spy, or assassin. Like *A Case of Exploding Mangoes*, *The Reluctant Fundamentalist* defines the post-2001 era as one of mutual and sustained mistrust. However, by framing the story as an unresolved encounter and leaving the ending open, the novel also asks larger metafictional questions about how readers relate to certain characters and not to others, which characters we empathise with and how that empathy shapes the story, and the centrality of these questions to the category of the global novel (Anjaria 2016).

In contrast to *Moth Smoke*, which is absolutely a Lahore novel, *The Reluctant Fundamentalist* is set mostly in New York and follows Changez on his global travels, with only the frame taking place in Lahore. However, this elaboration of globality reads as a different project from Shamsie's discussed above, as here the global story is not one of hybridity and interchange but instead a story of the unitary homogenisation of global difference by the gavel of a hard-nosed, American capitalism. Lahore is significant in this story because it bears the double-brunt of American hegemony; the so-called war on terror is presented as the flip side of predatory capitalism. *The Reluctant Fundamentalist* is thus a Pakistani novel in a very different way from *Moth Smoke*; it is mostly set outside of Pakistan, but its entire vision of the world is filtered through the kind of global peripherality intensified in Pakistan following 9/11, in which capitalism and military force work together in increasingly terroristic ways.

Hamid seems to want to pursue this question of what it means to write a Pakistani novel in the post-9/11 world in his next two novels, both of which have no specified place setting. *How to Get Filthy Rich in Rising Asia* is a parody of a self-help book, told in the second person by an unnamed narrator. The narrator's story begins in what is clearly a Third World village, though few specifics are given, and then moves to an anonymous Third World city. In an interview about the novel, Hamid explained the decision to leave the setting unspecified by saying that 'the ingrained view is that South Asia is an exotic place, a peculiar place and a central place – [that] is a colonial mindset'.[4] Thus, it seems, removing place altogether is a rejoinder to that mindset. This sense of Pakistan's peculiarity has been even further intensified post-9/11, where 'Pakistan' has been overdetermined by the global language used to describe it, leaving very little space for alternative definitions. *Rising Asia* is a novel about aspiration and love, not terror and violence. Hamid suggests that if he had introduced the word 'Pakistan', those everyday stories would be overrun by pressing political concerns.

Hamid's most recent novel, *Exit West*, takes a similar approach, also refraining from naming the place of the story's origin even though, once again, it could easily be Pakistan. Here we have more direct references to religious nationalism and sectarian conflict as the reasons why the anonymous city erupts in war, but again the focus is on love and migration rather than on religion and conflict, and so the decision not to name the place seems a deliberate call for Pakistani writers to be able to tell *other* kinds of stories. While the Western marketplace for the global novel often calls for a certain kind of universal resonance (Rajan and Sharma 2006), Hamid's two most recent texts upend that formula by refusing to be educative and by pushing 'universalism' to its most extreme end, which is a denial of specificity altogether. This should not be read as a depoliticisation but as a rethinking of the very terminologies along which we imagine our political constructs: east vs west, universal vs particular, difference vs similarity. By undercutting our desire to specify and contextualise, Hamid's works stretch not only what the Pakistani novel does, but what the Pakistani novel *is*, after 9/11.[5]

Writing about Pakistani fiction in terms of 9/11 has the potential to recentre American exceptionalism (Singh 2012: 159) by focusing on a date that is important mostly in the US' own self-mythologising. This is far from my intention here. However, I suggest that the marker is useful insofar as it illuminates the renewed investment of Pakistani literature in questions of globality appropriate for a changing world order. In fact, as all these works show, cosmopolitanism, violence, Islamophobia, and cultural misunderstandings existed long before 9/11; however, the intensified cultural standoff that this event produced has the potential to shed light on Pakistan in new ways. 9/11 is not the defining point of Pakistani literature, nor will it be. But it is an optic that allows us to see certain trends in new ways.

It should also be stressed that the authors discussed here are three of Pakistan's most internationally recognised and do not represent the wide diversity of Pakistani fiction, not in English, let alone in Urdu, Punjabi, or other languages as well.[6] But as I have tried to show, their international recognition comes in part because they are all in different ways interested in the global *as a problem*, and they reflect that interest in their works. This seems to me as much an awareness of 'what sells' as a recognition that the problems of Pakistan are not Pakistan's alone, but are always mired in confluences of global, national, regional, and local concerns.

While Shamsie and Hamid have seemed to expand their scale as they continue to write (Shamsie's latest novel, *A God in Every Stone* (2014), also takes a broad historical and geographical sweep), Hanif has counterintuitively gone in the opposite direction with his second novel, *Our Lady of Alice Bhatti* (2011), which is set in Karachi and has intensely local concerns: daily violence, the state of Christian minorities, caste, and love. But the violence here is more on the level of the domestic and low-level urban warfare than the type of spectacular assassinations and global events discussed in his first book, in Hamid's *The Reluctant Fundamentalist*, and in Shamsie's *Burnt Shadows*. Hanif's trajectory from the global to the local suggests that no author or literary culture proceeds in a unidirectional trend. Rather than read these three authors as symptoms of a broad-sweeping trajectory of the transformation of Pakistani fiction, then, we might see them as extended experiments with particular questions relating to form, scale, and the global novel. From this perspective, *Our Lady of Alice Bhatti* is as much an experiment with localism as *Exit West* is with placelessness and the question of the universal.

Notes

1 The three authors discussed here have all lived abroad, and Shamsie continues to do so. I agree with Chambers that 'it is [...] untenable to impose a distinction between diasporic and Pakistani-resident authors writing in English' (2011: 124) and I hope the argument of this chapter shows why.
2 See Rahman (2011), Werbner (2013), and Yaqin (2013) for useful discussions of cosmopolitanism in recent Pakistani fiction.
3 The relationship between the Pakistani novel in English and its better-known Indian counterpart has been discussed by Cilano (2009: 185–186).
4 This is also cited in Anjaria (2013), from which some of this discussion of *How to Get Filthy Rich in Rising Asia* is taken.
5 See also Hamid's short story 'Terminator: Attack of the Drone' (2011), which similarly evacuates the specificity of place in the context of America's drone war.
6 Cilano records Kamila Shamsie's criticisms of a view on Pakistani literature that assumes that English-language writing is only an expression of a colonial mindset: 'Our [...] vexed relationship [...] with English is just not an issue' (2009: 192).

Bibliography

Anjaria, U. (2013) '"A True Lahori": Mohsin Hamid and the Problem of Place in Pakistani Fiction'. *Economic and Political Weekly* 48(25) [online]. Available from <www.epw.in/journal/2013/25/web-exclusives/true-lahori.html> [June 2017].

Anjaria, U. (2016) 'The Realist Impulse and the Future of Postcoloniality'. *NOVEL: A Forum on Fiction* 49(2), 278–294.

Bhabha, H.K. (1994) *The Location of Culture*. London: Routledge.

Chambers, C. (2011) 'A Comparative Approach to Pakistani Fiction in English'. *Journal of Postcolonial Writing* 47(2), 122–134.

Cilano, C. (2009) '"Writing from Extreme Edges": Pakistani English-Language Fiction'. *ARIEL* 40(2–3), 183–201.

CNN. (2001) 'You Are Either With Us or Against Us' [online]. Available from <http://edition.cnn.com/2001/US/11/06/gen.attack.on.terror/> [12 June 2017].

Crenshaw, M. (2001) 'Why America?: The Globalization of Civil War'. *Current History* 100(650), 425–432.

de Goede, M. (2012) 'Fighting the Network: A Critique of the Network as a Security Technology'. *Distinktion: Scandinavian Journal of Social Theory* 13(3), 215–232.

Hamid, M. (2000) *Moth Smoke*. London: Granta.

Hamid, M. (2007) *The Reluctant Fundamentalist*. New York: Houghton Mifflin Harcourt.

Hamid, M. (2011) 'Terminator: Attack of the Drone'. *Guardian* [online]. Available from <www.theguardian.com/books/2011/nov/07/short-story-mohsin-hamid> [13 June 2017].

Hamid, M. (2013) *How to Get Filthy Rich in Rising Asia*. New York: Riverhead.

Hamid, M. (2017) *Exit West*. London: Hamish Hamilton.

Hanif, M. (2008) *A Case of Exploding Mangoes*. New York: Vintage.

Hanif, M. (2011) *Our Lady of Alice Bhatti*. Toronto: Anchor.

Henry, M. (2017) *Narrative's Nuclear Spring: The South Asian Novel after the Nuclear Bomb*. Unpublished PhD thesis. Waltham: Brandeis University.

Imran, R. (2005) 'Legal Injustices: The Zina Hudood Ordinance of Pakistan and its Implications for Women'. *Journal of International Women's Studies* 7(2), 78–100.

Jani, P. (2010) *Decentering Rushdie: Cosmopolitanism and the Indian Novel in English*. Columbus: Ohio State University Press.

Luo, S.P. (2013) 'The Way of Words: Vernacular Cosmopolitanism in Amitav Ghosh's *Sea of Poppies*'. *Journal of Commonwealth Literature* 48(3), 377–392.

Rahman, S. (2011) 'Karachi, Turtles, and the Materiality of Place: Pakistani Eco-Cosmopolitanism in Uzma Aslam Khan's *Trespassing*'. *Interdisciplinary Studies of Literature and the Environment* 18(2), 261–282.

Rajan, G. and Sharma. S. (2006) 'Theorizing Recognition: South Asian Authors in a Global Milieu'. In *New Cosmopolitanisms: South Asians in the US*. Ed. by Rajan, G and Sharma, S. Stanford: Stanford University Press, 150–169.

Shamsie, K. (2002) *Kartography*. London: Bloomsbury.

Shamsie, K. (2009) *Burnt Shadows*. New York: Picador.

Shamsie, K. (2014) *A God in Every Stone*. New York: Bloomsbury.
Singh, H. (2012) 'A Legacy of Violence: Interview with Kamila Shamsie About *Burnt Shadows* (2009)'. *ARIEL* 42(2), 157–162.
Werbner, P. (2013) 'Paradoxes of Postcolonial Vernacular Cosmopolitanism in South Asia and the Diaspora'. In *Ashgate Research Companion to Cosmopolitanism*. Surrey: Ashgate, 107–124.
Yaqin, A. (2013) 'Cosmopolitan Ventures during Times of Crisis: A Postcolonial Reading of Faiz Ahmed Faiz's "Dasht-e tanhai" and Nadeem Aslam's *Maps for Lost Lovers*'. *Pakistaniaat: A Journal of Pakistan Studies* 5(1), 62–78.

5
PAKISTANI INOUTSIDERS AND THE DYNAMICS OF POST-9/11 DISSOCIATION IN PAKISTANI ANGLOPHONE FICTION

Claudia Nördinger

Globalised anglophone studies and inoutside perspectives

Since the 1990s, anglophone literature rooted in localities outside Great Britain and the USA has usually been considered within the framework of postcolonialism. Debates around the limitations of the postcolonial paradigm are almost as old as the field itself, but postcolonial theory has undeniably broadened the scope of analysis and inspired valuable scholarship over the decades. However, as more and more authors and literary texts seek to escape from the field through the cracks in its historical, cultural, and geographical implications, theories on transculturality and globalisation have suggested a multinodal approach to anglophone literature from around the globe. Meanwhile, 'postcolonial studies' has become well established as an institutional umbrella term that unites a large variety of scholarship under a recognisable – and marketable – label. In a field acutely aware of the power of naming and categorising, it seems only logical that there have been efforts to update and redefine the field, and recent works such as *The Postcolonial World* (Singh and Kim 2017) demonstrate the potential of postcolonial studies as a multidisciplinary and transcultural field.

I have argued in favour of 'globalised anglophone studies' elsewhere and tried to show what an analytic perspective considering the anglophone world as a whole and a cultural continuum might entail (Perner 2011). Of course, literary analysis should not be arbitrarily contained within 'linguistic containers' either. Many literary texts call for analysis that is prepared to step across linguistic divides. Like many scholars today, I am more interested in the manoeuvres of the literary text than in national, cultural, or even transcultural categorisation based on an author's heritage. Nevertheless, cultural and national categories remain significant reference points for literary texts and for the conflicts they represent, especially when those conflicts are fraught with complicated histories of interaction and domination. I will illustrate this point in the following as I examine two texts that engage with issues of cultural and religious membership: Mohsin Hamid's novel *The Reluctant Fundamentalist* (2007) and Ayad Akhtar's play *Disgraced* (2012). Both texts are part of the cultural continuum that connects Pakistan and the USA and carry transcultural echoes of the national paradigm.

In my analysis, I draw on my own conceptualisation of the 'inoutsider', an analytical category I have adapted from Obioma Nnaemeka's article on 'Feminism, Rebellious Women, and Cultural Boundaries'. Nnaemeka defines an insider as a person who has a birthright to national and cultural membership, while an outsider can merely acquire an empirical right of membership. Nnaemeka's argument targets a specific context, namely, the involvement of Western scholars in the interpretation of African cultural production. According to Nnaemeka, different combinations of birthright and empirical right produce 'different degrees of *cognitive right* to unlock cultural productions' (Nnaemeka 1995: 85; emphasis original). Nnaemeka conceded that it may be possible for outsiders to become 'inside outsiders' – or 'inoutsiders' – but emphasises that this 'requires a lot of hard work and a high dose of humility' (1995: 86). Nnaemeka's essentialist reliance on the notion of 'birthright' as the key to cognitive understanding is debatable, but it fulfils a strategic function: her aim is to avoid African literary and cultural studies being dominated and 'colonised' by Western scholars.

My reformulation of Nnaemeka's concept subjects it to a significant shift in focus: I have transferred the 'inoutsider' from the sphere of scholarly enquiry to the realm of creative production. The 'outsiders' whose work I have examined previously are authors engaging with the USA from a position outside the US-American mainstream. Stepping beyond questions of authorial biography, I have considered 'inoutsiders' in literary texts and analysed their encounters with the texts' fictional and factual US-American locations. In the context of this article, I apply my concept to Hamid's and Akhtar's literary encounters with the USA and with their protagonists' status of national and cultural membership. It is important to note that in contrast to the African scholars Nnaemeka had in mind, the USA hardly needs to be protected from the outsiders' colonising agendas or audacious judgements. US-American inside perspectives are commonly felt to have become something of a global cultural possession, available and decipherable to recipients worldwide. People who have never visited the USA feel that they know the country intimately. US-American settings and scenarios depicted in television shows, in Hollywood films, and on the news are more familiar to us than parts of our own home countries. In this respect, authors depicting the USA 'from the outside' might all be said to write from inoutsider perspectives. More importantly, both Hamid's novel and Akhtar's play demonstrate how fictional texts can simulate perspectives that propose alternative ways of thinking about the USA and its relations with the world, as well as about national and cultural affiliation in general.

I conceptualise the inoutsider as a person who has either acquired access to a sphere that is not originally his or her own (such as Hamid's Changez) or, alternatively, feels alienated in an environment that is his or hers by 'birthright' (as in the case of Akhtar's Amir). In the following, I will demonstrate how the inoutside perspectives articulated in *The Reluctant Fundamentalist* and *Disgraced* give expression to the precariousness of identity formation in a modern world of embattled absolutes and shifting boundaries.

The intricacy of Pakistan-US relations

The Reluctant Fundamentalist and *Disgraced* portray microcosms of a specific point in the relations between the USA and the world. They focus on events that take place shortly before, and in the immediate aftermath of, 9/11. Published in 2007 and 2012, respectively, they are products of a time in which relations between Pakistan and the USA were crucial for both sides, yet haunted by a complicated history and fraught with the challenges of a precarious present. The ambivalent nature of the relationship between the two countries may help to explain why identity appears to be a profoundly political matter in *The Reluctant Fundamentalist* and *Disgraced* and why both texts openly address issues that resonate within the theoretical framework of postcolonialism. At a time when other 'postcolonial authors' may choose to free themselves from what has been traditionally associated with the label, Hamid and Akhtar tap into discourses of mimicry, hybridity, domination, and (neo)colonialism.

Before turning to the aforementioned texts, let us briefly consider the cultural and geopolitical backdrop of the conflicts they portray. Long before compulsive tweeting from the White House became a major force in international relations, the relationship between Pakistan and the USA was crisis-ridden and difficult. At the surface level, Pakistan has been a strategically significant ally for the USA for decades. During the Soviet-Afghan War, the CIA channelled its support for the Afghan *mujahideen* through Pakistani intelligence forces, turning Pakistan into the USA's main partner in this proxy war extension of the Cold War. After 9/11, President Musharraf entered into an alliance with the USA that made Pakistan one of the front states of the so-called 'War on Terror'. This partnership has been very controversial in Pakistan and has contributed to an atmosphere of discord and instability (Zaidi 2013: 58ff.). The alliance has also been troubled by divergent objectives and a culture of mutual distrust since the beginning. One of the many grievances that Pakistanis hold against the USA is the country's refusal to take its ally's side in the conflict with India. Many Pakistanis are also critical of the USA's strong ties with Pakistan's military forces and accuse the USA of undermining the development of a stable democratic system. Anti-American sentiment has, furthermore, been fuelled by anti-Muslim rhetoric in US-American right-wing media and politics and by the rise in anti-Muslim sentiment among the US-American population, especially in the aftermath of the terrorist attacks. Of course, Pakistan has its own tradition of anti-Americanism, and anti-American rhetoric constitutes a powerful tool in political discourse, even while one continues to work with the USA behind the scenes.

All of the above is a relevant part of the backdrop of Pakistani writing engaging with the USA. However, when we look at Pakistani authors writing in English, we have to acknowledge that their perspective is hardly representative of Pakistani society as a whole. Many of them were educated in the West, most have lived and worked abroad at some point. This does not necessarily mean that they are less critical of the USA than Pakistanis more permanently settled in their home country, but it is likely that their perspective is informed by moving in and between different localities and views of the world. Whether their cosmopolitan outlook is always visible in their work is, of course, quite a different matter.

From American success story to cultural dissociation

I have chosen to discuss Hamid's novel *The Reluctant Fundamentalist* and Akhtar's play *Disgraced* side by side, because the basic setup of the two stories seems to be connected by a startling family resemblance. In both texts, the protagonist is a young man of Pakistani background who appears to have 'made it' in the USA. Hamid's Changez is raised in Pakistan and moves to the USA to study at Princeton. He then goes on to work for a prestigious valuation firm in New York. Like the play's author, Akhtar himself, Amir in *Disgraced* is a second-generation Pakistani-American. He is a successful corporate lawyer and lives a luxurious life on New York's Upper East Side. Changez and Amir are each romantically involved with a white American woman and seem to be well immersed in their US-American existence. For both of them, 9/11 is a turning point, the moment when their success story begins to crumble. Even their immediate responses to the terrorist attacks are strikingly similar. Changez, serving as the novel's first-person narrator, tells us that seeing the Twin Towers collapse on TV made him smile: 'Yes, despicable as it may sound, my initial reaction was to be remarkably pleased' (Hamid 2007: 72). In similar fashion, Amir confesses to having felt pride on the day of the attacks (Akhtar 2012: 39).

The main difference between Changez's and Amir's stories lies in where their estrangement from their US-American lives takes them. *The Reluctant Fundamentalist* chronicles a migrant's pursuit of the American dream, his hopes and aspirations, and his subsequent disappointment against the backdrop of the political and social climate brought about by the events of 9/11. The novel relates a perception of the USA which is dominated by the protagonist's realisation that, despite his immersion in a US-American life of privilege and success, he remains a Pakistani at heart. Thus Hamid persuasively labelled *The Reluctant Fundamentalist* an 'emigrant novel', a 'story of leaving America' (Yaqin 2008: 47). In this respect, Changez's Scheherazadic account of his 'rise and fall' offers a specific take on the inoutsider's perspective.

Hamid has stated that, after 9/11, it felt like a 'wall had suddenly come up between [his] American and Muslim worlds' (Solomon 2007: n.p.). His protagonist in *The Reluctant Fundamentalist* shares this sensation but his response to the attacks shows that this is not purely a matter of his adoptive country turning on him. Changez's smile marks him as an emotional outsider. It is a moment of revelation that, even before the rise of public hostility, makes clear that our narrator has not acquired an unproblematic sense of belonging in his US-American surroundings. His disenchantment with the USA, his 'emotional emigration' (even before his physical departure), is not only a response to the changing social and political climate. It also constitutes the recognition of an emotional partisanship that had been hidden beneath Changez's US-American success story all along. At a time when it holds obvious relevance to explain 'the other perspective', Hamid complicates notions of in- and outsiderdom.

As Changez comes to realise, he is 'a man lacking substance' (Hamid 2007: 125) and therefore easily influenced by his surroundings. His adaptability initially appears to be an advantage, even a skill, and it helps Changez to prosper in the USA. As a man without a 'stable core' (Hamid 2007: 148), he enacts the social scripts and stereotypes that his surroundings offer him, thus facilitating frictionless and satisfying social interaction. If considered in relation to Judith Butler's concept of performative identity construction,[1] *The Reluctant Fundamentalist* examines the question of what happens if a single event changes the scripts available and leaves you with no reliable role to enact, if your social existence can suddenly no longer be played out by the rulebook with which you are familiar. After 9/11, membership is defined by ethnic background, race, and religion. Whatever positive value flexibility of association may have held before, new and rigid lines are drawn. Beyond this, Changez's feelings of guilt demonstrate his schizophrenic dilemma: used to adapting to the role assigned to him, he suddenly finds himself being typecast as a threatening stranger, a potential terrorist. As he comes to understand his past role as a US-American *janissary* soldier, Changez appears to embrace the new script assigned to him: he assumes the role of a professed – and indeed rather reluctant – 'fundamentalist', withdrawing from his duties, growing a beard, and finally returning to his home country in anger.

In reconsidering Hamid's conception of the 'emigration novel', I would like to cite his remarks on the topic at some length:

> I suppose one of the things I was very concerned about in this novel was the immigrant novel about America – usually that's a story about coming to America, this magnet that pulls people, often poor, from all over the world to itself. There they have the American dream or the American nightmare. That is what I understand to be the typical American immigrant novel. Writing in the twenty-first century I was conscious of what happens to that dream after America's relationship to the world has radically changed. So this novel became an emigrant novel, a story of leaving America,

which I think is as much the immigrant novel of today as a story of going to the United States.

(qtd. in Yaqin 2008: 47)

The movement that Hamid describes proceeds outwards from a professed centre, away from the country that used to be the migrant's destination. Roots have been established in this country. A certain insider status has been acquired. Now our protagonist leaves behind his US-American aspirations and turns his back on the American dream. In such a scheme of national affiliation, the migrant is an inoutsider on account of having been settled in an US-American existence which is now consciously and – at least partly – voluntarily left behind.

When Changez returns to Pakistan for a visit, he is troubled that the Americanness of his own perception causes him to feel ashamed of the shabbiness of his parents' home. However, as soon as he becomes accustomed once more to his Pakistani surroundings, this experience only accelerates his conscious detachment from the US-American insider perspective. He is painfully aware of the shift in his frame of reference that has led him to regard his home with condescension (Hamid 2007: 124). Changez's temporary experience of defamiliarisation in his childhood home can be read as another instance of inoutsider perception. Darda has argued that it demonstrates the 'basic mechanism of critical global fiction': 'Once [Changez] sees the house not as an isolated entity but as conditioned by his family's history, it becomes more difficult to disdain or ignore it; it becomes intimate and recognizable as a site of precarious life' (2014: 114f.). Changez does not merely remove himself from the USA in a geographical sense but, more importantly, aims to reclaim a Pakistani perspective on the world, albeit a perspective informed by his encounter with other localities.

The small range of social roles available to Changez, both in the USA and back in Pakistan, suggests that his potential for subversive performative self-stylisation is meagre. In the USA, Changez's only choice is between sticking to the role assigned to him and rejecting it, thereby forfeiting social recognition, his job, and his right to stay in the country. When he returns to Pakistan, he becomes a university lecturer, teaching his students his 'ex-janissary's skills' (Hamid 2007: 181) and encouraging them to engage in campaigns and demonstrations demanding greater independence from the USA. As Gunning has pointed out, Changez's return to Pakistan

> is partly a nationalist redress to the global capitalist narratives he now identifies as so harmful, but the community he finds is not the traditional national body [...] but a coming together of people in reaction to the spread and callousness of American global power.
>
> (2013: 125)

Nevertheless, as Changez campaigns against US-American foreign policy, his public appearance continues to resonate within an Americentric frame of reference. He is a self-professed 'radical' delivering anti-American soundbites for international television, a mentor for a rising generation of 'fundamentalists' and thus, ultimately, has a media image that is used to heighten global paranoia and deepen the divide between his part of the world and the 'West'.

While, superficially, Amir's position in *Disgraced* appears both less precarious and less politically charged than that of Changez, his path of emotional dissociation is arguably even more painful. Amir's US-American self-conception at the beginning of the play is based not merely on his life, a second-generation migrant's version of the American dream, but on having cut his ties with what he considers the shameful Muslim heritage that governed his childhood. To Amir, it is a matter of intelligence and human progress to dissociate himself from the religion of his upbringing. However, in the aftermath of 9/11, it becomes clear that ties of religious membership cannot be chosen as freely as Amir would like to pretend. Amir experiences similar instances of mistrust and discrimination as Changez, but for him there is no home country to return to and no alternative community to claim membership of. The cultural and religious membership assigned to him is, tragically, one he has spent his adult life pathologising. The play's eruptive climax demonstrates the disorientation and psychological pain caused by Amir's predicament of being cast out of one culture while having learnt to hate the other. The man who seemed to have everything has become a man without a cultural home, with an identity painfully defined only by negatives. The play makes it patently clear that even for the most privileged second-generation Pakistani-American, there is no comfortable post-ethnic cosmopolitan space to inhabit, 9/11 having shattered the illusion that such a magical place might be more than a temporary delusion.

Of course, Amir's US-American identity may have always been more contested than his list of achievements implies. Everyday racism and his struggle not to be typecast as 'the Muslim attorney' serve as reminders of his inoutsider status. His wife's religious-themed art continuously forces Amir to reassert his position between a discarded Muslim past and his all-American success story. His absolute repudiation of Islam appears to be a defence mechanism and this poses the question of how he could have married a woman so invested in the tradition of Islamic art. The portrait that Emily paints of Amir, inspired by Diego Velázquez's painting of his slave assistant, Juan de Pareja, symbolises the ambivalent position that Amir occupies within US-American society and simultaneously appears to mirror his unacknowledged sense of uprootedness.

Interestingly enough, Pakistan is never invoked as a place Amir might turn to. In *Disgraced*, the country hardly features as a specific place at all. To Amir, it is merely the physical centre of a heritage he does not want to be associated with. In a bid to distance himself, he has even taken an Indian-sounding surname and pretended that his parents are Indian early in his career (Akhtar 2012: 22). Mirroring Amir's reluctance to disclose his Pakistani background, the play does not make mention of it until the moment his family's origin is unveiled at work. What is only alluded to through the debates on Islam at the beginning of the play is spelled out after 9/11, when Amir's US-American identity appears to be rescinded and the labels 'Muslim' and 'Pakistani' are assigned to him instead.

What Amir suffers from is the loss of a coherent self. His personality, convictions, and views are suited to a life that has been taken from him and do not match the new role he is cast in. In contrast to this, coherence between his identity and his cultural background is precisely what Changez appears to acquire in *The Reluctant Fundamentalist*. The novel leaves open whether this coherence culminates in the misguided absolutes of a fundamentalist world view. It is interesting to note that Changez's return to his cultural roots and traditional Pakistani values is mirrored by one of the minor characters in Akhtar's play. Amir's nephew, Abe, is Pakistani by birth, yet his appearance at the beginning of the play is described as 'as American as American gets' (Akhtar 2012: 11). In order to make things easier for himself in the USA he takes on the name 'Abe Jensen', but in contrast to Amir he still feels connected to his religious and cultural roots. Dressing in Western attire and choosing a Western name turns out to be little more than pragmatic play-acting, an inoutsider's performance that does not affect the core of Abe's identity. The events of 9/11 see him turning back to the culture he was raised in, and like Changez's, his story becomes a tale of post-9/11 dissociation from his US-American life. As he grows increasingly critical of the USA's position in the world, his assessment is remarkably similar to that of Changez. Abe's final conversation with his uncle demonstrates the philosophical gulf that divides them: when Amir maintains that the truth behind the US involvement in Afghanistan is 'a little more complicated' than Abe allows, Abe interrupts him, stating very simply and decisively: 'Actually, it's not, Uncle. Not really' (Akhtar 2012: 47).

My comparison of the characters of Changez, Amir, and Abe unveils an opposition between the processes of post-9/11 dissociation as experienced by the Pakistani migrant characters Changez and Abe and the second-generation Pakistani-American Amir. Changez's and Amir's lives in the US may be quite similar at the beginning, and all three men encounter the same attitude of racist distrust in the aftermath of 9/11, but it is Amir, American by birth, who ends up the most desperate and lost. He can no longer pretend to be simply 'an American', and he cannot take refuge in a Pakistani identity either, so the experience of being uprooted triggers the play's violent climax. Of course, the comforting absolutes of Changez's perspective may also be less than reliable. As I will show in the remaining pages of this article, both texts employ strategies of narrative ambivalence to deliver an unsettling portrayal of identity construction in the world after 9/11.

Narrating and debating culture, identity, and religion

A lot of the scholarly writing that deals with *The Reluctant Fundamentalist* focuses on the novel's first-person narrator and the ambivalence stemming from unreliable narration. This makes sense, as much of the novel's effect depends on its unusual narrative situation. Changez's recounting of his own story is delivered as a kind of dramatic monologue that implicates the listener – both a US-American in the novel and, by extension, the reader – but is restricted to Changez's part in the conversation. This narrative mode echoes the narrative voice of Jean-Baptiste Clamence in Albert Camus' *The Fall*, an intertextual reference that reinforces any reservations the reader may have about the reliability of Changez's narration. Of course, the fact that the narrator is unreliable does not necessarily imply that all of his statements and assessments are incorrect. Heidemann has suggested that Hamid's use of dramatic monologue 'serves as both a tactical and an ethical gesture towards a certain contrapuntal imagination in the face of post-9/11 partisanism' (2013: 158f.). The silencing of the American in the text allows a Pakistani perspective to take centre stage. At the same time, Changez's description of his response to, for instance, TV images of the US bombing of Afghanistan may well resonate with readers around the world. Thus, Changez's narration works to create fleeting moments of critical alliance, regardless of what we feel about Changez in the end.

Another textual feature that stands out is the lengthy description of Lahore's urban geography and Pakistani cultural history that Changez inserts into his narration. Peter Morey has persuasively argued that these passages do not merely serve the purpose of educating a Western readership, they also establish Pakistan as a tangible place rather than 'a strategic problem to be solved and a threat to [the West's] regional and international interests' (2011: 141). While Hamid's text clearly foregrounds such narrative manoeuvres, it may seem counterintuitive to consider the narrative strategies at play in *Disgraced*. However, a number of scholars have made a strong case for a narratological approach to dramatic text. As Ansgar Nünning and Roy Sommer have pointed out, 'plays do not only represent series of events, they also represent "acts of narration", with characters serving as intradiegetic storytellers' (2008: 337). This is particularly true for a play like *Disgraced*, which – in the tradition of Edward Albee's *Who's Afraid of Virginia Woolf?* – revolves around an emotionally charged dinner conversation. The play never moves beyond the spatial confines of Amir and Emily's apartment. Therefore, all the parts of the action that take place elsewhere need to be delivered by way of intradiegetic narration. This includes, for instance, the racist incidents experienced by several characters and the narrative act serves to highlight the subjectivity of perception. However, as is so often the case, the play's narrativity is also determined by the things that are left out. The past that haunts the whole play and appears to metaphorically and literally 'force the protagonist's hand' is crucially left off-stage. Amir's childhood in a migrant Pakistani community is a cipher. The only concrete account we are given is Amir's story about his infatuation with a Jewish girl and the way his mother made him turn on her (Akhtar 2012: 12f.). Amir introduces the story as paradigmatic of his relationship with Islam and – by extension and more problematically – of the nature of Islam.

In a subversion of dinner-party etiquette, large parts of the play's conversations are exchanges on Islam and its cultural politics. However, the play does not merely present opposing views but unveils many of the opinions expressed as acts of narrating identity.[2] At the same time, the conversational setup characterises the dramatic self-narration as essentially unreliable. In each of the conversations, potential truths about the self and the world compete with ulterior motives, social codes, emotional subtexts, personal adversity, vanity, and conversational competitiveness. Is it even possible to imagine a setup more detrimental to truth-speaking than an emotionally charged conversation at a dinner party? Isaac, one of the dinner guests, counters Amir's condemnation of Islam with commonplaces like 'Islam is rich and universal. Part of a spiritual and artistic heritage we can all draw from' (Akhtar 2012: 29). On the surface, Isaac appears to represent the jovial acceptance and liberal-mindedness of left-wing cosmopolitanism. Yet Amir's responses to Isaac's statements demonstrate how personal histories inform one's view of the world and that there is no superior standpoint from which to evaluate and speak objectively. In describing the ideological dynamic underlying Islam, Amir makes a persuasive intellectual argument, but we may doubt that the conclusions he draws from it are correct. The play deconstructs cosy left-wing wisdom, but then proceeds to discredit the ostensible truth-speaker.

The sense of uncertainty with which both *The Reluctant Fundamentalist* and *Disgraced* leave us is exemplified by the texts' endings. Both are intensely uncomfortable and destabilise our reading while holding up a mirror to the presuppositions and stereotypical notions that we may have brought to the text. In his lucid remarks on *The Reluctant Fundamentalist*, Tabish Khair argues that the novel 'works by way of revealing the gaps in the supposedly solid terrain of our beliefs and opinions, the silence in media speech on all sides. Aporia is essential to its purpose' (2011: 55). While the novel's ending has often been discussed as a question of 'either – or', it is also possible that Changez and his American listener are innocent (and/or guilty) in equal measure. The way we engage with the text's ending is informed by the way we perceive the world, and if we suspect sinister motives in what may be nothing but a conversation, we may well be, as Khair suggests, the 'reluctant fundamentalist' of the novel's title (2011: 55).

In similar fashion, Amir hitting his wife Emily at the end of *Disgraced* complicates our relationship with the play's cultural subtext. The text does not allow us to write off the incident as an isolated lapse. Echoing the voice of an omniscient narrator-director, the stage instructions tell us that Amir hits Emily repeatedly: 'In rapid succession. Uncontrolled violence as brutal as it needs to be in order to convey the discharge of a lifetime of discreetly building resentment' (Akhtar 2012: 45). Neither of the texts offers solid ground. There is no position that is purely right, no superior way of perceiving a world to withdraw to, and both withhold the presence of an omniscient narrator who might help us evaluate the protagonists' struggles. In an article on American prose writing after 9/11, Richard Gray criticised the way authors had taken to 'domesticating' the repercussions of 9/11 in their fictional writing:

> 'All life had become public,' that observation made by a central character in [Don DeLillo's novel] *Falling Man*, is not underwritten by the novel in which it occurs, nor in any of these novels. On the contrary, all life here is personal; cataclysmic public events are measured purely and simply in terms of their impact on the emotional entanglements of their protagonists.
>
> (2009: 134)

In response to Gray's poignant criticism of the books in question, I would argue that *The Reluctant Fundamentalist* and *Disgraced* establish connections between the personal, the public, and the global. To borrow from Morey's assessment of *The Reluctant Fundamentalist*, each text 'represents a sly intervention that destabilizes the dominant categories' of post-9/11 fiction by 'undercutting the impulse to national normalization' (2011: 136). Their enquiries into the repercussions of 9/11 also go beyond representing an outsider's perspective. Even while their protagonists appear to be typecast as 'the other side' in a clash of cultures and religions, both texts rely on complicated narrative strategies to delineate their protagonists' inoutsider positions in the USA, as well as in relation to Pakistan and within the globalised world.

While the terrorist attacks were clearly a shocking and extraordinary event, it may by now have become clear that for many US-Americans, even in New York City, they were probably less life-changing than was initially felt. My point is not that 9/11 was an insignificant event but that much of the debate after the attacks and many of the literary works that followed did not engage with the locations where the most drastic changes have taken place in the meantime, or with the people most inescapably affected. The repercussions for both global Islam and countries like Pakistan have certainly been immense, and fictional texts such as Hamid's and Akhtar's help us to understand what this might entail for the life of the individual, even on US-American soil. Darda has persuasively argued that *The Reluctant Fundamentalist* 'casts the United States and Pakistan in a global network of cultural […] interconnectedness' (2014: 118). It is only logical that Changez's return to Pakistan cannot be a return to his pre-American self. His 'fundamentalist' views are informed by his inoutsider perspective on the US, and his narration ultimately constitutes one side of a conversation with the world at large. For him, as much as for Amir and the reader, it would be perilous *not* to understand that, more than ever, the life of the individual is situated within and determined by complicated networks of interconnected ideas, agendas, and histories.

Notes

1. For an application of Butler's theory to the context of national and cultural identity, see my previous work on the topic (Perner 2011: 56ff.).
2. Akhtar's 'Note to Directors' in *Disgraced* reconfirms that conversation in the play is not meant to be read as opinion-based debating. It emphasises that the actors should not resort to 'playing the "ideas"' (Akhtar 2012: 6) contained in the play but should focus on the relationships portrayed instead.

Bibliography

Akhtar, A. (2012). *Disgraced*. New York: Dramatists Play Service.
Darda, J. (2014). 'Precarious World: Rethinking Global Fiction in Mohsin Hamid's *The Reluctant Fundamentalist*'. *Mosaic: An Interdisciplinary Critical Journal* 47, 107–122.
Gray, R. (2009) 'Open Doors, Closed Minds: American Prose Writing at a Time of Crisis'. *American Literary History* 21, 128–148.
Gunning, D. (2013) *Postcolonial Literature*. Edinburgh: Edinburgh University Press.
Hamid, M. (2007) *The Reluctant Fundamentalist*. London: Hamish Hamilton.
Heidemann, B. (2013) 'Embodiments of the West: Texture and Textuality of the Symbolic Body in Mohsin Hamid's *The Reluctant Fundamentalist*'. In *From Popular Goethe to Global Pop: The Idea of the West between Memory and (Dis)Empowerment*. Ed. by Detmers, I. and Heidemann, B. Amsterdam: Rodopi, 147–160.
Khair, T. (2011) 'Literature and the Limits of Language: An Essay on Silences and Gaps'. In *Reading Literature Today: Two Complementary Essays and a Conversation*. Ed. by Khair, T. and Doubinsky, S. New Delhi: Sage, 1–75.
Morey, P. (2011) 'The Rules of the Game Have Changed: Mohsin Hamid's *The Reluctant Fundamentalist* and Post-9/11 Fiction'. *Journal of Postcolonial Writing* 47, 135–146.

Nnaemeka, O. (1995) 'Feminism, Rebellious Women, and Cultural Boundaries: Rereading Flora Nwapa and her Compatriots'. *Research in African Literatures* 26, 80–113.

Nünning, A. and Sommer, R. (2008) 'Diegetic and Mimetic Narrativity: Some Further Steps Towards a Narratology of Drama'. In *Theorizing Narrativity*. Ed. Pier, J. and García Landa, J.A. New York: Walter de Gruyter, 331–354.

Perner, C. (2011) US-American Inoutside Perspectives in Globalized Anglophone Literatures. Unpublished PhD thesis. Available from <https://duepublico.uni-duisburg-essen.de/servlets/DerivateServlet/Derivate-33509/Claudia_Perner.pdf> [15 January 2018].

Singh, J.G. and Kim, D.D. (2017) *The Postcolonial World*. London: Routledge.

Solomon, D. (2007) '"The Stranger", Interview with Mohsin Hamid'. *New York Times* [online]. Available from <www.nytimes.com/2007/04/15/magazine/15wwlnQ4.t.html> [15 January 2018].

Yaqin, A. (2008) 'An Interview with Mohsin Hamid'. *Moving Worlds* 8, 111–119.

Zaidi, S.M.A. (2013) 'Factors of Anti-Americanism in Middle East and Pakistan'. *Conflict and Peace Studies: A PIPS Research Journal* 5, 51–68.

6

THE NUCLEAR NOVEL IN PAKISTAN

Michaela M. Henry

In an interview with the Booker Prize Foundation, Mohsin Hamid described his then latest novel, *The Reluctant Fundamentalist* (2007b), as reflecting back to its readers the political-emotional landscape in which they already find themselves. The interview quotes Hamid describing his novel: 'Many people have said it feels like a thriller. The reason for that is we are already afraid' (2007a: n.p.). This reflective process is especially fitting for *The Reluctant Fundamentalist* because the novel is written in the second person, addressing a disembodied 'you', allowing that pronoun to easily act as placeholder for a variety of readers. As the decade since 2007 has progressed, what remains clear is that culture continues to exist within Hamid's terms of, 'we are already afraid' (2007a: n.p.). For Hamid this is a statement of fact (though, importantly, the 'facts' used to support those fears are just as often closer to fiction), and yet he also comes to see his role as a novelist as not just reflecting that fear back to his readers but also as audaciously imagining hopeful futures – both for his home country of Pakistan and for the world. He articulates this mission in a 2016 *New Yorker* interview, stating that 'part of the great political crisis we face in the world today is a failure to imagine plausible desirable futures. We are surrounded by nostalgic visions, violently nostalgic visions. Fiction can imagine differently' (Leyshon 2016: n.p.).

This contentious mixture of pride, audacious hope, and fear, present over the course of Hamid's oeuvre, can also characterise Pakistan's relationship to nuclear weapons. Publicly crossing the nuclear threshold in 1998 – the only Muslim-majority country to successfully do so – elicited an amalgam of fear and pride in Pakistan. It brought fear of India, as the stronger military neighbour on the other side of the border, fear of the United States marching over Pakistan to serve its own needs – Ayesha Jalal remarks that 'the growing American presence in Afghanistan is a matter of great concern, as it is generally believed to be a prelude to a thrust into Pakistan and depriving it of its nuclear arsenal' (2011: 19) – or the inverse fear that the United States and US-backed institutions would march their aid money out of Pakistan. But nuclearisation also elicited pride in the technological achievement of producing the bomb, in the anticipated political clout of earning membership to 'the nuclear club', in the bomb buttressing the country's posture of self-defence, and perhaps in the satisfaction of a postcolonial coming of age for the nation.

The heterogeneous and ambivalent reactions to Pakistan's political complexity in general, and its nuclear weapons programme specifically, are ripe for literary response. As stated above,

Hamid puts great faith in literature's potential to imagine hopeful, liveable futures, and yet his nuclear novel, *Moth Smoke* (also his first novel) is perhaps his most cynical. In general, literary reactions to the bomb are various. They include terror, cynicism, and resignation, as well as pride, satisfaction, and flights of speculative imaginings. Accordingly, the presence of nuclear weapons presents a mass of potential literary material alongside a great literary challenge. On the one hand, the bomb as literary figure is capacious and generative. It provides powerful material for metaphor, imagery, and allegory, and it demands that tough ethical questions be asked. On the other hand, the bomb as a concept challenges textual representation because it pushes at the boundaries of the human ability to know. For example, access to actual nuclear weapons eludes all but a select group of people, and for all but a few significant exceptions, nuclear detonation exists as a threat, rather than a direct experience. This is all the more true since international treaties now demand that nuclear weapons testing only be conducted underground. When detonation does occur, though its effects are of course catastrophically explosive, the actual mechanism of the bomb operates beyond the reach of human senses, as Gabriel Hecht reminds us, splitting the 'most basic building blocks' of matter (2006: 321).

Therefore, the bomb ruptures the foundation of material existence at the scale of the infinitesimal to produce an explosion on the scale of the enormous, leaving behind residual effects that persist far beyond the duration of individual human lifetimes. The bomb pushes at the extremes of the human sensorium, the extremes of our ability to perceive and to know. This is complicated even more by the fact that after 1945, detonation has not occurred as an act of war. Instead, the general consensus internationally is that nuclear weapons are not tactical military weapons but rather political weapons, not intended for material use.[1] For most humans on this planet, both those who have direct access to nuclear weapons and most people who hopefully will never experience them first-hand, the bomb exists not as a material reality but rather as a figure in the realm of rhetoric, fantasy, and affect.

The nuclear bomb in its expansive capacity, materialises in a variety of ways in twenty-first-century Pakistani novels in English. As in most places in the world, it most frequently materialises in the novel as it does in life – as a lurking presence, generally in the background, occasionally making its way to the foreground in the form of threat. This chapter will consider a selection of novels from Pakistan and its diasporic writers that deal with nuclear weapons. These include two works of literary fiction, Hamid's *Moth Smoke* (2000) and Kamila Shamsie's *Burnt Shadows* (2009), and two more recent thrillers: Akbar Agha's *Juggernaut* (2015) and Munir Muhammad's *India Pakistan Nuclear War* (2016). Addressing the issue of nuclear weapons seems to cause writers of literary fiction, such as Hamid and Shamsie, to abandon, at least temporarily, their projects of imagining hopeful futures, other incarnations of the present world, or, as Shamsie says in a *New York Times Latitude* blogpost, to 'tell another story of Pakistan'. Instead, the bomb leads to the explorations of fairy tales, allegory, and other fictions we tell ourselves, individually and collectively, to process the 'unthinkability' of nuclear weapons. A nuclear novel of literary fiction seems to concern itself with finding ways to describe what exists in the world now, looking at that reality with a kind of blinking disbelief. Perhaps ironically, nuclear thrillers, on the other hand, are much more capable of indulging in audacious imagining, as their generic form allows them to put the greatest fears of the nuclear age into reality on the pages of the novel and then conjure up a hero to save the day.

Capaciousness of the nuclear question

The anglophone nuclear novel in Pakistan, in its various forms, demonstrates that the nuclear question in Pakistan always contains so many other concerns: Partition and the subsequent wars with India (often seen as unfinished business), growing fundamentalism, fears of so-called 'nuclear *jihadis*' hiding within military ranks, the US presence (ranging from intervention to malicious meddling), Kashmir, Kargil, Zia and the Bhuttos, and even 9/11. This phenomenon, on the one hand, speaks to Pakistan's historical and political realities. As Maleeha Lodhi argues in her introductory essay to *Beyond the Crisis State*, 'the external and internal have been so intertwined in Pakistan's history – as they are today – as to compound political challenges' (2011: 46). And nuclear weapons bring about unique transnational entanglements on top of the already intertwined 'external and internal' concerns within Pakistan. In addition to reflecting political realities, this level of entanglement is also consistent with the capaciousness of the bomb as a rhetorical figure and literary device.[2]

Part of the rhetorical power of the bomb, as Hecht reminds us, is that it is always singular. Hecht, drawing on Itty Abraham, calls the bomb 'the ultimate fetish object of our time' (2006: 100). She defines this singularity as enabling the capaciousness of the bomb as metonym, able to contain 'it all':

> Salvation and apocalypse, sacred and profane, sex and death: the bomb contains it all. World order has been imagined and challenged in its name and for its sake. Although well over twenty-eight thousand nuclear warheads populate the planet, they somehow maintain their singularity. It's always 'the' bomb.
>
> (Hecht 2007: 100)

'The bomb' as an image, in its enormous yet flexible scale, in its singularity and elusiveness, possesses the power to shape narrative, even when (or perhaps especially when) no individual or actual bomb is detonated. Hecht writes of 'nuclearity' as a capacious concept that 'depends on history and geography, science and technology, bodies and politics, radiation and race, states and capitalism. It is not so much an essential property of things, as it is distributed *in* things' (2007: 100). The bomb's lurking potentiality, its scale that exceeds the human sensorium on macro and micro levels, has hero-making and hero-defaming capabilities in literature as in life.

Each of the nuclear novels referenced in this chapter see the nuclear question as 'distributed' across – and inseparable from – a variety of the categories named above. For example, literary and genre fiction alike contextualise their nuclear plots in terms of corruption at home in Pakistan. And each novel contextualises that corruption in terms of corruption at the highest levels of the world's most respected institutions. They thereby make the argument that Pakistan is more alike the other nations in the world than aberrant, countering the perception that the nation is an abject outsider, merely a failed state. For example, Hamid's protagonist in *Moth Smoke*, Daru, uses examples of corruption in Pakistan and around the world to justify the increasingly volatile and self-serving nature of his own actions. He insists that he finally refuses to serve, saying, 'I'm ready to take' (2000: 247). *Moth Smoke* does not valorise Daru for turning to drugs and robbery, nor does it absolve him of his selfishness, but it does have empathy for him and his exhaustion. Moreover, the novel's narration places him directly in the company of the Nobel and the Rhodes families, responsible for money laundering and horrific colonial violence but now known for financing the worlds' most prestigious prizes for research, arts, and world peace in the case of the Nobels, and one of the world's most prestigious scholarship institutions in the case of the Rhodes. According to Hamid and his compatriot nuclear novelists, Pakistan is a part of a complex economy of global wrongdoing, but like Daru, it lacks the cash and the clout to launder its image in the way more affluent people and countries can. *Moth Smoke* does not absolve its characters involved in their different levels of corruption but places them in terms of history and current events on a global scale.

Nuclear armament in Pakistan

The nuclear novel in Pakistan, much like the nation itself, can be characterised by syntactical relations – accidents of geography and temporality, consequences of living in 'the neighbourhood' (Hamid 2000: 129) where it is caught between India, China, and Afghanistan, and swimming in a history of unresolved conflicts. As a consequence, from its birth in independence movements, the anglophone Pakistani novel has always been already transnational or, as Lodhi says, 'intertwined'. Pakistan's birth as an independent nation occurred simultaneously with India's, and its nuclearisation (at least in public form) was twinned with India's too. On its other border, Pakistani writers figure their nation as being penetrated by US forces, overt and covert, and, similarly to the India case, this is a consequence of geographic proximity, this time to Afghanistan.

The anglophone novel holds a complicated position in Pakistan – as the novel form does throughout the postcolony, since its form and language are inherited from colonising cultures. Earlier twentieth-century writers of the subcontinent, some of whom would become Pakistani and some Indian,[3] chose the novel form as one expansive enough to contain the social and psychological complexities of a nation in the process of becoming. Others chose the novel, especially in English, as a way of communicating to the rest of the English-speaking world, especially in the West, the capacity of India/Pakistan to produce the art form most associated with becoming, thereby making a case for the justice of independence. In its variety of forms, the anglophone novel in what would become Pakistan largely came to be as a part of Indian/Pakistani independence movements.

In India and Pakistan alike, the novel in English became a way to think through the development of the new nation, with a full range of emotions, from hope to discontent and disillusionment. Although this historical inheritance remains in twenty-first-century texts, enough time has passed to dull its determining weight over new novels being written. This brings about the question of how to think the new novel and of what a novelist writes when she writes of Pakistan now. Nuclear novels, because of their relationship to actual nuclear weapons' capabilities of the state, coupled with the metaphoric capacity of the image of the bomb, offer one of several answers to these questions.

Fifty-one years after their twinned independence and the violence of Partition, India and Pakistan each crossed the threshold of nuclear armament – India's test on 11 May 1998 was quickly followed by Pakistan on 28 May 1998. Prime Minister Nawaz Sharif was quoted at the time of the Pakistani tests as saying that 'Today, we have evened the score with India' (Burns 1998: n.p.). With such a statement, Sharif claimed the need to avenge historical inequities and restore national pride, because of both the recent nuclear test and the list of ways in which Pakistan figures itself as having been unevenly treated. For example, Akbar Ahmed describes Jinnah's plan for Pakistan as an independent Muslim state as a seemingly impossible achievement, but one aimed at 'restoring Muslim pride' (2011: 20). And yet this achievement at the time of independence was already, by Jinnah's own words, 'truncated' and 'moth-eaten' (Ahmed 2011: 20). By 1971, with the war with India and the creation of Bangladesh, Pakistan's territory was further eroded to the point of existential fear. Many saw the bomb as a long-awaited assertion that Pakistan could not be pushed around.

Declarations of 'We are a nuclear power' were proudly made by government and civilians alike. Meanwhile, the Pakistani government simultaneously declared a state of emergency, fearing military confrontation with India. The *New York Times* quoted then US President Bill Clinton as saying:

> I cannot believe [...] that we are about to start the twenty-first century by having the Indian subcontinent repeat the worst mistakes of the twentieth century, when we know it is not necessary to peace, to security, to prosperity, to national greatness, or to personal fulfilment.
>
> (Burns 1998: n.p.)

Clinton's words highlight a few significant details of the 1998 South Asian arms race: the degree to which India's and Pakistan's nuclear tests were out of sync with the general trends of the world's most powerful nations, and the way in which the actions and fate of Pakistan and India continued to be linked both in the realm of concrete actions being taken and in the international rhetoric and imaginary.

Even more significantly, when Clinton listed all the things that the bomb 'is not necessary for', he in fact highlighted all the hopes with which the bomb was and is imbued. Clinton stated that it was a mistake of the twentieth century to think that possessing nuclear capability would lead to 'peace' and 'security', even though this was the primary stated motivation behind the United States' decisions to continue to pursue a nuclear programme after the end of the Second World War. By stating the characteristics of the bomb in the negative, Clinton paradoxically identified the still strongly held beliefs that nuclear weapons would lead to things like 'prosperity', 'national greatness', and 'personal fulfilment'. Sharif, among others, characterised the tests 'as a national rite of passage', as inevitable as a God-given 'opportunity to take critical steps for the country's defence' (Burns 1998: n.p.). As an act of justification, he connected the 1998 tests to what he saw as India's expansionist tendencies, claiming that India had started each of the three wars between the two nations and therefore positioning Pakistan's bomb as merely an assertion of self-respect and self-defence. As the *New York Times* reported, an Agence France-Presse report quoted a Pakistani student claiming that the bomb was a worthwhile sacrifice that would allow Pakistan 'to live as a self-respecting nation' (Burns 1998: n.p.).

Addressing the fairy tale of American exceptionalism

In 1998, the bomb was characterised as a material-martial manifestation of national self-esteem. It was characterised as a national coming of age, both keeping pace with India and demanding a seat at the international 'adult's table'. Pakistan figured its public nuclear weaponisation as a taking of power, justified by its perception of Indian aggression and demonstrated in the material form of the test. And yet, as Clinton's comments show, the international community's collective narrative of national power and development by 1998, just prior to the turn of the twenty-first century, had moved on from this understanding of nuclear weapons as something that commanded respect. Insisting on nuclear armament was not seen on the international stage as an assertion of self-respect, one which the rest of the world could not help but follow. Instead, it was seen as a perversion of the hoped-for narrative of national becoming. Clinton clearly characterised Pakistan's nuclearisation as a sort of temper tantrum worthy of sanctions (which had also been applied to India following their nuclear tests) that repeated mistakes long recognised as such by Western powers. Such a statement is at least in part rooted in American exceptionalist beliefs that nuclear weapons are most safe in the hands of the American government and least safe in the hands of anyone else.

Pakistani nuclear fiction written in English harnesses such American historical short-sightedness, not to absolve Pakistan from the violence of nuclear armament, or its own corruption, but to place those actions without a broader international view. Novels like Shamsie's *Burnt Shadows* (as well as the more recent thrillers, *Juggernaut* from 2015 and *India Pakistan Nuclear War* from 2016) insist that Pakistan's difficult intimacy with the US is inextricable from the nation's nuclear story. *Burnt Shadows*, for example, examines the way in which the US figures itself as purveyor and protector of justice and peace in the world, stating that American affect works to obscure (to the world and especially to the American people) American acts of violence. Shamsie insists that kindness, familial affinity, and interpersonal intimacy, in the last instance, generally do not prevent violence. Rather, American self-narratives – both individual and collective – of their own righteousness and benign desire to help are extremely effective in justifying violent exercises of power, whether that be the dropping of atomic bombs on Hiroshima and Nagasaki in 1945 or detaining masses of people without sufficient evidence or due process during the post-9/11 securitisation and the ongoing 'war on terror'. The power of such narratives lies in their inability to acknowledge the partiality of the individual's or the group's perspective and the prejudices therein.

Jack Zipes' language of fairy tale's political dimension helps frame these narrative practices of US exceptionalism. In *Fairy Tales and the Art of Subversion*, Zipes focuses on the utopic potential of fairy tales, but he helpfully identifies the use value of the fairy tale form to being in the world and shaping the world to suit one's needs. Zipes writes that 'Fairy tales are predicated on a human disposition to social action – to transform the world and make it more adaptable to human needs while we try to change and make ourselves fit for the world' (1999: ix). As I will show below, Shamsie's engagement with nuclear war in *Burnt Shadows*, in actuality (Nagasaki in 1945) and threat (Pakistan in 2001–2002), demonstrates the use of fairy tale's storytelling mechanisms towards any kind of 'social action' that suits the personal-political needs of the storyteller. This, according to Shamsie, can serve a variety of needs, from processing memories of nuclear detonation towards personal healing, to justifying callous acts in the name of American security. For Zipes, fairy tales' 'disposition to social action' is located in 'their focus […] on the struggle to find magical instruments, extraordinary technologies, or helpful people and animals that will enable protagonists to transform themselves and their environment and make the world more suitable for living in peace and contentment. (1999: ix–x). Shamsie offers a variety of scenes where fairy tales are read or told, and she also shows how the mechanism of fairy tales towards 'magical instruments' or magical mechanism of simplification can be used in real life to commit acts of violence regardless of good or ill will. The protagonist of *Burnt Shadows*, Hiroko Tanaka-Ashraf, is a survivor of the nuclear bomb in Nagasaki who finds herself in Delhi in 1946 and in Karachi from 1947 to 2001, when she moves to New York, running away from the threat of nuclear war on the subcontinent. In her past, she had invented fairy tales to explain to her son what it had been like living through the nuclear explosion in Nagasaki and its aftermath. Her husband had used the story of the Prophet Muhammad being protected by the spider as an allegory to explain the unlikely but mutually protective friendship between their family, the Tanaka-Ashrafs, and another transnational family with whom their lives were intertwined, the German-British-American Weiss-Burtons. However, Hiroko's final scenes demonstrate the insidious possibilities of fairy tale's 'disposition to social action' seen through the lens of the form's narrative practice of using magical mechanisms of simplification.

In the case of American action in the larger world, Hiroko names this practice the deployment of 'the big picture'. Upon hearing of her son Raza's detainment under vague suspicion of terrorism, Hiroko identifies a common American practice, repeated often, from the bombing of Nagasaki to the indiscriminate detention or murder of Afghans after 9/11. According to Hiroko, this practice does not, for example, disregard or erase human rights of its target populations (or any populations caught in the line of fire, for that matter), but merely reduces the focus on individuals in service of 'the big picture'. Shamsie writes:

> Hiroko spoke [...] 'When Konrad first heard of the concentration camps he said you have to deny people their humanity in order to decimate them [...] You just have to put them in a little corner of the big picture. In the big picture of the Second World War, what was seventy-five thousand more Japanese dead? Acceptable, that's what it was. In the big picture of threats to America, what is one Afghan? Expendable. Maybe he's guilty, maybe not. Why risk it? Kim, you are the kindest, most generous woman I know. But right now, because of you, I understand for the first time how nations can applaud when their governments drop a second nuclear bomb.'
>
> (2009: 370)

In these, some her final words in the novel, Hiroko connects and indicts US practices from 1945 to 2001. As she states, the US' strategy of expansive nationalism – zooming out to the big picture – does not need to 'deny the humanity' of those individuals or populations obstructing its chosen mission. It does not need to exterminate a demonised population, nor does it need to expel groups of foreigners publicly and outright. Instead, the US needs only expand the frame of the story it tells of itself, putting undesired elements, human or otherwise, in the corner, out of the way.

This narrative practice of deploying the (at times) hidden nationalist narrative of 'the big picture' secured US military victory and global hegemony at the end of the Second World War and perpetuates US moral dominance into the post-9/11 twenty-first century. *Burnt Shadows* argues for the omnipresence of this narrative practice by demonstrating the inability of personal friendship to overcome it. At the beginning of the novel, at the very end of the Second World War, Hiroko is caught in the invisible and inconsequential corner of the big picture on the impersonal world-historical scale, when the Americans happen to drop the second atomic bomb on Nagasaki, the city of her birth. At the end of the novel, Hiroko is caught in the invisible corner of the big picture on the personal scale when Kim Burton, her roommate and companion, the granddaughter of her nearly life-long closest friend, unwittingly betrays her son, Raza. Hiroko's close proximity to Kim does not allow her to escape to the refuge of the big picture with clear 'good guys' and 'bad guys', just as, over fifty years before, Hiroko's husband Sajjad's proximity to Kim's grandfather, James Burton, did not spare him the violence and heartbreak of Partition, even when it allowed him to escape physical harm.

Shamsie shows the haphazard narrative mechanism that undergirds the US' world-dominating force that wins out over other empires by telling fairy tales about itself to its own people. The novel links the nuclear bomb in 1945 to an unnamed detainee in an identified location that could be any black site, and links CIA involvement in Pakistan and Afghanistan over three decades to the same, by showing the mechanism of shifting narrative scale that produces the fairy tale of its own benevolence that America as a nation and Americans as individuals must repeatedly tell and retell to themselves. The novel identifies American individual friendliness and affability – Americans' willingness to mix with others around the world – as a means of solidifying their dominance, buttressing their illusion of benevolence, an illusion that does not need to fool dominated peoples nearly as much as it must convince Americans themselves in order to be effective. According to *Burnt Shadows*, it is America's (and Americans') belief in its benevolence and its good intentions that makes it most capable of doing harm.

In short, Shamsie's novel puts forth a long view of US neo-imperialism that begins with the bomb being dropped on Nagasaki in 1945 and continues through the US 'war on terror' in the first decade of the twenty-first century. Hiroko shows that regard for others on the individual scale – when pressed – is not a prophylactic against violence, whether individual, structural, or mass. The text ends with Hiroko's resignation, perhaps even despair: 'outside at least, the world went on' (Shamsie 2009: 370). Thus, for Shamsie's protagonist, Pakistan's nuclear weaponisation is just another example of misguided nationalist storytelling that leads to violence. For Shamsie, Pakistan's first nuclear decade cannot be separated from a global history of violence that precedes the nuclear age and exceeds the specifics of nuclear weapons.

Moth Smoke: regionality and allegory

In Hamid's *Moth Smoke*, the bomb features in the background – it is the backdrop to two-thirds of his novel about the deterioration of a protagonist, Daru, once a promising student of development studies (a field emblematic of hope in the possibility of positive change) turned disaffected banker. *Moth Smoke* is most often characterised as a drug novel. However, it also invites us to read the story of its protagonist as an allegory of contemporary Pakistan's coming of age with extraordinary potential. He is dangerously smart and irreverent, but seeks to quickly acquire the spoils of wealth; hating the super-rich party class of Lahore, while coveting their drugs, money, ease of life, and fancy lifestyle.

Interestingly, both *Moth Smoke* and *Juggernaut*, discussed below, feature once-staunchly ethical, idealist academics who forgo those ethics and ideals in favour of corruption and self-interest – blaming the tides of the country and absolving themselves. *Moth Smoke* is in some ways more cynical, positioning such a figure as its young protagonist, while *Juggernaut* positions a similar figure as an older, dim-witted side character who causes problems but is too peripheral to be either sympathetic or truly villainous. Both novels show this figure as dulling his morals and intellects with alcohol, drugs, and sex. Only one, *Juggernaut*, passes judgement on that degeneracy, however. The other, *Moth Smoke*, seems to view it as an unfortunate accident of fate, and some arrogance.

Among other things, Hamid's *Moth Smoke* tracks the various reactions of Lahoris as they learn of Pakistan's nuclear weaponisation in real time in 1998, and the great variety of responses of citizens across class lines, demonstrating the difficulty of pinning down a single literary use of the bomb. In one moment, the novel reduces the bomb to the digestive tract – as something that undergirds everything, but remains untalked about in polite company:

> It was the summer of great rumblings in the belly of the earth, of atomic flatulence and geopolitical indigestion, consequences of the consumption of sectarian chickpeas by our famished and increasingly incontinent subcontinent. Clenched beneath the tightened sphincters of the test sites and silos, the pressure of superheated gasses was registering in spasms on the Richter scale.
>
> (Hamid 2000: 79)

At the same time as it mocks the nuclear test as delivering real power in the world, the novel recognises the bomb's subject-forming power for Pakistan's exhausted or jaded citizens. For example, *Moth Smoke*'s narration exclaims: 'We've done it! [...] We've exploded the bomb', and this spirit affects even the cynical Lahoris, fulfilling some national psychological chasm. Even Daru narrates, 'I feel something straighten my back, a strange excitement, the posture-correcting force of pride' (2000: 148). Clinton's statement above – naming all the things the bomb is not – fails to recognise the subject-creating power of the nuclear bomb as symbolic weapon, while *Moth Smoke* recognises it immediately.

In *Moth Smoke* Pakistan's test leads to morbid speculation by various Lahoris. They worry about India, wondering whether 'they' will 'nuke' Lahore, Karachi, or Islamabad first. This worry is quickly mixed with cockiness and blustering – 'we'll nuke them first' (2000: 124). The tests also evoke a secretive fascination among Lahoris – the sense that they have witnessed something that should be forbidden. The novel shows teenage boys (Daru's nephew and his friend) watching nuclear test videos like they might huddle together and watch pornography (not videos of either the Indian or Pakistani tests because these were conducted below ground, but of earlier above-ground tests on the internet).

At this point in the story, Hamid uses language that emphasises the regionality of Pakistan's nuclear situation: 'the neighborhood's nuclear test count is up to five' (2000: 113). Soon, however, the bomb becomes an all-encompassing image, available to be used for whatever need arises. For example, when Daru is at the police station, he walks by an interrogation room where 'an old man is screaming that an atomic bomb incinerated his wife' (2000: 120). Speculation continues and issues vague, metaphorical material that could be applied multiply, to Daru and other characters, to the country overall, perhaps: 'They say the nuclear tests released no radioactivity into the atmosphere. Each a huge gasp, smothered unsatisfied' (2000: 122–123). In this description, the bomb, like Daru, perhaps like Pakistan, remains in a state of waiting, satisfaction repeatedly denied.

Moth Smoke's title imagery, the remnants of the moth drawn to the flame, resists simple coding into celebration or condemnation. Hamid invites comparison between Pakistan's nuclear quest to his protagonists' descent into self-destruction and violence, and implicitly likens both to the moth obsessively seeking the flame. Hamid all but wonders on the page if the state is on the edge of a passion leading to self-immolation: overcome by fascination and desire, it is the moth drawn to the flame. The moth may escape incineration for a while but eventually will go up in smoke. Hamid describes Daru consumed with watching the moth persist towards its death:

> The moth takes off again [...] A few times he seems to touch the flame, but dances off unhurt [...] Then he ignites like a ball of hair, curling into an oily puff of fumes with a hiss. The candle flame flickers and dims for a moment, then burns as bright as before.
> (2000: 168)

The image of the self-immolating moth certainly references Daru's descent into heroin addiction and growing tolerance of violent acts. By placing this imagery within the backdrop of Pakistan's nuclear tests, Hamid links Daru's decline to the nation's flirtation with a substance that both satisfies a great yearning for self-esteem and a sense of empowerment at the same time as it heightens its risk of self-destruction.

Nuclear thrillers

Recently, in contrast to the ambivalence of Hamid and the outward indictments of Shamsie, a small group of nuclear thrillers have emerged, including Agha Akbar's *Juggernaut* and Munir Muhammad's self-published *India Pakistan Nuclear War*. These novels, more straightforward works of genre fiction, are at once more overtly apocalyptic and more hopeful than their counterparts in literary fiction. They tend to take a more masculine tone, common in the thriller genre, and emphasise the triumph of an everyman (although generally a military everyman) hero over internal threats of corruption and nuclear *jihad*, and external threats of Indian aggression and American interference. Thus, these thrillers present fantasies of an individual everyman – possessing the proper military or political credentials, appropriately masculine, neither over- nor undereducated, etc. – overcoming both American interference (in the case of *Juggernaut*, the protagonist turns the CIA's intimacy with Pakistan into a sexual conquest of a Pakistani soldier over a female CIA agent) and internal corruption to save the country and the world from nuclear disaster.

The plots of both *Juggernaut* and *India-Pakistan Nuclear War* feature the worst fears of people on both the Indian and Pakistani sides – the possibility of 'nuclear *jihadis*' lurking among the ranks of Pakistan's most powerful generals – those who wish to bring about the end of the world because, as Muslims, they will be rewarded in heaven. Rather than simply linking contemporary nuclear events to a global network of historical entanglements and wrongdoings, recent nuclear thrillers imagine specific historical wrongs leading directly to an apocalyptic nuclear crisis: *Juggernaut* builds a story about PTSD (though not in name) and deeply rooted hatred of India and Hindus resulting from imprisonment during the war in 1971; *India-Pakistan Nuclear War* builds on the smouldering resentment of US drone strikes and violations of Pakistani sovereignty to motivate bringing about nuclear war. In both cases, a home-grown hero averts the crisis (either partially or fully), allowing the historic wrong to remain highlighted while simultaneously restoring peace and power to Pakistan.

Juggernaut's army captain protagonist, Gul, after thwarting an assassination attempt on one general, is sent by another to question several others as part of an investigation into a missing and eventually murdered army psychiatrist. Specifically, Gul is sent by a General Shah to question three high-ranking generals who were all forced into the psychiatrist's treatment when they became part of the strategic nuclear response team. Supposedly, it was the psychiatrist's job to root out possible residual issues and treat them to facilitate the greatest possible nuclear safety – ensuring that all future nuclear decisions would be made rationally, rather than emotionally. However, we come to know that General Shah interfered with the treatment, hoping to force the generals to access and exacerbate their anger, fear, and hatred at having been imprisoned and badly treated by India in POW camps, and thus push them over the edge. This, he hopes, *will* incite a subcontinental nuclear war, bringing about the destruction of both countries. Bringing about the end of the world is his goal as it means that Muslims will be ushered into Paradise.

Captain Gul, as the novel's true patriot, is not apocalyptically minded and manages to thwart Shah's plan. In this way, he provides Pakistan with the perfect nuclear-era hero. He embodies the power and self-esteem which the bomb was hoped to bring to the nation, but he has the ethics and savvy to root out the enemies within. In *India Pakistan Nuclear War*, a single bomb is detonated over Mumbai, but not only are a dozen other warheads neutralised, the first detonation causes regional disarmament *and* long-sought peace in Kashmir.

Returning to his 2016 *New Yorker* interview, Hamid writes about his hope for fiction:

> maybe our children and grandchildren can still inhabit a world where they have a chance at hope and optimism. Fiction can explore this possibility, it can make us feel something other than the sense of either doom or denial that is so prevalent in our nonfiction discourse.
>
> (Leyshon 2016: n.p.)

Recent nuclear thrillers seem to do a kind of fictional imagining, offering 'a chance at hope and optimism' but wrapped within existing narratives of the bomb as the embodiment of national self-assertion and self-esteem, narratives questioned long before the nation joined the nuclear club.

It is now nearly twenty years after South Asian nuclearisation. The question of nuclear war remains pressing, perhaps increasingly so, and the appearances of several new nuclear thrillers indicate that the possibility remains compelling, at least in narrative form.[4] Arundhati Roy famously called the twinned Indian and Pakistani nuclearisation 'the end of imagination', claiming that the bomb, as the ever-present threat of total war, is too expansive to allow anyone to think outside of it (1998). Twenty years later, the bomb seems not to have brought about an end of imagination, at least not in the simplest terms. There has been a proliferation of narrative and great exercise of imagination. But perhaps even more dangerously, a tendency has crept up to let the bomb slide into the corner of the big picture. While it remains an ever-lurking threat, its rhetorical nature risks forgetting its enormous materiality – ready at any moment. In 2017, the international nuclear temperature is rising once again, and Pakistani novelists are, as ever, aware of the intertwining of their nation with the outside world.

Notes

1 See Joseph Masco's *The Nuclear Borderlands* (2006) for further reference to nuclear weapons as 'technoaesthetics', rather than material military weapons.
2 I theorise this idea further in my unpublished dissertation, *Narrative's Nuclear Spring: The Anglophone Novel after the Nuclear Bomb* (2017). There, I posit that a subset of anglophone novels in South Asia – those written after the twinned armament of its two largest nations – coalesced around the task of thinking through what the novel is after the region joined the so-called 'nuclear club'. I identify these texts as deploying a nuclear literary method – a collection of trends, rather than hard and fast rules. I argue that the repetition of these trends demonstrates that the novel shifts once 'the bomb' enters the collective imaginary of a nation. In order to make this argument, I draw upon, though not in a straight line, Arundhati Roy's assertion that the bomb led to 'the end of imagination' in South Asia because of its enormity of scale and the Indian and Pakistani governments' linking the bomb to their respective nationalist (and specifically religious-nationalist) narratives.
3 I am referring to certain members of the All India and later All Pakistan Progressive Writer's Associations (AIPWS and APWS), perhaps most famously Ahmed Ali and Mulk Raj Anand, as well as others who never joined the groups or split from them, such as Raja Rao.
4 Other nuclear thrillers include Vikram Chandra's *Sacred Games* (2006), Mainak Dhar's *Line of Control* (2008), and Vivek Ahuja's *Fenix* (2015).

Bibliography

Agha, A. (2015) *Juggernaut*. New Delhi: 4 Hour Books/Tara Press.
Ahmed, A. (2011) 'Why Jinnah Matters'. In *Pakistan Beyond the Crisis State*. Ed. by Lodhi, M. New Delhi: Rupa, 21–34.
Burns, J. (1998) 'Nuclear Anxiety: The Overview; Pakistan, Answering India, Carries out Nuclear Tests; Clinton's Appeal Rejected'. *New York Times* [online]. Available from <www.nytimes.com/1998/05/29/world/nuclear-anxiety-overview-pakistan-answering-india-carries-nuclear-tests-clinton.html?mcubz=1> [12 August 2017].
Derrida, J. (1984) 'No Apocalypse, Not Now (Full Speed Ahead, Seven Missiles, Seven Missives)'. *Diacritics* 14(2), 20–31.
Hamid, M. (2000) *Moth Smoke*. New Delhi: Penguin.
Hamid, M. (2007a) 'Interviews' [online]. Available from <www.mohsinhamid.com/interviews.html> [6 July 2017].
Hamid, M. (2007b) *The Reluctant Fundamentalist*. New Delhi: Penguin.
Hecht, G. (2006) 'Nuclear Ontologies'. *Constellations* 13(3), 320–331.
Hecht, G. (2007) 'A Cosmogram for Nuclear Things'. *Isis* 98(1), 100–108.
Jalal, A. (2011) 'The Past as Present'. In *Pakistan Beyond the Crisis State*. Ed. by Lodhi, M. New Delhi: Rupa, 7–21.

Leyshon, C. (2016) 'This Week in Fiction: Hamid on the Migrants in all of Us'. *The New Yorker* [online]. Available from <www.newyorker.com/books/page-turner/this-week-in-fiction-mohsin-hamid-2016-11-14> [August 2017].

Lodhi, M. (2011) 'Beyond the Crisis State'. In *Pakistan Beyond the Crisis State*. Ed. by Lodhi, M. New Delhi: Rupa, 45–78.

Masco, J. (2006) *The Nuclear Borderlands: The Manhattan Project in Post-Cold War New Mexico*. Princeton: Princeton University Press.

Muhammad, M. (2016) *India Pakistan Nuclear War*. Charleston: CreateSpace.

Roy, A. (1998) 'The End of Imagination'. *Outlook Magazine* [online]. Available from <www.outlookindia.com/magazine/story/the-end-of-imagination/205932> [August 2012].

Shamsie, K. (2009) *Burnt Shadows*. New York: Picador.

Shamsie, K. (2012) 'The Softer Side of Peshawar'. *Latitude, New York Times* [online]. Available from <http://nyti.ms/2f3sQQj> [23 February 2012].

Zipes, J. (1999) *Fairy Tales and the Art of Subversion: The Classical Genre for Children and the Process of Civilization*. New York: Routledge.

7

USES OF HUMOUR IN POST-9/11 PAKISTANI ANGLOPHONE FICTION

H.M. Naqvi's *Home Boy* and Mohammed Hanif's *A Case of Exploding Mangoes*

Ambreen Hai

Humour is perhaps not the first thing most people associate with Pakistani fiction. This chapter will argue, nonetheless, that humour is an essential component, indeed a driving force, for a significant strain of twenty-first-century anglophone fiction produced by a new generation of Pakistani writers, central to the cultural and political work that they undertake, and to the formal aesthetic that structures their writing. Focusing on two novels as examples – H.M. Naqvi's *Home Boy* (2009) and Mohammed Hanif's *A Case of Exploding Mangoes* (2008) – I explore how, in a post-9/11 context of globalised Islamophobia, each deploys various strategies and forms of humour.[1] Humour serves multiple purposes in both novels: to contest the claim that Muslims do not have a sense of humour and to hence establish the humanity denied to Muslims by this logic;[2] to challenge oppressive forms of dominance or state power; to subvert by exposing and rendering absurd certain forms of authority; and, via the pleasure and bonhomie created by humour, to reach a broader audience and suggest persuasive alternatives to binary and prejudiced thinking. Naqvi uses humour to build trust and understanding, and to push back against racist or Islamophobic ideologies and practices in the US; Hanif to satirise and assert a lively resistance to, and refusal to be vanquished by, the deeply oppressive, corrupt nexus of military government and American involvement in Pakistan.

In Europe and America, minority or 'ethnic' comedians have long used humour to defuse tension, to challenge dominant discourses, and to present alternative non-normative viewpoints and frameworks. Since 9/11, Muslim comedians have intensified this cultural work. Sociologist Mucahit Bilici argues that:

> Muslim ethnic comedy [in the US] is a form of code-switching in the face of situations where the language of reason is overtaken by a wrong common sense or a common wrong sense. […] It redefines the common sense […] to disclose the rock

bottom of our identities as 'human', to re-establish the humanity of those 'othered.' [...] [It] is the world of Islamophobia turned upside down.

(2010: 207)

Humour does cultural work in multiple ways, and goes beyond simple reversal or inversion. Ideally, argues Rainer Emig (regarding the British-Asian television sitcom *Goodness Gracious Me*), hybrid humour can create an in-between 'third space' and 'double vision' to expose stereotypes and unsettle 'identities and authorities' in both majority and minority groups (2010: 178, 188).

It is important, however, to distinguish between malign and benign humour, for not all humour does the positive, constructive work of re-establishing humanity or undoing prejudice. Clearly, some negative kinds of humour reaffirm prejudice and social hierarchies: mean-spirited mockery and racist, sexist, or homophobic jokes are well-known examples of such 'punch-down' humour, where laughter asserts superiority over those laughed at. But humour is not always or only malign, though it does always involve some exertion of power. Benign or socially constructive forms of humour can engage in healthy pushback or punch *up*; or, by laughing *with*, not *at*, its target or audience, they can reach out, be inclusive, and create a sense of community or sense of connection even across lines of difference and inequality. Some non-Muslim audience members' responses to US Muslim stand-up comedians attest to these effects: 'You can't hate the person you've laughed with'; 'I didn't see you as a Muslim, I saw you as a human being' (Bilici 2010: 207).

Prominent theories of humour do not always acknowledge both malign and benign kinds of humour, though they can be used to explain both. The superiority theory of humour recognises the relations of power inherent in the act of evoking, and responding with, laughter. From Plato onwards, many thinkers and cultural traditions have regarded humour as derisive, as exerting superiority over others. But humour can be used both to reinforce and to challenge dominance and power. The 'marginal humor [of those in socially disadvantaged positions] may empower the powerless, may invert and subvert the status quo' (Gilbert 2004: xv). The superiority theory can thus also explain benign or socially beneficial humour: those laughing can push back against what threatens them, asserting resistance or refusal of defeat, and thus regain some psychological control over oppressive conditions. Authoritarian regimes often forbid laughter to the disempowered because they recognise it as a challenge to authority.[3] Psychologist Rod Martin notes, 'Humor is inherently neither friendly nor aggressive: it is a means of deriving emotional pleasure that can be used for both amiable and antagonistic purposes. This is the paradox of humor' (2007: 18). Both Naqvi and Hanif use humour for benign purposes, either to assert resistance and push back against wrongful uses of power, or to reach out to more dominant groups to educate and enable better understanding of those who are maligned and disempowered.

Two other influential theories of humour explain different dimensions of humour and its psychological and sociopolitical functions.[4] The relief theory, based on Freudian psychoanalysis, explains humour as a 'cathartic release from repression', a reversion to the 'pleasure principle' that allows escape from 'the reality principle' or 'the psychic cost of civilization' (Bilici 2010: 202). Humour can enable relief from repression in both malign and benign forms; malign humour can enable escape from social censors, allowing the otherwise unsayable to be said, even if it vilifies the weak and buttresses the power of the dominant; benign humour can enable resistance, coping, or healing for those experiencing disempowerment by allowing them to feel less oppressed by what threatens them. Laughing at a problem can reduce it by making it feel less overpowering, and demonstrate to others one's relative control over it. As I will show, this positive psychic effect of humour works for both the characters and the readers of the novels discussed below.

The incongruity theory, proposed by Schopenhauer and others, argues that humour is a surprise reaction to the incongruous or absurd, the result of a cognitive 'conceptual shift' upon discovery of the mismatch between expectation and reality (Morreall 1987: 4). Perhaps humour brings pleasure because it occasions the recognition of something known but suppressed, the uncanny or (un)familiar, the unhomely that brings us home to ourselves. For malign humour, the cognitive shift can occasion reaffirmation of a desire for mastery over those targeted and laughed down, the pleasure of (re)discovery of what one wished for. For benign humour, the incongruity theory offers different benefits. If humour occasions a recognition of something unknown yet known, a discovery of one's own misconceptions, then Bilici's point about Muslim ethnic hybrid humourists becomes highly significant. Because such humourists inhabit two worlds, bridging dominant and minority groups, and can 'code-switch', they can speak the language of the majority, establish belonging in both groups, and translate from the 'othered' group to enable re-education of the dominant group. The 'essence of humor' is 'the simultaneous activation of two contradictory perceptions' or 'bisociation', when 'two self-consistent but normally incompatible or disparate frames of reference', 'both X and not-X', are seen or brought together (Martin 2007: 63). Incongruity theory thus explains how the benign humour of the oppressed can work to speak to the oppressor group(s), to bring about recognition of misconception, to redress misconception, and enable greater understanding and trust across difference. Incongruity theory explains how pushback humour like Naqvi's and Hanif's can be educational: by making explicit the absurdity of certain assumptions, preconceptions, or biases, it can provoke laughter at oneself for holding them, and promote the rethinking of those assumptions. Humour depends on and enables a shift in ways of seeing: 'Applying humor to a situation is like applying lateral thinking – it allows you to see things from a new angle' (Barreca 1991: 126).

Humour in Naqvi's *Home Boy*

Scholars have rightly approached *Home Boy* as a counter-discursive critique of dominant American political and cultural responses to the events of 9/11, an ironic coming-of-age story where growing up involves the shattering of the American dream. Most view its young Pakistani Muslim narrator-protagonist, Chuck, as a casualty of racial profiling and Islamophobia as his early effervescent cosmopolitanism and sense of self declines – after he is detained by the FBI under wrongful suspicion of terrorism – into identity crisis, paranoia, and suicidal depression (see Heidemann 2012). Daily-Bruckner reads the novel as an 'ethnic bildungsroman' that disrupts and revises American literary tradition to present Chuck's rejection of and disaffiliation from America when the 'promise of America' is violated post-9/11 (2016: 223, 219). Roy critiques it for focusing on a culturally hybrid figure 'that may appeal to a white audience' and failing to address broader systemic realities and forms of difference (2011: 14). No critic, however, addresses the novel's multiple uses of humour, perhaps because humour is not understood as doing serious work.

To begin with, Naqvi uses Chuck's colloquial, ebullient humour and first-person voice to establish this narrator-protagonist's engaging, disarming personality and to win the sympathy of potentially suspicious Western readers. Chuck's confidence, cultural conversance, and claim to belonging as a New Yorker, as a Westernised, secular, hybrid cosmopolitan, are established though his voice – peppy, funny, at times crude, and anything but threatening. However goofy or clueless he is, this style suggests, Chuck is not a terrorist (nor a potential one).[5] At age twenty-one, just graduated from NYU, an English major turned investment banker, he has taken to taxi-driving in New York since he was laid off in July 2001, unbeknownst to his widowed mother in Pakistan. Early on, when he introduces his cohort of 'home boy' Pakistani-American friends, Chuck suggests how top-down malign humour is used to stereotype, homogenise, and put down minorities, against which he pushes back:

> Though we shared a common denominator and were told jokingly, *Oh, all you Pakistanis are alike*, we weren't the same, AC, Jimbo, and me. AC – a cryptonym, short in part for Ali Chaudhry – was a charming rogue, an intellectual dandy, a man of theatrical presence. […] Jamshed Khan, known universally as Jimbo, was a different cat altogether, a gentle, moon-faced man-mountain with kinky dreadlocks and a Semitic nose which, according to AC, affirmed anthropological speculation that Pathans are the Lost Tribe of Israel. […] As for me, they called me Chuck and it stuck. I was growing up but thought I was grown up.
>
> (Naqvi 2009: 2–3)

This stylistic mix of knowing, self-ironising, intellectual sophistication, word-play, and jauntiness works to upend binary assumptions, to demonstrate control through mastery of language and humour, and to showcase the diversity and heterogeneity *among* Pakistanis, as well as their affiliations *across* national boundaries to various ethnic formations that have resulted from migrations and cultural exchanges over centuries.[6]

Chuck's feisty humour also exposes and pushes back against common white American misconceptions about South Asians. Soon after 9/11, Chuck and his friends go to a nightclub – they 'were getting cabin fever watching CNN 24-7' and 'there was something heroic in persisting, carrying on, in returning to routine, revelry', he explains – where a white American 'carrying on bombastically' at the bar mistakes them for Indians (2009: 7–8, 9): 'Turning around, the Bombaster asked, "So lemme get this straight: you guys aren't Indian?" "We're too handsome, chum! You can call us Metrostanis! Cheers! Skål! Adab!"' (2009: 14).

Chuck's light, deft comeback is at once funny because it is silly (claiming that Pakistani men are better looking than Indian),[7] clever (coining the portmanteau neologism 'Metrostani' from metropolitan/cosmopolitan Pakistani), and smart as it establishes his multilingualism, witty verbal ability, and intellectual superiority to the American he cornily dubs 'the Bombaster', whose mistaken assumptions and inferior language skills are exposed in his speech.

But Chuck's persona is also self-undercutting, not set up as an infallible ideal. His flippant city boy lingo accompanies a certain naiveté. 'In the four years I had been in the city, in the twenty-one and half years that comprised my life, I fell in love routinely. It went almost entirely unrequited', Chuck reports with bathos (2009: 15). Naqvi's own humour thus subtly invites (gentle) laughter at Chuck's expense, often via verbal play and plot twists. At the same nightclub, Chuck tries to pick up a Venezuelan (whom he dubs 'the girl from Ipanema', referencing the Brazilian international hit song) with whom he instantly imagines a future and shared immigrant American dream – 'if I married her, I too would become a bonafide American. In a sense, we were peas in a pod, she and I, denizens of the Third World turned economic refugees turned scenesters by fate' – until he hears her say, 'Jou haf a nice ass' (2009: 16). Realising he has misheard her accented English – her compliment turns out to be about his *eyes* – Chuck's gratification and notion of Third World solidarity are shattered by his discovery that they literally cannot understand each other, and by her rejection when she finds out that he is from Pakistan. This double-edged humour targets not the Venezuelan's accent, but Chuck's foolish idealism, and the prejudice that he faces; its effect is not to mock Chuck, but to render him endearingly inexperienced, vulnerable, and harmless. It also exemplifies Naqvi's double language, or code-switching, as he uses the knowledge of the dominant group to speak to them about the injustices suffered by the non-dominant.

Naqvi's humour thus goes beyond Chuck's, and works with it to delineate and contest the increasing racism that Chuck and his friends face after 9/11. Right after the episode above, Chuck and his friends go to Jake's, their favourite nightclub and refuge, and have a run-in with two drunken white racists:

> Brawler No. 1 hissed, 'A-*rabs*.'
> Repeating the word in my head, I realized it was the first time I'd heard it spoken that way, like a dagger thrust and turned, the first time anything like this had happened to us at all. [...] 'We're not the same,' Jimbo protested.
> 'Moslems, Mo-hicans, whatever,' Brawler No. 2 snapped.
> 'I'm from Jersey, dude!' [replies Jimbo].
>
> (2009: 30)

Significantly, Naqvi represents the three men of Pakistani origin as non-violent, even placatory in the face of open aggression, and the violent attack on Chuck as initiated by the 'brawlers'. (When they fight back, they get kicked out.) In fact, Jimbo is Pakistani-American, born in New Jersey, AC is the 'only immigrant', and Chuck is Pakistani, on a temporary H-1B 'work visa' (2009: 2, 116). In the humorous play on 'Moslems, Mo-hicans', Naqvi invokes James Fennimore Cooper to link nineteenth century-white supremacy and imperialism to the present day; he thus exposes the American ignorance or prejudice that, despite clarification, does not care about conflating Arabs and Muslims, or Muslims and Native Americans (or American Indians). In so doing, Naqvi strategically separates those he critiques from his potential American readers, whom he seeks to reach and educate. The comic presentation of this episode in Chuck's tongue-in-cheek style contributes to this positive effect. This humour is benign, I would argue, because it is not punching down those already disempowered; instead it pushes back and seeks to communicate and build understanding via the community-building work of sharing laughter *about* misconception (not *at* a stigmatised group).

This use of humour as pushback and relief intensifies as Naqvi highlights the increasing racial suspicion and danger that besets these young men because of their appearance and accents. As Chuck and his friends drive to Connecticut to check on 'the Shaman', a Pakistani friend they have not heard from since before 9/11, they are stopped by police officers who question Chuck for wearing the dark glasses that he is using (ironically) to cover up the bruise he got from the racist 'brawlers'. Suddenly aware that they are '*a bunch of brown men in a car, the night of heightened security in the city*', Chuck realises that his former sense of ease in America is gone, that he feels newly 'uneasy, guilty, criminal' (2009: 97). When AC tries to intervene calmly in fluent English, the officers act as if he is speaking a foreign language: '[Officer] Brophy processed the information slowly, as if AC had just gushed a verse of Urdu poetry' (2009: 97). Chuck's comical comment punctures the rising tension (for readers) as it suggests that the slow-witted American officer cannot understand the sophistication or language of Urdu poetry, and reverses assumptions of Western cultural superiority. This humour pushes back against and diminishes the power of the police officer, rendering it ridiculous; it demonstrates Chuck's ability to maintain control of the situation precisely because he is able to use humour; and it offers relief to readers who are thus nudged towards further good will and sympathy with Chuck and his friends and against alignment with the officers.

This dynamic is repeated in the crisis of the novel, when Chuck and his friends are wrongly arrested by the FBI under suspicion of terrorism, handcuffed at gunpoint, and taken to the

Metropolitan Detention Center (MDC), where 'the worst abuses in the American prison system took place after 9/11', and where many Muslim men were in fact detained and their civil rights suspended under the Patriot Act (2009: 133). Significantly, at this pivotal point of the narrative, located at its centre, Chuck's humour disappears, as if he is overwhelmed by the terror of what is happening to him. Humour here seems reserved – as a malign, punch-down tactic – for the agents of power, who use it to establish their superiority. Chuck is stripped, humiliated, denied his rights, almost starved, subjected to Islamophobic verbal abuse ('sand nigger') and sexual mockery (for his circumcision), and thrown into a solitary cell (2009: 137). When he asks for a phone call, he is told, 'You aren't American! [...] You got no fucking rights', and threatened with deportation to 'Bumfuckistan' (2009: 135). But even when Chuck is unable to use humour, and sensible enough not to try it, Naqvi uses humour to deflate the power of these officials, and to demonstrate Chuck the narrator's retrospective control over the situation via his humorous retelling and deadpan style. When Chuck the character is afraid he will vomit in the police car, Chuck the narrator describes his captor, whom he could not see, as sounding 'small and dumpy, like Mickey Rooney', or (later at the MDC) his second interrogator as a 'graying, fiftysomething grizzly bear of a man', naming him 'Grizzly' (suggesting he is both bear-like and grey-haired) (2009: 143). This use of creative, comical nicknames punctures the power of these figures and the fear they induce, and asserts Chuck's refusal to be conquered by that fear, even though with the interrogator he remains polite and cooperative.

Chuck the narrator's humour returns as Grizzly begins to soften (upon discovering that Chuck majored in English literature and was an investment banker). Asked to explain 'why Muslims terrorize', Chuck uses humorous analogy to expose (to his readers) the absurdity of the very premises of such a question:

> As a Muslim, he figured, I would have special insight into the phenomenon [...] just like a black man, any black man, should be privy to black-on-black violence [...] But like everybody, I figured the hijackers were a bunch of crazy Saudi bastards.
>
> (2009: 146)

If it is not clear to readers that the question is essentialist and racist because it lumps all Muslims and Arabs together and assumes they have insider knowledge of terrorism, the analogy to similar assumptions about black men makes it clearer. Chuck's colloquial language and youthful slang further expose the question as ridiculous, as he distances himself from the 9/11 attackers and points out, through his casual generalisation about what 'everybody' knows (except, apparently, Grizzly), that the hijackers were Saudi, and that most Muslims do not condone terrorism.

But Chuck is careful not to use humour on Grizzly, for in such a fraught situation, it would only be understood as non-cooperation, or a challenge to authority. Only when Grizzly rephrases his questions ('why the hell did they have to blow up the Twin Towers'), showing that he is less hostile, Chuck pushes back with increasing gutsiness ('Your guess, sir, is as good as mine'; to Grizzly's question, 'Can't you put yourself in their shoes?' he responds, 'No, can you?') (2009: 147). Chuck challenges both Grizzly's alignment of him with terrorists and the assumption that he can imaginatively understand them any more than Grizzly can himself. Rhetorically, he switches roles, turning the question on the interrogator, as if turning the mirror upon him to see himself. Chuck is the only one of his friends to be released from the MDC without outside intervention, as if his cooperative demeanour, ready tongue, use of logic, knowledge of history, and exposé of the incongruity of Grizzly's assumptions together undo Grizzly's suspicions and effect Chuck's release. However, while in this situation Chuck the character maintains a tone of deference and cooperation even as he questions his interrogator's questions, Chuck the retrospective narrator continues to use humour for his readers (continuing to describe his interrogator as 'Grizzly', inserting editorial remarks), splitting the narrating from the narrated self, and separating his readers from the suspicious mindset of the detention officials, realigning himself, through the use of humour, with the former against the latter.

As the rest of the novel describes Chuck's return from detention, his budding romance with Jimbo's sister Amo, his successful negotiation of a new job offer, and his ultimate inability to stay in an America that has traumatised him, humour remains an important tool that serves to lighten grim moments and maintain sympathy with Chuck without diminishing the seriousness of the critique that Naqvi presents. For American readers, it also serves to make more receivable the dark counter-narrative *Home Boy* presents of American prejudice and official and unofficial mistreatment of Muslims after 9/11. This is not to say that Chuck's (or Jimbo's or Naqvi's) use of humour is not at times distasteful or puerile. It is not above targeting women or working-class individuals: Jimbo's overweight American girlfriend is dubbed 'the Duck' because she waddles; Jimbo claims she wants marriage and children because her ovaries are 'drying up'; the Moroccan who helps Chuck as a fellow Muslim says, 'I brayed for you' (2009: 6, 70, 258). But perhaps this is precisely the point: that Chuck and his friends are not perfect or even admirable human beings, but they are not deserving of persecution or relegation to the category of potential terrorist. As if speaking for Naqvi, at a key moment in the novel Chuck addresses a gathering of 'Puppies' (a humorous play on Yuppies, for children of Pakistani Urban Professionals): 'We're not model citizens – I'm not a citizen at all – but I can tell you this much: we've done nothing wrong. This is no way to treat human beings, and this is no way to achieve security' (2009: 172). These claims to humanity and efforts to educate, in the hope of ameliorating hostility and misconception, are the basis for the humour in *Home Boy*. Humour serves to establish the humanity and intelligence of the youthful Chuck and his cohort, and to *appeal* (in every sense: to please; and to make an urgent request or plea) to readers, not to pander, but to arouse sympathy and empathy, and to prepare readers to be more open to the counter-story it tells, to be able to hear the debunking of the pernicious myths and prejudices that have been used to dehumanise and demonise Muslims and Pakistanis after 9/11. In this sense, humour in Naqvi's work acts as a bridge-builder, not to appease or placate, but to do the important cultural and political work of reaching out to those who might otherwise see only through the dangerous frameworks of a single story – I refer here to Adichie's famous TED talk, 'The Danger of a Single Story' (2009).

A comparison with *A Case of Exploding Mangoes*

As yet, only a handful of scholars have attended to this dazzling first novel, and fewer even mention Hanif's humour.[8] In alternating chapters, the novel follows two narrative threads – the story of Junior Under Officer Ali Shigri, a trainee in the Pakistani Air Force, who is imprisoned and tortured by the military and secret service when his gay friend and lover disappears in a stolen airplane; and the story of the historical figure President Zia-ul-Haq (Martial Law Administrator and President of Pakistan, 1977–1988) and his associates in the months before Zia's plane mysteriously exploded on 17 August 1988 – that converge on the day of the crash. The title itself puns on 'case' as a mystery to be solved (the cause of the explosion remains unknown) and a container of fruit (the mangoes that were later suspected of containing explosives). Though set in a pre-9/11 world, the novel looks back with a post-9/11 geopolitical understanding to a time when the US supported a military dictator in Pakistan to train the Taliban to fight Russians in Afghanistan – the very Taliban who would later turn against the US.

Given the limited space of this essay, I will highlight some brief comparative points. To begin with form: unlike *Home Boy*, which is narrated throughout by one first-person narrator (Chuck), *Exploding Mangoes* alternates between a first-person male narrator-protagonist (Ali Shigri) and a third-person omniscient narrator (unnamed). These two alternating voices together offer more varied modes of humour and a range of humorous effects. Shigri's voice, like Chuck's, is young, insouciant, and similarly uses verbal humour (wit, jokes, puns, word-play, irreverent comments, comic rhetoric such as understatement and exaggeration) to debunk authority, to undercut the oppressive force of power, and to establish Shigri's resilience, his refusal to succumb to the horrors that afflict him as he is (also) wrongly imprisoned and tortured. The third-person narrator's voice is different, however: satiric, deadpan, reductive, more knowing; in addition to absurdist narration and commentary, it uses free indirect discourse (and the liberties of historical fiction) to describe the inner thoughts and emotions of General Zia-ul-Haq, his wife (described as the 'First Lady'), and their subordinates. This narrator's humour includes Bakhtinian scatological references, a sardonic tone, comic description, ridiculous analogy, and absurdity of detail that all serve to deflate the pompous stature of powerful officials, to demystify their power, and to expose the corruption of his network of allies and rivals. Beyond these two different narrative voices and their different modes of humour, I would distinguish the humour of the author, who deploys absurdities of plot and symbolism, and comparative juxtapositions (of event, scene, character, voice) to bring out incongruities that produce comic effects.

The Prologue opens with Shigri's irreverent voice, describing himself as 'the one who got away', the only one to have boarded the doomed plane and survived (because he was 'off-loaded' to make room for more important passengers), audaciously addressing the reader as 'you', pulling us in to participate from his perspective (Hanif 2008: 5, 309). Claiming a brief background presence in the last TV clip showing Zia alive, Shigri presents the great man walking to the plane as follows:

> For a brief moment you can see General Zia's face in the clip, the last recorded memory of a much-photographed man. The middle parting in his hair glints under the sun, his unnaturally white teeth flash, his moustache does its customary little dance for the camera, but as the camera pulls out, you can see that he is not smiling. If you watch closely, you can probably tell that he is in some discomfort. He is walking the walk of a constipated man.
>
> The man walking on his right is the US ambassador to Pakistan, Arnold Raphel, whose shiny bald head and carefully groomed moustache give him the air of a respectable homosexual businessman from small-town America.
>
> (2008: 3–4)

With the 'middle parting' (a possible allusion to Rushdie's description of Indira Gandhi in *Midnight's Children*, suggestive of the divisiveness of these tyrannical rulers), Shigri begins by breaking down Zia's face into its component parts – hairstyle, teeth, moustache – all of which are disaggregated and rendered somewhat ridiculous. The moustache dances as if to appease onlookers, the teeth flash unnaturally as if again to reveal Zia as insecure, trying too hard, putting undue effort into his appearance. The description next uses Rabelaisian humour, focusing on Zia's bowels and dysfunctional digestive system (suggestive of Zia as a blockage himself, an obstruction to the nation), a known strategy of bringing the high low.[9] Such descriptions reduce the mighty and dispel awe (for readers as well as for the narrator). Shigri similarly describes the US ambassador as comically hairless (perhaps signifying reduced virility or manliness), equally 'carefully groomed', focused on maintaining a public façade, and, with the unexpected combination of 'respectable' with 'homosexual businessman', as absurdly incongruous. Via inversion, the joke also calls out American homophobia, especially in 'small-town America', and commercialism, that lies beneath the diplomatic exterior and interference in other nations' autonomy.

The Prologue thus sets up this tongue-in-cheek style and attitude that undercuts the powerful and establishes Shigri's humour and verbal dexterity. 'There is poetry in committing a crime after you have served your sentence', Shigri remarks: 'punishment before a crime does have a certain singsong quality to it. The guilty commit the crime; the innocent are punished. That's the world we live in' (2008: 6). With such wit and aphoristic brevity, Shigri begins his story, how he woke to find his roommate Obaid gone: 'the buggers would obviously suspect me. You can blame our men in uniform for anything, but you can never accuse them of being imaginative' (2008: 7). Hidden in this obvious put-down of army officials is perhaps an ironic reference to Hanif himself, who was trained in the Pakistani Air Force, and, contrary to expectation, has written this brilliantly imaginative novel (Filkins 2016).

Hanif's own humour is evinced as he juxtaposes for comparison, in the next section, Shigri's controlled official 'Statement'. This is addressed to Shigri's military superiors, and though also in Shigri's voice, presents an entirely different persona. Shigri turns banal detail into subversive, hilarious absurdity as he recounts the minutiae of his day to claim that he knew nothing of his friend Obaid going 'AWOL'. Performing dutiful subordination, quite unlike his voice as narrator, Shigri writes: 'As I was inspecting the second row, I realized that the sash on my belt was loose. I tried to tighten it. The sash came off in my hand. I ran towards my barracks to get a replacement' (2008: 9). The simple, factual sentences combine with mundane detail to poke fun at army discipline and dress: 'I noticed that Cadet Obaid's cupboard was open. [...] I didn't notice anything unlawful in the cupboard' (2008: 9). Humour creeps in as Shigri connects the official term 'unlawful' with 'cupboard', parodying the surveillance he is under and is required to enact. Noting the absence of the poems Obaid often taped inside his cupboard, Shigri again covertly makes fun of military regimen as he asserts his own innocence:

> Since the Academy's standard operating procedures do not touch upon the subject of posting poetry in dorm cupboards, I had not reported this matter earlier. I arrived back at 0643, to find that the entire squadron was in Indian position. I immediately told them to stand up and come to attention and reminded Cadet Atiq that the Indian position was unlawful as a punishment.
>
> (2008: 10)

As a subordinate empowered to exert discipline on his own subordinates, Shigri sends up the Pakistani military's disciplinary regime and its paranoid rivalry with India, and ridicules the ritual violence and humiliation enacted upon junior trainees: 'I caught one first-termer with a slice of French toast in his uniform shirt pocket. I stuffed the toast into his mouth and ordered him to start front-rolling' (the first-termer subsequently vomits the toast all down his uniform) (2008: 11–12). This debunking humour at the minute tonal and verbal level is augmented by our knowledge that Shigri is performing subservience, as he is required to do. The contrast Hanif sets up with Shigri's voice as narrator makes evident that underlying this façade of subservience is a comic subversion of the very regime Shigri purports to uphold.

Shigri's humour later also becomes a tool for relief (for himself and readers) and a sign of his resilience when he is imprisoned and subjected to starvation and torture. After an excruciating night spent dozing standing up locked in a toilet full of excrement, for example, he sees the graffiti left on the walls by previous prisoners with nails and possibly in blood: 'I think about contributing my own two bits. Something like [...] "On a very hot evening, Under Officer Shigri had a flash of brilliance." Not enough space on the wall' (2008: 97). The third-person self-description and the droll, offhand, understated thought of adding his 'own two bits' is paired with the laconic comment that cuts it off; both suggest Shigri's irrepressibility and refusal to be cowed. Later, threatened with a hot iron by two interrogators, Shigri uses witty obscenity to brace himself: 'Don't listen to him, I tell myself. It's the same old good cop/bad cop bullshit. They are all sons of the same bitch' (2008: 116). Even when Shigri's humour disappears at terrible moments, when he is truly overwhelmed, such as when a general describes how he allowed a train full of Hindus to be massacred during the 1947 Partition, it returns, if only in retrospect, 'I have quietly pushed my plate away, the bird intact except for one half-chewed leg' (2008: 210). As in *Home Boy*, the occasional disappearance of humour intensifies the horror faced by the young narrator, and its reappearance suggests his resilience and effort to recover.

The humour of the third-person narrator, by contrast, works consistently throughout the novel, and deploys different strategies. It targets the powerful, and produces an overall tonality of the absurd, even when describing the horrific, as if to help readers cope with that horror. The second chapter opens with the narrator's deft, satiric portrayal of Zia as insecure, absurd, even pathetic. Zia hesitates over a translation of the Qur'an, rattled by Jonah's admission that he 'was wrong' (2008: 31). This reference to Jonah inside the whale inaugurates a network of bodily tropes of containment and rupture – including bulging bellies, intestinal disorders, and the case of exploding mangoes itself – that structures the Zia narrative. We see Zia 'Absent-mindedly, he [...] scratched his left buttock on the prayer mat', undercutting the religiosity he zealously self-advertises (2008: 31). Later, we learn, Zia's 'itsy-bitsy itch' is diagnosed as an intestinal system riddled with tapeworms (2008: 91). The narrator's incongruous coupling of deadpan, matter-of-fact tonality with a Rabelaisian focus on bottoms and bodily detail induces laughter, and serves both to deflate this presidential figure's self-importance and to suggest metaphorically that the nation (as body politic) too is riddled by parasites eating it from within, working their way out. Through ironic humour, Hanif also suggests Zia's extraordinary self-delusion, hubris, and hypocrisy in imagining he would receive the Nobel Peace Prize, as Zia uses the Qur'an to 'prepare for his acceptance speech at the Nobel Prize presentation ceremony' (2008: 31).

Hanif's third-person narrator uses multiple humorous tactics to diminish Zia and render him absurd: verbal choices to describe humiliating details, such as Zia's failed masculinity on his wedding night, when he could not 'kill the cat' or dominate his wife (2008: 37), or his weeping during the mosque prayers, which is attributed to 'another tongue-lashing from the First Lady' (2008: 43); absurd analogy ('like a child taking a peek, [...] General Zia could not resist the temptation) (2008: 34); deflating symbolic descriptions ('startled' by the thump of a salute, he stumbles (2008: 35). Zia's more Westernised, snobbish generals look down scathingly on him and his religiosity, revealing class differences between them: 'A country that thinks it was created by God has finally found what it deserves: a blabbering idiot' (2008: 40). All this is compounded by the narrator's droll voice, which is also used to describe the army and Zia's associates. Sprayed with a rose-scented air freshener, an important conference room 'smelled like a freshly sealed coffin', ironically undermining the army takeover of democracy (2008: 37). In a bilingual pun, a sycophantic general is named 'Beg' (pronounced to rhyme with 'vague') (2008: 37). Soldiers joke that another sycophant, General Akhtar, 'could wipe out a whole enemy unit by kissing their asses' (2008: 41).

In addition to these two narrators' voices, Hanif's own humour in this novel deploys symbolism, folktale, and absurd plotting. Blind Zainab (based on an actual case of a blind pregnant woman who was sentenced to death by stoning for fornication because, under the infamous Zia-authorised *sharia* law, the Hudood Ordinance, she could not identify her rapists), is one of the few women in this novel. Sentenced to death for being gang-raped, she curses Zia: 'May worms eat the innards of the person who is taking me away from my home' (2008: 169). Unknown to her, her curse has the power to destroy her destroyer. Hanif's plot, as if to offset and critique Pakistan's explicitly male-dominated world, centres on this blind woman's curse, delivered to Zia by the crow that ultimately flies into his plane, and leads to his death. The third-person narrator first describes curses as folkloric and ridiculous, known to work only 'if a crow hears a curse from someone who has fed him to a full stomach and then carries it to the person cursed' (2008: 188). But Hanif as author turns the joke upon such urban scepticism via a plot that achieves precisely this improbability, validating the wisdom and power of this demotic belief. Through the hilarious success of Zainab's curse and the angry First Lady's absurd domestic manoeuvres, Hanif both highlights the disempowerment of women under Zia's 'Islamic' regime and suggests the covert ways that women can deploy power in response. In Hanif's narrative logic, Zia's misogyny and gender discrimination comically come back to bite him. This undoing of Zia too is rendered through the serious use of humour and absurdity. The crow that carries Zainab's curse to Zia is ready to burst from over-feeding on ripe mangoes; it literally becomes a container of exploding mangoes that crashes into, and explodes, the plane.

Yet another tactic of Hanif's humour is the use of ribald symbolism, such as the farcical situation when Zia is caught literally with his pants down, as he bends over so that the Saudi's prince's personal physician can inspect his bleeding anal cavity. Submitting to the discomfort of this undignified posture (suggestive of the disease and homoerotic relations between Saudi and Pakistani rulers) while 'the Royal Dick Doctor' probes his 'private things', Zia places his head on a table and realises he is stuck 'between two flags' – Pakistan's green and white national flag 'on one side' and the flag of the Pakistan Army on the other (2008: 93–94). In this powerful, comical moment, Hanif uses multiple symbolisms, not only to ridicule the figure of Zia and to suggest his damaging, divided loyalties, but also, more importantly, to suggest the conflictual relationship between the nation and the army designed to keep that nation safe, when martial law and dictatorship suspend democracy.

Sadia Abbas describes the humour in Hanif's work as an 'ethical and destabilizing tool' designed to create an overall distancing effect and to disallow easy identification or sympathy:

> The absurdism, farce, and humor in the novel are part of Hanif's mechanisms for describing the phenomenological encounter with horror too difficult to assimilate. [...] These features work with the anger, restrained and tightened in Hanif's work [...] Comedy in Hanif's work enables an alienation effect that allows a critical distance from the characters and events [...] without too sentimental and morally paralyzing an empathy.
>
> (2014: 168–169)

While this is true of the third-person Zia narrative, I would add, as demonstrated above, that Hanif's humour works in multiple ways, and has multiple effects. We need to separate the two narrators' voices and distinguish between their different modes of humour, which are in turn separate from the tactics of Hanif's authorial humour. Shigri's first-person narrative (like Chuck's in *Home Boy*) invites empathy through its engaging first-person narrator, whereas the third-person narrative voice invites alignment with its critical perspective and disalignment from the powerful figures it debunks. I would argue instead that the *combination* of Hanif's two narrators, their different humouristic modes, and different narratives works *contrapuntally*, to produce *both* distance and closeness, *both* horror and engagement, inviting readers into both a critical and caring relation with what is described, and, by enabling them to cope with the horror of what is described, to continue reading. In the face of grim horror and abuses of power, humour serves to take that power down a notch, not to vanquish it, but to diminish its force, to undercut it. Without humour, the horror would be unrelenting, leading to readers' disengagement; humour serves to pull readers in, to build community through shared laughter; it does not alleviate the horror, but enables learning, and engagement with, rather than disengagement from what it describes. Hanif's humour thus also reaches out to a broad audience to enhance understanding and critique of the difficult geopolitical, national, and cultural problems he takes on.

Unlike *Home Boy*, which focuses primarily on benign humour, *Exploding Mangoes* also explores more fully the workings of malign, punch-down humour. Official superiors and powerful men often use negative humour to put down and further oppress those below them. General Zia and the Saudi prince, for instance, joke about the 'huge organs' and 'huge derrières of their women' (Hanif 2008: 34). Or, in his 'Statement', Shigri reports how his superiors use sexual jokes to mock him: 'the 2nd OIC [officer in command] did not return my salute and made a joke about my sword and two legs. The joke cannot be reproduced in this statement' (2008: 10). By noting what he must leave out of his statement, marking the gap that signifies enforced self-censorship, Shigri both demonstrates his own conformity with military decorum and reports on the violation of that decorum by the officer who victimises him. Later, Shigri repeats this move when he describes the response to his question of whether he was being placed in detention: '[the OIC] laughed and made a joke about the cell mattress having too many holes. The joke cannot be reproduced in this statement' (2008: 13). Hanif thus engages in a broader exploration than Naqvi of how humour works with power: it is used both as a weapon by the powerful to further empower themselves and abuse those below, and as a tool of resistance by the disempowered against oppression or aggression.

Hanif also describes how powerful men use jokes to build camaraderie, to perform to each other their sense of ease with each other, especially when that is in question. Ominously, as Zia and the American ambassador walk arm in arm towards the doomed plane, Shigri notes that 'There is an air of important men sharing a joke, spreading goodwill' (2008: 312). Earlier, the Saudi prince and Zia joke with each other to establish their (male) bonding. The prince presents Zia with a prayer mat, saying, 'This will point you towards Mecca even if you are in space', and Zia replies 'with humor characteristic of their relationship, "if wishes were Aladdin's carpets, sinners like me would always be flying to Mecca"' (2008: 31). In reporting these jokes, Hanif adds another layer of satiric irony: Zia will soon die in the 'space' of an airplane pointed anywhere but Mecca, and Zia is indeed a sinner, more than he acknowledges. Hanif's humour undercuts Zia's, as he delineates both Zia's understanding that joking is a sign of confidence, power, and intelligence, and Zia's failed, anxious efforts to tell a joke. Zia mishears the American ambassador as saying that Zia would be remembered as 'a bit of a bore' (2008: 311). In a 'panic', he tries to tell a joke, struggling to remember the 'hundreds of one-liners' he has painfully rehearsed but, aware that 'jokes are all about timing', he cannot recall or understand a joke he has heard (about himself in paradise with seventy *houris*, who are thus condemned to a hellish eternity) that in fact ridicules Zia himself (2008: 311). Hanif thus uses a range of modes of humour and abstains from others, as he explores broadly how humour can be used for both constructive and destructive purposes.[10]

Humour has been used by a new generation of Pakistani anglophone (predominantly male) writers, especially since 9/11, for a range of important purposes: from satire, pushback, demystification, and relief to assertion of humanity, resilience, and intelligence, to building community and fostering rethinking. Salman Rushdie is an important precursor, especially in his comic satire of Pakistan's politics in *Shame*. Hence it is important to consider how the use of humour is itself gendered. Muslim women writers certainly can and do use humour – Firoozeh Dumas from neighbouring Iran is an important example – but Pakistani anglophone women writers seem to use it less. Perhaps this is because deploying humour involves a certain cultural privilege and room to take risks. Since women's humour is perceived differently from men's, and is more fraught with the danger of being misread, women writers who use humour face arguably greater, different risks and gender biases. The uses of humour in women's writing and their implications are thus very different, and will be the subject, I hope, of future exploration.

Notes

1 I understand Islamophobia as not just a fear of Islam or Muslims, but as 'a new form of racism, based on assumptions about (and attributions of) inherent characteristics linked with national origin, or other markers such as names, forms of dress' (Naber 2008: 303), and as a new mutation of orientalism, 'an ideological formation' emergent from post-Cold War politics, that has accompanied and enabled the rise of US imperialism and globalisation (Sheehi 2011: 31).
2 For example, the Danish cartoon controversy showcased Western assumptions that Muslims lacked a sense of humour; the inability to generate or laugh in response to humour supposedly signified Muslims' 'cultural inferiority' and lack of humanity (Bilici 2010: 195–196).
3 In many patriarchal systems, for instance, women's laughter has been seen as threatening or irreverent (Parvulescu 2010: 17, 26). Since 9/11, 'making jokes in the security check area at the airport is strictly prohibited and punishable by law' (Bilici 2010: 206).
4 For a fuller account of these theories, see Morreall (1987: 3–7), (1983: 4–37), Martin (2007: 20–26), Bilici (2010: 201–203).
5 While I agree with Roy that this tactic of seeking belonging is risky, because it asks for understanding on the basis of sameness, not difference, I disagree that Naqvi fails to address the complexity or variety of Muslims who are against both terrorism and 'the Americanized worldview' of Chuck (Roy 2011: 12). First, to assume a singular 'Americanized worldview' is to risk homogenising all Americans; second, Chuck and his friends are themselves heterogeneous and over the course of the novel change and learn from each other and their experiences; third, the novel includes a variety of Muslim figures from different classes and nations, who manifest varying degrees of devotion, and an array of positions (Old Man Khan, Abdul Karim, the Moroccan well-wisher, etc.). I would argue instead that Naqvi uses Chuck's putative sameness as a bridge to difference, and thus to invite non-Muslim American or global readers to start to see as human the range of figures that Chuck sees as human. Thus, Naqvi seeks to reduce distrust by starting with the engaging figure of Chuck, and then inviting readers to move to others.
6 It is important that Chuck begins by emphasising the cosmopolitan, national, and gendered (but not religious) aspects of his identity. Identities are intersectional; identity categories are interlocking and mutually constitutive – Chuck is at once Pakistani, male, middle-class, Muslim, post-adolescent – but it is not until after 9/11 that his Muslimness is thrust upon him, that he begins to recognise religious affiliation as a dimension of his identity. His religious belief, in contrast with his religious identity, is minimal when the novel begins; by the end he turns to prayer when he learns of a friend's death in the Twin Towers, but whether he has now become a full-fledged believing 'Muslim' (whatever that means) is an open question.
7 Of course, it is funny on many counts: as an absurd self-compliment; as patently false; as evoking the rivalry between the two countries on the ridiculous scale of masculine looks.
8 For an important exception and account of the novel's politics, critique, and formal strategies, see Chapter 5 of Abbas (2014). Mukherjee (2009) and Shamsie (2009) discuss the novel briefly in comparison to two others (regarding, respectively, the use of global postcolonial English and US-Pakistan involvement in Afghanistan). Waterman (2015) discusses the novel as historical fiction.
9 Bakhtin's theory of carnivalesque humour describes the laughter that diminishes the pretensions of the socially powerful by focusing on the (often naked) bodies they share with all humans and animals, and on their lower bodily functions (sex, excretion): 'Festive folk laughter presents an element of victory not only over supernatural awe, over the sacred, over death; it also means the defeat of power, of earthly kings, of the earthly upper classes, of all that oppresses and restricts' (1968: 92). The grotesque body, and the nether regions, are key to this 'debasement [which] is the fundamental artistic principle of grotesque

realism; all that is sacred and exalted is rethought on the level of the material bodily stratum or else combined and mixed with its images' (Bakhtin 1968: 370).

10 Hanif's humour in his second novel, *Our Lady of Alice Bhatti*, is equally powerful and important, but uses different strategies, which cannot be elaborated upon within the scope of this chapter.

Bibliography

Abbas, S.A. (2014) *At Freedom's Limit: Islam and the Postcolonial Predicament*. New York: Fordham University Press.

Adichie, C.N. (2009) 'The Danger of a Single Story' [online]. Available from <www.ted.com/talks/chimamanda_adichie_the_danger_of_a_single_story/transcript?language=en> [30 May 2017].

Bakhtin, M. (1968) *Rabelais and his World*. Cambridge, MA: MIT Press.

Bilici, M. (2010) 'Muslim Ethnic Comedy: Inversions of Islamophobia'. In *Islamophobia/Islamophilia: Beyond the Politics of Enemy and Friend*. Ed. by Shryock, A. Bloomington: Indiana University Press, 195–208.

Barreca, R. (1991) *They Used to Call me Snow White: Women's Strategic Use of Humor*. New York: Penguin.

Daily-Bruckner, K. (2016) 'Reimagining Genre in the Contemporary Immigrant Novel'. In *The Poetics of Genre in the Contemporary Novel*. Ed. by Lanzendörfer, L. New York: Lexington, 219–235.

Emig, R. (2010) 'The Empire Tickles Back: Hybrid Humor (and its Problems) in Contemporary Asian-British Comedy'. In *Hybrid Humor: Comedy in Transnational Perspectives*. Ed. by Dunphy, G. and Emig, R. Amsterdam: Rodopi, 169–190.

Filkins, D. (2016) 'Dangerous Fictions: The Writer Mohammed Hanif Probes for Truth in Pakistan'. *New Yorker* [online]. Available from <www.newyorker.com/magazine/2016/05/09/a-pakistani-novelist-tests-the-limits> [7 June 2017].

Gilbert, J.R. (2004) *Performing Marginality: Humor, Gender, and Cultural Critique*. Detroit: Wayne State University Press.

Golimowska, K. (2016) *The Post-9/11 City in Novels: Literary Remappings of New York and London*. Jefferson: McFarland.

Hanif, M. (2008) *A Case of Exploding Mangoes*. New York: Knopf.

Hanif, M. (2011) *Our Lady of Alice Bhatti*. London: Random House.

Heidemann, B. (2012) '"We are the glue keeping civilization together": Post-Orientalism and Counter-Orientalism in H.M. Naqvi's *Home Boy*'. *Journal of Postcolonial Writing* 48(3), 289–298.

Martin, R.A. (2007) *The Psychology of Humor: An Integrative Approach*. Burlington: Elsevier Academic Press.

Morreall, J. (1983) *Taking Laughter Seriously*. Albany: SUNY Press.

Morreall, J. (ed.) (1987) *The Philosophy of Laughter and Humor*. Albany: SUNY Press.

Mukherjee, A. (2009) '"Yes, Sir, I Was the One Who Got Away": Postcolonial Emergence and the Question of Global English'. *Etudes Anglaises* 62(3), 280–291.

Naber, N. (2008) '"Look, Mohammed the Terrorist is Coming!": Cultural Racism, Nation-based Racism, and the Intersectionality of Oppressions after 9/11'. In *Race and Arab Americans Before and After 9/11: From Invisible Citizens to Visible Subjects*. Ed. by Jamal, A. and Naber, N. Syracuse: Syracuse University Press, 276–304.

Naqvi, H.M. (2009) *Home Boy*. New York: Random House.

Parvulescu, A. (2010) *Laughter: Notes on a Passion*. Cambridge: MIT Press.

Roy, C.B. (2011) 'The Tragic Mulatto Revisited: Post 9/11 Pakistani-American Identities in H.M. Naqvi's *Home Boy* and Mohsin Hamid's *Reluctant Fundamentalist*'. *Reconstruction: Studies in Contemporary Culture* 11(2), n.p.

Shamsie, M. (2009) 'Covert Operations in Contemporary Pakistani Fiction'. *Commonwealth Essays and Studies* 31(2), 15–25.

Sheehi, S. (2011) *Islamophobia: The Ideological Campaign Against Muslims*. Atlanta: Clarity.

Waterman, D. (2015) *Where Worlds Collide: Pakistani Fiction in the New Millennium*. Karachi: Oxford University Press.

8
COMIC AFFILIATIONS/COMIC SUBVERSIONS
The use of humour in contemporary British-Pakistani fiction

Sarah Ilott

'Yes I'm Muslim, Please Get Over It' is the title of Sofia Khan's blog. Sofia is the titular protagonist of Ayisha Malik's *Sofia Khan is Not Obliged* (2015) and its sequel *The Other Half of Happiness* (2017). Appearing at the top of the first page of the first novel, alongside the title of the particular entry – 'Fight the Good Fight' (2015: 3) – the blog's title foregrounds the tension between affiliation and conflict which the novels' humour goes on to negotiate. The assumption of a conflict of perspectives that might lead to shock that the blog's author is Muslim, or mistrust, is immediately countered by the colloquial instruction to 'get over it', which implies a level of familiarity and establishes a closer relationship between the author/protagonist and reader. This chapter explores the use of humour to create new affiliative networks and subvert power hierarchies in the work of British Muslim Pakistani-heritage author, Ayisha Malik. Frequently dubbed the 'Muslim Bridget Jones', Sofia Khan's comical adventures in the world of dating and publishing engage with the cultural contexts of a white-dominated publishing industry, trips to Karachi, and the generation gap between first-generation Pakistani immigrant parents and their second-generation offspring.

There is little work to date that explores the role of comedy in relation to Pakistani and/or Muslim cultural texts. A notable exception is Mucahit Bilici's chapter on 'Muslim Ethnic Comedy', in which he explores stand-up comedy in the context of an increasingly Islamophobic America. There are parallels to be drawn between the cultural contexts of Britain and the US and the work required of comic utterances in their various forms, yet the relationship constructed between author/comedian and audience is markedly different for fictional uses of humour. Whilst stand-up comedy operates in the public domain and elicits an immediate response, relying on laughter to drive a comparatively short performance, fictional narratives operate primarily in the private realm over a long period of time and do not require readers to confront the author of the humour face-to-face. Unlike in stand-up comedy, moments of audible laughter are not prerequisites for the success of the comic fiction text. Bilici references the paradigm for 'Muslim ethnic comedy in the United States', in which 'a series of inversions [are] played out against a backdrop of Islamophobia' as a means of uniting an otherwise divided populace (2010: 196). This is comparable to occasional moments in Malik's work, such as when

Sofia's mum forgets white people's names, and Sofia's white friend Katie couches her friend's embarrassment by saying, 'To be fair, Sweetu – we do all sound the same' (Malik 2017: 144), playing upon and inverting racist stereotypes regarding Asians all looking the same. However, this comic paradigm is largely inapplicable to Malik's body of work. Though Islamophobia and racism are referenced in the novels, most notably when Sofia is called a terrorist and later a 'Paki bitch' (Malik 2015: 406) whilst travelling on the London Underground, the way that the audience is constructed through the texts works on the prioritisation of similarity over difference. It assumes a set of shared values whilst acknowledging but often downplaying the effects of difference (rather than exaggerating them to comic effect).

Stand-up comedy, such as that explored by Bilici, often operates according to the principles of the relief theory of comedy, as proposed by Sigmund Freud, in which laughter functions as a cathartic release of repressed emotions, enabling a temporary liberation from the reality principle as the pleasure principle takes over; there is an 'expenditure of psychic energy' – often taking the form of audible laughter – as the manifest content of the jokes 'yield pleasure through their disguised expression of unconscious wishes' (Freud qtd. in Bergmann 1999: 3). However, freed of the necessity of outbursts of laughter driven by the expression of otherwise repressed cultural taboos, such as Islamophobic beliefs, the humour of Malik's novels is better interpreted through the superiority and incongruity theories of comedy which acknowledge and engage with a set of cultural norms without relying on the more extreme subjects of cultural taboo. Premised upon the assumption of a series of cultural hierarchies and a set of acknowledged differences between 'others' and 'ourselves', the superiority theory of comedy, as proposed by Thomas Hobbes, states that 'Laughter is nothing else but a sudden glory arising from some sudden conception of some eminency in ourselves, by comparison with the infirmity of others' (1840: 46). Dangerously conflating normativity with superiority, this form of comedy laughs down at others perceived as inferior due to a deviation from a preconceived set of norms. Malik's work engages with this brand of humour insomuch as it tackles stereotypes that serve the dominant group in constructing Muslims or Pakistanis as Other. In so doing, it follows Homi Bhabha's imperative to engage with the '*effectivity*' of stereotypes in order to displace rather than simply dismiss them (2000: 67; emphasis original). However, the dominant comic mode of Malik's work is that of incongruity, serving to highlight and derive humour from the gap between expectations and reality through the juxtaposition of conflicting discourses and the representation of voices in dialogue. For Mikhail Bakhtin, whose theory of the carnivalesque engages with instances of incongruity, the type of laughter engendered through this form of comedy is inclusive: it 'expresses the view point of the whole world' and 'he who is laughing also belongs to it' (1994: 201). There is no outside to the kind of carnival laughter that Bakhtin envisions, as individuals are joined together through laughter at a ridiculous world. Bakhtin's work demonstrates the potential for laughter to create new affiliative networks, or what Marie Gillespie refers to as the (temporary) community created by 'people alike enough in outlook and feeling to be joined in sharing a joke' (2003: 93). The remainder of this chapter engages with the ways in which Malik's novels subvert existing hierarchies (imagined and sociopolitically actualised) through an engagement with stereotypes and adoption of the position of butt of the joke, before moving on to consider ways in which new affiliative networks are created through the means by which the ideal reading audience is constructed by the novel and through intertextual affiliations that create and/or parody fields of reference.

In the author blurb at the start of both novels, Malik describes herself as a 'British Muslim, lifelong Londoner and lover of books', a tagline that could easily extend to her protagonist, Sofia Khan, a Londoner and practising Muslim working in a publishing house and living with her Pakistani immigrant parents. The narrative starts *in medias res* as Sofia confides, 'You'd have thought that a break-up just before Ramadan would have inspired some kind of empathy from extended family members' (Malik 2015: 3). Inviting laughter at the absurd ending to her previous relationship, she goes on:

> 'O-ho,' one auntie might've said. 'I'm sorry that your potential husband wanted you to live with his family and a hole-in-the-wall.'
> Perhaps even a show of shock – a gasp, a hand to the chest or to the mouth …
> 'Hain? A *hole-in-the-wall*? What is this?'
> Nope.
>
> (2015: 3)

Encouraging readers to empathise with her situation and join in her incredulity at the aunties' inappropriate responses to her misery, Sofia recounts her woes in a melodramatic tone that sets the novel firmly in the genre of comedy rather than tragedy. *Sofia Khan is Not Obliged* and its sequel follow the protagonist's personal and professional forays into romantic adventure as she takes a practical approach towards researching a book on Muslim dating that leaves her with a converted husband-to-be and a book under her belt at the end of the first novel. Picking up shortly after the previous novel left off, *The Other Half of Happiness* opens following Sofia's elopement with her convert husband to Pakistan, as she balances marital bliss with a level of disdain for her Karachi surroundings and domestic boredom that leads her to return, alone, to London for work. The novel deals with life after marriage, and her husband Conall lives up to his name (Con-all) in revealing on their wedding day (arranged by her mother to make up for her elopement) that he is a divorcee with an ex-wife and child in Ireland, facts that he had previously neglected to tell his wife. The remainder of the novel sees Sofia taking comfort regarding their increasing estrangement in her friends (each of whom are struggling with their own romantic entanglements), her family, and an attractive colleague called Sakib in whom she deludes herself that she is not interested. The novel ends in Tooba Mosque, Karachi, where Sofia and Conall meet for a bittersweet divorce before Sofia returns home and – it is implied – to Sakib.

Part of the implicit work of the novels is to engage with and subvert stereotypes associated with Muslims and Pakistanis, identity categories that are conflated or made interchangeable in racist and Islamophobic rhetoric, particularly in the British context in which racism towards Pakistanis has quickly been superseded by – yet directed at the same groups as – Islamophobic utterances and attacks. Particular stereotypes countered by the novel relate to allegations that Pakistanis and Muslims are not funny – the objects of humour but never the authors – and that the practice of veiling signifies that Islam is a patriarchal religion and its female practitioners naïve and/or oppressed. The novels also function to resist homogenising discourses through Sofia's varied modes of identification (as Muslim, as Pakistani, as a Londoner, as a woman) and an internal othering of certain Asians and Muslims through Sofia's gentle mockery.

Writing in the long aftermath of the Rushdie and Danish Cartoon affairs, and in the midst of the *Charlie Hebdo* shooting in France, Malik would have been forced to resist and write back to the notion that Muslims lack a sense of humour. Citing the post-9/11 context, Bilici states that 'The simplistic idea that Muslims "hate us" has simultaneously produced rigid stereotypes and a countering desire to discover what those stereotypes deny: among other things, a Muslim sense of humor' (2010: 195). He emphasises the importance of acknowledging a sense of humour, as 'humor usually stands for humanity' and if 'someone has a sense of humor, then he is just like us: likeable' (2010: 195). He goes on to state that things like the Danish Cartoon affair exacerbated this problem, as despite the contestable 'degree to which the cartoons were actually funny or offensive, to whom, and for what reasons', the affair was constructed as demonstrating a 'Muslim intolerance of humor' (2010: 195–196). In a European context, the recent surge in Islamophobia also piggybacks on a far longer history of racism towards Pakistanis, which often led to comedy in which Pakistanis were the butts of jokes. In the British sitcom *Curry and Chips* (1969), for example, white British Spike Milligan 'blacked up' to play an Asian immigrant called Kevin O'Grady, referred to by the racial slur 'Paki Paddy'. Despite the show's cancellation for its racism (director Johnny Speight defended it as highlighting rather than promoting discrimination to no avail), Milligan was invited to repeat his role twice in Speight's hugely popular *Till Death Us Do Part* (1965–1975). These are brief examples taken from a long history in Britain of constructing Pakistanis as people to be laughed at rather than laughed with.

In this manner, Pakistanis and Muslims have been constructed as Other through racist and Islamophobic discourses that have had currency in Britain since the British Raj but gained steam following mass migration to the United Kingdom and then again following the Rushdie affair and 9/11. For Bilici, referring to the American context, 'Because the everyday world has become extraordinary, the Muslim [...] becomes an oddity when he appears "ordinary"' (2010: 205). The solution that he puts forward is that 'Those whose reality is already distorted because of stereotypes resort to humor to rectify and reassert their own sense of what is real' (2010: 205). Malik's work effectively asks readers to 'get over' any preconceptions about Muslims in the first line of *Sofia Khan is Not Obliged*, and to accept the humour on her own terms. In addition, much of the humour of the novels functions to undermine expectations of po-faced seriousness associated with Muslim faith. In *The Other Half of Happiness*, the seriousness of the questions that the Imam asks as part of the marriage ceremony in Karachi are undermined through the interpolation of Sofia's inner monologue: 'Imam asked Conall in English: "You tell people? '*I am Muslim. I believe*'?" He furrowed his dark brows. I resisted the urge to sing "In a Thing Called Love"' (2017: 4). This juxtaposition of the ceremonial rites of marriage and lyrics from a song by a ludicrous, spandex-clad British rock band called The Darkness both removes the possibility of undue seriousness and redraws the frame of reference to construct Britons familiar with contemporary rock as insiders on the joke.

Beyond the fairly obvious demonstration that Muslim faith is not limited to humourless expressions of devotion, there is also a regular confluence of the sacred and profane. For humour theorists such as Bakhtin, the incongruous convergence of the sacred and the profane in a carnivalesque inversion of hierarchies through the debasement of the spiritual to the mundane and grotesque serves to bring the high low and to strip it of its power. It involves the 'lowering of all that is high, spiritual, ideal abstract; it is a transfer to the material level, to the sphere of the earth and body in their indissoluble unity' (1994: 205). For Bakhtin, this carnivalesque inversion has a political function as the temporary erosion of boundaries between the sacred and profane means that institutions lose their power. Much of the humour of Salman Rushdie's *The Satanic Verses* (1988) performs this function, as the Prophet Muhammad and his wives are mimicked by a harem of prostitutes who adopt the identities of the Prophet's wives for the sexual gratification of their clients, marrying the poet Baal in an act of bawdy parody. As such, the irreverent humour of Rushdie's novel functions to undermine the religion and religious believers. However, for Malik the confluence of the sacred and the profane comes *alongside* her devout protagonist's expressions of faith: the humour functions to demystify Muslim practices without undermining the religion.

A focus on Sofia Khan's bodily functions – 'the human body with its food, drink, defecation, and sexual life' (Bakhtin 1994: 204) – serves to ensure that the character is humanised, rather than placed on a pedestal as an infallible representative of her religion. Sofia often does the work of introducing the bathetic plunge from spiritual ideal to grotesque reality herself. Swiftly on the heels of accusing her sister of failing to 'understand the spiritual transformation of the past month', Sofia admits that 'Images of Dairy Milk only occasionally punctuated the formation of my new Zen-like personality' (Malik 2015: 7). Similarly directing a shift in focus from matters of the mind to matters of the body, Sofia interrupts a discussion about *kismet* – destiny – to inform her mother that 'Kismet, right now, tells me I need the toilet' (2015: 9). Sofia even associates her prayers with her tendency to overeat, joking that 'It's probably a good thing' that there are no biscuits in the house, as otherwise she would 'end up eating an entire packet and then spend the next three days wasting prayer time on asking for a stomach bug' (2015: 43). Sofia frequently presents religious practices in secular terms, such as describing *iftari* as the 'fast-breaking ritual of stuffing gob' (2017: 279) and comparing the practice of fasting to being 'on the 5:2 diet' (2015: 245). In this manner, Malik draws attention to Sofia's physicality, depicting her as a creature of appetites and desires rather than ideals alone.

Malik's novels also function to challenge and engage stereotypes regarding the practice of veiling, through their deployment of humour. Anxieties about veiling in a British context are evident in high-profile cases that received a huge amount of media attention in the decade leading up to the publication of *Sofia Khan is Not Obliged*, such as Shabina Begum's lengthy court battle for the right to wear the *jilbab* to school (BBC 2006a), MP Jack Straw's expressions of discomfort regarding the face-veiling practised by his Blackburn constituents (BBC 2006b), and Aishah Azmi's dismissal from her position as a teaching assistant for her insistence on wearing a *niqab* (BBC 2006c). Such expressions of anxiety often take the form of a white saviour narrative, in which the Muslim woman is cast as the oppressed victim of a patriarchal religion in need of rescue by liberated Westerners, a discourse famously summarised by Gayatri Spivak as 'white men [...] saving brown women from brown men' (1994: 93). It is thus important that veiling is presented in Malik's novels as Sofia's decision, in line with (rather than in opposition to) her feminism. With reference to Shelina Zahra Janmohamed's *Love in a Headscarf* (2009), a humorous memoir by a British Muslim with an East-African Asian diasporic background that similarly deals with the romantic life of a *hijabi*, Rehana Ahmed argues that:

> The insertion of a veiled Islamic subjectivity into a post-feminist chick-lit femininity is an important political gesture [...] The narrative facilitates identification with the cultural Other while preventing the absorption of the (veiled) Other into the Self by making visible the former's significant difference.
>
> (2015: 209)

Malik comparably redraws lines of identification through her protagonist, encouraging readers to laugh at stereotypes about veiled Muslim women as they are redeployed jokingly, as when Sofia redeploys the stereotype in a tongue-in-cheek retort to justify her momentary grumpiness to Sakib: 'I'm a hijabi. I'm meant to look sullen and severe' (2017: 283).

The subversion of stereotypes regarding veiling as symptomatic of a religion constructed as patriarchal and illiberal is partly enacted through the opposition that Sofia encounters to her decision. Whilst her father supports Sofia in her decision, made in the immediate aftermath of 9/11, to adopt the *hijab*, her mother, who does not herself practise veiling, objects on the grounds that it will make her less desirable to future husbands. Her mother jokes that she looks 'like one of those *Gontonomo* Bay wives', with the exception, from which she derives much mirth, that 'at least they have husbands' (Malik 2015: 11). In so doing she both plays into patriarchal discourses that construct women in terms of their sexual desirability to men and, as a Muslim herself, demonstrates that there is a spectrum of religious beliefs and practices. A British Muslim BBC correspondent whom Sofia meets through online dating constructs his objection as follows: 'A hijab???? Seriously??!! You're living in the West!!!!', a position that is undermined when Sofia ridicules his 'punctuation hysteria' (2015: 40). As a representative of the BBC, this view demonstrates the problem which secular liberalism has with religious belief and the notion that Islam and the West are mutually opposed (cf. Ahmed 2015). Finally, it is implied that Sofia's identifiable Muslim-ness motivates the Islamophobic and racist abuse that she receives at two instances from the same man when travelling on the London Underground, demonstrating that the principle of opposing the practice of veiling on the grounds of opposition to a patriarchal system is too easily co-opted by racists and Islamophobes. As such, the characteristics represented by those opposing Sofia's decision are made extreme and absurd in various ways through both the novels' humour and their more sombre moments.

In addition, suggestions of a correspondence between religious dress and seriousness are undercut by jokes that Sofia makes at the expense of her *hijab*. At Conall's question as to her omission of an umbrella on a rainy day, Sofia responds, 'Why do you think I wear a hijab? Part religious reasons, part good sense', reiterating that she is joking by recording Conall's inappropriate response: 'He put his umbrella over my head, not a flicker of a smile. Tough crowd' (2015: 200). Sofia maintains control over her decision by defining the parameters of discussion around her *hijab*. Tired of questions, she jokingly justifies her decision to veil as deriving from 'George [...] Michael. Gotta have faith', once again associating her religious beliefs with popular song lyrics and promising to give a 'normal response' only 'when the question is interesting' (2015: 329). In this manner, Sofia is represented as maintaining agency and control over the discourse by embodying the active role of joker. If her immediate audience fails to acknowledge her jokes, a stronger collusion is achieved with the wider reading audience through the former's exclusion from the bond created between teller and audience of the joke.

In addition to engaging and combating particular stereotypes, Malik reworks the roles of teller, audience, and butt negotiated in a joking exchange. Racist/Islamophobic jokes and stereotypes combine to cast Muslim women in passive roles, excluded from the joking exchange as the butts of jokes in a manner that simultaneously confirms the superiority and collusion of the joker and teller, and rendered passive through the anxious repetition of the stereotype that functions to 'fix' those constructed as culturally Other (cf. Bhabha 2000: 66). However, Sofia's character deconstructs this situation by merging the positions of teller and butt, poking fun at herself whilst maintaining authorial power in her self-mockery. Comparable to Helen Fielding's character, Bridget Jones (to whom I return later), Sofia Khan encounters her friends' gentle derision for her inability to cook (she is always asked to bring the salad), whilst manifesting through her diary entries a comical gap between aspirations and reality. The goals Sofia sets herself oscillate between the ambitious and mundane to comic effect:

Things to do: Finish book. Find next bestseller and become editorial star. Sort out Mum's love life. Give up biscuits. Fill each second of each day with forward momentum. DON'T LOOK BACK.

(2017: 307)

Furthermore, her target-setting is frequently undercut by an observation that demonstrates her immediate failure. Following a self-directed exhortation to 'maintain focus', for example, the following line reads, 'Ooh, Naim calling' (2015: 111). Sofia invites readers to join in self-deprecating laughter at her figure as she vows to 'avoid any [...] *ho*jabi tendencies. I.e. stay away from jersey, Lycra, tight-knit material that leaves little to the imagination, and expose what can only be described as the *wrong* type of lady-lumps' (a decision that she suggests demonstrates her 'community spirit') (2015: 6). Whilst she sets her own figure up as a source of ridicule, she nevertheless retains power through the verbal dexterity of her jokes, as indicated through the *hijabi/hojabi* wordplay. The combination of self-deprecation, lack of self-awareness, and inability to fulfil some of the impossible goals that she sets herself are represented as the source of humour, yet the manner in which Sofia narrates the book through her diary entries ensures that the laughter engendered is complicit and inclusive, rather than placing readers in a position of superiority over the character.

In this and other ways, Malik's novels employ humour to create a new community. The temporary spaces carved out through joking utterances and their attendant power structures are heterotopic in the sense conveyed by Michel Foucault, as they represent, contest, and distort contemporary social worlds (1997: 333). This is evident in the reconfigured power dynamic created when Sofia first meets Conall's father, Colm:

> 'Well,' he said, turning to look at me. 'Let's see what my son married without so much as an invite to his parents.'
> His eyes took in my scarf; his face red and rugged and the distinct smell of alcohol emanating from his mouth. He took me by the shoulders and I saw Conall step forward.
> 'Colm, best you sleep this off,' said Mary.
> 'Be good to sleep off this whole nightmare, don't you think?' he said, leaning towards me.
> I glanced at Conall. 'A coma right now wouldn't be a bad thing,' I replied.
> His grip loosened a little as his eyes bored into mine. A few seconds passed as he burst into laughter, putting his arm around me as we walked to the table.
>
> (2017: 208–209)

The quotidian response to Sofia's unwelcome presence is registered in the increasing sense of physical threat indexed through Colm's aggressive language and stance. An implicit binary is created between the alcoholic father-in-law and the daughter-in-law who makes her religious beliefs (which include abstention from alcohol) public in her choice of dress. However, the nature of the scenario shifts when Sofia jokingly and unexpectedly colludes with Colm's view, as the joke does the work of bridging the implied cultural divide. The humour is derived from the juxtaposition of the two worlds created in the scenario: Colm's animosity, which voices the Islamophobia and racism of the contemporary moment (Sofia is referred to in dehumanising terms as an object rather than a subject through the pronoun 'what', whilst the gaze directed at her scarf positions it as the cause of offence) is both registered and contested through the work of Sofia's joke.

Malik's creation of a new community based on shared laughter functions to rework the 'staged marginality' that Graham Huggan finds to be inherent in postcolonial literature. For Huggan, postcolonial literature is frequently complicit with 'the booming "alterity industry" that it at once serves and resists' by virtue of its status as commodity in the 'global late-capitalist system' in which works are produced and consumed (2001: vii). He defines 'staged marginality' as 'the process by which marginalised individuals or social groups are moved to dramatise their "subordinate" status for the benefit of a majority or mainstream audience', clarifying that this is 'not necessarily an exercise in self-abasement; it may, and often does, have a critical or even a subversive function' (2001: 87). Examples are drawn from a variety of works including Hanif Kureishi's *The Buddha of Suburbia* (1990), another novel by a Pakistani-British author in which, Huggan suggests, 'Minorities are encouraged, in some cases obliged, to stage their racial/ethnic identities in keeping with white stereotypical perceptions of an exotic cultural other' (2001: 95). As I have argued elsewhere, Kureishi foregrounds questions of audience through his protagonist's occupation as an actor, meaning that 'Theatre becomes […] an allegory for society, where the processes of casting and staging, and the composition of the audience ("four hundred white English people") are writ large' (Ilott 2015: 105). It is implied that the audience for the protagonist's plays is comparable with the audience imagined for (and through) the novel, meaning that the humour of Kureishi's novel functions predominantly to parody white expectations and poke fun at those who would seek to position protagonist Karim and his father – the eponymous 'Buddha of Suburbia' – as exotic Others.

Questions of audience are similarly important in Malik's work; however, through the juxtaposition of different modes of writing, it is made apparent that the novels' imagined audiences will be sympathetic to – and understand – Sofia and her way of life. In a manoeuvre similar to Kureishi's, Malik creates a foil for the reader, in this case through the world of publishing – 'quite possibly the most white-centric, middle-class industry there is' – which Sofia negotiates first as publicist then as author (2015: 18). Interrupted from a daydream in a meeting, Sofia finds herself inadvertently pitching a book about 'her string of God-awful dates' (2015: 7). There is a general air of awkwardness and lack of understanding amongst the majority of her colleagues, while her boss, Brammers, functions to voice any stereotypes that people might have about Sofia's book on Muslim dating (which stands in for Malik's book on Muslim dating). Engaging questions of audience, Brammers gushes, 'It'd give a fascinating insight into modern Muslim dating and marriage', imagining its coverage of 'all types of things – forced marriages, honour killings' (2015: 19, 20). Brammers' senior, Trumps, reinforces the idea that Muslims are exotic Others about whom the white majority knows little to nothing, stating, 'Muslim dating? Well, I had no idea you were allowed to date', asking whether her parents are disappointed, suggesting that 'It's all very *western*, isn't it?', and voicing his concern that she will 'get *stoned* to death for this' (2015: 29–30). However, the asides that Sofia makes to readers imply that she imagines a different audience for the book she is writing, as illustrated in the following passage: '"Sex?" I asked. "What's that?" Apparently this wasn't funny because only Katie let out a stifled laugh, whilst the others weren't sure whether to laugh or be shocked. Indeed, my friends, indeed' (2015: 20). The implication is that whilst the people present in the meeting might not understand that she is joking, the reading audience will. Referencing readers as 'my friends' at this significant juncture early in the novel constructs the reading audience as complicit with Sofia in her incredulity at her colleagues' inability to acknowledge the joke for what it is.

Malik cleverly negotiates the fact that not all readers will be cognisant of the various cultural and religious practices that Sofia describes through the different modes of writing which the novels incorporate. The novels are predominantly comprised of Sofia's diary entries, which allow readers access to a personal and unfiltered account. Also included are blog entries, which are more stylised but nevertheless similarly assume an audience of insiders, or people with shared beliefs. Finally, the first novel in the series includes excerpts from Sofia's draft 'Muslim Dating Book'. These excerpts are presented as works in progress with long passages *sous rature*; this implies that the readership has privileged access to Sofia's inner workings, but also allows certain points to be explained – such as common confusions between Muslim and Asian dating practices – without giving the impression of patronising the audience. In one entry, Sofia writes:

> *Yes, we are devout, but don't we have the same struggles as most other girls? (With the additional pressure of keeping God on side for the afterlife.) We smoke behind closed doors, don't always tell our families who we're seeing that evening, but never forget to set the alarm to wake up for morning prayers. [...] Faithful, flawed, trying to learn the true meaning of jihad as we teach it, we're also girls who wouldn't have it any other way.*
>
> (2015: 216)

This passage reads as a manifesto for the novel that Malik has written, but rendered in cheesier one-liners. It takes the same subject matter as the content of Sofia's blog and diary entries but presents it as if for an audience of outsiders. The key difference in mode is that whilst this passage is written in earnest, Sofia's more personalised accounts create the impression of experiences shared through the inclusive environment created by humour.

Part of the work of creating new affiliative networks is enacted through the field of reference that Malik creates through her use of intertexts and what Hans Robert Jauss has termed the 'horizon of expectations' created by the genre (1999: 131). For Malik's works, this has involved a process of distancing from the 'veiled bestseller' (Whitlock 2010) or misery memoir genre, her protagonist explicitly stating at one point in a note for the book she is planning: '*Whatever you do – if writing a guide to marriage, don't end up penning your very own misery memoir*' (2017: 40). The misery memoir genre is characterised by harrowing tales of forced marriage accompanied by the iconic cover imagery of a veiled woman gazing wistfully past the camera or with eyes modestly averted.[1] Instead, the paratexts of Malik's novels point to their inclusion in the chick lit genre.[2] The cover art of *Sofia Khan is Not Obliged* incorporates red looping script and figures rendered in cartoon silhouette, boasts endorsements from popular novelist Mhairi McFarlane and the 'Chicklit Club', and heralds its modernity and status in a consumer culture through the inclusion of a hashtag for the novel's protagonist (#SofiaKhan) and Malik's Twitter handle. *The Other Half of Happiness* sports on its cover a pair of perfectly manicured hands – one white, one brown – holding opposite ends of a winding silk scarf. The visual iconography and subject matter of Malik's novels situate them firmly in the emerging tradition of what Lucinda Newns terms 'Muslim Chick Lit', encompassing works such as Shelina Zahra Janmohamed's memoir *Love in a Headscarf*, whose cover art is similarly designed to distinguish it from 'one of the many veiled memoirs circulating in the marketplace' and to shape the reading experience differently: 'rather than reading *Love in a Headscarf* through a jumble of orientalist tropes, we are instructed to read it through the feminine and fashionable "cool" of chick lit, with its message of liberal consumerism and female empowerment' (Newns 2017: 10).

Helen Fielding's *Bridget Jones's Diary* (1996) – the 'most canonical of chick lit titles' (Harzewski 2011: 58) – functions as a key intertext for Malik's first novel, and popular reviews of *Sofia Khan is Not Obliged* frequently refer to it as the 'Muslim Bridget Jones', signifying its successful incorporation into the chick lit genre. *Bridget Jones's Diary*, itself a rewriting of Jane Austen's *Pride and Prejudice* (1813), is emulated in Malik's work, through a post-feminist celebration of choice (in this case with reference to the marriage 'market') as the hallmark of liberation, through the protagonist's endearing combination of a humorous lack of self-awareness and self-deprecation, and through minutiae such as the protagonists' shared failings in the domestic space and anxieties over fluctuating weight coupled with a love of food. Where Bridget has a tendency towards uncensored outbursts that demonstrate her true feelings, Sofia's directness makes her incapable of couching the truth regarding her friends' relationships, refusing to sugarcoat her opinions that, for example, her friend Foz is 'throwing [her] life away to an unworthy cause' (Malik 2017: 310). Like Bridget, Sofia surrounds herself with a close group of friends who meet for regular coffee dates to discuss their various romantic adventures. Comparable to parody of the 'smug marrieds' in Fielding's novel, Sofia is sceptical about the forms that married life can take, despite her own romantic ideals. Malik's first novel begins, as does Fielding's, with the protagonist's list of resolutions. Sofia's mother's insistence on referring to her son-in-law as Colin (rather than Conall) might even be read as an intertextual allusion to Colin Firth, the actor who plays the romantic lead in both the BBC adaptation of *Pride and Prejudice* and the film adaptations of Fielding's novels. Finally, Sofia's story also has a sequel that – like *Bridget Jones: The Edge of Reason* (2000) – 'indirectly problematizes the neat endings of Austen's marriage plots'

(Harzewski 2011: 59), in this case through an exploration of the lies and failed compromises on which a marriage falls apart.

What Stephanie Harzewski identifies as central to the chick lit genre in which Malik's novels participate is their humour, and the marketability that has meant that 'In the past decade major publishers have launched imprints capitalizing on a particular kind of feminine angst, fictionally rendered humorous or, as some readers have claimed, archetypal' (2011: 3). This humour involves elements of self-deprecation, accompanied by Austen's legacy in 'the satiric aspects of the novel of manners' (Harzewski 2011: 3), a 'caricatured portrait' of the protagonist's shortcomings that reflects back onto the reader (Harzewski 2011: 62), and, perhaps most significantly in this case, a parodic, ironic, or mocking stance towards the *Bildungsroman* genre (Harzewski 2011: 60–62). Each of these elements is undoubtedly evident in Malik's novels, as this chapter has demonstrated. However, one topic that escapes the novels' parodic gaze – which rests alternatively on family life, dating rituals, gender norms, and the internet-dependency of millennial life – is Sofia's Muslim faith. Whilst, as I have demonstrated previously, there is a blurring of the sacred and the secular/profane in a manner that encourages readers not to place the protagonist on a pedestal as an exemplar of the religion she practises, and fun is made of ceremonial rituals tied to cultural interpretations of the religion, there is no comparable ironic detachment from her faith itself, as it remains the one constant force in her life in the midst of tribulations and upheavals that range from disastrous dates, to her father's death, to the collapse of her marriage. In Harzewski's summary of Fielding's novel, she gestures towards the failure or limitation of the novel's humour, suggesting that it 'may succeed at lightheartedness, but this does not make for a spiritually uplifting reading experience. While through blunders she surpasses her predecessor [Elizabeth Bennet] on the point of endearing vulnerability, Bridget evokes not inspiration, but merely sympathetic laughter' (2011: 66). This, I would argue, is where Malik's novels differ: because the parody of the *Bildungsroman* form does not extend to the protagonist's spiritual maturation and development, the novels maintain a glimmer of hope that is premised on strength of faith rather than the promise of romantic fulfilment. Like *Love in a Headscarf*, in which Newns reads 'faith and spirituality, rather than media-driven consumption, as an alternative "solution" to the malaise left behind once the romantic myths can no longer hold water' (2017: 13), Malik's novels merge some of the hope inherent in the narrative of self-improvement or self-actualisation offered by the *Bildungsroman* with the light-heartedness and parodic gaze of chick lit.

Malik is not alone in her appropriation of the chick lit genre to centralise Pakistani/Muslim protagonists and position arranged marriages or the hunt for a husband in a tradition of literary romance dating back to Austen.[3] Rekha Waheed's *The A–Z of Arranged Marriage* (2005) proclaims its generic affiliations through a cartoon image of a woman on the front cover and an unaccredited promise that it is 'unapologetically sassy'. Located in London, New York, and Dhaka, the trials of finding a husband amidst a diminishing stock of eligible bachelors are rendered by Waheed in a tone of comic glee. Nasreen Akhtar's *Catch a Fish from the Sea (Using the Internet)* (2008) sees its protagonist turn to the web after an excruciating interview for an arranged marriage. A number of other authors locate similar novels in a Pakistani, often Karachi, setting. Blending the romantic with the political in a manoeuvre familiar to this Pakistani/Muslim subgenre of chick lit, Maha Khan Phillips' *Beautiful from this Angle* (2010) promises an intoxicating cocktail of 'Chanel and cocaine, fundoos and feudalism' on the journey to love and happiness. Saba Imtiaz's *Karachi, You're Killing Me* (2014) takes a comic approach to the crime genre, and has also been compared to *Bridget Jones's Diary*. Also Karachi-based, Shazaf Fatima Haider's *How it Happened* (2013) has drawn responses that focus on 'family comedy' and associate it with Austen's legacy through its description as 'Lizzie Bennett comes to Karachi'

(Soofi 2013). Moni Mohsin's trilogy *Duty Free* (formerly *Tender Hooks*, 2012), *The Diary of a Social Butterfly* (2013), and *The Return of the Butterfly* (2014) comes emblazoned with *Glamour* magazine's endorsement: 'Jane Austen meets Bridget Jones' (apparently oblivious to the fact that Austen and Jones have already 'met' in an intertextual sense).

In sum, Malik's appropriation of the chick lit genre to engage a Muslim protagonist enables a redeployment of the genre's humour to a variety of purposes. Creating a heterotopic space through her humour, social norms that work to stereotype and other Pakistanis and Muslims are acknowledged and subverted. Through the inclusive environment created by the novel's humour, which positions readers as insiders on the various jokes, Malik creates a British-Pakistani Muslim everywoman. Deviating from common media and literary representations of Muslim women's oppression through patriarchal systems and forced marriages, problems that Sofia suffers in her romantic life are not exoticised or presented as stemming from her religious or ethnic identity. Largely conforming to norms of the chick lit genre, the limits of the humour in leaving Sofia's faith unscathed by the parodic/ironic gaze employed elsewhere mean that Malik can demonstrate what is missing when fulfilment is sought – in true post-feminist fashion – in sex and shopping alone.

Notes

1. Newns cites Jean Sasson's *Princess* trilogy (1992, 1994, 2000), Latifa's *My Forbidden Face* (1985), and Betty Mahmoody's *Not Without My Daughter* (1978) in her discussion (2017: 2).
2. I do not employ the 'Chick Lit' classification as a slur, but to designate a popular and critically maligned genre that has a rich potential for social commentary. I nevertheless recognise the negative connotations that this post-feminist genre has accrued for being frothy, un-literary, or even debilitating to the feminist movement (see Harzewski 2011).
3. Thanks go to Rabaha Arshad, Claire Chambers, Aroosa Kanwal, Ayisha Malik and Shelina Zahra Janmohamed for their recommendations of similar books in this genre.

Bibliography

Ahmed, R. (2015) *Writing British Muslims: Religion, Class and Multiculturalism*. Manchester: Manchester University Press.
Akhtar, N. (2008) *Catch a Fish from the Sea (Using the Internet)*. London: Greenbirds.
Austin, J. (1813) *Pride and Prejudice*. London: T. Egerton.
Bakhtin, M. (1994) 'Rabelais and his World'. In *The Bakhtin Reader*. Ed. by Morris, P. London: Edward Arnold, 194–244.
BBC. (2006a) 'School Wins Muslim Dress Appeal'. *BBC News* [online]. Available from <http://news.bbc.co.uk/1/hi/education/4832072.stm> [15 December 2017] .
BBC. (2006b) 'Straw's Veil Comments Spark Anger'. *BBC News* [online]. Available from <http://news.bbc.co.uk/1/hi/uk_politics/5410472.stm> [15 December 2017].
BBC. (2006c) 'The Woman at Centre of Veil Case'. *BBC News* [online]. Available from <http://news.bbc.co.uk/1/hi/uk/6068408.stm> [15 December 2017].
Bergmann, M. (1999) 'The Psychoanalysis of Humour and Humour in Psychoanalysis'. In *Humor and Psyche: Psychoanalytic Perspectives*. Ed. by Barron, J.W. Hillsdale: Analytic Press.
Bhabha, H. (2000) *The Location of Culture*. London: Routledge.
Bilici, M. (2010) 'Muslim Ethnic Comedy: Inversions of Islamophobia'. In *Islamophobia/Islamophilia: Beyond the Politics of Enemy and Friend*. Ed. by Shyrock, A. Bloomington: Indiana University Press, 195–208.
Fielding, H. (1996) *Bridget Jones's Diary*. London: Picador.
Fielding, H. (2000) *Bridget Jones: The Edge of Reason*. London: Picador.
Foucault, M. (1997) 'Of Other Spaces: Utopias and Heterotopias'. Trans. by Miskowiec, J. In *Rethinking Architecture: A Reader in Cultural Theory*. Ed. by Leach, N. New York: Routledge, 330–336.

Gillespie, M. (2003) 'From Comic Asians to Asian Comics: *Goodness Gracious Me*, British Television Comedy and Representations of Ethnicity'. In *Group Identities on French and British Television*. Ed. by Scriven, M. and Roberts, E. New York: Berghahn, 93–107.

Haider, S.F. (2013) *How it Happened*. New Delhi: Viking Penguin.

Harzewski, S. (2011) *Chick Lit and Postfeminism*. Charlottesville: University of Virginia Press.

Hobbes, T. (1840) *The English Works of Thomas Hobbes Volume 4*. Ed. by Molesworth, W. London: John Bohn.

Huggan, G. (2001) *The Postcolonial Exotic: Marketing the Margins*. London: Routledge.

Ilott, S. (2015) *New Postcolonial British Genres: Shifting the Boundaries*. Basingstoke: Palgrave Macmillan.

Imtiaz, S. (2014) *Karachi, You're Killing Me*. Noida: Random House.

Janmohamed, S.Z. (2009) *Love in a Headscarf*. London: Aurum Press Ltd.

Jauss, H.R. (1999) 'Theory of Genres and Medieval Literature'. In *Modern Genre Theory*. Ed. by Duff, D. London: Longman, 127–147.

Kureishi, H. (1990) *The Buddha of Suburbia*. New York: Viking.

Malik, A. (2015) *Sofia Khan is Not Obliged*. London: Twenty7.

Malik, A. (2017) *The Other Half of Happiness*. London: Zaffre.

Modood, T. (1990) 'British Asian Muslims and the Rushdie Affair'. *Political Quarterly* 61(2), 143–160.

Mohsin, M. (2012) *Duty Free*. London: Vintage.

Mohsin, M. (2013) *The Diary of a Social Butterfly*. London: Vintage.

Mohsin, M. (2014) *The Return of the Butterfly*. London: Vintage.

Newns, L. (2017) 'Renegotiating Romantic Genres: Textual Resistance and Muslim Chick Lit'. *Journal of Commonwealth Literature* [online]. Available from <http://journals.sagepub.com.ezproxy.lancs.ac.uk/doi/pdf/10.1177/0021989416686156> [15 December 2017].

Phillips, M.K. (2010) *Beautiful from this Angle*. New Delhi: Penguin.

Soofi, M.A. (2010) 'Book Review: How it Happened'. *Live Mint* [online]. Available from <www.livemint.com/Leisure/PMpZmxUK7hoD2WMegjqlBK/Book-Review--How-It-Happened.html> [15 December 2017].

Spivak, G.C. (1994) 'Can the Subaltern Speak'. In *Colonial Discourse and Post-Colonial Theory: A Reader*. Ed. by Williams, P. and Chrisman, L. Hemel Hempstead: Harvester, 90–105.

Waheed, R. (2005) *The A–Z Guide to Arranged Marriage*. London: Monsoon Press.

Whitlock, G. (2010) *Soft Weapons: Autobiography in Transit*. Chicago: University of Chicago Press.

9
RESISTANCE AND REDEFINITION

Theatre of the Pakistani diaspora in the UK and the US

Suhaan Mehta

The playwright Wajahat Ali opened his talk at Google by saying:

> Today's [...] speech [...] has solidified my worth as a human being for my family members who in their typical South Asian bluntness see my professional career as a writer as [...] useless. Today they said, 'Try to get a job at Google!' And I told them, '[...] Google invited me to speak for them', and they said, 'Yes, yes! But after the speech get a job. Stop being useless'.
>
> (2012: n.p.)

The dismissive attitude of Ali's Pakistani immigrant parents is central to his play *The Domestic Crusaders* (2004). The character Ghafur, who had been the apple of his parents' eye, leaves them aghast when he says that he no longer plans to become a doctor (51–52). Ghafur's parents cannot understand why he wants to pursue Middle Eastern history, Islam, and Arabic (54–55). Their angry reaction to Ghafur's revelation in Ali's post-9/11 play is reminiscent of the ending of Ayub Khan-Din's *East is East* (1996) set in 1970s Salford, England. While the authoritarian patriarch George Khan thinks that his son Saleem is studying engineering, in reality he is pursuing art; Saleem has been working on a 'model [...] of a vagina complete with pubic hair', rather than building machines (1996: 70). Ali and Khan-Din draw on their experiences growing up in immigrant Pakistani households to show how families limit the career choices of second-generation Pakistani youth.

Besides these internal restrictions, playwrights of Pakistani origin have struggled to find audiences in America and the UK. One of Ali's motives for writing *The Domestic Crusaders* was to counter the cartoonish representation of Muslim-Americans (Illumemedia 2009: n.p.). In a conversation with Al-Jazeera, Ali said:

> Mainstream theatres were not ready for [*The Domestic Crusaders*]; they were afraid. They thought 'What will people say?' Here is a Muslim-American with a multi-syllabic, Arabic name showing Muslim-American characters talking freely about religion

and politics and race very honestly and bluntly. 'What will people say?' Eight years later there is a change. [...] *The Domestic Crusaders* is written, and it is on in New York. It wouldn't have happened eight years ago.

(Nichena 2009: n.p.)[1]

There is a longer tradition of Pakistani-British drama, but contemporary playwrights also comment on their relative invisibility. In an online interview, the playwright Avaes Mohammad said that:

One of the major reasons I started writing was the events around summer of 2001 where in the North there were riots between young British-Asian youth and the far right which also spilled onto the police. That spread like a flame actually from Oldham to Bradford to Burnley. [...] It started going off like matchboxes, really just all over and then 9/11 happened at the end of that.

(FIPA Arts 2014: n.p.)

Mohammad was disturbed by the skewed representations of British-Asian youth in these eruptions as 'terrorists', 'rioters', and 'disaffected youth' and remarked to his flatmate at the time, 'We need to talk about us' (FIPA Arts 2014: n.p.).

In this chapter I study playwrights from the Pakistani diaspora in the UK and the United States, all of whom have at least one parent born in Pakistan (for a comprehensive account of theatre in Pakistan, see Mundrawalla 2014). Pnina Werbner writes that while Muslims in England were seen 'as a law-abiding minority', starting with the Rushdie Affair a number of them developed an 'oppositional consciousness' (2005: 480–481). While younger generations of Pakistani-British immigrants continue to feel alienated from the mainstream, they also interrogate their parents' 'culture', 'custom', and 'tradition', either through 'reformist Islam' or 'satirical artistic works' (Werbner 2005: 483). This dual alienation of individuals from their country and family is seen in several contemporary Pakistani-British plays. The creative output from the Pakistani-American diaspora is partly a response to being 'othered' after the events of September 11. In his essay 'The Pakistani Diaspora in North America', Iftikhar Dadi writes that no existing creative work provides 'insight into the dilemmas of Pakistani American identity, culture, and politics' (2006: 55). This may have little to do with the merit of the plays and more with the lack of recognition given to minority playwrights. For instance, Fawzia Afzal-Khan points to the paucity of critical commentary on the playwright Bina Sharif, who has published twenty-four plays over a career spanning three decades (Afzal-Khan, Khoury, and Bose 2016: 51). Sharif's *An Afghan Woman* (2002) is a powerful commentary on the post-9/11 world wherein the speaker, a veiled woman, is communicating to an imagined audience of American women looking at images of her on their television screens. The speaker chronicles the many acts of violence by the Taliban and by her American liberators but still reimagines a life where she can 'talk', 'laugh', and 'be free' (Sharif 2002: 251–252). It is true, however, that after 9/11 more Pakistani-American voices have emerged as Dadi predicted (2006: 56, 63). Within a decade of the publication of Dadi's article, a handful of playwrights attained national prominence: Rohina Malik's *Unveiled* premiered at the 16th Street Theatre and received wide critical acclaim; Rehana Lew-Mirza's *Barriers*, published in 2002, is taught in several American universities; Ali's *The Domestic Crusaders* debuted in California in 2005 and premiered on Broadway in 2009; and Ayad Akhtar won a Pulitzer for his first play *Disgraced* (2012) in 2013. These playwrights provide rich alternatives to one-dimensional representations of Muslim-Americans.

Drama from the South Asian diaspora in the UK and America has been receiving increasing critical scrutiny, but the output by playwrights of Pakistani origin has not yet been studied as an independent body of work. Neilesh Bose's *Beyond Bollywood and Broadway* (2009) is the first critical anthology of plays from the diaspora based in three continents. In a summative comment, Bose writes that the 'theater of the South Asian Diaspora reflects a highly diverse set of sociopolitical and aesthetic concerns, such as the engagement with classics of various forms as well as explorations of questions of the "homeland"' (2009: n.p.). The British and American diasporas have been studied independently, too. Sarah Dadswell and Graham Ley write that the emerging scholarship on British South Asian theatre has documented this new body of work, presented 'theoretical and critical assessments', provided 'historical' readings of the plays, and paid 'attention to [elements of] performance and production' (2012: 2–3).[2] Despite being in its infancy, South Asian American drama has also started to attract academic interest. Ashis Sengupta argues that contemporary South Asian American plays combine 'Western performance aesthetics with innovative South Asian dramaturgies and popular performance culture' (2012: 838, 853). Rohini Chaki's doctoral dissertation *Desis in the House* is the first full-length study of South Asian American theatre. Chaki examines how the possibilities and limitations of 'belonging [are] embodied differently [in South Asian American plays] across structures of class, gender and sexuality, and religion' (2016: 41). The journal *Performing Islam* devoted an entire issue to critically reflect on the success of Akhtar's *Disgraced* and its position in Muslim-American theatre (Afzal-Khan et al. 2016: 5). This chapter is the first study wholly devoted to the theatre of the Pakistani diaspora in America and the UK. It presents an overview without attempting to be comprehensive, and unlike many of the scholars referenced here, offers textual analyses of the plays. My argument is that Pakistani-American and Pakistani-British playwrights create characters that are constrained by forces within and outside their communities. These fictional characters cope with constraints and deal with prejudices by refashioning their identities to creative or destructive ends.

A recurring theme in this body of work is how familial and community expectations restrict the individual's professional options. In Ali's *The Domestic Crusaders*, the parents, Salman and Khulsoom, have dreams for their children, and every one has disappointed them in one way or another. Salman is especially horrified that his youngest son, Ghafur, who had such a promising future, 'is going to become some third-rate, penniless professor teaching little kids grammar and sentence-vocabulary structure' (Ali 2004: 53). Khusloom is worried about what Ghafur's decision will do to their status among the Muslim-American community: 'Our nose is cut. I brag and brag about you gaining admission to the top university, scholarships […] They will be rich in ten years, and you'll be getting apples from two-year olds' (2004: 53–54). Not unlike Saleem in Ayub Khan-Din's *East is East*, Ghafur's defiance of his father earns him a loud slap (Ali 2004: 57). Though more than three decades and an ocean separate George Khan and Salman, their tunnel vision is linked to their desire for upward mobility and social respectability in their adopted homelands. The psychological stress on Ghafur and Saleem shows how those who opt out of 'respected' career paths risk being ostracised.

Characters also face ostracism owing to prejudice towards non-normative sexualities. Alia Bano's *Shades* (2009) highlights the challenges facing queer Pakistani-British Muslim men. *Shades* opens with a speed dating event for Muslims and introduces two lead characters, Sabrina (Sab for short) and her queer friend and roommate Zain. While Sab does not find a date she subsequently falls in love with a religious scholar's son named Reza, whom she meets at a fundraising event for the Palestinian cause. In her analysis, Ariane De Waal argues that Bano's play challenges several assumptions regarding British Muslims, but ultimately rehashes dichotomies such as 'fundamentalism versus secularism, self-determination versus oppression, homosexuality versus heterosexuality' (2017: 77, 80). De Waal offers a particularly trenchant analysis of the character of Reza, who is both a devout Muslim and a British citizen (2017: 79). She also critiques the play for its uncritical 'bourgeois', 'heteronormative', and 'cosmopolitan' world view and suggests that the homosexual characters, Zain and Mark, do not subvert it in a meaningful way (2017: 80–83). I would argue, however, that Zain is not just an enabler of heteronormativity. Through Zain's character, Bano exposes the homophobia among sections of Pakistani-British society. When Zain informs Reza and Reza's friend Ali that he is gay, Ali makes some virulent homophobic comments: 'B-b-but, b-b-but you're Muslim […] This is worse than we thought […] You're so much better without her. [Reza, look] at who [Sab] would have brought into your home. You were spared' (Bano 2009: 77). Zain challenges Ali by presenting a more humane and profound understanding of Islam: 'God does not judge according to your bodies and appearance, but He scans your hearts and looks into your deeds […] Maybe if we listened to [the Prophet Muhammad] we wouldn't be so quick to try and judge each other' (2009: 79). Zain plays an important role in reconciling queer, British, and Muslim identities. While Ghafur and Zain do not conform to normative ideas of masculinity, playwrights of Pakistani origin also examine the distinctive struggles of young women.

Shades represents the hurdles before single young British Muslim women looking for meaningful relationships.[3] De Waal reads the opening speed dating scene as highlighting Sab's freedom of choice in the face of patriarchal misgivings regarding 'Muslim women's (in)appropriate behavior' (2017: 78). De Waal's claim is borne out through the words of a potential date, Ali. Once Ali learns about Sab's profession as an events manager, he starts making unfounded assumptions about her personal life (Bano 2009: 5–6). He turns out to be sanctimonious, making public noises about piety on the one hand and trying to have a fling with Sab on the other. De Waal argues that Reza is wrongly typecast as a fundamentalist by Zain; Reza actually has a sophisticated take on Islamic traditions (2017: 78). De Waal, however, does not explore how Zain's mischaracterisation of Reza exposes the limitations of his liberalism. Without really knowing Reza, Zain believes that he is a bad suitor for Sab and will subject her 'to the whims of the community auntie' (Bano 2009: 47). While, as a queer Muslim, Zain is mostly terrified of losing Sab to homophobic men; he does not trust her to make decisions. In this instance, Bano presents a feminist critique of the queer, liberal Muslim male.

Pakistani-American playwrights also reveal how Muslim women cope with familial pressures. In Ali's *The Domestic Crusaders*, Khulsoom is upset with Fatima for 'still [being] single' (2004: 7). Fatima is dating a devout African-American Muslim named Aziz, but she knows that her parents will never accept him. As Fatima says to her brother Ghafur, 'They'd rather I married a Hindu, as long as he's relatively brown', pointing to the anti-black racism of South Asian Americans (2004: 69; for a detailed treatment of this subject see Prashad 2000). The intrusiveness in women's personal lives takes a comical turn in Akhtar's play *The Who & the What* (2014). The protagonist Zarina's father, Afzal, creates a profile for her on an online dating site and meets young men on her behalf. When Zarina is flabbergasted, Afzal rationalises his actions saying, 'All I care about is the two of you [Zarina and her sister]. Your happiness' (2014: 25). Unlike Zarina's non-Muslim boyfriend Ryan, Afzal approves of Eli, a convert to Islam who 'runs a soup kitchen and a masjid on the Northside […] [making] people's lives better' (2014: 24). Much against her initial judgement, Zarina ends up marrying Eli, whose company she enjoys, thereby striking a compromise. The situations discussed above illustrate the internal pressures on young Muslims who also have to deal with religious and racial discrimination outside their homes.

In the aftermath of 9/11 and 7/7, Muslims of South Asian and Middle Eastern background have seen an alarming rise in hate crimes; however, anti-Muslim sentiment is not new in the UK or America. The spike in Islamophobia in the UK after 9/11 was an aggravation 'of existing

[...] everyday racism, both before [the first Gulf war] in 1991 and in the intervening period' (Mason and Poynting 2007: 81).[4] In the United States too, Islamophobia is not a twenty-first-century phenomenon; Khambiz Ghanea Bassiri writes that Muslims are only the most recent group to have experienced discrimination (2006: 70).[5] Anti-Muslim sentiment in both North America and the UK is linked to fear of the outsider. British-Pakistani drama has not shied away from the topic of race relations. The 1979 Southall riots, for instance, serve as the backdrop to Hanif Kureishi's play *Borderline* (1992). Bart Moore-Gilbert writes that *Borderline* shows British-Asian characters resisting racism in different ways (2001: 45). Anwar and Yasmin are passionate members of the anti-racist Asian Youth Movement, and have little faith in the Labour Party to speak on their behalf (Moore-Gilbert 2001: 45). On the other hand, their friend Haroon believes that the way to be 'properly influential' is to '[join] parties, sit on committees, work for papers' (Kureishi 1992: 150). Furthermore, Moore-Gilbert notes that 'Kureishi's attempt to rebut the host culture's misconceptions about Asian Britain does not entail the production of a series of naively celebratory and compensatory counter-images of "his" community' (2001: 45). As a case in point, Anwar and Yasmin are critical of Haroon's father for his exploitation of British-Asian workers, making him 'the first of many ruthless British-Asian bosses in Kureishi's work' (Moore-Gilbert 2001: 46). Avaes Mohammad's play *Hurling Rubble at the Moon*, published along with *Hurling Rubble at the Sun* in 2015, takes a similarly nuanced perspective.

Set over a four-year period from June 2001 to July 2005, *Hurling Rubble at the Moon* examines racism against British-Asians without dehumanising racists. The actions of the white working-class British characters Skef and Dean reveal the deep resentment that some locals feel towards South Asian immigrants. The play opens with Skef being laid off by his employer and feeling that he was singled out for being white. He says, 'D'you know what I feel like? Do yer? [...] Token fuckin' white guy in my own 'ome-town. D'you lot even realize this is fuckin' England?!' (Mohammad 2015: 48). A disaffected youth, Skef is particularly susceptible to white nationalist politics espoused by his father, Dean (Mohammad 2015: 58–61). At the same time, Skef is also critical of white nationalism and courageously stands up to Dean – 'This is where [British-Asian minorities] come from. This is their fuckin' home' (2015: 75). However, before questioning the aims of white nationalists Skef participates in a march and intimidates a British Muslim character named Taufeeq. Taufeeq is more central to *Hurling Rubble at the Sun*, which is set in July 2005. He is deeply embittered by injustices suffered by Muslims in the UK and overseas. He sees the anti-Muslim violence in Britain and the 'war on terror' on a continuum: 'Here they break two, three, four mosque windows so shards carpet our prayer hall, but Amma in Iraq they're bombing whole buildings, right now, one after the other so the entire city is carpeted to dust' (2015: 21). He exacts revenge on his adopted country by blowing himself up on a London bus on 7/7. Taufeeq's alienation is also felt by characters in Rehana Lew Mirza's aptly titled *Barriers*.

Mirza's *Barriers* reminds audiences of the deep sense of mistrust between Muslim and non-Muslim Americans in the immediate aftermath of 9/11. A Pakistani-Chinese-American family is haunted by the memory of their oldest son, Nabhil, who was last seen at the World Trade Center on 9/11. In one of the most poignant moments of the play, Nabhil's father Khalil laments that holes had been burned into the eyes and mouth of his son's photograph on a flier circulated after he went missing. In her analysis, Rohini Chaki writes that the image of the burnt holes 'indicates the double victimization – angry racists may have burnt holes into Nabhil's picture, but it is the fanatic Muslim terrorists who have burnt holes into his actual body' (2016: 168). Khalil observes that when some Americans 'read a Muslim name, they don't want to see kind eyes staring back at them' (Mirza 2002: n.p.). As Chaki notes, Khalil's family members are 'perceived as perpetrators and not victims by the outside world' (2016: 168). This episode in *Barriers* is somewhat reminiscent of Mira Nair's untitled short film in the collection

11'09"01. Nair's film is based on the true story of a Pakistani-American named Mohammad Salman Hamdani. Hamdani died after he tried to save victims of 9/11, but for a certain time was suspected of being a terrorist. At his funeral, Hamdani's mother says that her son sacrificed his life for fellow Americans because he was a devout Muslim (Nair 2004: n.p.). *Barriers* also offers a critique of liberal America (Sengupta 2012: 849). Khalil's daughter, Sunima, is engaged to a white art history professor named Roger. Roger's initial sympathy for an Indian guy who is nervous around him paves the way for feelings of animosity towards that 'fucking brown piece of shit' (Mirza 2002: n.p.). As Sengupta writes, despite Roger's ostensibly liberal outlook, 'prejudice lies hidden deep down in the human psyche and can surface at the smallest of excuses' (2012: 849). Post-9/11 Islamophobia directly affects Sunima's brother, Shehry, whose Muslim classmate, Shafiq, is brutally attacked and called 'Bin Laden Cousin' (Mirza 2002: n.p.). Shehry initially resents Roger for being white, illustrating that his 'fear [transforms] into paranoia' (Sengupta 2012: 849). There is a suggestion that some of these divides can be bridged as the white art history professor, his Pakistani-Chinese-American fiancée, and her brother share a quiet moment at the end of the play.

Muslim characters like Sunima, Shehry, Nabhil, and Taufeeq are constrained by multiple forces; however, in most cases, they do not allow these constraints to overdetermine their lives. Rather characters defy restrictive norms and prejudices by making bold choices, interrogating traditions, and standing up to injustice. In Aisha Zia's *No Guts No Heart No Glory* (2014), women opt for an 'unsafe' career option. The play, with Muslim female boxers in the lead, gives greater interpretive latitude by imposing few stage directions (2014: 22). *No Guts No Heart No Glory* also departs from conventional choices by being set in a boxing facility and permitting free movement of attendees (2014: 22). The collective manifesto of the boxers is to '[get] out a bit; see the world ask some questions' (2014: 43). Zia's play opens with characters' accounts of overcoming shyness, of having the courage of their convictions, and of being open about their passion for boxing (2014: 23–25). Over the duration of the play, as the young women practise their routines, they recount struggling with body image issues, avoiding nosy members of the community, and even being optimistic about marriage (2014: 26, 31, 38–42). At times, the characters address the audience as if they are members of their extended families: 'Am I embarrassing you? Are you embarrassed? [...] My mum doesn't mind, my dad doesn't care, they're cool with it. So why can't you be?' (2014: 37). Just like the women in Zia's play, who choose an 'unconventional' career, the protagonist of Akhtar's *The Who & the What* attempts to break new ground in her debut novel. Zarina is writing a work of fiction about the Prophet in which she revisits a contentious event in his life – his marriage to Zaynab bint Jash (2014: 36). Afzal-Khan analyses Zarina's attempt to undermine the interpretive consensus around this episode, as it relates to the Prophet's desires and the question of veiling. Drawing on Fatima Mernissi's study *The Veil and the Male Elite* (1991), Afzal-Khan argues that Zarina offers a feminist take on Quranic verse 33:53 by reading the veil as a metaphorical 'barrier' separating 'two men' rather than 'a man and a woman' (2014: n.p.; Mernissi 1991: 85). Zarina believes that 'contradictions only make [the Prophet] more human' and refuses to jettison her book project, despite her father Afzal's angry protests (Akhtar 2014: 36). Zarina's metaphorical reading of the scriptures is at odds with her sister Mahwish's uncritical acceptance. Mahwish refuses to leave a young man named Haroon, with whom she is no longer in love, because she sees herself as a contemporary incarnation of Aisha, the Prophet's youngest wife: 'I got it in my head that when I was nine, I was going to become the Prophet's favorite wife, too [...] if it wasn't meant to be then everything in between has just been wasted time' (Akhtar 2014: 64–65). Mawish finds herself in an unhappy situation because she reads the religious texts too literally and is unable to draw relevant moral lessons from them.

Where the feisty characters in *No Guts No Heart No Glory* and *The Who & the What* largely respond to pressures from within the domestic sphere, several others stand up to anti-Muslim bigotry outside their homes. In Ali's *The Domestic Crusaders*, Fatima misses school to participate in activism; in Bano's *Shades*, Zain, Mark, and Sab organise an event to create awareness of the situation in the West Bank; in Kureishi's *Borderline*, Anwar and Yasmin join the Asian Youth Movement to combat white nationalists. While characters in *Borderline* refrain from violent resistance, there are plays where the quest for justice takes a destructive turn. The protagonists of Akhtar's *Disgraced* and Mohammad's *Hurling Rubble at the Sun* respond to the collective humiliation of Muslims through violence.[6] The reinvention of the protagonist's identity in *Disgraced* has been analysed in detail (Basu 2016: 92; Chaki 2016: 173–176).[7] Consequently, in the following paragraphs I focus on the central character of *Hurling Rubble at the Sun*.

In *Hurling Rubble at the Sun*, the principal character Taufeeq refashions himself after the hip-hop star Tupac Shakur and, in keeping with Shakur's public persona, invites ambivalent responses (Quinn 2005). The play traces the footsteps of the 22-year-old Taufeeq from the time he starts assembling a bomb in his apartment to the moment he blows himself up on a London bus. Mohammad's play opens with lines from Shakur's song 'Ambitionz az a Rider' playing in the background. Shakur was a practitioner of gangsta rap which, according to Eithne Quinn, obtains its 'cultural and political force' through a 'double vision' whereby 'artists spout [and critique] angry and exploitative views' (2005: n.p.).[8] As Quinn writes, however, 'Ambitionz az a Rider' emerges from the latter phase of Shakur's career, when he had moved 'from a stance of political and communal engagement to one of nihilistic disengagement' (2005: n.p.). Taufeeq, much like Shakur, sees his death coming and wants to script his ending: 'When it's time to die to be a man you pick the way you leave' (Shakur qtd. in Mohammad 2015: 11). Taufeeq, though, struggles with the idea of going through with the suicide mission when he sees people from various backgrounds on the train (2015: 36). After his bomb does not go off the first time, he gets on a bus and a 51-year-old lady named Mary – tellingly Taufeeq's girlfriend is also named Mary – sits next to him. While Mary opens up to him about her family, Taufeeq struggles to convince himself that she and the other passengers are no different from the media pundits who demonise Muslims. Despite his inner turmoil, he has gone too far down the road to change course and ultimately detonates the bomb. Although Taufeeq's actions are political, like the end of Tupac's career, rather than resuscitating the self, his story ends on a nihilistic note. At the same time, Mohammad humanises Taufeeq by devoting Act 1 Scene ii entirely to his meeting with his mother, Noor 'Amma' Sultan. When Taufeeq visits Noor the night before his mission she is visibly disappointed in him for not assuming the role of a community leader. What follows is a moving encounter between mother and son as they have dinner, make plans for his future, and pray together. Importantly, their conversation also foregrounds how South Asian British Muslims are consistently targeted by racist groups. Taufeeq's attempt to reach out to his mother has a parallel in Shakur's 'Ambitionz' as the speaker implores his mother 'to come rescue [him]' (1996: n.p).

Taufeeq's identification with a gangsta rap artist while lashing out against the dominant group is comparable to how hip-hop assumes an anti-establishment dimension in Pakistani author H.M. Naqvi's novel *Home Boy*. Protagonists Chuck, A.C., and Jimbo frequently belt out the rap group NWA's song 'Straight Outta Compton', but without grasping its political message. NWA's single assumes true significance for them after they are racially profiled in post-9/11 New York. Once Chuck has been tortured, the 'anthem's resonance was no longer mere novelty or a boyish sense of affinity with the hood; no, it put things in perspective' (Naqvi 2009: 138). Naqvi and Mohammad repurpose gangsta rap to point out how young

Resistance and redefinition

South Asian Muslim men are radicalised partly as they face individual and collective acts of humiliation.

In the preceding pages, I have argued how playwrights from the Pakistani diaspora in the UK and North America create characters that reconfigure their identities in the wake of internal pressures and external prejudices. The theme of reinventing the self is hardly unique to these plays, but its rendition by playwrights of Pakistani origin takes on urgency in today's climate. I hope that this study will be followed by detailed analyses of individual plays and further investigations into connections with other media. Additionally, my textual focus would be enriched by studies that consider the performative aspects of the theatre of the Pakistani diaspora.

Notes

1 Ali's comment has been echoed by more established figures in other media. In a television interview, the film-maker Mira Nair remarked that it was 'enormously challenging' to secure financial support for her adaptation of Mohsin Hamid's novel *The Reluctant Fundamentalist*. The protagonist of Hamid's novel, Changez, is a Pakistani who graduates from Princeton and works at a firm called Underwood Samson before growing disillusioned with the United States. Nair was told by a financier that 'if you have a Muslim hero' you are worth only about two million dollars (NDTV 2012).

2 Dadswell and Ley (2012) refer to the following studies in their excellent summary: Godiwala, *Alternatives within the Mainstream* (2006); Hingorani, *British Asian Theatre: Dramaturgy, Process and Performance* (2010); Davis and Fuchs (eds.), *Staging New Britain: Aspects of Black and South Asian British Theater Practice* (2006); Griffin, *Contemporary Black and Asian Women Playwrights in Britain* (2003); Chambers *Black and Asian Theatre in Britain* (2011).

3 Rukhsana Ahmad's seminal play on domestic violence, *Song for a Sanctuary*, reveals how the attempt to legislate a Muslim (and non-Muslim) woman's choices persists even after marriage. Ahmad's play has received significant critical commentary. See especially Scholte (2015: 66–78); Griffin (2003: 138–169); and Bose (2009).

4 See Abbas (2005) for a historical perspective on Islamophobia in the UK. Abbas writes that while citizens of formerly colonised countries filled England's labour shortage after the Second World War, the latter was offset by a recession in 'the late 1950s'. These migrant workers were grudgingly tolerated on the assumption that they would leave; they 'were placed at the bottom of the labor market, disdained by the host society, and systematically ethnicized and racialized in the sphere of capitalist accumulation' (Abbas 2005: 9).

5 See Bassiri (2006) for the historical reasons behind anti-Muslim sentiment in the United States. Bassiri argues that the rise of nativist sentiment in America has always been preceded by an erosion of trust in the ability of 'national institutions to mediate ethnic and religious conflicts', and that Protestant Christianity shapes the collective American political sense of self and other (2006: 60). As a result, 'religious minorities [are seen] not only [as] theologically but also politically suspect as doubts are raised about their national loyalties and adherence to democratic principles' (2006: 61).

6 *Disgraced* was the subject of an illuminating conversation between Fawzia Afzal-Khan, Neilesh Bose, and Jamil Khoury that was published in a special issue of *Performing Islam*. They talk about their collective disquiet with the themes and reception of Akhtar's play (2016: 9). They are critical of Akhtar's trivialisation of 'Palestinian suffering', his misrepresentation of anti-Semitism, the problematic pursuit of 'whiteness' by Akhtar's male protagonist and his fuelling of his audience's 'Islamophobic anxieties' (2016: 12–14).

7 Lopamudra Basu presents a rich study of *Othello*'s influence on *Disgraced*. Basu argues that, like Othello, the protagonist Amir Kapoor '[strives] very hard to assimilate into the dominant white culture and consciously [effaces] ethnic and religious markers of his identity' (2016: 92). In her analysis, Rohini Chaki applies Mahmood Mamdani's categories of 'good Muslims' and 'bad Muslims' to demonstrate Kapoor's failed attempt at becoming a model neoliberal citizen by denying his Pakistani-Muslim background (2016: 173–175).

8 Eithne Quinn (2005) writes that the term 'gangsta rap' originated in 1989 with the success of NWA's single 'Gangsta Gangsta', which 'deals with gang conflict, the pursuit of young women, male group bonding, and a strong sense of place'.

Bibliography

Abbas, T. (ed.) (2005) 'British South Asian Muslims: Before and after September 11'. *Muslim Britain: Communities under Pressure*. London: Zed Books, 3–17.

Afzal-Khan, F. (2014) 'A Feminist Reclamation of Islam?' [online]. Available from <www.counterpunch.org/2014/07/04/a-feminist-reclamation-of-islam/> [25 July 2017].

Afzal-Khan, F., Khoury, J., and Bose, N. (2016) 'Editorial'. *Performing Islam* 5(1–2), 5.

Afzal-Khan, F., Khoury, J., and Bose, N. (2016) 'Expansions of the Dramaturgy of Political Violence: Snapshots of Three Muslim American Playwrights'. *Performing Islam* 5(1–2), 49–64.

Afzal-Khan, F., Khoury, J., and Bose, N. (2016) 'Roundtable: Ayad Akhtar and the Politics of Representation and Reception of Muslims on American Stages'. *Performing Islam* 5(1–2), 7–27.

Ahmad, R. (1993) *Song for a Sanctuary*. In *Six Plays by Black and Asian Women Writers*. Ed. by George, K. London: Aurora Metro Press, 159–186.

Ahmad, R. (2017) '"I'll explain what I can": A Conversation with Avaes Mohammad'. *The Journal of Commonwealth Studies* [online]. Available from <http://journals.sagepub.com/doi/pdf/10.1177/0021989416684184> [4 June 2017].

Akhtar, A. (2012) *Disgraced*. New York: Back Bay.

Akhtar, A. (2014) *The Who & the What*. New York: Back Bay.

Ali, W. (2004) *The Domestic Crusaders*. San Francisco: McSweeney's.

Ali, W. (2012) *From Chaiwallah to Playwright*. [online]. <www.youtube.com/watch?v=GqpC3aP_6qg> [14 June 2017].

Bano, A. (2009) *Shades*. London: Methuen.

Bassiri, I. (2006) 'Islamophobia and American History: Religious Stereotyping and Out-grouping of Muslims in the United States'. In *Islamophobia in America: The Anatomy of Intolerance*. Ed. by Ernst, C. New York: Palgrave Macmillan, 53–74.

Basu, L. (2016) 'Between Performativity and Representation: Post-9/11 Muslim Masculinity in Ayad Akhtar's *Disgraced*'. In *South Asian Racialization and Belonging after 9/11*. Ed. by De, A. New York: Lexington, 83–101.

Bose, N. (2009) *Beyond Bollywood and Broadway: Plays from the South Asian Diaspora*. Indiana: Indiana University Press.

Chaki, R. (2016) *Desis in the House: South Asian American Theatre and the Politics of Belonging*. Unpublished PhD thesis. Pittsburgh: University of Pittsburgh [online]. Available from <http://d-scholarship.pitt.edu/27822/> [3 June 2017].

Dadi, I. (2006) 'The Pakistani Diaspora in North America'. In *New Cosmopolitanisms*. Ed. by Rajan, G. and Sharma, S. Stanford, California: Stanford University Press, 37–70.

Dadswell, S. and Ley, G. (2012) 'Introduction'. In *Critical Essays on British South Asian Theatre*. Ed. by Dadswell, S. and Ley, G. Exeter: University of Exeter Press, 1–6.

De Waal, A. (2017) 'Home Front Plays: Subject Positions in the British Terror City'. In *Theatre on Terror: Subject Positions in British Drama*. Berlin: Walter de Gruyter, 48–150.

FIPA Arts. (2014) British South Asian Theatre Memories: Avaes Mohammad [online]. Available from <www.youtube.com/watch?v=l3SiVynIzRY> [10 June 2017].

Godiwala, D. (ed.) (2006) 'Introduction'. In *Alternatives within the Mainstream: British Black and Asian Theatres*. Newcastle: Cambridge Scholars Publishing, 1–20.

Griffin, G. (2003) 'Culture Clashes'. In *Contemporary Black and Asian Women Playwrights in Britain*. Cambridge: Cambridge University Press, 138–169.

Hamid, M. (2007) *The Reluctant Fundamentalist*. Orlando: Harvest.

Illumemedia. (2009) Interview with Playwright Wajahat Ali [online]. Available from <www.youtube.com/watch?v=Ue3ua3Odhzc&t=96s> [14 June 2017].

Khan, N. (2012) 'British Asian Theatre: The Long Road to Now, and the Barriers In-between'. In *Critical Essays on British South Asian Theatre*. Ed. by Dadswell, S. and Ley, G. Exeter: University of Exeter Press, 7–19.

Khan-Din, A. (1996) *East is East*. London: Jerwood.

Kureishi, H. (1992) *Borderline*. In *Hanif Kureishi: Plays 1*. London: Faber, 91–168.

Mason, V. and Poynting, S. (2007) 'The Resistible Rise of Islamophobia Anti-Muslim Racism in the UK and Australia Before 11 September 2001'. *Journal of Sociology* 43(1), 61–86 [online]. Available from <http://journals.sagepub.com/doi/pdf/10.1177/1440783307073935> [4 June 2017].

Mernissi, F. (1991) *The Veil and the Male Elite: A Feminist Interpretation of Women's Rights in Islam*. Reading, MA: Addison-Wesley.

Mirza, R. (2002) *Barriers*. New York: Indie Theater Now [online]. Available from <www.indietheaternow.com/> [15 May 2017].

Moore-Gilbert, B. (2001) 'Plays'. In *Hanif Kureishi*. Manchester: Manchester University Press, 33–66.

Mundrawalla, A. (2014) 'Theatre Chronicles: Framing Theatre Narratives in Pakistan's Sociopolitical Context'. In *Mapping South Asia Through Contemporary Theatre*. Ed. by Sengupta, A. Basingstoke: Palgrave Macmillan, 103–134.

Nair, M. (dir.) (2004) *11'09 "01 September 11: India*. Film. First Run Features.

Naqvi, H.M. (2009) *Home Boy*. New York: Shaye Areheart.

NDTV. (2012) The Reluctant Fundamentalist is not about US Bashing: Mira Nair [online]. Available from <www.youtube.com/watch?v=93-u017RFkM> [15 May 2017].

Nichena. (2009) The Domestic Crusaders: Al-Jazeera English Interview with Playwright Wajahat Ali [online]. Available from <www.youtube.com/watch?v=6G47brjCDJA> [14 June 2017].

Prashad, V. (2000) 'Of Antiblack Racism'. In *The Karma of Brown Folk*. Minneapolis: University of Minnesota Press, 157–183.

Quinn, E. (2005) *Nuthin' but a "G" Thang*. New York: Columbia University Press [online]. Available from <http://web.b.ebscohost.com/ehost/ebookviewer/ebook/bmxlYmtfXzIyNDU5Ml9fQU41?sid=5739ca26-ae65-4ffb-91c7-670df3f1a76a@pdc-v-sessmgr01&vid=0&format=EK&rid=1> [1 June 2017].

Scholte, C. (2015) 'Dramatising Refuge(e)s: Rukhsana Ahmad's *Song for a Sanctuary* and Tanika Gupta's Sanctuary'. In *Critical Essays on British South Asian Theatre*. Ed. by Dadswell, S and Ley, G. Exeter: University of Exeter Press, 66–132.

Sengupta, A. (2012) 'Staging Diaspora: South Asian American Theater Today'. *Journal of American Studies* 46(4), 831–854 [online]. Available from <http://rave.ohiolink.edu/ejournals/article/313710438> [18 May 2017].

Shakur, T. (1996) 'Ambitionz az a Rider'. On *All Eyez on Me*. Los Angeles: Polygram [online]. Available from <https://play.google.com> [23 September 2017].

Sharif, B. (2002) *An Afghan Woman*. In *Shattering the Stereotypes: Muslim Women Speak Out*. Ed. by Afzal-Khan, F. Northampton, MA: Olive Branch Press, 246–253.

Werbner, P. (2005) 'Pakistani Migration and Diaspora Religious Politics in a Global Age'. In *Encyclopedia of Diasporas: Immigrant and Refugee Cultures Around the World*. Ed. by Ember, M., Ember, C., and Skoggard, I. New York: Springer, 475–484.

Zia, A. (2014) *No Guts No Heart No Glory*. London: Oberon.

10
HISTORIOGRAPHIC METAFICTION AND RENARRATING HISTORY

Nisreen T. Yousef

This chapter examines representations of Islamic cultures in two Pakistani anglophone historical novels: *The Book of Saladin* (1998) by Tariq Ali and *Shadow of the Swords* (2010) by Kamran Pasha. It considers Ali's and Pasha's deployment of historiographic metafiction as a means of complicating, refuting, or reinforcing established present-day ideas about Islam and the West. I argue that Ali, as a Pakistani-British novelist and writer, and Pasha, as a Pakistani-American novelist concerned with the postcolonial world, show a keen interest in rewriting Arab/Islamic history from a Muslim perspective. Ali and Pasha endeavour to present images of twelfth-century Islamic societies that challenge persistent stereotypes of Muslims as uncivilised and Muslim women as passive and oppressed. Drawing on theories of historiographic metafiction, I argue that both authors attempt to eliminate the boundaries between what is fictional and what is real in order to defy the ability of history to provide ultimate truth and thereby challenge historical narratives that are narrated from the standpoint of the West. In presenting fictional accounts of the Third Crusade, both Ali and Pasha reconstruct Islamic cultures as civilised and compatible with Western cultures in ways that defy their representations in Western media and complicate Samuel Huntington's thesis of 'Clash of Civilizations'. Furthermore, both authors grant a voice to Muslim women, who are absent from historical sources. Such representations, I contend, are meant to undermine ongoing political discourse on the necessity of Western military interference in Muslim-majority countries.

In his book *Orientalism* (2003), Edward Said argues that the West's 'structured archive' about the East was built up as early as the Middle Ages. He mentions the Crusades as one of the West's early sources of knowledge about the East. As Said points out, Islam was associated with 'terror, devastation, the demonic, hordes of hated barbarians' (2003: 58). He contends that this record of representations constructed the Orient as a 'great complementary opposite' to the Occident and served as a means of controlling it (1978: 59). In his book *Covering Islam: How the Media and the Experts Determine How We See the Rest of the World* (1997), Said demonstrates how Islam, Muslims, and Arabs have been portrayed in the Western media in recent decades, particularly in American media, and how they are often associated with violence, terrorism, and war. Islam, he argues, is portrayed as a religion of violence and trouble, a menace and a threat to the West (1997: xi–xxii).

Both Ali and Pasha, I argue, deploy historiographic metafiction to serve a postcolonial objective. The ability of history to present truth and the division between history and fiction have been controversial in postmodern times. In her book *Metafiction* (1984), Patricia Waugh argues that postmodern fiction questions the relation between story and history; that the main assertions of postmodern novels are the plurality of truth and the difficulty of separating history from fiction, as history itself is a fictional construct. She maintains that 'Metafictional texts show that literary fiction can never imitate or "present" the world but always imitates or "represents" the discourses which in turn construct that world' (1984: 100–108). Accordingly, historiographic metafiction challenges the ability of history to provide ultimate truth. In a brief author's preface to *The Book of Saladin*, Ali explains his method of giving priority to historical evidence over the writing of a good story:

> Any fictional reconstruction of the life of a historical figure poses a problem for the writer. Should actual historical evidence be disregarded in the interest of a good story? I think not. In fact the more one explores the imagined inner life of the characters, the more important it becomes to remain loyal to historical facts and events, even in the case of the Crusades, where Christian and Muslim chroniclers often provided different interpretations of what actually happened.
>
> (1998: xiii)

Ali's statement indicates that his fictional account of the Third Crusade aims to provide his own version of the truth in which he contests the dichotomy between history and fiction. As we see, the novel is narrated by a Jewish character, Ibn Yakub, whom Saladin has entrusted to write his biography. Although he is the chief narrator, Ibn Yakub does not produce much direct commentary himself, leaving space for the characters to speak for themselves and about Saladin's life. The narrative constantly fluctuates between the present and the past, giving a detailed description of Saladin's life as well as Arab and Islamicate communities during the Middle Ages. Questioned by Saladin about the heterogeneous nature of narratives about the Sultan's boyhood, the scribe replies: 'Your Majesty is talking about facts. I am talking about history' (1998: 12). The narrator problematises the ability of history to present a fixed reality. His statement implies that historical accounts do not convey ultimate truth as they combine the subjective and the objective, the real and the fictional. Thus, Ali eliminates the boundaries between what is historical and what is imaginary. I contend that this juxtaposition of the historical and the fictional in the narrative serves a revisionist purpose.

In this vein, Avrom Fleishman argues that the major resemblance between the historian and the historical novelist lies in their use of imagination. Examining how real events are transformed into a narrative (1972: 6), White too problematises the ability of historical accounts to truthfully represent real events. For him, history is a type of literature that differs from other types in content rather than form, and thus claims for the ability of history to represent historical events truthfully become problematic. History, just like literature, is a kind of narrative. As Hayden White notes, a narrative is a form of discourse that is determined by the end it serves. For him, the term 'history' is rather ambiguous as it combines both the objective and the subjective (1995: 105, 107). Accordingly, the tasks of Ali as a historical-novel author and of Ibn Yakub as a historian have much in common. Both are free to exercise their imagination. In view of Fleishman's and White's arguments, I contend that Ali's fictional account of Islamic history in *The Book of Saladin* is connected to a postcolonial objective. In constructing his fictional account of the Third Crusade, Ali tries to renarrate history from a Muslim viewpoint, by challenging ongoing political discourses that support military interventionism in Muslim-majority countries.

Drawing on theories of historiographic metafiction, Ahmed Gamal argues that *The Book of Saladin* can be read as a postcolonial metafictional work as it aims to rewrite the discourse of colonial history. He notes that metafiction is a 'postcolonial act of rewriting and hence recuperate[s] the history of the colonized' (2010: 27). Gamal explains that the novel contests the dichotomy between what is historical and what is fictional. He notes that the term 'postcolonial metafiction' was first used by Timothy Brennan to describe Salman Rushdie's *Midnight's Children* (1981). Gamal indicates that postcolonial metafiction allows a space for the voice of the 'subaltern' to be heard, and that postcolonial metafiction has thus been utilised to rewrite the history of the Middle East. In light of this, Gamal argues, Ali's *The Book of Saladin* is a metafictional postcolonial narrative that re-narrates the history of the Western modernity and contests the Eurocentric narrative (2010: 1–5). My argument here expands on Gamal's work, particularly on representations of Saladin and the issue of Muslim women.

In an interview with Talat Ahmad, Ali states that his intention in writing the novel was to counteract the argument which claimed that 'the Arabs are people without political culture'. Ali points out that such claims were made by professors on TV during the first Gulf War in 1991. He adds that he wrote the novel to challenge the claims of the media and the political discourse that 'Islamic culture is backward and its politics are despotic' and 'Islam is a religion characterized by intolerance' (2006: n.p.). It is important to note that the novel's publication was followed by the release of Huntington's article 'A Clash of Civilizations?' in 1993, and later his book *The Clash of Civilizations and the Remaking of World Order* in 1996. In parts of this book, Huntington argues that Islamic cultures are incompatible with Western values, in particular with Western principles of democracy (1996: 29). Andrew Goldsmith and Colleen Lewis observe that, in the 1990s, democratising Arab and Islamic countries was seen as essential. They add that Islamic countries' political cultures were viewed as weak and lacking in harmony (2000: 313). Thus, the overall picture that we get of Islamic cultures as depicted in *The Book of Saladin* is one of political maturity.

In the novel, Saladin, the central character, is portrayed as a man with a solid political culture. As a political and a military leader, he is presented as a shrewd planner and a subtle strategist who concentrates all his energies and efforts on materialising clearly envisioned objectives. This is clearly manifested in his determined endeavours to recapture Jerusalem. The novel charts the rise of Saladin as Sultan of Egypt and Syria and follows him as he arranges to take back Jerusalem and other occupied cities from the Crusaders. Saladin appears to be a smart strategist: his move on Jerusalem comes late in his war agenda because he believes that coastal towns should be taken first. He guarantees that his soldiers arrive at Lake Tiberias in order to deprive the Crusaders' army of access to water sources, which will weaken them (Ali 1998: 273). Saladin's strategies reflect mature political and military planning.

As noted in the novel, Saladin has various diplomatic relations with different leading figures. In addition to two major Western historical figures, King Richard of England and King Philip of France, several other Crusaders are introduced into the narrative, including Raymond of Tripoli, Bertrand of Toulouse, King Amalric of Jerusalem, Balian of Ibelin, and King Guy of Jerusalem. Raymond is shown as being on good terms with Saladin, who sometimes considers him an ally rather than an opponent. Saladin is ready to save Raymond's face by refraining from attacking Tripoli, where Raymond rules, because he does not want to insult his friend and he knows that any successful attack would require either taking Raymond prisoner or killing him: 'I still feel close to him. Friendship is a sacred trust' (1998: 293). This reflects Saladin's sincerity as well as his ability to keep his word and maintain diplomatic relations with the leaders of the Crusades. By the same token, Saladin has a diplomatic relationship with Bertrand of Toulouse, a member of the Knights Templar and a heretic who escaped from the Kingdom of Jerusalem, ruled by King Amalric, joined the Muslim camp, and was immediately 'taken on trust' (1998: 113). Though Bertrand's scepticism and blasphemous views extend to criticising both Christianity and Islam, Saladin listens to him with an open mind and a genuine humanistic understanding (Ali 1998: 118). There is also a mention of al-Farabi in the novel. The choice of al-Farabi, I suggest, is significant. He is introduced as the founder of political philosophy within Islamic cultural traditions and being 'the second teacher' of philosophy after Aristotle (Al-Farabi 2004: ix). This indicates that Muslims in the medieval period were aware of political science, had their own views and theories on it, and made their own contributions to the field. Again, Ali seeks to challenge the persistent claims about Arab and Islamic communities lacking political culture.

As Peter Morey and Amina Yaqin argue, after 9/11, Western media endeavoured to create a dichotomy between Islamic and Western cultures. This supposed dichotomy was essential to promoting military action after the 9/11 attacks (2001: 1). According to Huntington, Islamic-Western relations have been problematic since the emergence of Islam:

> Conflict along the fault line between Western and Islamic civilizations has been going on for 1,300 years. After the founding of Islam, the Arab and the Moorish surge west and north only ended at Tours in 732. From the eleventh to the thirteenth century the Crusaders attempted with temporary success to bring Christianity and Christian rule to the Holy Land.
>
> (1993: 31)

In addition, in *The Clash of Civilizations and the Remaking of World Order* (1996), Huntington argues that the relationships between groups from different civilisations are usually aggressive. He maintains that relations between Islam and Christianity have often been hostile, despite the fact that there have been periods of peaceful coexistence (1996: 207, 209).

Ervand Abrahamian argues that American media have framed the 9/11 attacks in line with Huntington's 'Clash of Civilizations'. He goes on to argue that Huntington's thesis has triumphed: mainstream newspapers and journals that are read by the 'attentive public', such as the *New York Times*, *Wall Street Journal*, *Washington Post*, *Time*, and *Newsweek*, adopted Huntington's theory. Abrahamian also notes that this view was keenly embraced by television and radio networks, and that after the 9/11 attacks, Huntington's *The Clash of Civilizations and the Remaking of World Order* became a bestseller (2003: 529–530). Similarly, Fazal Rizvi argues that although Huntington's thesis has been demolished in the academic sphere, it is still influential in popular media; the 9/11 attacks were viewed by many Americans as the embodiment of a cultural and religious conflict between Islam and the West. He maintains that Huntington's frequently criticised thesis has become 'a successful political myth' which has become part of the 'social imaginary' (Rizvi 2011: 227–229). Hence, the American media played a significant role in propagating Huntington's theory, trying to present the 9/11 attacks as a civilisational clash between Islam and the West.

In his article 'The Clash of Ignorance', Said counter-argues that while Huntington succeeds in creating a binary opposition between Islam and the West, he fails to admit that the West is indebted to medieval Islamic civilisation in various disciplines of knowledge, such as humanism, science, philosophy, sociology, and historiography (2001: 197). As Jim Al-Khalili points out, in the Middle Ages, the Islamic world was at its peak in terms of scientific advancement and the period is referred to as the Golden Age of Islamic history. Europe, he clarifies, is indebted to Islamic advances in medicine. For instance, al Zakariya Razi's *al-Hawi* (925) and Avicenna's *Canon of Medicine* (1025) were translated into Latin and drawn upon in the medical field in Europe during the fifteenth and sixteenth centuries (2012: 197).

As a Muslim-American author concerned about representations of the Islamic world in Western media, Pasha, like Ali, is keen to present Islamic cultures as sophisticated and enlightened.

In *Shadow of the Swords*, Pasha provides an account that mixes the historical and the fictional in order to fulfil a postcolonial mission. This takes us to Linda Hutcheon's argument in *A Poetics of Postmodernism* (1988). Hutcheon contends that postmodernism questions the dichotomy between history and fiction and focuses on what they share rather on how they differ. For her, both history and fiction are linguistic constructs that 'derive their force [more] from verisimilitude than from any objective truth' (1988: 105). She points out that historiographic metafiction 'plays upon the truth and lies of the historical record' (1988: 114). As Hutcheon indicates, historiographic metafiction subverts the established views of history and fiction by challenging what the historical novel takes for granted. She indicates that postmodern fiction contests the ability of both history and fiction to convey truth; that it seeks to determine whose version of the truth is told (Hutcheon 1988: 105, 114, 120, 123).

In light of Hutcheon's argument, I contend that Pasha creates fictional characters such as Sir William and Miriam, who play major roles in Saladin's political and personal lives in order to contest the dichotomy between the historical and the fictional. Pasha offers his own version of the past. Pasha's fictional account of the Third Crusade constructs Islamic cultures as civilised and, furthermore, as compatible with Western cultures in ways that challenge the Western media's attempts to create an artificial division between a 'backward' Islamic world and a 'civilised' West, especially following the 9/11 attacks.

Pasha shows Saladin and Sir William establish a solid friendship. Sir William stays in Saladin's camp and develops an admiration for Islamic culture (Pasha 2010: 159). This fictionalised friendship between Saladin and Sir William, I argue, is an attempt to eliminate the boundaries between history and fiction. Pasha constructs a fictional account of Saladin's private life for postcolonial ends. In providing a mixture of the historical and the fictional, Pasha challenges the ability of history to present ultimate truth and offers a version of history that challenges historically established images of Islamic cultures as backward. To deconstruct the colonial discourse, he undermines the ideas behind Huntington's thesis of the 'Clash of Civilizations'. Ultimately, Pasha, like Ali, challenges political discourses that promote the war option in our present time.

In the novel, King Henry II is critical of his son Richard labelling Muslims as 'barbarians'. For him, 'a day in the school of Cordova would shame the greatest scholars of the Christian courts' (Pasha 2010: 56). Such a statement associates Islamic culture with knowledge and enlightenment. Moreover, after staying at the Muslims' camp and being exposed to Islamic civilisation, Sir William shows appreciation for Muslims' codes of chivalry and honour (2010: 356), and he points out that the Muslim army possesses more advanced arms than its European counterpart (2010: 106). According to the narrator, 'The soldiers knew that victory today meant triumph over the forces of barbarism and ignorance that threatened to plunge the civilized world back into the illiterate darkness that still covered Europe' (2010: 16). Through his narrator's voice, Pasha tries to put Europe and the Islamic world in sharp contrast.

Furthermore, the author suggests that Islam and the West had collaborated in trade in the past. As Ahmed Essa and Othman Ali indicate, when the Crusaders first arrived in Syria, they focused a great deal on trade. They also benefited from goods that were in high demand in Europe, such as sugar. He notes further that the Crusaders bought from Muslims icons and lapidaries that were used in churches. For Essa, trade with Muslims drew Europe's attention to the need to engage in trading activities beyond the continent, as Europe had nothing to export (2010: 57–58). In *Shadow of the Swords*, the narrator points out that Italian jewellery and French pots are available for purchase in the markets of Jerusalem; he also indicates that the Franks in the Holy Land are conducting trade with their homelands (Pasha 2010: 80–81). According to Miriam, this intercultural trade marked 'the beginnings of cultural awareness among the infidels' (2010: 81). This observation alludes to the contribution of Islamic cultures to the later rise of

Historiographic metafiction

the European Renaissance, as discussed earlier by Essa. Thus, Pasha, like Ali, seeks to defy the Western media's depictions of Muslims as backward and uncivilised.

As argued earlier in this chapter, the juxtaposition of the historical and the fictional in Ali's *The Book of Saladin* serves a revisionist purpose. By presenting the fictionalised private life of Saladin, Ali brings to light the issue of Muslim women, who are marginalised, if not completely absent from history. Ali imagines alternative historical narratives of medieval Muslim women and his fictional construct of this history serves an ideological end. This brings us to Jerome de Groot's argument about the functions of historical fiction. De Groot contends that the historical novel can challenge the subjectivity of history by providing multiple possibilities and narratives. Moreover, it functions as a postcolonial tool as it rewrites Eurocentric versions of history (2009: 139, 159). Ali, I argue, attempts to rewrite history in a way that defies assumptions that Islam is a patriarchal religion. He finds a voice for Muslim women and gives an important postcolonial revisionist impetus to the task of writing historical fiction. As Ali writes in his preface, 'Women are a subject on which medieval history is usually silent. Salah al-Din, we are told, had sixteen sons, but nothing has been written about their sisters or mothers' (1998: xiv, xvii–xviii). It is also easily observed that all the women depicted in the novel are fictional, as opposed to the men, who are a mixture of historical and fictional figures. This indicates the lack of historical evidence of women's affairs in Saladin's time. Amira el-Azhary Sonbol argues that women's status in Islamic societies is still not comprehensive and that thorough research is still required to uncover the realities of Muslim women's histories. This lack of knowledge about women in the Islamic world has resulted in exotic stereotypes (2005: xvii–xviii).

However, Gavin Hambly provides instances of real pivotal Muslim women in the medieval period who had great influence on public life in Islamicate communities, including queens, poets, and patrons. In addition, he offers instances of significant characters in Arabic, Persian, and Turkish literature and art. For him, the West has misrepresented medieval Muslim women by instantly associating them with the veil and the harem. Hambly explains that nineteenth- and twentieth-century European travellers made a significant contribution to viewing Muslim women as submissive, and maintains that these explorers only had contact with servant and slave women, and thereby drew generalised pictures of oppressed Muslim women (1998: 4).

As concluded from these works, some Muslim women in the medieval period were not submissive but rather took part in public life and played influential roles. Through representations of his two fictional female characters, Jamila and Halima, Ali presents a complex reality about living in 'harems' and royal courts. They are often portrayed in *The Book of Saladin* as enjoying a social life of their own, one that is highly developed on both intellectual and cultural levels. For example, Jamila, one of Saladin's wives, is a free, open-minded and secular-oriented woman. She is a sceptic who is intelligent enough to understand the philosophical ideas and concepts of the famous Islamic philosopher Ibn Rushd, who favoured reason over mysteries, and to teach her ideology to other women (Ali 1998: 152, 184). Jamila also adheres to al-Farabi's view that 'human reason is superior to all religious faiths' (Ali 1998: 221–222).

As the novel is a fictionalised version of a possible past reality, Jamila's interest in al-Farabi and Ibn Rushd suggests that Muslim harem women in the medieval period were sophisticated enough to understand such complicated philosophies: they were philosophically dissident and opposed to the religious mainstream. However, these women are only shown as influential, free, and strong-willed behind the scenes. Although Jamila is aware of existing political theories, she is unable to take part in public political affairs. In this regard, Ibn Yakub is critical of the fact that Jamila is prevented from participating in the public sphere, particularly in commerce and state affairs (Ali 1998: 189).

Jamila's interest in Ibn Rushd's philosophy is highly significant. Ali's mention of it is meant to suggest that there was a keen interest in gender perspectives in the twelfth century. This submits that, in contrast to clear signs of gender bias in Islamicate communities manifested in the exclusion of women from the public sphere, there was also a philosophical probing of such gender inequality. Ibn Rushd argues that women are equal to men in intellectual capacity and that if women were granted the same education and opportunities to engage in the public sphere, they would perform their roles as skilfully as men. For him, women's exclusion from the public domain is what makes them inferior to men (Sonneborn 2006: 632–661). The philosophical views of Ibn Rushd indicate that there was gender inequality after the rule of Prophet Mohammad and the Rashidun Caliphs. According to Ibn Rushd, the reign of the Arabs under the rule of the Prophet Mohammad and the Rashidun Caliphs, his immediate successors, was an imitation of Plato's republic, and that the start of the Umayyad Dynasty marked the end of it (Ali 1998: 121).

Ali reinforces a more gender-balanced approach to women in the Islamic past through Saladin's explanation that Islam permits women to learn, work, and even fight:

> There are some who argued this during the time of the Caliph Omar. They told him that our Prophet's first wife, Khadija, was a trader in her own right and she hired the Prophet to work for her, some time before she wed him. After the Prophet departed, his wife Aisha took up arms and fought, and this was accepted at the time.
>
> (1998: 127)

As can be noted, women here play a significant role in public life and nothing in Islam stops them from engaging in the social, economic, and military domains. Ibn Rushd's standpoint on gender inequality, which dates back to the twelfth century, still has resonance in contemporary Islamicate communities. Mehrunisha Suleman and Afaaf Rajbee note that women played a major role in sustaining and developing Islamic learning after the emergence of Islam in the seventh century. They indicate that women were jurists, trusty narrators of *hadith*, and teachers of *hadith*, philosophy, logic, and calligraphy. In light of this, they explain that the teachings of Islam did not lead to the subjugation of Muslim women in Islamicate societies. They argue that some Muslim men's tendency to 'overprotect' Muslim women and eliminate them from public life led to Islamicate communities losing much of their potential (Suleman and Rajbee 2017: n.p.). Ali's revisionist history has an ideological end. He provides a multifaceted image of women in the harem and challenges assumptions that Islam is backward and deprives women of the right to participate in the public sphere. He implies that the teachings of Islam allow women to participate in public life and blames communities dominated by patriarchal ideologies and values for disqualifying women from taking part, in both the past and the present. Ultimately, I argue that Ali suggests that Islamicate communities could be more just to women, similar to the way things were during the rule of the Prophet Mohammad and the Rashidun Caliphs, and tries to undermine political discourse that Western interventionism is essential to enabling women's participation in the public domain.

By presenting an account of the past that mixes history with fiction and by means of creating historical analogies between the Third Crusade and the ongoing Western military interference in Muslim-majority countries, Pasha highlights the terrible consequences of war on women. He establishes this notion as crucial in the opening episode of the novel. The narrative begins with the story of the fictional Miriam. The third-person narrator informs us that Miriam and her mother have both been raped by Crusaders and that her mother was then killed (Ali 1998: 3–5). Miriam is later captured by Richard's army on her way to Cairo (1998: 278). As Sadia Abbas argues, the emancipation of Muslim women in Islamic cultures has been used as a pretext for the ongoing 'War on Terror' (2014: 44). Morey and Yaqin observe that wives of prominent politicians in the West, including Laura Bush and Cherie Blair, used the discourse of protecting Muslim women in Afghanistan to justify the moral objectives of the 'War on Terror' (2011: 178). Nevertheless, in her paper 'Sexualized Violence Against Iraqi Women by US Occupying Forces', McNutt reported incidents of rape and sexual violence by US military personnel in a presentation made to the United Nations Commission on Human Rights 2005 Session in Geneva. She referred to a letter smuggled from inside Abu Ghraib Prison by an Iraqi woman in December 2003 who reported that women detainees were raped by American guards. Kristen McNutt further noted that President Bush had insisted that these actions could not be said to be the outcome of military action and were only perpetrated by a few recruits (2005: n.p.). Accordingly, I argue that Pasha deploys representations of the Third Crusade to reinforce the notion that the 'War on Terror' has had a negative impact on women in Muslim-majority countries, although the objective of protecting Arab and Muslim women was among the supposed objectives of the mission. Ultimately, Pasha tries to undermine the political discourse that Western military interventionism aims to save women in Muslim-majority countries.

Ali and Pasha both endeavour to discourage the ongoing political discourse proclaiming the necessity of Western military interventionism. They seek to challenge the Western media's representations of Muslims and to undermine Huntington's thesis of the 'Clash of Civilizations'. With his fictionalised account of the Third Crusade, Ali presents nuanced depictions of life under Islam. He depicts Muslims as enjoying a sophisticated political culture in ways that defy their image in the Western imaginary. Moreover, by creating Muslim female characters who are intellectually sophisticated, Ali performs a revision of colonial history and complicates the ongoing Western discourse that Muslim women are passive and thus in need of emancipation. Ultimately, Ali presents a solid anti-war stance. In a similar fashion, in *Shadow of the Swords* Pasha provides alternative images of Islamic and European civilisations, in contrast to those routinely presented by Western media following the 9/11 attacks. As opposed to media attempts to create a presumed dichotomy between 'backward' Islamic and 'advanced' Western civilisation, Pasha presents Islamic cultures as more advanced in different scientific fields. He also depicts Islamic and European cultures as enjoying a healthy relationship based on fruitful scientific and cultural interaction when Europe drew on the advances of Islamic civilisation in various domains. Pasha presents characters who are interested in building intercultural relations and mutual understanding, and notes the negative impact of war on women. Through such representations, he undermines political discourses arguing for the necessity of Western intervention in Muslim-majority countries.

Bibliography

Abbas, S. (2014) *A Freedom's Limit: Islam and the Postcolonial Predicament*. New York: Fordham University Press.

Abrahamian, E. (2003) 'The US Media, Huntington and September 11'. *Third World Quarterly* 24(3), 529–544.

Ahmad, T. (2006) 'Interview: Tariq Ali'. *Socialist Review* [online]. Available from <http://socialistreview.org.uk/311/interview-tariq-ali> [15 June 2017].

Al-Farabi. (2004) *The Political Writings: Selected Aphorisms and Other Texts*. Trans. by Butterworth, C.E. New York: Cornell University.

Al-Khalili, J. (2012) *Pathfinders: The Golden Age of Arabic Science*. London: Penguin.

Ali, T. (1998) *The Book of Saladin*. London: Verso.

De Groot, J. (2009) *The Historical Novel*. London: Routledge.

Essa, A. and Ali, O. (2010). *Studies in Islamic Civilization: The Muslim Contribution to the Renaissance*. Herndon: The International Institute of Islamic Thought.

Fleishman, A. (1972) *The English Historical Novel: Walter Scott to Virginia Woolf*. Baltimore: Hopkins.
Gamal, A. (2010) 'Rewriting Strategies in Tariq Ali's Postcolonial Metafiction'. *South Asian Review* 31(2), 27–50.
Goldsmith, A. and Lewis, C. (eds.) (2000) *Civilian Oversight of Policing: Governance, Democracy and Human Rights*. Oxford: Hart Publishing.
Hambly, G. (ed.) (1998) *Women in the Medieval Islamic World*. Houndmills: Macmillan.
Hutcheon, L. (1984) *Narcissistic Narrative: The Metafictional Paradox*. New York: Methuen.
Hutcheon, L. (1988) *A Poetics of Postmodernism: History, Theory, Fiction*. New York: Routledge.
Hutcheon, L. (2003). *The Politics of Postmodernism*. New York: Routledge.
Huntington, S.P. (1993) 'The Clash of Civilizations?' *Foreign Affairs* 72(3), 22–49 [online] <www.foreignaffairs.com/articles/united-states/1993-06-01/clash-civilizations> [3 July 2015].
Huntington, S.P. (1996) *The Clash of Civilizations and the Remaking of World Order*. New York: Simon & Schuster.
McNutt, K. (2005) 'Sexualized Violence against Iraqi Women by US Occupying Forces'. In *A Briefing Paper of International Educational Development, Presented to the UN Commission on Human Rights*. Geneva: UN Commission on Human Rights.
Morey, P. and Yaqin, A. (2011) *Framing Muslims: Stereotyping and Representation after 9/11*. Cambridge, MA: Harvard University Press.
Pasha, K. (2010) *Shadow of the Swords*. New York: Washington Square Press.
Rizvi, F. (2011) 'Beyond the Social Imaginary of "Clash of Civilizations"?' *Educational Philosophy and Theory* 43(3), 225–235.
Said, E.W. (1997) *Covering Islam: How the Media and the Experts Determine How We See the Rest of the World*. London: Routledge & Kegan Paul.
Said, E.W. (2001) 'The Clash of Ignorance'. *The Nation* [online]. Available from <www.thenation.com/article/clash-ignorance/> [3 July 2015].
Said, E.W. (2003) *Orientalism*. London: Penguin Books.
Sonbol, A. (2005) *Beyond the Exotic: Women's Histories in Islamic Societies*. New York: Syracuse University Press.
Sonneborn, L. (2006). *Averroes (Ibn Rushd): Muslim Scholar, Philosopher, and Physician of the Twelfth Century*. New York: Rosen Publishing Group.
Suleman, M. and Rajbee, A. 'The Lost Female Scholars of Islam'. *Emel* [online]. Available from <www.emel.com/article?id&a_id=828> [2 July 2015].
Waugh, P. (1984) *Metafiction: The Theory and Practice of Self-Conscious Fiction*. London: Methuen.
White, H. (1995) 'The Question of Narrative in Contemporary Historical Theory'. In *Metafiction*. Ed. by Currie, M. New York: Longman, 104–144.

PART III

The dialectics of human rights

Politics, positionality, controversies

11
PAKISTANI FICTION AND HUMAN RIGHTS

Esra Mirze Santesso

The earliest works of post-Partition Pakistani anglophone fiction tended to focus on two subject groups: British colonialists (as in Zulfikar Ghose's first novel, *The Contradictions*, 1966) and the emerging elite class of the new country (as in his second novel, *The Murder of Aziz Khan*, 1967). More recent literature coming out of Pakistan, in contrast, presents a striking thematic and aesthetic diversity that echoes the country's 'plurality and cultural commingling', which Muneeza Shamsie describes as essential to numerous 'dimensions of Pakistani life: from the structures of power and class, to natural disasters, daily struggles and cricket' (2010: 649). This emphasis on heterogeneity has generally been examined in the context of a departure from the traditional formal realism of the Western novel, or else in the context of an ongoing effort to complicate the representation of the South Asian experience by moving away from colonial stereotypes. I wish to examine Pakistani literary pluralism instead as evidence of a growing interest in scrutinising the nation's record of human rights violations under political Islam. As several scholars have noted, the relationship between theology and politics has never been well-defined in the Islamic tradition, just as the divide between the secular and non-secular has never been self-evident in the Qur'an – many revelations are fundamentally legalistic and clearly paved the way towards developing *sharia*-based law in Muslim societies. Therefore, the Islamisation of civic and political life in many Muslim states – what is commonly referred to as 'Islamopolitics' – has presented significant technical and legal problems for emerging democracies such as Pakistan.

The relevance of plurality and discourses of human rights to Pakistani literature is partly a legacy of the nation's long engagement with religious nationalism and authoritarianism. The era of Zia-ul-Haq's regime (1977–1988) was a particularly crucial and bitter one, marked by an unprecedented degree of despotism (with links to religious fundamentalism, moral corruption, economic disenfranchisement, and political suppression). Zia named himself head of the state after a military coup, and ushered in a series of *sharia*-based laws that threatened the secular structure of the post-Partition state in an effort to reignite Islamopolitics. Islamopolitics, or political Islam, 'draws on that inseparable link between religion and politics by endorsing a fundamentalist interpretation of the Qur'an and accepting *sharia* decrees as the legal basis for state power' (Santesso 2017: 8). While it would be short-sighted to assume that Islam is permanently incompatible with secular governance, it would be equally unwise to ignore the fuller connotations of Islam as *din*, which signifies an entire way of life with no differentiation between the spiritual and the political – an idea which Zia exploited fully in redefining Pakistani citizenship.

Zia's reign marked a turning point in Pakistani literary history as well: for numerous authors, his repression of Pakistan's inherent diversity, his closing of cinemas and banning of Western culture, and his introduction of Hudood and blasphemy ordinances demanded the adoption of a new approach to literary fiction. Traditional realism would no longer do; now, styles that lent themselves more easily to absurdist representation (magic realism, etc.) seemed to be called for. Salman Rushdie's *Shame* (1983), written during Zia's regime, for example, employs magic realism, perhaps to enforce the idea that 'the art of governmentality in Pakistan is a form of magic, in which people mysteriously vanish in a puff of smoke' (Morton 2007: 54). Rushdie focuses upon the disconnect between Zia's ruthless and ultra-pragmatic approach to geopolitics and his carefully constructed religious persona. Yet he adopts a more sombre attitude – similar to the style of poets such as Habib Jalib and Faiz Ahmed Faiz, known to be vocal critics of Zia – when he condemns the tyrant as a hypocrite; in the novel, Hyder (representing Zia) appears on TV the day after the coup as part of a well-orchestrated political theatre:

> On the morning after the coup Raza Hyder appeared on national television. He was kneeling on a prayer-mat, holding his ears and reciting Quranic verses; then he rose from his devotions to address the nation. [...] What, leatherbound and wrapped in silk, lent credibility to his oath that all political parties, including the Popular Front of 'that pluckiest fighter and great politician' Iskander Harappa, would be allowed to contest the rerun poll? [...] Raza Hyder, Harappa's protégé', became his executioner, but he also broke his sacred oath, and he was a religious man.
>
> (1983: 235)

The novel illustrates the link between despotism and religious fundamentalism based on visual and linguistic engineering, which turns politics into a kind of well-crafted performance art. Here, Islam is used strategically to silence, to demand not only the spiritual but also the political surrender of the individual. In this production staged for the masses, the Qur'an becomes a prop to convey Hyder's moral and political authority – but as a servile disciple rather than a menacing dictator. His meticulously tailored image as a religious devotee is essentially 'an editorial project of culture' aimed at increasing his credibility as a morally righteous leader (Abbas 2014). Such self-fashioning captures not only Zia's determination to redefine citizenship on the basis of religious belonging, but also the deeper insinuation that Pakistani individual consciousness can no longer be separate from the religious *ummah*.[1] More recently, in *A Case of Exploding Mangoes* (2008) Mohammed Hanif similarly captures the theatricality of politics as he describes Zia by way of a visual conceit. The character studies a portrait of himself that conveys his virtues as a Muslim – but a Muslim with military power at his command:

> *I am a soldier of Islam* appeared under his official portrait, in which he was wearing his four-star general's uniform. *And then, as an elected head of the Muslim state, I am a servant of my people* was the caption for the third picture.
>
> (2008: 102)

Sadia Abbas describes this self-aggrandisement as an aggressive image-building campaign 'executed through the control of language, and more significantly, through an attempted transformation of forms of devotion – forms fully entangled with the most ordinary actions and objects of life' (2014: 151). Zia's self-invention is motivated by a desire to homogenise the population and quash democratic dialogue: politics is now no longer a sphere for debate. By transmuting and suspending the law, he hopes to bolster his own autocratic rule. In *Shame*, Rushdie also picks up on this alliance between Islamisation and despotism:

> people respect [religious] language, [and] are reluctant to oppose it. This is how religions shore up dictators; by encircling them with words of power, words which the people are reluctant to see discredited, disenfranchised, mocked.
>
> (1983: 266)

As religious language oozes into the political discourse in the form of fundamentalism (which ironically suggests a direct and literal reading of the sacred text – even in nations where literacy rates are particularly low), it threatens individual autonomy and erases political agency. Opting out of the divine law, to put it differently, necessitates the suspension of secular law, and repudiates the rights of the individual to privilege a majoritarian and populist will.

It is perhaps because of the centrality of Zia's regime in the philosophical reimagining of Pakistani identity, rights, and individuality that more recent authors continue to return to this period. Both Hanif's *A Case of Exploding Mangoes* and Kamila Shamsie's *Broken Verses* (2005) choose this particular era in order to scrutinise the government's complicity in human rights abuses. Portraying Zia's rule as a period of repression, they highlight the marginalisation and victimisation of the dissident individual, who refuses to be interpellated into 'a population infused with a particular kind of piety through the implementation of punitive laws' (Abbas 2014: 164). This new generation of authors (which includes also Mohsin Hamid and Nadeem Aslam to name two) participates in the new, global literary tradition of 'human rights narratives' – narratives that convey 'particular kinds of stories – strong emotive stories often chronicling degradation, brutalization, exploitation, and physical violence' (Schaffer and Smith 2004: 4). These narratives treat human rights as 'a subset of individual moral rights which are distinguished in terms of their connection to basic human needs, are connected to political legitimacy, and place constraints on the permissible exercise of power by states' (Zoana 2011: 198). Both Shamsie and Hanif partake in a rights-oriented form of storytelling, which 'functions as a crucial element in establishing new identities' based on resistance (Schaffer and Smith 2004: 19). They ultimately characterise Islamopolitics as a threat against democratic ideals outlined in the 1956 constitution as well as a disavowal of human rights issues based on a narrow definition of citizenship that serves to intensify the fault lines between secular and non-secular factions of society.

Central to this rethinking of identity in the context of human rights is the notion and symbol of silence. By drawing attention to the experiences of the 'violated' as a way to recognise their struggles, Shamsie and Hanif both imagine Islamopolitics as a form of political theatre that essentially legitimises and codifies fundamentalism. This validation of literalism in Islam transforms the subaltern class by integrating them into the national sphere – giving them a voice – while silencing the middle-class, secular elites as threats and targets. The triangulation between dialogue, language, and violence in both narratives points to the state's transgressions in the degradation and dehumanisation of the individual for political capital. In creating these stories as narrative petitions with the intent to establish an ethics of recognition of those abandoned by the law, both authors put forward an argument that Pakistan – a society which at a certain point stopped building bridges between its diverse communities – needs a new type of literature to aid in rebuilding those bridges for the future.

'Silence' is Shamsie's muse in *Broken Verses*. Inspired by Azhar Jaffery's black-and-white photographs of members of the Women's Action Forum (WAF) marching against the newly passed 'Law of Evidence' in 1983, Shamsie 'piece[s] together a collage of different images' (2013: 12) to create a larger-than-life female heroine:

> As a novelist, I was interested in silences – those periods of history that don't enter official narratives or are pushed to the margins – but thereafter I started to say that I was interested in the missing pictures [...] pictures that exist but weren't in the newspapers at the time they should have been the main story. [...] I could swear that it was in the moment of looking at those images that the character of the activist mother in my novel *Broken Verses* started to form.
>
> (2013: 11)

Broken Verses focuses primarily on the silencing of women by a regime that authorises patriarchal repression. While the Universal Declaration of Human Rights does not include specific language about women's rights, Article 2 guarantees that everyone is 'entitled to all the rights and freedoms set forth in this Declaration, without distinction of any kind, such as race, colour, sex, language, religion, political or other opinion, national or social origin, property, birth or other status' (1948 n.p.). As Charlotte Bunch notes,

> feminists redefine human rights abuses to include the degradation and violation of women. The specific experiences of women must be added to traditional approaches to human rights in order to make women more visible and to transform the concept and practice of human rights in our culture so that it takes better account of women's lives.
>
> (1990: 487)

Shamsie captures this spirit by giving an account of a female political activist, Samina Akram, whose personal and political life mark her as a feminist; not only does she defy state authority by organising women's protests, she also goes against social expectations by entering into a highly public post-divorce relationship with a dissident poet, Ashiq. Her story is relayed posthumously through the first-person narration of her daughter, Aasmaani, who is forced to confront her past after receiving a series of cryptic letters. Remembering Samina's legacy fuels an ethics of recognition initially denied to the women protesters in the photographs. Such an homage is testament to the novel's desire to act as a narrative petition, to destabilise official history and make room for women victimised by the patriarchal order. Their refusal to be silenced essentially reflects their desire to establish women's rights as human rights.

Thematically, Shamsie approaches the concept of 'silence' by complicating Gayatri Spivak's earlier theorisations of 'speaking' as a way to discover one's voice or agency in entering into a dialogic exchange. In her influential essay 'Can the Subaltern Speak?', Spivak famously examines the way the 'third-world subject is represented within Western discourse'; paying specific attention to the subaltern subject, the economically dispossessed and politically disenfranchised peasant, she attests that even though the subaltern can *talk*, they cannot *speak*. *Speaking*, in her terminology, is 'a transaction between speaker and listener' (2010: 49): subaltern *talk* does not attain what she calls the dialogic level of utterance. *Broken Verses* expands on the idea of transmission, arguing that when theological language becomes the medium of exchange, the power dynamics shift in a way that makes it possible for the subaltern classes to gain greater visibility in the national sphere. In an ironic reversal, under Islamic regimes, it is the uneducated, often illiterate, subaltern classes who find their fundamentalist views legitimised and authorised by the state: in the new Pakistan, Shamsie writes, 'religion [comes] out from behind its veil of privacy and into the realm of politics' (2005: 91). Shamsie describes the *ummah* as consisting mostly of 'young, idealistic, confused, angry, devout, ready-to-be-brainwashed boys', who become pawns to be disposed of in the war in Afghanistan – a military campaign presented to the pious as 'a matter of religious duty' (2005: 285). State-sponsored Islamisation succeeds in giving voice to the subalterns by hailing them as agents of change; as the novel illustrates, Islamopolitics mobilises historically marginalised social and economic groups by appealing directly to identity politics. Indeed, the calculated valorisation of the subaltern classes carried Zia to victory in the 1984 referendum, where 94% of the voters expressed support for the government's Islamic agenda.

In contrast, the educated elite, shocked by the desecularisation of the constitution and wary of expressing any objections, is condemned to silence. Indeed, for Shamsie the silencing of the traditional ruling groups is so complete that even the language of democracy is taken away from them, co-opted by those who ultimately wish to end it:

> The battle-lines were so clearly drawn then with the military and the religious groups firmly allied, neatly bundling together all that the progressive democratic forces fought against. Now it was all in disarray, the religious right talking democracy better than anyone else.
>
> (2005: 73)

The nation has in effect erected a 'democratic façade', reinforcing the idea of Islamopolitics as political theatre with only certain characters allotted speaking roles (2005: 73). By empowering the subaltern classes at the expanse of the secular elite, Islamopolitics blocks any possibility of dialogue between different segments of the society: 'This move towards theocracy sent violent tremors down the spine of the women's movement, which knew that Zia's Islam concerned itself primarily with striking down the rights of women and befriending fundamentalists' (2005: 138). After she witnesses the introduction of Hudood in 1977, which criminalised 'immoral' behaviour by women (by making offences such as fornication and adultery punishable by stoning to death and amputation), Samina realises that women of all walks of life will be robbed of their ability to speak for themselves.[2] This is consistent with what Bunch describes as a fear-mongering tactic for the gendered body: 'The message is domination: stay in your place or be afraid' (1990: 491). When Samina finds out about the imprisonment of Safia Bibi, a thirteen-year-old rape victim who could not prove her assault due to her blindness, she understands that women are to be reduced to an utterly abject position not just beyond expression, but beyond choice and will.[3]

Silence eventually leads to violence, which finds its grimmest expression in the torture and killing of Ashiq. The literal silencing of the poet – who was known, ironically, as 'the voice of resistance' – shows how individuals in this new and silenced version of Pakistan morph into mere bodies to be disciplined, re-educated, and exterminated once they become threats. Aasmaani recalls reading about the poet's torture and death in the tabloids:

> Here were details, graphic details, of the broken bones, the features smashed beyond recognition, the purple bruise that his face had become.
> No teeth remained inside his mouth.
> His tongue was a stump of muscle.
> [...]
> Smashed beyond recognition.
>
> (2005: 168)

The individual stripped of rights becomes an inanimate, fragmented, and mutilated body. The violated body as spectacle showcases the calculating and dispassionate banality of state brutality as a control mechanism – what Marjorie Agosin and Janice Molloy describe as 'The body in pain as property of state' (1988: 181). This type of brutality is clearly a sign of 'the structural relationships of power [and] domination' symptomatic of government corruption (Bunch 1990: 491).

More intriguing is the way silence is presented as contagious. Violent silencing, in other words, begets more, self-inflicted silence as a response: Samina, unable to cope with the death of the poet, commits suicide. Her self-willed silence spreads to her daughter as Aasmaani distances herself from her mother's world by embracing an apolitical, apathetic persona – her numb, robotic detailing of Ashiq's killing further signals her emotive disentanglement. Rather than idealising the previous generation's ambitions and emulating them, she perceives them as 'victims of a mullah dictator' (Kanwal 2015: 138) whose lives present 'a lesson in futility' (Shamsie 2005: 287). If her narrative is supposed to provide a testimony to the insuperable idealism of Zia's victims, Aasmaani comes across as an unwilling pseudo-witness.[4] Such detachment points to 'the total usurpation of one's personal life by the dictatorship in an atmosphere of asphyxia and terror. The individual exists or ceases to exist according to the whim of the state' (Agosin and Molloy 1988: 187). Redemption is only available through an acknowledgement of her own voice: Aasmaani ends her silence only when she is able to come to terms with her mother's suicide, and work towards making that voice public by speaking about her mother's story in a documentary.[5] Her recuperated agency asserts the idea that 'words continue [...] to be both the battleground and the weapon' (Shamsie 2005: 222).

Silence plays a similarly potent role in Hanif's *A Case of Exploding Mangoes*. Obsessed with Zia's death in a plane explosion, Hanif, then a news correspondent working for BBC London, starts investigating the President's assassination as a journalist. When he realises that he will be unable to solve the crime due to the reluctance of eyewitnesses, he turns to fiction: 'What if, fictionally, I raise my hand and say, "Look, I did it"?' (Filkins 2016: 31). This role-playing is the premise behind the author's 'satirical thriller' in which Zia appears as a self-aggrandising narcissist (as opposed to fear-inducing despot). Shamsie describes Hanif's belittlement as poetic retribution: 'Hanif is essentially saying, let's not see Zia as a big man, as a monster – let's see him as a pathetic man. [...] This book feels like revenge' (2013: 32). The plot, switching between first- and third-person narration, thickens as more potential murder suspects materialise – including not only plausible aspirants such as political rivals, a rape victim named blind Zainab (a nod to Safia Bibi), or the members of the sweepers union, but also magic realist avatars including a crow and 'tunneling' worms (Hanif 2008: 95).

The protagonist of the novel, Ali Shigri, closely resembles Aasmaani – a disillusioned army recruit plagued by his father's suspicious death. Suspecting Zia of orchestrating his father's suicide, he resolves to poison the general during a ceremonial military exercise. Cognisant of Ali's plans, Obaid, a close confidant and love interest, steals a plane in the hopes of delaying Zia's visit to the base. Set in 'a cocooned military world', the novel gestures towards a Gramscian idea of the subaltern, placing various military personnel in plainly subordinate and voiceless positions (Shamsie 2009: 17). The symbolic silencing of the militarised subaltern is reinforced by the two characters' involvement with the 'Silent Drill Squad', in which commands are given non-verbally. Silence is introduced as a form of self-restraint and, ultimately, power: according to the lieutenant, 'A drill without commands is an art. When you deliver a command at the top of your voice, only the boys in your squadron listen. But when your inner cadence whispers, the gods take notice' (2008: 21). At the same time, those at the bottom of the hierarchy are denied their right to remain silent: both Ali and Obaid find themselves prisoners in a state facility used for torture. There, they are forced to confess to whatever 'the gods' desire – and revert back to silence once they fulfil their part. The military and the prison are the ultimate spaces in which silent obedience is required of all individuals – to the extent that the individual is defined no longer on the basis of agency but on the basis of their complicity with the rituals imposed by the higher-ups.

The prison, a space removed from normal human rights expectations and structures, ultimately complicates the basic idea of silence and introduces the idea of 'unspeakability' – a concept that obfuscates the line between humanity and monstrosity. Hanif's detailed description of the state's torture chambers at the fort, a historical site turned into a secret government facility, effectively unveils the 'traumatic side of history' (Kozol 2012: 175). Ali finds himself in a group of detainees whose rights have been suspended indefinitely as they await charges for their alleged crimes. His anticipation of torture normalises the state's lawlessness: he accepts that it will treat the prisoners as punishable and perishable bodies to be disciplined and, if necessary, exterminated. Ali's torture begins in a filthy bathroom:

> That terrible smell of the closed toilet, which has not seen a drop of water for ages, welcomes me, my head hits the wall, and a thousand-watt bulb is switched on. So bright is the light, so over-powering the stench, that I cannot see anything for the first few moments. [...] There is a hole in the ground so full of indistinguishable faeces that bubbles are forming on its surface.
>
> (2008: 87)

Hanif skilfully uses sensory images to convey this form of 'soft' torture in which the reader 'becomes a participant' by 'enter[ing] into a world of human brutality and violence' (Agosin and Molloy 1988: 191). In this environment, Ali is reduced to mere animal biology as he struggles to remain in charge of his bodily functions surrounded by excrement. Despite his drowsiness, he forces himself to remain on his feet so that he does not 'give these butchers the pleasure of watching [him] lie down in this pool of piss' (2008: 88). Even though he is determined to appear in control – just enough to preserve his autonomy and dignity – his physical needs soon take over: first, he urinates in his pants ('soaking wet'), then, as fatigue takes over, he is subsumed by the environment, becoming indistinguishable from the filth.

Unlike Shamsie's poet, who is physically tortured beyond recognition, Ali is tormented through wordless degradation; his symbolic transformation into waste not only signals his dehumanisation but also his delegitimisation as a citizen under the protection of the state. Hanif is careful to present a form of torture that specifically targets Ali's dignity, denying him the human quality that requires the preservation of moral and legal rights.[6] As tortured bodies, the prisoners at the fort remain outside the protection of the law; thus, they are disqualified from their status as citizens. Reduced to a subhuman category incapable of political exchange, these prisoners are discarded by the state as unfit for assimilation. Torture, the very act that forces people to speak to implicate others, is also a way of silencing the suspect, and robbing him/her of humanity by denying a voice. And of course torture removes the victim's ability to determine the nature of his/her own narrative: the subject of torture ultimately ends up voicing whatever story their torturers wish them to articulate. Removing one's ability to narrate one's own story is like removing one's connection with humanity; for Maria Gabriela Zoana, 'Human dignity consists in having one's own story to tell and in not subsuming one's own point of view to the impersonal needs of the legal system' (2011: 197).

As in *Broken Verses*, silencing as an act of exclusion proves contagious: like Aasmaani, Ali eventually embraces a self-willed silence, a form of escape and a strategy to avoid confronting his complicity in another's pain. In an unexpected twist, when Ali is released from his cell, and is invited to have tea in the garden of the fort, he sees Obaid in the distance with the other detainees. The physical signs of torture are evident on Obaid's body: 'the fuckers ironed his head' (2008: 224). Trapped inside his deformed body, Obaid is no longer a human being but a spectacle; not a sovereign subject, but an object to be manipulated by the state. Still, it is not the embodied experience of torture or the corporal infliction of pain that immediately triggers Ali's desperation. Rather, it is the psychological torment that stems from his own treachery: 'I signed a fucking statement because you were dead. I cut a bloody deal because you were supposed to have been blown to bits because of your own stupidity' (2008: 224). Knowing that he betrayed Obaid under pressure augments Ali's sense of dehumanisation as he becomes complicit in the torture of another. Unable to confess his remorse, Ali is condemned to a guilt-ridden silence.

Ultimately, the motif of silencing has ramifications beyond the suppression of individual agency; it is also a repressive state apparatus used to reinforce an anti-intellectual climate in which science is cast aside for the benefit of religion – a point elegantly explored in Uzma Aslam Khan's *The Geometry of God* (2009). In the novel, Khan introduces multiple narrative voices to depict national fractures and conflicted allegiances: a scientifically minded young woman, Amal; her blind, highly intuitive sister, Mehwish; and their admirer, Noman, who is burdened by his father's political ambitions to expose Zahoor (the girls' grandfather) as a heretic due to his propagation of Darwinism. Amal fears that her grandfather's obsession with palaeontology will make him a target:

> Nana has been angering a lot of people at the university where he teaches. He points out what others overlook. While the Soviets bomb Afghanistan for the seventh year, Pakistan Television no longer broadcasts weather forecasts because predictions of rain have become witchery. Science and history books are being rewritten. Teaching evolution is banned. Nana says to learn is to search for what isn't written, or rewritten. He has become a dangerous man.
>
> (Khan 2009: 41)

The state's 'cultural war' against secular intellectuals, who are invested in articulating a cosmopolitan Pakistani identity backed up by archaeological evidence, is an attempt at flattening the national history (2009: 115). Zahoor understands that Zia's Islamisation of civic and political life will essentially 'change knowledge [...] irreversibly' and redefine public memory to render it consistent with religious nationalism (2009: 15). The juxtaposition between 'the scientific methods of palaeontology and religious obscurantism' essentially masks the state's 'deeper anxiety' about cultivating a multidimensional Pakistani identity that negates religious purity (Kabir 2011: 175). As Ananya Jahanara Kabir notes, 'Through *prehistory*, [...], Aslam Khan navigates an identity politics beset with violence and uncertainty. Palaeontology, an intellectual endeavour, becomes the means of extracting this knowledge' vital in producing 'counter-Islamic' foresight (2011: 180). Extracting unbiased, scientific knowledge, then, is the true antidote to silencing.

When the Universal Declaration of Human Rights was ratified by the United Nations General Assembly in 1948, Pakistan not only sided with the original majority and signed the declaration, but also openly disagreed with Saudi Arabia's early critique of Article 18 (which affords the individual the right 'to change his religion or belief') as violating basic tenets of *sharia* law. With that agreement came a commitment from member states to recognise that 'the inherent dignity and [...] the equal and inalienable rights of all members of the human family is the foundation of freedom, justice and peace in the world' (1948 n.p.). Indeed, the 1956 constitution embraced life and liberty as paramount values of civil rights, and included clauses on freedom of speech and expression, as well as assembly and association. It was not until 1973 that the early signs of Islam's impact on the law became clear; Article 19 made provisions on the freedom of speech, stating:

> Every citizen shall have the right to freedom of speech and expression, and there shall be freedom of the press, subject to any reasonable restrictions imposed by law in the interest of the glory of Islam or the integrity, security or defence of Pakistan or any part thereof, friendly relations with foreign States, public order, decency or morality, or in relation to contempt of court.
> (Constitution of the Islamic Republic of Pakistan, art. 19 1973)

Pakistan's support of the Universal Declaration of Human Rights continued to waver over the years as a result of Zia's influence, eventually culminating in the signing of the 'Cairo Declaration on Human Rights in Islam' in 1990. This new agreement affirmed Islamic law's primacy in matters of religious freedom and gender equality, launching an alternative set of rights based on *sharia* ethics.

What is abandoned by the law is preserved in the works of fiction writers. Hanif's Ali wonders how he will be able to leave his prison cell as he is being fed: 'You want freedom and they give you chicken korma' (2008: 147). But that food symbolises the uncertainty of his fate, and the indefinite duration of his incarceration. Contemplating his situation with his next-door neighbour, he observes:

> We sit in silence for a while. The absence of any prospects of freedom in the near future hangs heavy in the air. Suddenly, this plate of rich, hot food seems like the promise of a long sentence. I feel the walls of this dungeon closing in on me.
> (2008: 156)

Similarly, Aasmaani reflects on the meaning of freedom by showing the disconnect between what the constitution says and how it is implemented by the state: 'Freedom of speech was all very well, but there was no need to exercise it against a government that was helping in the fight against Communism' (Shamsie 2005: 54). In his meeting with an old acquaintance, the value of freedom is reiterated: 'You must have freedom, even in times of war and barbarity' (217). Both Shamsie and Hanif show the challenges of incorporating the subaltern class into the national sphere via the state's populist politicisation of religion. In many ways, their efforts express a desire to define the modern individual by articulating the relationship between one's body and autonomy. As Judith Butler reminds us, 'essential to so many political movements is the claim of bodily integrity and self-determination. It is important to claim that our bodies are in a sense our own and that we are entitled to claim rights of autonomy over our bodies' (2004: 25).[7] At the same time, Shamsie and Hanif make the case that a direct consequence of Zia's regime is the refocusing of Islamophobia within the Muslim homeland: in this context, Islamophobia becomes the province of the secular elite, who care little about heresy, but fear that their basic rights as citizens are under attack – as we see in the case of Zahoor, who does not oppose religion but fears its manipulation under corrupt regimes.

If in totalitarian regimes the individual loses the ability to defend him/herself against injustices, the task falls to the writer to expose the state's wrongdoings and to create a forum in which the victims can speak. In this regard, storytelling becomes a way of questioning the legitimacy of the state. If there is no accountability, if there is no way of restoring the positive rights of the individual when those rights are violated in the name of religion, then, in Hannah Arendt's words, we face 'expulsion from humanity altogether' (1976: 297).

Notes

1 As Kanwal notes, 'There is no denying that Islamic radicalism and the culture of intolerance inaugurated by Zia continue to have significant social, cultural and political momentum in contemporary Pakistan' (2015: 8).
2 According to Maleeha Aslam, 'Misogyny was institutionalized in law […]. The state started promoting *ulema* for political gains and to give Islam an "official" face. Maceration of the feminine side of Islam was indirectly allowed by a state that was driven by "militaristic machismo" and interested in promoting an "*ulemasculinised* theology" that was primarily "aggressive and violent"' (2012: 158).
3 The law that states 'an accusation of rape could only be proved in a court of law if there were four pious, male Muslim adults willing to give eye-witness testimony' (Shamsie 2005: 92).
4 Aasmaani writes: 'All those years she had fought against Zia's government – she and the poet – with rallies and speeches and poems. And it had got them nowhere. It had got him tortured and killed; it had got her – well, there were no words for that either' (Shamsie 2005: 139). This passage clearly reveals Aasmaani's inability to employ language to describe her mother's agony. But it also shows her reluctance get involved emotionally.
5 Madeline Clements argues that 'It is the living, spoken word, as expressed through contemporary and populist media – documentaries, drama, poetry, song – in which *Broken Verses*' strong-minded female characters invest greatest hope' (2016: 140).
6 As David Luban writes, 'Torture is among the most fundamental affronts to human dignity', which is essential in the preservation of moral and legal rights in democratic societies (2007: 163).
7 As Ignatieff notes, 'Human rights is a language of individual empowerment, and empowerment for individuals is desirable because when individuals have agency, they can protect themselves against injustice' (2001: 57).

Bibliography

Abbas, S. (2014) *At Freedom's Limit: Islam and the Postcolonial Predicament*. New York: Oxford University Press.
Agosin, M. (1987) 'So We Will Not Forget: "Literature and Human Rights in Latin America"'. Trans. by Molloy, J. *Human Rights Quarterly* 10(2), 177–192.
Arendt, H. (1976) *The Origins of Totalitarianism*. Orlando: A Harvest Book.
Aslam, M. (2012) *Gender-based Explosions: The Nexus between Muslim Masculinities, Jihadist Islamism and Terrorism*. New York: United Nations University Press.
Bunch, C. (1990) 'Women's Rights as Human Rights: Toward a Re-vision of Human Rights'. *Human Rights Quarterly* 12(4), 486–498.
Butler, J. (2004) *Precarious Life: The Powers of Mourning and Violence*. London: Verso.
Clements, M. (2016) *Writing Islam from a South Asian Muslim Perspective: Rushdie, Hamid, Aslam, Shamsie*. Basingstoke: Palgrave Macmillan.
Constitution of the Islamic Republic of Pakistan. 10 April 1973. Available from <www.pakistani.org/pakistan/constitution/> [26 June 2017].
Filkins, D. (2016) 'Dangerous Fictions'. *The New Yorker* [online]. Available from <www.newyorker.com/magazine/2016/05/09/a-pakistani-novelist-tests-the-limits> [10 July 2017].
Ghose, Z. (1966) *The Contradictions*. London: Macmillan.
Ghose, Z. (1967) *The Murder of Aziz Khan*. London: Macmillan.
Hanif, M. (2008). *A Case of Exploding Mangos*. New York: Vintage Books.
Ignatieff, M. (2001) 'Human Rights as Politics and Idolatry'. In *Human Rights as Politics and Idolatry*. Ed. by Gutmann, A. Princeton: Princeton University Press, 3–98.
Kabir, A.J. (2011) 'Deep Topographies in the Fiction of Uzma Aslam Khan'. *Journal of Postcolonial Writing* 47(2), 173–185.
Kanwal, A. (2015) *Rethinking Identities in Contemporary Pakistani Fiction: Beyond 9/11*. Basingstoke: Palgrave.
Khan, U.A. (2009) *The Geometry of God*. Northampton, MA: Clockroot Books.
Kozol, W. (2012) 'Complicities of Witnessing in Joe Sacco's *Palestine*'. In *Theoretical Perspectives on Human Rights and Literature*. Ed. by Goldberg, E.S. and Moore, A.S. New York: Routledge, 165–179.
Luban, D. (2007) *Legal Ethics and Human Dignity*. New York: Cambridge University Press.
Morton, S. (2007) *Salman Rushdie: Fictions of Postcolonial Modernity*. London: Palgrave.
Rushdie, S. (1983) *Shame*. New York: Picador.

Santesso, E.M. (2017) 'Introduction'. In *Islam and Postcolonial Discourse*. Ed. by Santesso, E.M. and McClung, J. London: Routledge, 1–12.

Schaffer, K. and Smith, S. (2004) *Human Rights and Narrated Lives: The Ethics of Recognition*. New York: Palgrave.

Shamsie, K. (2005) *Broken Verses*. Orlando: A Harvest Original.

Shamsie, K (2013) 'The Missing Picture'. *World Literature Today* 87(2), 10–13.

Shamsie, M. (2009) 'Covert Operations in Pakistani Fiction'. *Commonwealth* 31(2), 15–25.

Shamsie, M. (2010) 'Pakistan'. *The Journal of Commonwealth Literature* 45(4), 641–658.

Spivak, G. (2010) 'Can the Subaltern Speak?' In *Can the Subaltern Speak? Reflections on the History of an Idea*. Ed. by Morris, R.C. New York: Columbia University Press, 21–78.

The United Nations. (1948) Universal Declaration of Human Rights [online]. Available from <www.un.org/en/universal-declaration-human-rights/> [26 June 2017].

Zoana, M.G. (2011) 'Torture, Ill-treatment, and Human Rights'. *Review of Contemporary Philosophy* 10, 196–201.

12
DIVERGENT DISCOURSES
Human rights and contemporary Pakistani anglophone literature

Shazia Sadaf

The rise of human rights literature

Pakistani anglophone literature has come of age at a very crucial point in the geopolitical history of modern civilisations. The role of these writings is both valuable and disputable, as is reflected in its widely divergent reception by global and local audiences, and in its ambivalent position *vis-à-vis* universal human rights debates. Therefore, an examination of how Pakistani anglophone literature speaks to the global reader is not only timely, but valuable for its insights.

After the events of 11 September 2001, human rights have become an increasingly important area of enquiry with changing perceptions of the US involvement in the War on Terror and the ensuing global questions about the human cost of this project. This has led to a simultaneous rise of three areas of scholarly interest: 9/11 literature, human rights discourse and War on Terror studies. The resulting intersections between literature and human rights, foregrounded by an overarching narrative of terror, have opened a new line of interdisciplinary enquiry broadly classed under the label 'human rights literature'.

Lynn Hunt's (2007) historiography of human rights as an 'invention' stemming from the Western literary tradition, Joseph Slaughter's (2007) work on the relationship between law and literature, and Elizabeth Anker's (2012) views on human rights discourses that validate Western values are recent theoretical works that have urged an exploration of the complications that arise when the postcolonial *Bildungsroman* becomes complicit in the projects of globalisation and neo-imperialism. Besides fiction, non-fictional genres like memoirs have prompted readings of 'life narratives and human rights campaigns as multidimensional domains that merge and intersect at critical points, unfolding within and enfolding one another in an ethical relationship that is simultaneously productive of claims for social justice and problematic for the furtherance of this goal' (Schaffer & Smith 2004: 2). Such diverse and complex readings of both fiction and non-fiction writings have required academics to address urgently the pedagogical challenges in the effective utilisation of this literature in the classroom (Moore and Goldberg 2015).

Anker's recent essay 'Teaching the Legal Imperialism Debate over Human Rights' calls attention to the increasing focus on the postcolonial world in human rights discourse, which makes humanitarianism and human rights activism synonymous with Western foreign aid projects. By extension, it judges postcolonial nation states' respect for human rights as a measurement of their civilisational progress (2015: 39). Anker warns that challenging human rights in a literature classroom requires the instructor to be unusually circumspect because of the general resistance to a critique of its motives, and that a delicate balance must be maintained between the interrogation of rights and larger considerations of social justice (2015: 40). One of the techniques she proposes is to introduce students to the cultural imperialism[1] debate in human rights, and to frame texts within a history of colonisation (2015: 41).

A broader contextualisation of contemporary literary texts within the colonial history of the Indian subcontinent can yield important insights into the current contradictions within human rights debates in the post-9/11 period: for example, the contradiction of how the logic of universal human rights discourse can coexist in a world in which undefinable[2] enemies are excluded from the same rights through legal codification. The continuity of such 'states of exception'[3] can be traced in the usage of terms like 'Subjects' instead of 'Citizens' during empire, to 'illegal enemy combatants'[4] instead of 'prisoners of war (POW)' in the recent War on Terror. In both cases, human rights exceptions have been justified: on moral grounds of the civilising mission in the former case, and in the interest of national security in the latter. Therefore, in response to these suggestions, it is important to foster a nuanced approach for the teaching of Pakistani literature through a human rights lens, in the light of the geopolitical history that complicates its role in the global War on Terror.

A helpful introductory note for intersectional scholarship in human rights literature, 9/11 writing and War on Terror studies is the idea of human empathy. It is interesting that the English term 'empathy' has its origins only in the early twentieth century. From its initial usage in the field of psychology, the word entered popular vocabulary around the same time as the formal articulation of human rights in the 1940s. British psychologist Edward Bradford Titchener first translated the word from the German *Einfühlung* ('in-feeling')[5] as 'empathy' in 1909.[6] The shift from the concept of sympathy, which stood for 'aesthetic feeling' in the nineteenth century, to the coining of the term 'empathy' in the twentieth, which is associated with 'social understanding', has meant that the latter is used synonymously with altruism and social justice (Swanson 2013: 128). The application of this word has also expanded from psychology into social sciences and the humanities.

Literature's capacity to evoke empathy in readers has been identified as a key factor in the recognition of human dignity and humanitarian action (Hunt 2007; Slaughter 2007, 2012; Barnett 2011; Anker 2012; O'Gorman 2015). As Amy Kaminsky reminds us, 'the right to produce, circulate, and read literary texts is a subset of human rights, literature constitutes a piece of the very stuff of human rights' (2009: 44). Article 19 of the Universal Declaration of Human Rights guarantees freedom of expression and the right to 'receive and impart information and ideas through any media and regardless of frontiers' (1948: n.p.). In a fractured post-9/11 world, literature has the potential to re-establish humanitarian connections. Mohsin Hamid's belief that 'the core skill of a novelist is empathy', because 'the world is suffering from a deficit of empathy at the moment' (2007: n.p.) reflects the conscious movement of new Pakistani writers towards bridging cultural divisions through fiction. Nadeem Aslam shows a similar commitment when he says, 'I must find what I have in common with others. Not what sets me apart […] then the book will have a better chance of connecting with others' (2010: n.p.). This heightened sense of responsibility to emphasise sameness rather than difference is a key feature of contemporary Pakistani fiction.

The rising interest in this area can be gauged from a recent scientific experiment carried out at the University of Toronto to investigate literature's potential to increase empathy in readers (Djikic, Oatley, and Moldoveanu 2013). The results, published in *Scientific Study of Literature*, suggest a positive role for literature in facilitating the development of empathy. Yet, human rights literature sets itself a difficult task simply because human rights concerns can have shifting perspectives in a culturally diverse world under the pressures of globalisation. Despite the post-Cold War era being dubbed the period of 'solidarity' in human rights, and despite all efforts to promote a global human rights awareness, international forums are still divided about what these rights are, and how they will be enforced. To date, the largest obstacle to attaining human rights ideals is different interpretations of the term in various regions around the world.

Historians and writers, however, have responded differently to the stalemate. Unlike political theorists and activists, who champion cultural relativism and level charges of cultural imperialism against human rights discourse, the onset of globalisation has spurred literary historians to look beyond the particular/universal divide by focusing on the nuances of the political language of human rights in different cultural contexts (Cmiel 2004: 119–120). The point is to look at local histories of human rights that make 'universal claims'. Taken in this sense, 'human rights talk communicates across cultures in ways similar to money, statistics, pidgin English, or a discussion of soccer' (Cmiel 2004: 126). As far as writers' contribution to these debates is concerned, the future of international human rights can only be meaningful if there is a careful balance between representations of local cultures and the globalised world, and if regional political movements are not completely neglected in the face of larger political claims.

A new turn in Pakistani anglophone fiction[7]

It is perhaps significant that concurrently with the development of human rights literature as a distinct field, a new wave of Pakistani writing emerged on the anglophone literary scene. Indeed, authors including Kamila Shamsie, Hamid, Aslam, Daniyal Mueenuddin, Muhammad Hanif, and Jamil Ahmad have attracted significant international accolades and literary prizes. These emerging writers, jokingly dubbed the 'Pak Pack' by Shamsie (quoted in Shah 2010), have captured more attention post-9/11 than at any prior time, mainly because the event caused an identity crisis within the country which the Pakistani intelligentsia has felt a responsibility to address in a more globally accessible language medium; but also, with international focus turning to Pakistan's role in the War on Terror, Pakistani anglophone writers have found a more receptive publishing industry in the West that is ready to capitalise on the global curiosity about Pakistan and neighbouring Afghanistan. Even though his tongue-in-cheek exasperation is clear, Mueenuddin realises the benefits of seizing the world market:

> When it comes to Pakistani writing, I would encourage us all to remember the brand. We are custodians of brand Pakistan. And beneficiaries. The brand slaps an extra zero onto our advances, if not more. Branding can be the difference between a novel about brown people and a best-selling novel about brown people. It is our duty to maintain and build that brand [...] people from all over the world have come to know and love brand Pakistan for its ability to scare the shit out of them. Whatever you write, please respect this legacy. We're providing a service here. We're a twenty-storey straight-down vertical-dropping roller coaster for the mind. Yes, love etcetera is permissible. But bear in mind that Pakistan is a market-leader. The Most Dangerous Place in the World™.
>
> (2010a: n.p.)

Mueenuddin's dark humour, however, does not undercut the seriousness with which fiction writers have taken this opportunity to produce narratives that offer an alternative approach to 9/11-related themes and which shift perspectives on human rights in relation to the War on Terror.

Any critical engagement with this new wave of Pakistani fiction must address three areas in which it makes a significant contribution. Besides its role as a valuable counter-narrative to 9/11 writings in the West, and its position in the War on Terror debates, Pakistani fiction seeks alignments of vision towards a future beyond recent events. This shifts the focus from 9/11 as a site for trauma writing, to include the equally calamitous issues of human rights that have resulted in its global aftermath. Fiction has the potential to achieve these ends by evoking empathy and encouraging a broader contextual understanding of past events leading to the current situation. At the same time, it must also counter the unidirectional creation of knowledge about Pakistan and Islam by the larger volume of Western 9/11 narratives available to a global readership.

A pertinent point here is to delineate the two different kinds of anglophone writings by Pakistani authors that have met with an avid reception in the Western literary market in the post-9/11 period. Both strains connect with human rights discourse, in divergent ways. Firstly, there are biographical works, mostly by women, often written in collaboration with journalists, which are intentionally geared towards rights awareness; secondly, there are works of fiction which have the potential to be read as rights narratives that problematise commonly understood interpretations of human rights. The fact that these publications have elicited very different responses at home and abroad epitomises the ideological divide of Pakistani society caught in a flux between a nationalistic defensiveness and the pressures of globalisation.

In the post-9/11 period, forces of cultural imperialism have inspired a pronounced nationalist reaction in Pakistan, because of which reading locally produced works of fiction as human rights narratives has become doubly problematic. Pakistani authors find themselves navigating the paradox of conflicting responsibilities: to write about present-day injustices caused by the failure of the state without being accused of subscribing to Western agendas that promote the same instances of violence to justify military aggression in Pakistan.

The reaction of readers in Pakistan to recent fiction has been complicated by the rise of a nationalist sentiment precipitated by the 'us vs them' rhetoric of the Bush administration in the wake of 9/11. Pakistani authors, on the other hand, are not only sensitive to reader's sentiment in Pakistan, but also demonstrate an awareness of their responsibility to bridge cultural barriers through the written word, increasingly making a mark in global academia. Novels like Hamid's *The Reluctant Fundamentalist* (2013) are read in postcolonial courses at universities around the world as an example of 'writing back' to the West, and as such are classed in the confrontational postcolonial category. Others, like *The Wasted Vigil* (2008) by Aslam, or *Burnt Shadows* (2009) by Shamsie, which speak directly to the War on Terror and its effect on Pakistani identity, are read as examples of contemporary transnational literature emerging from countries previously grouped as 'postcolonial'. Because the move from the term 'postcolonial' to 'transnational' as a course title for global anglophone literature study favours a 'bridging' role of works from countries with a colonial past, it problematises the role of Pakistani writers in that their fiction oscillates between a defensive tone and one of optimism about overcoming differences in a period marked as a 'clash of civilisations'. Their writings are, consequently, divergent discourses.

From Hamid's *The Reluctant Fundamentalist* to his recent novel *Exit West* (2017), the effort to both write back and write beyond 9/11 is evident. In his latest work of speculative fiction, through the story of Saeed and Nadia, who are citizens of an unknown country, Hamid moves beyond a clinging colonial past and hurtles into an immigrant future. What is interesting in this fairy-tale world is the presence of magical 'doors' that open into destinations around the world, literally defying the 'borders' that divide people today. These doors that allow access, unchecked by barbed wire and walls, are wormholes through the border security concerns that have hampered cross-cultural understanding in recent years.

Hamid himself points to the importance of Pakistani literature's unique offering, in that it is location-specific yet pluralistic, in contrast to the dominant discourses of globalisation:

> I think Pakistan matters, not just to myself and other Pakistanis, nor only because it is beset with terrorism and possesses nuclear weapons, but because Pakistan is a test bed for pluralism on a globalizing planet that desperately needs more pluralism. Pakistan's uncertain democracy and unsteady attempt to fashion a future in which its citizens can live together in peace are an experiment that mirrors our global experiment as human beings on a shared Earth. The world will not fail if Pakistan fails, but the world will be healthier if Pakistan is healthy.
>
> (Hamid 2014: 5)

Yet, at the same time, Hamid also feels that it is time for writers' attention to turn to the future:

> I think we need to radically reimagine the future. Citizens, artist, writers, politicians, everyone. What's happening now is our failure to come up with radical new futures that we think could maybe come in to [sic] existence. If we don't, then that space is abandoned to people who are peddling nostalgic disasters.
>
> (Hamid qtd. in Milo 2017: n.p.)

It is interesting that Hamid's idea of a radical change is to stop writing cyclically from within a disaster site, which is primarily what 9/11 literature does.

Perhaps the first novelist to lay the groundwork for what fiction written after 9/11 was to achieve was Ian McEwan. Just a few days after the events of 11 September 2001, he wrote about the loss of life in the attacks for the *Guardian* (15 September 2001), making the connection between creative empathy and being human, the main characteristic of human rights literature: 'Imagining what it is like to be someone other than yourself is at the core of our humanity. It is the essence of compassion, and it is the beginning of morality' (2001: n.p.). He also made another important point about the failure of the American public to look beyond their personal and national traumas to the 'policy failures, or geopolitical strategy' that may have led to this catastrophic event. Despite the importance of his points, McEwan attributes the power of empathy only to the American victims, for whom he uses the pronoun 'we' in the essay. He distinctly excludes the attackers from this capacity because of what he sees as their 'dehumanising hatred to purge themselves of the human instinct for empathy'(2001: n.p.). McEwan's approach thus curtails the very use of empathy in overcoming differences by making it exclusive to one side of the Us versus Them divide. Similarly, 9/11 fiction in the West invites a one-way empathy towards American victims, while denying a claim to empathy to the victims of the global reverberations of the consequent War on Terror.

One of the reasons why contemporary Pakistani writers like Shamsie are important in this regard is that their writings make a more balanced appeal to humanity. In *Burnt Shadows*, Shamsie defends the bleak view of all nation states, including America, that justify horrors through a rhetoric of war:

> Too many people seem to think I'm making a particular comment on America, but really I'm talking [sic] about nations in wartime and the particular inhuman logic they start to follow when they decide what is an acceptable price for some other nation's people to pay.
>
> (Shamsie interviewed by Singh 2012: 160)

As Daniel O'Gorman points out, writers from countries like Pakistan have attempted 'blurring the boundaries between the domestic and the foreign in a way that draws attention to the element of the other within the self, as well as the self within the other' (2015: 6). They invite more than just a unidirectional empathy that only perpetuates difference; instead, they draw a pluralistic response that questions the very existence of these divisions.

Thus, Shamsie reminds readers that there is a prior history that feeds into the events of 9/11 and that she has striven to write a novel that does not regard 'that one date as if history proceeds from it but doesn't precede it' (Shamsie interviewed by Singh 2012: 158). Instead of being limited to the cinematic trope of the falling tower popular in the American 9/11 novel, Shamsie's work is what can be termed a 'widescreen'[8] novel, which stretches out horizontally across a wider historical timeline. From the Nagasaki bombings of 1945 to the Partition of India in 1947; from post-Partition Karachi to the 1980s Soviet-Afghan war, *Burnt Shadows* builds up to the attacks in New York in 2001. Significantly, instead of ending there, the narrative engages with the War on Terror and takes the reader to Guantanamo Bay prison in Cuba and the present day. Through a widescreen technique Shamsie stretches the canvas for a historicised perspective on the attacks.

The prologue to Shamsie's *Burnt Shadows* starts with a nameless character in Guantanamo Bay prison, stripped simultaneously of his clothes and his human dignity. His desperate rhetorical question, 'How did it come to this?' (2009: 1) reflects the disconnectedness of people, and the loss of human empathy in the world. The divergent answers to this question offered by different characters in the novel, caught in a sway between optimism and pessimism, represent the ambivalence of Pakistani anglophone writers regarding the geopolitical future of the world beyond 9/11. Indeed, there is a sense of desperation in the hyphenated identities of Shamsie's characters and in their musing like, 'Whatever might be happening in the wider world, at least the Weiss-Burtons and the Tanaka-Ashrafs had finally found spaces to cohabit in, complicated shared history giving nothing but depth to the reservoir of their friendships' (2009: 282). Even in the protagonist Raza's fluid identity, Shamsie tries to cast a wider net for empathy, and emphasises the futility of nationalist identities by making him a biracial child who looks confusingly like a Hazara, is mistaken for an Afghan, and who is a polyglot speaking the languages of the world. The wish to bridge gaps and the nod to transnationalism are obvious.

Although it is in an altogether different style to Shamsie's, Jamil Ahmad's *The Wandering Falcon* (2011) is largely driven by a similar commitment to historicity. However, Ahmad's work is retrospective[9] in its method and content. His interconnected short story collection highlights a long-continuing trend of misunderstanding regarding the ancient tribal ways, from the colonial ways of the British Raj to a postcolonial, post-Partition Pakistan, and beyond to the neo-imperialist US interference in the Soviet-Afghan war. Ahmad's main purpose in writing these stories was to bring about an awareness of the need to preserve these traditional communities against modern warfare, succinctly dubbed 'Global War on the Tribes' by Akbar Ahmed (2013). Ahmad thinks that in sweepingly grouping all tribal people of Pakistan as extremists, the West has only done itself a disservice:

> One thing is very clear, that you see a lot of mistakes have been made in the recent past. [The drone attacks] are, in a way, destroying a system which was a strong countervailing system to [...] [terrorism and] all [that] [...] is happening today.
> (*NPR* interview 2011: n.p.)

Although Ahmad refrains from making direct political statements, he feels disappointed about the destruction of the tribal leadership as a result of Pakistan's and the United States' sponsorship of the Afghan *mujahideen* against the Soviet occupation. In his opinion, this lies at the very root of the escalating problems in this region today: 'I'm angry about it. I could call them [the *mujahideen*] Frankensteins, these monsters who were created and they stood by and watched the tribes being decimated' (*The Nation* 2012).

Ahmad's stories restore the dignity of the ancient communal ways of life seen in the West as uncivilised. By providing a historical understanding of the tarnished tribal belt that is now widely popularised in the Western world as a hub of the Taliban leadership, high-tech warfare, and the target for US drone strikes, the stories offer rare insight into the Pashtun tribal principles that have puzzled the West. These tribal areas bordering Iran and Afghanistan are often reported as 'lawless' and dangerous in the international media. Ahmad's depiction reveals that the nomadic code of life values the collective tribal community over individual identity. This is the main cause of the clash between tribal honour codes and state laws, and the collision between tradition and modernity.

Ahmad's stories, which are based in his real experiences living amongst the tribes as a civil officer, respond to the demonisation of the tribal areas in Pakistan in the post-9/11 period in three significant ways. Firstly, the stories reveal that the history of Pashtun[10] resistance to Western interference is older than their defensive stance on the War on Terror, and their extreme antagonism needs to be contextualised to facilitate better understanding and effective reconciliation. Secondly, that the locals of tribal areas in Pakistan are not radical Islamists. Their allegiance is to the code of *pashtunwali*[11] before religion. Contrary to Western understanding, the ancient code of *pashtunwali* is not directly connected to Islam, but is much older. In fact, the *jirga* system of justice at times contradicts *sharia* law. The third point that Ahmad makes is that, contrary to the view propagated by the UNESCO Charter of the Book, which equates illiteracy with backwardness and places the 'writing man's burden' on the civilised world to educate the non-reading nations (Brouillette 2012: n.p.), the oral traditions of the 'illiterate' tribal groups are grounded in a different, yet highly sophisticated sense of justice that has been practised successfully for centuries. The stories exemplify the complex unwritten laws of the tribes.

It is important to mention that fiction writers in Pakistan have taken a two-pronged approach to human rights in their work: to highlight violations of Pakistani citizens arising from international geopolitical interferences (Shamsie, Aslam, and Hamid), but also to expose failures of the Pakistani state to protect the rights of its citizens, especially women, the underprivileged, and minorities. Examples of the latter would be Hanif's *Our Lady of Alice Bhatti* (2012) and Mueenuddin's *In Other Rooms, Other Wonders* (2010b). Both these works of fiction lay bare issues like acid attacks against women, power politics, police incompetence, gross neglect of patients in hospitals, discrimination against minorities, and rampant corruption. This work is important for its representations of Pakistani women, their rights, and the limitations of their agency.

In his latest novel, *Our Lady of Alice Bhatti*, Hanif says he wanted to create a 'female superhero flying around and kicking ass' but soon felt uncomfortable with the idea (Hanif interviewed by Filkins 2016: n.p.). His wish to create a powerful woman figure reflects recent conceptual developments about female identity in the Pakistani imagination. One example is the success of the animated TV serial of well-known singer Haroon, which is also about a Pakistani super-heroine, a schoolteacher who turns into Burka Avenger to fight the Taliban, who stand against female education. Another parallel is the recent induction of fully veiled women commandos by the Pakistan army, trained to fight terrorists. Contesting views about these veiled figures offer insights into the difficulty of legitimising a Pakistani super-heroine figure, one that fits within the religious and nationalist ideologies of post-9/11 Pakistan. That is why, in trying to find a more relatable Pakistani female figure whose dedication in the face of adversity and hardship appeared to Hanif to be equally heroic, and why he fashioned the eponymous Alice after the nurses he had seen take care of his ill mother in a Karachi hospital.

One wonders if Hanif was being sarcastic when he said he wanted to write about a superwoman figure when he so obviously ends up creating a female saint. Or perhaps he started out with this aim, but discovered during the process the difficulty of such a project. The latter is more likely since the novel shows how Alice is systematically crushed, and Hanif himself comments, 'Alice may have been a superhero, but in Pakistan not even female superheroes can prevail' (Filkins 2016: n.p.). As far as the connection between human rights and literature is concerned, the novel simultaneously succeeds and fails. It succeeds in giving the poor and disadvantaged Alice-the-woman the capability and drive to do what she wants, which challenges the stereotypical image of the subaltern Pakistani woman, while at the same time demonstrating male insecurity through Teddy-Butt-the-Pakistani-man's precarious position in a traditionally patriarchal nation. But the novel fails in that Alice's success is passive and does not derive any action or change through the novel's plot that might stimulate Pakistani readers towards taking concrete steps in real life. Neither does it successfully agitate the universal human rights idiom for Western readers by proposing particular solutions, or local resistance to violence through other characters.

The interlinked stories of Mueenuddin's *In Other Rooms, Other Wonders* open a door into contemporary Pakistan. The female characters come from a broad cross-section of the Pakistani society and do not portray their subjugation under a patriarchal system in isolation, but balance it with the many ways in which they practise their agency within the class divisions. By extension, these stories reflect a society shaped by a traditionally understood concept of masculinity faced with conditions of rapid social and political change. In Mueenuddin's work there is a subtle undercurrent of a threat to this sustained sense of masculinity.[12] Through the complex dynamics between male and female characters, these stories communicate a slow erosion of Pakistani masculinity and highlight the resistance of women to patriarchy within the societal limitations they face. The portrayal of strong women in these contemporary stories challenges the post-9/11 stereotyping of Pakistani women as non-agentic and controlled by men, which is often projected in popular media reporting on the war on terror campaigns in this region, and through literature that sustains these views.[13] International human rights reports have repeatedly presented instances of violence against women as failures of Pakistan's government (Human Rights Watch (2015; 2016). Instead of a sweeping condemnation of state policies that overlooks most underlying causes of human rights violations, Mueenuddin's stories point at the recent precariousness of masculine identity in Pakistan as a factor which has contributed to increased violence and failure to protect the rights of women and the underprivileged in society.

The controversy of memoirs by Pakistani women

Compared to fiction, biographical works published after 9/11 are more contentious in their articulation of human rights. In the case of memoirs,[14] increasingly regarded as the most effective conduits for human rights awareness because of their testimonial value (Schaffer and Smith 2004), recent Pakistani works have generated the most debate. Biographical works, specifically directed at a particular cause, makes them not only political but often controversial in nature, because there are contesting claims about human rights that emerge from their writing and circulation. Therefore, making a general case for contemporary post-9/11 life writing as a straightforward instrument for the promotion of human rights is not only simplistic, but dangerously optimistic in a period touched by the War on Terror. It is mainly for this reason that memoirs like Malala Yousafzai's *I Am Malala* (2015) and Mukhtaran Mai's *In the Name of Honour* (2007), despite their wide international acclaim, have garnered a largely negative reaction among the general population in Pakistan.

Such memoirs, mostly written in collaboration with Western journalists, have been criticised by Pakistani fiction writers like Fatima Bhutto (2013) because one is 'never sure whose voice is leading whose', or whether its 'message will be colonised by one power or other for its own insidious agendas' (2013: n.p.). Often read by Western readers in a prescriptive manner dictated by school curriculum outcomes, or end-of-book-discussion questions popular at book clubs, these memoirs influence the shaping of public opinion by limiting knowledge about Pakistan to its most negative aspects. The reader[15] thus becomes unwittingly embroiled in configuring what Lila Abu-Lughod calls a 'new common sense about going to war for women' (2013: 81), which gains its authority by employing a human rights idiom that has been affirmed internationally and made synonymous with freedom of choice and its value. The language of human rights has become so important in defining a 'universal metric of humanity', that drawing upon women's rights discourse brings validation to other public discourses in America and Europe through its strong emotional appeal (Abu-Lughod 2013: 81). Academics have voiced concern about this trend:

> Since 9/11 and the ongoing 'war on terror', narratives by and about Muslim women have been increasingly commodified, circulated and uncritically consumed, particularly in the West. As part of this process, a proliferation of books promising to take the Western reader 'behind' or 'beyond' the veil of Muslim society and 'demystify' the lives of Muslim women have been fodder for a fetishistic voyeurism rooted in the Orientalist and Western feminist preoccupation with 'unveiling' Muslim women's bodies and lives. Of particular interest and concern to this special issue [of *Intercultural Education*] is the predominant paradigm framing the production, circulation and reception of these narratives.
>
> (Zine et al. 2007: 272)

A Pakistani woman who ventures to write a memoir, especially if it reflects her experiences as a person facing restrictions on her freedom, or indeed physical or emotional violence, faces a daunting prospect. To project her voice beyond the society that is the primary source of her oppression, she needs to have the language and means to reach an international audience. This need places her in a vulnerable position, one that accentuates her already precarious condition. The problem of such a woman is complex because she 'enters a commercial book industry that on the one hand has begun to treat her texts as a hot commodity, and on the other hand has a limited repertoire for placing her work' (Kahf 2006: 78). In the post-9/11 market, there are only two 'Eurocentrically slanted slots' for Muslim women:

> No matter how much a Muslim woman may have something different to say, by the time it goes through the 'machine' of the publishing industry, it is likely to come out the other end packaged as either a 'Victim Story' or 'Escapee Story.'
>
> (Kahf 2006: 78)

To counter the appropriation of these life narratives by the West, several reading strategies have been put forward that suggest more cognisant ways of interpreting memoirs like *I Am Malala* (Khoja-Moolji 2015; Ryder 2015; Fitzpatrick 2017). While the critics generally agree that the publication and circulation of memoirs and biographies by Muslim women are politically driven, they all suggest more nuanced readings that move beyond what fuels global narratives of power. Both Khoja-Moolji and Fitzpatrick believe that attention should be drawn to other issues like class division, corruption, and power which are revealed through Malala's story, while Phyllis Mentzell Ryder stresses that readers pay attention to Malala's comments about Islamisation as a political movement rather than a religious one. In Ryder's opinion, Malala consistently disrupts the appropriation of her story, even while she uses the Western media to relay her message, and that critics should pay attention to these disruptions (2015: 176).

Although strategies that encourage reading between the lines are likely to be more constructive, unless these memoirs are examined as testimonies as well as commodities that can be marketed in complex ways, their contribution to the universalisation of human rights remains questionable. To this end, it is crucial to highlight the ideological and geopolitical positions of the local versus the global readership in an effort to bridge these divisions. The recent volume by Alexandra Schultheis Moore and Elizabeth Swanson Goldberg makes important advances in the pedagogical field of human rights literature, suggesting that 'Teachers in human rights and literature classrooms […] must present human rights through the scope of their own doubled optic: as a discourse and practice of social justice and as a vehicle or alibi for militaristic neo-imperialism' (2015: 5).

In conclusion, because Pakistani anglophone literature has begun to come into its own in the last two decades, there is a need for cogent study of these works in postcolonial and transnational literature courses because of their relevance to the most recent challenges faced by a global human rights vision. Due to their historical and political complexity, these writings can be most productively utilised in a cross-disciplinary classroom if students are encouraged to read them more perceptively from multiple perspectives, and they are taught within a contextual framework that allows contesting interpretations to emerge. Pakistani fiction and memoirs are important in their very ambivalence because they have the potential to identify the challenges faced by a universal vision of human rights in a post-9/11 world; only then can progress be made.

Notes

1 Universalism vs cultural relativism is a long-standing debate in human rights discourse. The universalist stance treats human rights as universal and applicable to all human beings equally. Cultural relativism argues that human rights are dependent on culture, and therefore no single definition of moral principles can be applied to all cultures across the globe. The general concern of relativists arises from the view that the principles upon which the Universal Declaration of Human Rights (1948) is structured stem from Western political history. In response, Jack Donnelly proposes a multidimensional space that accommodates elements from both universality and relativity, which he terms 'relatively universal' (2013: 105). He believes that in the contemporary world relativity operates within the boundaries drawn by universal human rights.
2 Friedman writes: 'The individuals with whom the United States and its allies are currently at war defy easy definition, much less understanding' (2011). The 'enemy' in the War on Terror is an elusive entity defined by the United States' *Authorization for Use of Military Force* signed on 14 September 2001 as 'those nations, organizations, or persons he determines planned, authorized, committed, or aided the terrorist attacks that occurred on September 11, 2001, or harbored such organizations or persons, in order to prevent any future acts of international terrorism against the United States by such nations, organizations or persons' (Congress 2001).
3 A 'state of exception' gives a government, or a sovereign, the power to transcend the rule of law in the name of the public good. It is increasingly becoming the norm, turning democratic states into totalitarian states. See Agamben's *State of Exception* (2005) for an examination of 'states of exception' in the post-9/11 period.
4 William J. Haynes II, JD, General Counsel of the US Department of Defence, wrote in a 12 December 2002 memo to the Council on Foreign Relations that: '"Enemy combatant" is a general category that subsumes two sub-categories: lawful and unlawful combatants […] Lawful combatants receive prisoner of war (POW) status and the protections of the Third Geneva Convention. Unlawful combatants do not receive POW status and do not receive the full protections of the Third Geneva Convention.

The President has determined that al Qaida members are unlawful combatants because (among other reasons) they are members of a non-state actor terrorist group that does not receive the protections of the Third Geneva Convention. He additionally determined that the Taliban detainees are unlawful combatants because they do not satisfy the criteria for POW status set out in Article 4 of the Third Geneva Convention' (ProCon 2008).

5 See Mallgrave and Ikonomou (1994), eds. *Empathy, Form, and Space: Problems in German Aesthetics*, 1873–1893.
6 See Mallgrave and Ikonomou (1994). Greiner (1909) offers a detailed etymological examination of the difference in meaning between 'sympathy' and 'empathy'. See also Jahoda (2005).
7 For a more detailed discussion of the critical views in this section, please see: Sadaf, S. (2018) 'Human Dignity, the War on Terror, and Post-9/11 Literature.' Special issue Global Responses to War on Terror. *European Journal of English Studies*, 22.2.
8 Increasingly, the term 'widescreen' is being used to describe trends in recent comic books. For the use of this term regarding novels, see MacConnell (2015).
9 In *Rethinking Identities in Contemporary Pakistani Fiction: Beyond 9/11*, Aroosa Kanwal categorises fiction produced by Pakistani writers in the aftermath of the September 11 attacks as 'post-9/11 fiction' and 'retrospective prologues to post-9/11 fiction'. The first category foregrounds the 'repercussions of the September 11 terrorist attacks on the lives of Pakistanis in the diaspora and at home', and writings in the latter category 'look at political decisions and social factors in Pakistan from the late 1970s onwards that have contributed towards Pakistan's image as a terrorist land, particularly after 9/11' (2015: 7). Shamsie's novel falls in the first category, while Ahmad's novel falls close to, if not perfectly within, the second. Ahmad's stories are set in pre-1970s Pakistan, but identify an important connecting thread with a colonial past that still reverberates in tribal lives today.
10 Pushtun, Pukhtun, and Pathan refer to the same tribe, whose ancient mother tongue is Pushto (or Pushtu). This ethnic group is native to Afghanistan and Northern Pakistan.
11 For a detailed report on the Pashtunwali code as distinct from the Islamic *sharia*, see *The Economist* (2006) and Community Appraisal and Motivation Programme and Saferworld (2012: 7).
12 Maleeha Aslam's *Gender-based Explosions* (2012) is perhaps the only work offering a definition of Pakistani masculinity in a contemporary context by analysing qualitative data collected from samples taken from three social strata: low socioeconomic group, socially stigmatised and distressed, and university students and professionals. Chapter 7 of the book, 'Self-image, Social Expectations and Pressures', is about the self-sustained pressures and expectations to which Pakistani men subject themselves in order to uphold their masculinity. This role is increasingly hard to maintain as more women start to work outside the home. For a more detailed examination of Pakistani masculinity in Mueenuddin's *In Other Rooms, Other Wonders*, see Sadaf (2014).
13 Elizabeth Anker writes that 'Certain human rights best sellers, such as any of Khalid Husseini's novels, provide case studies that disclose how popular fiction both exoticizes the non-Western world and promotes coercive Western intervention within its crises', and are a part of 'the self-indulgent and consumer-based "armchair activism" fashionably marketed at the Western women's book club circuit' (2015: 42).
14 Some parts of this chapter are taken from my article, 'I Am Malala' (2017).
15 For the most part in this chapter, my use of the term 'readers' does not imply that there is always an 'ideal' (Culler 2006) or 'model' (Eco 1979) reader of human rights narratives in whom 'empathy' is evoked as a necessary response to stories of suffering. I also want to avoid the neat (though sometimes contested) distinction between 'lay' and 'professional' readers (Guillory 2000) of literary texts. I use the term for readers with preconceived notions that affect the reception of the book. Notions of 'location' and 'identity' (see Procter 2009), are important in this case, because they do influence reader response, hence the use of 'Western' and 'Pakistani' readers as a broad (if rather simplistic) distinction.

Bibliography

Abu-Lughod, L. (2013) *Do Muslim Women Need Saving?* Cambridge, MA: Harvard University Press.
Agamben, G. (2005) *State of Exception*. Chicago: University of Chicago Press.
Ahmed, A.S. (2013) *The Thistle and the Drone: How America's War on Terror Became a Global War on Tribal Islam*. Washington, DC: Brookings Institution Press.
Ahmad, J. (2011) *The Wandering Falcon*. New York: Riverhead Books.
Ahmad, J. (2011) 'Wandering Falcon Describes Pakistan's Tribal Areas'. Transcript of an interview with Jamil Ahmad, *NPR* 16 June [online]. Available from <www.npr.org/2011/06/16/137216570/wandering-falcon-describes-pakistans-tribal-areas> [2 February 2017].

Anker, E.S. (2012) *Fictions of Dignity: Embodying Human Rights in World Literature*. New York: Cornell University Press.
Anker, E.S. (2015) 'Teaching the Legal Imperialism Debate over Human Rights'. In *Teaching Human Rights in Literary and Cultural Studies Vol. 38*. Ed. by Moore, A.S. and Elizabeth, S.G. New York: The Modern Language Association of America.
Aslam, M. (2012) *Gender-based Explosions: The Nexus Between Muslim Masculinities, Jihadist Islamism and Terrorism*. New York: United Nations University Press.
Aslam, N. (2009) *The Wasted Vigil*. New York: Vintage.
Aslam, N. (2010) 'Where to Begin'. *Granta* [online]. Available from <https://granta.com/where-to-begin/> [2 February 2017].
Barnett, M. (2011) *Empire of Humanity: A History of Humanitarianism*. New York: Cornell University Press.
Bhutto, F. (2013) '*I Am Malala* by Malala Yousafzai – review'. *Guardian* [online]. Available from <www.theguardian.com/books/2013/oct/30/malala-yousafzai-fatima-bhutto-review> [2 February 2017].
Brouillette, S. (2012) 'UNESCO and Book Development'. *Maple Tree Literary Supplement* 13 [online]. Available from <www.mtls.ca/issue13/impressions/> [20 May 2016].
Cmiel, K. (2004) 'The Recent History of Human Rights'. *The American Historical Review* 109(1), 117–135.
Community Appraisal and Motivation Programme and Saferworld. (2007) The Jirga: Justice and Conflict Transformation [online]. Available from <www.saferworld.org.uk/resources/publications/647-the-jirga-justice-and-conflict-transformation> [20 May 2016].
Congress. (2001) Authorization for Use of Military Force [online]. Available from <www.congress.gov/bill/107th-congress/senate-joint-resolution/23/text/enr> [20 May 2016].
Culler, J. (2006) *The Pursuit of Signs*. London: Routledge.
Djikic, M., Oatley J., and Moldoveanu. M.C. (2013) 'Reading Other Minds: Effects of Literature on Empathy'. *Scientific Study of Literature* 3(1), 28–47.
Donnelly, J. (2013) *Universal Human Rights*. New York: Cornell University Press.
Eco, U. (1979) *The Role of the Reader: Explorations in the Semiotics of Texts*. Bloomington: Indiana University Press.
The Economist. (2006) 'Pushtunwali: Honour among Them' [online]. Available from <www.economist.com/special-report/2006/12/19/honour-among-them> [4 June 2017].
Filkins, D.F. (2016) 'Dangerous Fictions'. *The New Yorker* [online]. Available from <www.newyorker.com/magazine/2016/05/09/a-pakistani-novelist-tests-the-limits> [20 May 2016].
Fitzpatrick, C. (2017) 'Malala in Context'. *Contemporary Literary Criticism* 403, n.p.
Friedman, L.M. (2011) 'Who Are We Fighting? Conceptions of the Enemy in the War on Terror'. *Ohio Northern University Law Review* 37(1), 11–22.
Greiner, R. (1909) 'The Introduction of the Word "Empathy" into English'. In *BRANCH: Britain, Representation and Nineteenth-Century History*. Ed. by Felluga, D.F. Extension of Romanticism and Victorianism on the Net. available from <www.branchcollective.org/?ps_articles=rae-greiner-1909-the-introduction-of-the-word-empathy-into-english> [29 July 2017].
Guillory, J. (2000) 'The Ethical Practice of Modernity: The Example of Reading'. In *The Turn to Ethics*. Ed. by Garber, M., Hanssen, B., and Walkowitz, R.L. New York: Routledge, 29–46.
Hamid, M. (2007) 'Harcourt interview on *The Reluctant Fundamentalist*' [online]. Available from <www.mohsinhamid.com/interviewharcourt2007.html> [4 June 2017].
Hamid, M. (2013) *The Reluctant Fundamentalist*. Toronto: Anchor Canada.
Hamid, M. (2014) 'It Had to Be a Sign'. *Discontent and its Civilizations: Dispatches from Lahore*. London: Hamish Hamilton.
Hamid, M. (2017) *Exit West*. London: Penguin.
Hanif, M. (2012) *Our Lady of Alice Bhatti*. Toronto: Bond Street Books.
Human Rights Watch. (2015) *World Report 2015: Pakistan* [online]. Available from <www.hrw.org/world-report/2015/country-chapters/pakistan#49dda6> [10 February 2017].
Human Rights Watch. (2016) *World Report 2016: Pakistan* [online]. Available from <www.hrw.org/world-report/2016/country-chapters/pakistan> [10 February 2017].
Hunt, L. (2007) *Inventing Human Rights*. New York: W.W. Norton.
Jahoda, G. (2005) 'Theodor Lipps and the Shift from "Sympathy" to "Empathy"'. *Journal of the History of the Behavioral Sciences* 41(2), 151–163.
Kahf, M. (2006) 'On Being a Muslim Woman Writer in the West'. *Amman: Islamica Magazine* 17, 78–85.
Kaminsky, A. (2009) 'Densely Woven Skeins: When Literature is a Practice of Human Rights'. *Hispanic Issues On Line* 4, 44–57.

Kanwal, A. (2015) *Rethinking Identities in Contemporary Pakistani Fiction: Beyond 9/11*. London: Palgrave Macmillan.

Khoja-Moolji, S. (2015) 'Reading Malala: (De)(Re)Territorialization of Muslim Collectivities'. *Comparative Studies of South Asia, Africa and the Middle East* 35(3), 539–556.

MacConnell, K. (2015) 'Widescreen Sci-Fi Novels' [online]. Available from <http://ken-mcconnell.com/2012/06/09/widescreen-sci-fi-novel/> [10 February 2017].

Mai, M. and Cuny, M. (2007) *In the Name of Honor: A Memoir*. Trans. by Coverdale, L. New York: Washington Square Press.

Mallgrave, H.F. and Ikonomou, E. (eds.) (1994) *Empathy, Form, and Space: Problems in German Aesthetics, 1873–1893*. Santa Monica: Getty Center.

McEwan, I. (2001) 'Only Love and then Oblivion'. *Guardian* [online]. Available from <www.theguardian.com/world/2001/sep/15/september11.politicsphilosophyandsociety2> [10 February 2017].

Milo, J. (2017) '"We Are All Migrants": Mohsin Hamid Talks his New Novel, *Exit West*'. [online]. Available from <www.pastemagazine.com/articles/2017/03/mohsin-hamid-exit-west.html> [8 June 2017].

Moore, A.S. and Goldberg, E.S. (eds.) (2015) *Teaching Human Rights in Literary and Cultural Studies*. New York: The Modern Language Association of America.

Mueenuddin, D. (2010a) 'How to Write about Pakistan' *Granta* [online]. Available from <https://granta.com/how-to-write-about-pakistan/> [10 February 2017].

Mueenuddin, D. (2010b) *In Other Rooms, Other Wonders*. London: Bloomsbury.

The Nation. (2011) 'Wandering Falcon Captures Raw Romance of Badlands' [online]. Available from <https://nation.com.pk/17-Oct-2011/wandering-falcon-captures-raw-romance-of-badlands> [20 August 2016].

O'Gorman, D. (2015) *Fictions of the War on Terror: Difference and the Transnational 9/11 Novel*. London: Palgrave Macmillan.

ProCon (2008) *What is the Difference between an Enemy Combatant, an Unlawful Combatant, and a Prisoner of War?* [online]. Available from <http://usiraq.procon.org/view.answers.php?questionID=000934> [22 February 2017].

Procter, J. (2009) 'Reading, Taste and Postcolonial Studies: Professional and Lay Readers of Things Fall Apart'. *Interventions* 11(2), 180–198.

Ryder, P.M. (2015) 'Beyond Critique: Global Activism and the Case of Malala Yousafzai'. *Literacy in Composition Studies* 3(1), 175–187.

Sadaf, S. (2014) 'Daniyal Mueenuddin's Dying Men'. *South Asian History and Culture*. Special Issue: *Mapping South Asian Masculinities: Men and Political Crises* 5(4), 490–504.

Sadaf, S. (2017) 'I Am Malala: Human Rights, and the Politics of Production, Marketing, and Reception of the Post-9/11 Memoir'. *Interventions: International Journal of Postcolonial Studies* 19(6), 855–871.

Schaffer, K. and Smith, S. (2004) *Human Rights and Narrated Lives: The Ethics of Recognition*. New York: Palgrave.

Shah, B. (2010) 'The Pak Pack Takes over the Literary World?' *The Hindustan Times* [online]. Available from <www.hindustantimes.com/books/the-pak-pack-takes-over-the-literary-world/story-qElm4U4NLcjasMUv6gZZIK.html> [22 February 2017].

Shamsie, K. (2009) *Burnt Shadows*. London: Bloomsbury.

Singh, H. (2012) 'A Legacy of Violence: Interview with Kamila Shamsie about *Burnt Shadows* Conducted via e-mail on October 26, 2010'. *Ariel: A Review of International English Literature* 42(2), 157–162.

Slaughter, J.R. (2007) *Human Rights, Inc.: The World Novel, Narrative Form, and International Law*. New York: Fordham University Press.

Slaughter, J.R. (2012) 'Enabling Fictions and Novel Subjects: The *Bildungsroman* and International Human Rights Law'. In *Theoretical Perspectives on Human Rights and Literature*. Ed. by Goldberg, E.S. and Moore, A.S. New York: Routledge, 41–64.

Swanson, G. (2013) '"The Tender Instinct is the Hope of the World': Human Feeling and Social Change Before Empathy'. *New Formations* 79, 126–148.

The United Nations. (1948) Universal Declaration of Human Rights [online]. Available from <www.un.org/en/universal-declaration-human-rights/> [26 June 2017].

Yousafzai, M. and Lamb, C. (2015) *I Am Malala*. London: Back Bay/Little, Brown and Company.

Zine, J., Lisa, K.T., and Hilary, E.D. (2007) 'Reading Muslim Women and Muslim Women Reading Back: Transnational Feminist Reading Practices, Pedagogy and Ethical Concerns'. *Intercultural Education* 18(4), 271–280.

13

THE TAMING OF THE TRIBAL WITHIN PAKISTANI NARRATIVES OF PROGRESS, CONFLICT, AND ROMANCE

Uzma Abid Ansari

This chapter analyses representations of tribal identity in Pakistani anglophone works of fiction and examines how the tribal are 'tamed' by reducing the complexity of their social system to a simplified image which is easily judged and 'othered' by mainstream populations both in Pakistan and abroad. It demonstrates how tribal identities and their cultures are perceived and represented in such a way as to be made to perform the function of an imaginary 'nomadic regime', a concept from Gilles Deleuze and Felix Guattari's thesis on nomadology that signifies disruptive assemblages that counter the reified structures of the state, and shows how the tribal regions are rendered into a 'smooth space' that serves the purpose of warding off repressive state apparatuses (Deleuze and Guattari 2010).

'Smooth space' and 'nomadic regime' are concepts drawn from 'Nomadology', a section of Deleuze and Guattari's *A Thousand Plateaus*. 'Smooth space' refers to the space occupied by the 'counter-signifying regime' of certain elements in and around the state that work in opposition to its apparatuses, in a metaphoric exteriority to it. Collectively these elements are called the 'Nomadic War-Machine', which occupies the spaces outside the 'signifying regime' of the state and is not stratified (i.e. it is free of the hierarchies and stratifications of the state model). By deploying this conceptualisation of an anti-state assemblage, I will critically interrogate three narratives by 'progressivist'[1] Pakistani writers who have engaged with tribal identity in Pakistan. In the first narrative, tribal identity is romanticised as nomadic and peripheral; in the second, it is placed at the centre of conflict within the state of Pakistan in the post-9/11 era; and in the third narrative it is pitted against 'progressivist discourse', which juxtaposes Western feminism with tribalism in Pakistan. The novels selected for this analysis – *The Wandering Falcon* (2011) by Jamil Ahmad, *The Shadow of the Crescent Moon* (2013) by Fatima Bhutto, and *A God in Every Stone* (2014) by Kamila Shamsie – have purportedly made interventions in the field of cultural identity in the Pakistani context, but I contend that by framing tribal cultures within narratives of romance, conflict, and progress, their human and lived realities are skewed and simultaneously augment these narratives as internalised orientalist representations by authors whose subject positions reinforce the power structures put in place by the modern state of Pakistan.

These cultural representations of tribal ways of life are informed by prevalent hegemonic discourses, and in turn help to accumulate images of the tribal that support such discourses. In a symbiotic relationship with the dominant discourses of their time, they reinforce the image of the tribal as an outsider to city life, as a potential militant, and the trajectory of their life ways as running against the grain of progressivism and modernity. The following sections look at each narrative separately but with a view to underscoring the representation of tribal identities as 'nomadic' and occupying a smooth space outside the state model and progressivist discourse, which includes Western feminism and nationalism.

Narrative of romance

Ahmad's *The Wandering Falcon* is a compelling narrative fiction in terms of its representation of tribal culture and also the historical time frame it represents. Written in the 1970s, when Ahmad was serving as a government representative in the tribal belt of the then North West Frontier Province, present-day Khyber Pakhtunkhwa, and Baluchistan, *The Wandering Falcon* was published almost forty years later, in 2011. The significance of this detail lies in the fact that the novella, or collection of interconnected short stories, was released for public consumption a decade after the damaging events of 9/11, which were followed by an international military intervention in those very tribal areas that Ahmad had so affectionately depicted in 1974.

The result of this gap between writing and publication created an interesting anachronistic perspective on tribal representation, one which marks a shift from images of conflict-ridden and war-torn landscapes to a more romanticised visualisation of tribal culture that seeks to situate it in a conceptual smooth space outside the administrative apparatus of the Pakistani state. The novella sheds light on how tribal identity had been perceived prior to the many wars the region witnessed, and it demonstrates how this periphery was romanticised and even 'othered' by the 'centre' (i.e. the federal government of Pakistan). In this regard, Ahmad's subject position and agency as author and invisible third-person narrator are important points of departure for this cultural analysis, because they inform and provide the conditions for knowledge production related to tribal identity that had been relegated to the periphery. His social status during the two decades he spent in the Federally Administered Tribal Areas and Baluchistan as a government representative and bureaucrat was without question a political position, which implicated him in the dynamics of power and knowledge production of the regions under his administrative control.[2] Ahmad's agency as author and third-person narrator of the novella is thus closely tied to the power relations and disciplinary techniques adopted by the postcolonial nation state from the colonial era, for the administration of the so-called 'Pashtun problem' in the Pakistani state's 'wild west', a space on the western borders notorious for its lawlessness. The role of the government representative, who exercised considerable authority in the tribal regions, was to implement the Frontier Crimes Regulation law among other disciplinary laws which were drawn up by the British Raj to control the 'martial' and unruly Pashtun tribes on the western borders of British India (Tripodi 2011: 8).

The evident institutional connection with the colonial era, due to the transference of the state apparatus from the British colonists to the newly founded state of Pakistan, has not moderated the discourse surrounding the administration of the tribal regions. The anti-colonial resistance encountered by the British in the border regions was translated and depicted by them as romanticised battles fought valiantly by a British army who had finally met its match in the tribals. By reifying Pashtun character traits, they diminished the element of human mutability and adaptation to new and changed environmental and social circumstances of the Pashtun stereotype, mounting him as the quintessential noble savage on their colonial wall of fame

(Tripodi 2011: 3, 43). In what follows, I demonstrate how Ahmad, with his subject position embedded in a colonialist and ultimately orientalist discourse of the legacy of the British Raj, deploys the tribal stereotype to produce a romanticised narrative about what can be read as the smooth space of the nomadic regime which counters the state apparatus.

Ahmad's *The Wandering Falcon* is a collection of nine short stories loosely based around the figure of Tor Baz, or 'black falcon', a wanderer of Baluchi origins who ekes out a livelihood roaming among the various tribes of the rugged regions in the western borders of the state of Pakistan. The first story or chapter of the novella tells the tragic tale of Tor Baz's conception, his parents being eloping lovers who were hunted down and ruthlessly murdered in the name of honour by his mother's father, a tribal chief, and her fiancé (who then proceeded to kill the tribal chief as well). From then on, the novella follows Tor Baz's passage through life in the rugged landscape between Afghanistan and Pakistan. The remaining eight chapters or short stories depict major and minor life events in the various tribes among whom Tor Baz happens to pass. The reader soon realises that the novella isn't particularly about Tor Baz, but he is a point of reference creating an itinerary across the tribal belt and a means of loosely linking the short stories together. He constitutes this space, yet at the same time he is external to it because he doesn't belong to any of the tribes. His character is embedded in what Mieke Bal terms the hidden or naturalised ideology of a narrative representation (2009: 31), consolidating a *mise-en-scène* of a smooth 'nomadic space' external to the state but passively constituted by the 'noble savage', represented as violent yet domesticated. The externality of the tribal region to the state is established early on in the narrative:

> This way of life had endured for centuries, but it would not last forever. It constituted defiance to certain concepts, which the world was beginning to associate with civilization itself. Concepts such as statehood, citizenship, undivided loyalty to one state, settled life as opposed to nomadic life, and the writ of the state as opposed to tribal discipline. The pressures were inexorable. One set of values, one way of life, had to die. In this clash, the state, as always, proved stronger than the individual. The new way of life triumphed over the old.
>
> (Ahmad 2011: 8)

In the above excerpt, Ahmad pits the state against the individual instead of the communal collective of nomadic society. This reduction of a pastoral community to a single individual opposed to the state is an interesting perspective on what is a semi-nomadic and pastoral social system which transacts with the state, and whose members are extremely communal and interdependent. Although he does point out the incongruous association of civilisation with sedentary urban life, in referring to the juxtaposition of civilisation with the nomadic 'individual', Ahmad reiterates the binary opposition of civilisation/nature, with the idyllic tribal individual falling neatly into the category of nature. The tribal discipline by which this individual abides lends him humanity and primitive clarity, so that despite being close to 'nature' (i.e. far from civilised), he nevertheless possesses an appreciable degree of dignity and nobility. This individual, isolated from communal contingencies, is pitted against the state, creating a romantic image of a noble savage, to be respected yet recognised as the Other who cannot be assimilated into the urban or civilised milieu, because his lifestyle in the present is relegated to an old, more 'natural' lifestyle, incompatible with the new values of 'civilised' life.

The key idea in such a romanticised conceptualisation of the individual versus the state is that of the 'nomad', an exonym with which the tribes in question do not identify (Tapper 2008: 98–99). Nomadism is a concept that covers a wide range of social mobilities and transnationalism, and the 'nomadism' represented in Ahmad's short story is identified as the *powinda*s, which he translates as 'people on foot'. But a more accurate translation would be 'grazers', implying pastoralism (Tapper 2008: 98). In addition, the migratory tribes who self-identify as *powinda*s cannot be isolated from their historical geopolitical importance in the region in a simplistic way, nor from the role they play in the political economy of a country like Afghanistan. Historically, these tribes, who are pastoral Pashtuns, have held important military and political positions in the largely Pashtun-dominated history of the region (Titus 1998: 670), and they still contribute to the economy of Afghanistan to a considerable extent, which arguably suggests interdependence between the state and the pastoral social structure.[3] Therefore, to say that the nomad is a creature of the past who could not fit into the modern political scheme of the state is to fall into a binary logic which overlooks the complexities of the pastoral lifestyle on the frontier between Afghanistan and Pakistan, one which is firmly rooted in the geopolitics of the region.

While pastoral tribes are depicted as the passive victims of a modern state defined by a heavily militarised frontier, the more sedentary tribes come across as groups of swashbuckling trigger-happy men whose basic means of subsistence is banditry on the frontiers of the state. They are described in a manner which merges them with their 'habitat', so to speak, so that there is little difference between them and an exotic animal species:

> The Mahsuds, because they always hunt in groups, are known as the wolves of Waziristan. A Wazir hunts alone. He is known as 'the leopard' to other men [...] Nature has bred in both an unusual abundance of anger, enormous resilience, and a total refusal to accept their fate [...] To both tribes, survival is the ultimate virtue. In neither community is any stigma attached to a hired assassin, a thief, a kidnapper, or an informer.
>
> (Ahmad 2011: 20)

These semi-pastoral tribes historically inhabited the mountain passes between the Delhi Sultanate and Afghanistan, and later British India and Afghanistan. Opinions on their conduct towards outsiders are part of a colonial discourse that has been passed on to the Pakistani state's administrative authorities who politically represent the central federal government. Ahmad's description of the Mahsuds and Wazirs as 'wolves' and 'panthers' is part of this colonial orientalist discourse, and has been deployed as a truism since the account of Waziristan by the last British governor, Sir Olaf Caroe, in his book *The Pathans*, which was published in 1965 (Ahmad 2004). Paul Titus has pointed out that the massive armed uprising on the frontiers faced by the British in India shaped their perception of the Baluch and Pashtun tribes there, but individually their views on the tribes 'ranged from romantic admiration to utter revulsion' (Titus 1998: 662). According to Titus, such views depended on the nature of their holders' interactions with the tribes: the more administrative their interactions, the friendlier their relations were, and the more confrontational their interactions due to the aggressive 'forward policy', which involved military intervention in the region, the more negative the attitudes developed towards the tribals. Although these are seemingly anthropological observations, they were not conducted by academics but by government representatives and administrators during the British colonial era (Titus 1998: 663).[4] And they too relied heavily on previous accounts by colonial officials who mostly wrote down their observations of the region and tribal inhabitants in travel journals and correspondence. Nevertheless, this created a discourse which has lasted to this day.

A similar ambivalence of romantic admiration and revulsion is present in Ahmad's fictionalised representation of the frontier region's various tribes. The narrative representations of the various tribes, which include the Baluch, pastoral Pashtuns, sedentary Pashtuns, and Gujjars, are based on Ahmad's observations of and interactions with them as a bureaucrat who held office as a government representative in Baluchistan and the Federally Administered Tribal Areas (FATA). And, not unlike the British predecessors of this government instrument, his observations, as a non-academic, are peppered with stories of violence as well as admiration for a lifestyle that defies the dictates of the state. Revulsion at the acts of violence is evident in the depiction of ruthless honour killings and infringement of the state's laws; admiration is evidenced by the sympathy shown for the non-nationalist sentiments of the tribes. This ambivalence present in the narrative voice is denotative of the relegation of tribal society and individuals to a dual temporality, that is, they exist and represent for the narrator an originary past and a present, so that their originary characteristics are permanent fixtures in the present, thus perpetuating a stereotype that embodies a violent primitivism at the same time as an admirable individualism that refuses to merge with the modern state. In *Orientalism* Edward Said speaks of a similar bureaucratic Western observer of natives who categorises them into fixed types of communities like Aryans, Semites, etc., thus:

> [F]unctionally speaking this came to mean that for the Orientalist no modern Semite, however much he may have believed himself to be modern, could ever outdistance the organising claims on him of his origins. This functional role worked on the temporal and spatial levels together. No Semite advanced in time beyond the development of a 'classical' period; no Semite could ever shake loose the pastoral, desert environment of his tent and tribe.
>
> (Said 2001: 234)

By the same token, no tribal in Ahmad's narrative representation can distance him or herself from their pastoral, desert environment. Even though the novella was written in the mid-1970s, there are references to the pre-Partition period, since which time the Pashtuns and Baluch have seemingly remained unchanged in their originary societal design, with no mention of internal mobilisation due to large-scale urbanisation and their role in the political economy of Pakistan. This has only led to a reiteration of the colonial discourse on warfaring tribes, which subsist on either illegal or nomadic activities in order to survive in the vast hinterland on the peripheries of the much more stable federal centre of the state.

Narrative of conflict

In a much more contemporary setting, Bhutto's *The Shadow of the Crescent Moon* is a riveting narrative of a family from Mir Ali, a town in North Waziristan, recuperating from the war on terror and the marginalisation of their home town and people by the federal government of Pakistan. Although it is a relevant and even timely projection of the socially marginalised region of North Waziristan, the novel's contextualisation appears misplaced as it instrumentalises the actuality of the region and its nominal space in the geopolitics of Pakistan as a mere prop in the narrative. I contend that Mir Ali is factual only in name and its representation in the narrative relies heavily on the narrative agent's subject position in a discourse of separatism that emerged in the political and feudal culture of southern Pakistan in Sindh, with its leftist intelligentsia and political workers based in the urban centre of Karachi, rather than Waziristan in the north of the country.

This is Bhutto's first work of fiction, her previous literary works include a compilation of poems, *Whispers of the Desert*, and the biographical *Songs of Blood and Sword* about her father, Mir Ghulam Murtaza Bhutto, who was killed in an encounter with police in front of his house in Karachi. Both of these works are touching reflections of the dramatic history of the Bhutto clan, from the time when Zulfiqar Ali Bhutto was executed by a military regime and the tragic events that unfolded in its wake in the lives of his children. Fatima Bhutto's childhood was spent in exile in Damascus with her father after his leftist insurgent activities with a terrorist organisation by the name of al-Zulfiqar led him to hijack a PIA aeroplane to Kabul, in which an army major was shot and killed. Although Mir Murtaza's involvement with al-Zulfiqar predated her birth in 1982, Bhutto grew up in exile, and on their return to Pakistan she was a witness to her father's work for the Movement for the Restoration of Democracy (MRD), a left-wing political alliance with communist leanings. Despite being an alliance of political parties from all over Pakistan, it nevertheless remained active mostly in the south of the country, where the Bhutto family had a large following in Sindh province.

This brief background of *The Shadow of the Crescent Moon* is important because it helps place Bhutto as author in a wider historical context, which in turn is of paramount significance for assessing the political basis of the established cultural hegemony of the centre over the periphery. Interpreting the author's subject position in a discursive field is thus important, as Mieke Bal points out in *Narratology*, so as 'to develop a politics of reading that draws its legitimacy from political positions, not from any fictitious "real" knowledge' (2009: 16). In this case, even though she does not claim a commitment to any political party, Bhutto has a strong political position, more so than Ahmad, because she writes from a position steeped in power relations between state and leftist insurgents from, ironically enough, a feudal cultural background. Having grown up almost stateless in exile with her father, Western educated, and transnational in outlook and lifestyle, Bhutto writes from this subject position for an international and urban readership which has access only to anglophone works such as hers, and hence she has the privilege to claim knowledge of a region invisible to this readership.

In the representation of the small North Waziristani town of Mir Ali, a narrative of conflict and sedition frames the actuality of the region. Bhutto literally produces knowledge about a geopolitical space that had until recently been visible to the public as a hinterland breeding violence and terrorist activity, because of its proximity to the war-torn country of Afghanistan. The geographical location of Waziristan, on the borders of the state and visible only in the peripheral vision of mainstream media, has made it a smooth space external to the state and its apparatuses, and thus the object of a leftist discourse that projects a narrative of sedition onto the region, producing 'real' knowledge for the centre's consumption. By 'centre', I refer to the mainstream and urban population, which is far removed from the border regions of FATA, where North Waziristan is located. Being a citizen of Pakistan and a journalist allows Bhutto access to such areas, but then the knowledge she produces as a narrative agent is filtered by their cultural representation in her narrative fiction. Revolving around the lives of three brothers in the town of Mir Ali, *Shadow of the Crescent Moon* depicts the traumas inflicted on a Shia Pashtun family who grapple with the takeover by the fanatical Sunni Taliban, as well as the injustices of the state meted out in their region as the military apparatus brings down a heavy hand in order to quell any and all insurgencies along the border. The three brothers, Aman Erum, Sikander, and Hayat, have chosen different paths in life: Aman moves to the United States for a better future, leaving behind his childhood love, Samarra Afridi; Sikander becomes a doctor and marries Mina; and finally the youngest, Hayat, runs a covert leftist political organisation from his university with the help of Samarra, carrying out small-scale insurgent activities against the military presence in their region.

The scenario depicted in this narrative fiction brings to light the heavy military intervention and its complicity with drone attacks carried out by NATO forces in North Waziristan from across the border with Afghanistan. But apart from this detail, the entire context is fabricated as an urban setting where the characters are not only unaffiliated with the dominant tribes of the region, but also display urban features like having a local university in their midst and a young girl riding a motorbike in public. Such scenes are completely removed from the reality of the region, which is inhabited only by the Mahsud and Wazir tribes, with the Shia Pashtun population settled in Parachinar district and the Afridis around the Khyber Agency and Kohat. This point is important because the areas affected by military action against the Taliban were not Parachinar and Kohat; consequently, the inhabitants of these areas, the Shia Pashtuns and the Afridis, were not displaced, and nor were they involved in seditious activities against the state. This seemingly minor detail leads one to question the representation of North Waziristan in Bhutto's narrative as a region whose primary inhabitants, Wazirs and Mahsuds who were displaced from their villages and towns in huge numbers during the war on terror, are conspicuously absent along with an authentic depiction of their plight. On the contrary, the town of Mir Ali, where military action did take place in 2007, is represented as a small, almost modern town replete with a local university where a small group of students is planning and carrying out anti-state activities in the style of Cuban revolutionary guerrilla warfare:

> Hayat remembers comrades, men who had devoted their lives to the cause of Mir Ali, abandoning their careers, money and families. Those men sat at desks all night and smoked and typed leaflets and posters and articles. They recited poetry because no one heard them when they used their own words.
>
> (Bhutto 2013: 17)

The fact of the matter is that no such insurgent activities were ever planned or carried out by the locals of North Waziristan, who are mostly poor farmers, and certainly not by the Pashtun Shia population who live in and around Parachinar, or by the Afridis who historically helped the newly founded state of Pakistan in its war against India over Kashmir in 1948 (Tucker 2010: 2109).

So why does Bhutto take such liberties with the cultural representation of Mir Ali and its inhabitants? Given her subject position and her target audience, she relies on a hegemonic discourse concerning the region. This discourse reiterates that the region harbours, as it has always done in the past, militant tribals of local origin because they have not been assimilated into the mainstream population. The dominant discourse is perpetuated by the mass media and consumed by urban populations, rendering the lived realities of the locals of North Waziristan invisible and distant, both culturally and physically. Because of its invisibility to mainstream vision, the region has come to serve the purpose of a smooth space for an urban leftist intelligentsia that exists outside the oppressive regime of the state and functions as a 'war-machine' that has the potential to disrupt state apparatuses, such as the military. But the narrative of the novel focuses only on the spatio-geographical aspect of the 'war-machine', chiefly because it exists on the peripheries of the state as well as in the peripheral vision of the centre, and it is therefore easier to ignore the lived reality of the tribes who are not an eclectic mix of urbanised Pashtun families but are rather small-scale landowners who subsist on agricultural activity. Hence, this underdeveloped area becomes a convenient conceptual smooth space upon whose surface a leftist subject position can project its discursive construct. Bhutto has essentially done the same by projecting her Westernised, urban, albeit leftist, discourse onto this space existing outside the urban centres of the state of Pakistan. By harnessing the unrest in North Waziristan and FATA generally over not being assimilated into the provincial jurisdiction, and representing it as seditious activity, the novel's narrative caters to a Westernised and anglophone readership who have internalised an orientalist outlook that lets them view the tribal regions as an exotic 'other'. This tribal 'other' not only allows them to define themselves in a certain way (i.e. progressive, urbanised, transnational etc.), but in sympathetic accounts of this 'other' they project their self-image onto tribal regions' representations in various media, thus effectively erasing the culture and identity of the tribals.

In Bhutto's case, being of Pakistani origin and a journalist has built her image as an authentic voice from a global periphery in her transnational circuit. But this perception tends to overlook the diversity of the region in which Pakistan is situated, which includes not only disparities between urban and rural populations but also various ethnicities, linguistic groups, and communal structures, of which disparities Bhutto is a part since she comes from a privileged feudal background. In her first fiction, Bhutto has effectively utilised a socially marginalised frontier region to project her narrative of conflict which is based on personal memories and experiences of her father's Marxist activism in Karachi, and in the process facilitated the erasure of cultural awareness of the Wazir and Mahsud tribes, who are the indigenous inhabitants of Waziristan.

Narrative of progress

As the world moves on from 9/11, writers from Pakistan are beginning to explore alternative themes from those areas affected by the US-led war on terror in order to create a counter-narrative that is more empathetic towards local sensibilities but does not lose sight of the global context. Shamsie's latest novel, *A God in Every Stone*, is such a narrative fiction that places the much-hyped but little understood Pashtun tribal region in a global historical context, highlighting the complexities of historical transculturalism and inter-civilisational ties that have made the region what it is today. This work aims to present a nuanced narrative which explores meetings of cultures over time and space, and their effects on intra-cultural dynamics by inducing change and sociocultural metamorphosis. The narrative highlights spatio-temporal complexity by moving from a distant past to a specific modern historical moment when anti-colonial movements were gaining momentum, and issues of identity and loyalty to one's 'land' had taken on nationalist overtones. Shamsie highlights social change in two social milieus, in Britain as women became more aware of their rights and began asserting themselves politically, and in the subcontinent as Indians began demanding their political rights against the British Raj. With this approach, Shamsie takes the focus away from a discourse of Islamist extremism and instead steers the narrative within a discourse of progress, teasing out issues of feminism, nationalism, and inter- and intra-cultural relationships. Hence, feminism and nationalism, which are constitutive of progressivism, are juxtaposed with raw tribalism, which is represented as regressive and, again, exterior to the politically correct discursive space occupied by progressivist ideologues such as Ghaffar Khan.

The plot of *A God in Every Stone* straddles two narratives, one that begins with a young British woman, Vivienne Rose Spencer, apprenticing as an archaeologist in Turkey, and the other involving a young Pashtun man from Peshawar, Qayyum Gul, serving in a British regiment as a *sepoy* stationed in Marseilles, France, and to later fight in the battle of Ypres. After losing an eye in the battle, he returns home to Peshawar, where he briefly crosses paths with Vivienne, who is in Peshawar in search of an ancient artefact belonging to a Carian called Scylax from 515 BCE. Although the two narratives merge eventually, they remain distinct in their representation of a young British woman's growth into a feminist during the heyday of the suffrage movement in Europe and the USA, and of a Pashtun man's reprioritisation of loyalties and reconstitution of selfhood on the lines of the non-violence movement. As these two narratives merge, Shamsie raises the issue of Vivienne's European or white feminism as an exclusivist yet universalising movement that tends to overlook women's struggles in other global, especially postcolonial, contexts. In parallel to this but worlds apart, the other narrative develops around Qayyum's recognition of the vicious cycle of violence and revenge inherent in his culture, and his initiative to overcome this by joining the Khudai Khidmatgar movement, a non-violent nationalist struggle against British colonial rule. Both these parallel narratives are embedded in a discourse of progress from which proceed issues of feminism, nationalism, and cultural/political reform.

Focusing exclusively on the representation of Pashtun tribal identity, Shamsie frames it in a narrative of progress that attempts to make sense of it outside the discourse on Islamism[5] by envisioning it in a linear historical progression. The aim of this ambitious linear chronology is to touch upon the deep historical roots of the region and the presence of the 'Pactyikes', ancestors of the present-day Pashtuns, in the region and their civilisational interaction with the Greeks and Persians. By placing the Pashtun in a historical context, his essentialist traits are made to appear ontologically inherent and to perpetually define his identity. For instance, while Qayyum endeavours to adopt the moderate ideology of Ghaffar Khan, founder of the Khudai Khidmatgar, his younger brother is being taught about his originary identity by Vivienne Rose: 'But we are Pactyike, the most warlike of the Indians' (Shamsie 2014: 204).

In Shamsie's narrative representation, two aspects of the Pashtun character emerge: they are more human than they are normally portrayed (i.e. as just one-dimensional fanatical tribals); and their masculinity, often seen as dominating their culture, tends to manifest itself as aggressive and sexually vigorous. Two pivotal scenes depicting violent confrontation, the battle of Ypres and the British attack on unarmed protesters of the Khudai Khidmatgar, are preceded and followed, respectively, by acts of sexual intercourse by Qayyum, the token Pashtun male representative in the novel. He is shown to be taken by French culture and the beauty of French women, and when an opportunity for intimacy with a French woman soon arises in the form of a prostitute, he avails himself just before his journey into battle against the Germans at Ypres. This double excitement of a sexual encounter followed by a bloody fight gives him an 'understanding at that moment [of] what it was to be a man – the wonder, the beauty of it' (Shamsie 2014: 57). In the encounter between the British and the unarmed protestors of the Khudai Khidmatgar, Qayyum is witness to the brutality of the soldiers and their indiscriminate killing of his fellow protestors, after which he hides with some other men in a nearby courtesan's house. On seeing a beautiful young prostitute in the house, the men are tempted to stay for the day, despite the strike on all businesses which they themselves had organised. Qayyum has recourse to his 'regular' woman, in whose room he has another insight into his maleness, in that 'he was a man, like all the other men who came here' (Shamsie 2014: 263). Once again, his essential maleness, like the other men with him, prevents him from acknowledging actions which could have been a source of shame when his comrades were dying on the streets, because this was something that was 'natural' to men, something that had to be done. Qayyum, a Pashtun man, thus becomes a quintessential, stereotypical male in a progressivist narrative with undertones of white feminism that tends to subject the Pashtun male to a European woman's gaze. Under this gaze, he appears as someone who cannot repress his overactive sexuality, even when not up in arms, which is an upshot of the rigid segregation between male and female spaces in the social structure. From a conceptual viewpoint, the Pashtun male and his tribal societal structure carry a potential for nomadism, which can disrupt the striated space of organised political movements for the political enfranchisement of English women and colonised subjects, as well as unsettle notions of sexual normalcy.

In fact, their overtly sexualised and violent masculinity is presented as an essential trait of Pashtun culture, one that needs to be restrained through more progressive means such as non-violent political movements that will help to bring about social reform of their strict tribal codes. These traits are also seen through the lens of a British feminist who, as a foreigner to the local culture, incidentally only sees that male behaviour which has been used to characterise Pashtun men as not only homosocial but overtly homoerotic and sexually fluid. In the marketplace, Vivienne sees men and boys walking 'hand in hand, flowers behind their ears and bandoliers across their chests. As if they had decided to be both man and woman at once, long of eyelash and broad of shoulder' (Shamsie 2014: 189). And in another place, when at the museum appraising Qayyum's younger brother's cataloguing of archaeological artefacts, she muses over his pairing of two stone heads, one Greek and one Indian:

> He had laid them down in profile so they looked each other in the eye, their mouths inches apart from each other. Was this an expression of his own proclivities or an acknowledgement of the passionate intimacy of Pathan men, sexual and otherwise?
> (298)

Representations such as these are indicative of orientalised stereotypes of Pashtun men, where their masculinity is fetishised as hypersexual with strong homoerotic tendencies. The explanation given for this usually points to their tribal structure, which segments their social spaces into strict public and private areas, rendering Pashtun women invisible in public spaces, so that Pashtun men have no other recourse to sexual intimacy than with their male companions. Such depictions of a Pashtun man's sexual preoccupations in narrative fiction are more than just 'realistic' cultural representations, they tap into the post-9/11 discourse on Afghan/Pashtun men's deviant sexuality which emerges from conditions of violence and regressive tribal laws (Manchanda 2014). In Shamsie's narrative, these essentialised characteristics are juxtaposed with a British woman's progressivist feminism so that they stand out in more vivid detail. Even though there are nuanced instances where Vivienne's 'civilising mission' to educate a young Pashtun man about his own identity is treated with slight irony, the essentialised Pashtun male traits remain a stronger motif throughout the novel, offset and framed within a narrative of progress which problematises the perceived and intense masculinity of the Pashtun man.

In all three types of narrative representation of tribal identity, the tribal is 'tamed' to fit the imagination and fantasy of the narrative agent or writer. As a concept, the tribal represents the smooth space outside the state apparatus, where the narrative representation can be projected and its fiction played out. In theory, the smooth spaces inhabited by the nomadic regime function to disrupt the oppressive regime of the state. In the above analysis I have shown how the periphery of the state is perceived as such a smooth space but is also deployed as a backdrop to the representation of tribal identity. And in each narrative, this identity takes on a different shape and different characteristics based on the discourse and historical framing of the narrative. The representational form of tribal identity, in turn, functions to support this very narrative framework, rather than saying anything about the lived realities of peripheral cultures in and around Pakistan.

The three narrative texts that have been critically examined in this chapter indicate a trend in anglophone Pakistani literature that engages with tribal identity as a perceived 'smooth space' or a space exterior to the state, which helps to underpin their respective narratives. The writers, in engaging with such identities, are neither themselves a part of this perceived smooth space, nor do they leave their privileged subject positions in the interiority of the state. It can therefore be concluded from this critical examination that when representing the culture of relatively peripheral communities in Pakistan, the anglophone writers discussed here maintain their subject positions in their respective discursive fields. Because none of the three, Ahmad, Bhutto, and Shamsie, identifies with any tribal community, their subject positions are embedded in political positions of privilege which validate any fictitious 'real' knowledge they produce about areas and communities existing on the peripheries of the state, based on an urban, Westernised third-person perspective, as well as an orientalist discourse which relegates the tribal to the category of the other. Hence, tribal identity can be compromised in their narrative fiction to accommodate an author's fiction.

Notes

1 Progressivism is the ideology of social reform in the areas of politics, the economy, and science; its basis is in the European Age of Enlightenment and the concept of modernity. Progressivist discourse advocates sociopolitical movements that seek to reform society on the lines of modernisation and Westernisation of state institutions by supplanting local and indigenous societal structures. It is not to be confused with, nor is it a reference to, the 'Progressive Writers' Movement' from the subcontinent, which was formed in 1936 in Lucknow.
2 In 'The Work of Representation' (1997), Hall explains Foucault's theory on the subject position in relation to discourse and the production of knowledge in a discursive field.
3 Titus (1998) discusses several aspects of Baloch and Pashtun tribes, one of which is the use of nomadism or pastoralism as a political strategy. According to Titus, historically, the Afghan leadership, in particular the Pashtun Durranies during the eighteenth century and a considerable part of the nineteenth, had pastoral elements and links.
4 Mountstuart Elphinstone, envoy to the court of Kabul in 1808, and then Governor of Bombay 1819–1827, is an example of such a government official. He is well known as a historian from the British Raj, and authored the famous book on Pashtuns *An Account of the Kingdom of Caubul and its Dependencies: Comprising a View of the Afghaun Nation, and a History of the Dooraunee Monarchy*, published in 1839 in London. Accounts such as Elphinstone's built up over the period of colonisation and relied on each other for validation. This created a certain discourse surrounding the Pashtuns which was based on observations by British political agents.
5 'Islamism' refers to political Islam, and in the context of the topic under discussion it refers to the instrumentalisation of Pashtun tribal elements by political Islamists to wage a war against unorthodox practices of Islam, as well as secular states.

Bibliography

Ahmad, A.S. (2004) *Resistance and Control in Pakistan*. New York: Routledge.
Ahmad, J. (2011) *The Wandering Falcon*. New York: Riverhead Books.
Bal, M. (2009) *Narratology: Introduction to the Theory of Narrative*. 3rd edn. Toronto: University of Toronto Press.
Bhutto, F. (2013) *The Shadow of the Crescent Moon*. London: Penguin Books.
Deleuze, G. and Guattari, F. (2010) 'Nomadology: The War Machine'. In *A Thousand Plateaus*. Seattle: Wormwood Distribution.
Hall, S. (1997) 'The Work of Representation'. In *Representation: Cultural Representations and Signifying Practices*. Ed. by Hall, S. Thousand Oaks: SAGE, 13–61.
Manchanda, N. (2014) 'Queering the Pashtun: Afghan Sexuality in the Homonationalist Imaginary'. *Third World Quarterly* 36(1), 130–146.
Said, E. (2001) *Orientalism: Western Conceptions of the Orient*. New Delhi: Penguin Books India.
Shamsie, K. (2014) *A God in Every Stone*. London: Bloomsbury.
Tapper, R. (2008) 'Who are the Kuchi? Nomad Self-Identities in Afghanistan'. *Journal of the Royal Anthropological Institute* 14(1), 97–116.
Titus, P. (1998) 'Honor the Baloch, Buy the Pushtun: Stereotypes, Social Organization and History in Western Pakistan'. *Modern Asian Studies* 32(3), 657–687.
Tripodi, C. (2011) *Edge of Empire: The British Political Officer and Tribal Administration on the North-West Frontier 1877–1947*. Farnham: Ashgate.
Tucker, S.C. (ed.) (2010) *A Global Chronology of Conflict: From the Ancient World to the Modern Middle East*. Santa Barbara: ABC-CLIO.

14
PHOENIX RISING
The West's use (and misuse) of anglophone memoirs by Pakistani women

Colleen Lutz Clemens

In 2014, I was invited to participate in a college's common reading programme by giving a lecture on Malala Yousafzai's book *I Am Malala* (2013). I took Malala everywhere with me that summer: the beach, coffee shops, doctors' offices, ballet classes. The cover is hard to miss: her bright pink scarf, her eyes looking right at the viewer. People comment on the book when they see it, as most people who follow the news know at least something of the young girl's story.

I start this chapter by sharing two stories of interactions – both with smart women who are readers and friends. In the first, I am sitting in a coffee shop in my town when a friend runs into me. She sees Malala smiling up from my table and begins to gush about how much she appreciated the book, having read it all in a few days. She felt grateful for how much she learnt about Afghanistan from reading it. The second story begins at the kitchen table of one of my tutoring clients. The mother is hovering, nervous about her daughter's upcoming SAT test. The mother sees Malala and begins to remind her daughter: 'Remember her, she was the girl in Afghanistan that the Taliban shot?' The daughter nods her head.

I do not recount these stories to disparage my friends, who are smart women who took the time to read the memoir. They are well-informed and care deeply about women's issues around the world. And yet even they had been lulled by the narrative that there is one essentialised version of the woman in the Muslim world, that all women from those regions have the same experience, and that they are powerless without the intercession of some element from the West. Books that reify these narratives are popular with the reading public in the 'West', a term I use with trepidation because of its slippery nature. This chapter will examine the phenomenon of what I term 'phoenix narratives' that are deployed to reify an essentialist notion of women in the 'East'. Phoenix narratives are the stories of young girls and women who have been beaten, tortured, and oppressed at the hands of misogynistic structures and risen out of the ashes of their suffering to find 'liberation'. Perhaps the most famous of these narratives is Yousafzai's, yet Mukhtar Mai's *In the Name of Honor* (2006) is an important predecessor to Yousafzai's memoir.

An essential notion generalises and limits simultaneously. For example, when one hears the platitude, 'If women were the rulers in the world, there would be no war', one is hearing an essential notion about gender and femininity in relation to violence. The idea behind this quote is that women are naturally not inclined to violence, that women are only soft and peaceful;

and when they are not, there must be a reason or reasons to explain why they are going against their 'natural' inclinations. Essentialist narratives are all around us, and we must unyoke ourselves from the powerful hold of essentialist narratives that hold us all in their grip and have the power to make people feel abnormal or diminished. These narratives – 'comforting myths', as Chinua Achebe calls them – must be deconstructed, and readers must work to create narratives that recognise diversity and the unique experience of the people around us in the world. Essentialism is the force that allows two very smart women who have spent considerable time thinking about Malala to conflate her with women in Afghanistan, even though Malala's story takes place in Pakistan, a country very different from Afghanistan. Do women in those countries share similar structural struggles? Yes. Does the United States have complicated geopolitical relationships with both? Yes. Comparisons can be made, but the conflation of nations and their peoples is a dangerous game.

This chapter will study closely a few of the moments that contributed to the construction of two essentialist narratives of women in the East that have overtaken the West's image of women from this region: the veiled woman and the 'phoenix', a term I apply to the genre of memoirs like Yousafzai's that shows a young woman emerging from the destruction wrought by the Taliban, a group that does not represent the majority of Muslims in the world.

Edward Said argues in the original introduction to *Orientalism* that 'without examining Orientalism as a discourse one cannot possibly understand the enormously systematic discipline by which European culture was able to manage – and even produce – the Orient politically, sociologically, militarily, ideologically, scientifically, and imaginatively' (1979: 3). This chapter works towards Said's original project of deconstructing orientalist narratives in order to understand how, in the twenty-first century, a single, narrow narrative of women in the Muslim world continues to be (mis)constructed, the impact of reorientalisation on those women, and the use – and often misuse – of these narratives within political discussions.

The 'veiled' woman in Western rhetoric and imagination

It should be no surprise that the narrative that leads to Yousafzai's memoir begins on 11 September 2001.

On that day, my second period Honours English class and I watched as planes flew into buildings. A roomful of seventeen-year-olds implored me to make sense of what was happening on the screen just as I had shepherded them through Hamlet's soliloquies and feminist readings of *Jane Eyre*. But I had nothing to offer them. That moment was too big for all of us, and only now are we starting to make sense of it and our response as a nation to what would become the moment by which many of us would measure our lives; from that morning on, many Americans lived in the 'post-9/11' world, and my research is one small piece of a larger body of work investigating this 'new' world and the ways we speak about each other in it.

After September 11, a trajectory of anti-Islamic sentiment began. Starting with an overt 'othering' of the Muslim faith, the US government under the purview of George W. Bush worked to focus attention on the oppression of Islamic women, a progression meant to provide a rationale for eventual military action taken in the name of the 'oppressed women' instead of in the name of US interests. Suddenly, names that had never entered the national discourse on a broad scale became household words uttered with a mix of contempt and confusion: al Qaeda, Osama bin Laden, Sunni and Shia. Areas of the world previously known for oil or unrest within their own borders – Iraq, Afghanistan, Pakistan – housed an enemy that professed a hatred for all things Western, a hatred about which those outside of academic or governmental circles knew little, up until 9/11. As Americans watched a new national department being created overnight, they began to speak about a world that, on 10 September 2001, had been of little interest to them.

An interest in the differences between the 'East' and the 'West' grew nationwide as people found these foreign words slipping off their tongues. I heed Said's warning against essential concepts such as 'East' and 'West' — that neither term 'has any ontological stability' — and recognise that no clear boundary exists between these two concepts (1979: xvii). He reminds readers that we must 'insist that the terrible reductive conflicts that herd people under falsely unifying rubrics like "America", "the West", or "Islam" and invent collective identities for large numbers of individuals who are actually quite diverse cannot remain as potent as they are', comments he makes in the new preface he added in 2003, after witnessing the 9/11 attacks and their political aftermath (1979: xxviii).

After the attacks, new images entered the living rooms of millions of Americans: bearded men in white turbans sat in caves and laughed at the unanticipated success of the attacks of 11 September, while women in light blue *burqas* wandered dusty streets between ruined buildings. Until that historical moment, many viewers had never considered the global tensions between East and West, between nationalist movements and fundamentalist religious factions. The events of 11 September forced the American population out of its ignorance as it witnessed on its own soil a tragic manifestation of a problem that certainly was not new to the rest of the world.

I witnessed a growing, rampant nationalism I had never seen before. Within days, reports of attacks against Muslims grew to higher numbers than ever before in this country. Anyone who could mistakenly be identified as a Muslim based on traditional garb was in danger, such as the Sikh Balbir Godhi, who was shot five times outside his gas station because his attacker, Frank Roque, assumed Godhi's turban meant he was a Muslim. Within the six days after the attacks, the Council on American-Islamic Relations received double the number of complaints about harassment than they had received during the entire year before. The Council estimated that, at that time, seven million Muslims lived in the United States. Though many of these millions of Muslims denounced the attacks, a fear of 'the Other' grew through binary rhetoric. Gender binaries and a Western attachment to female 'liberation' quickly found its signifier: the 'veil'.

Once Islam entered the US' national discourse, the 'veil' became a powerful symbol of women's oppression under the Taliban and in 'the East'. Images of veiled women ran on television and many public officials evoked the image to rationalise the War on Terror. Freeing women living 'under the veil' became a rallying cry to justify invasions to change the ideologies of nations. As President Bush stated just days after 9/11, 'This is the world's fight. This is civilization's fight. This is the fight of all who believe in progress and pluralism, tolerance and freedom' (2001: n.p.). The assumption follows that women living in countries where veiling is practised were not allowed 'freedom'.

Deployed by the Bush administration to gender the conflict, Laura Bush made similar rhetorical gestures in her Thanksgiving 2001 radio address focusing on women; she drew attention to the US' use of women's oppression to validate military action, thereby continuing to gender the ensuing conflicts:

> I'm delivering this week's radio address to kick off a world-wide effort to focus on the brutality against women and children by the al-Qaida terrorist network and the regime it supports in Afghanistan, the Taliban. That regime is now in retreat across much of the country, and the people of Afghanistan — especially women — are rejoicing. Afghan women know, through hard experience, what the rest of the world is discovering: the brutal oppression of women is a central goal of the terrorists.
>
> (2001: n.p.)

She then shifted to note that those in the Taliban are not civilised, alluding to the idea that it is the responsibility of the 'civilized' (read: 'the West') to police those who cannot live civilly (read: those in 'the East'). The latter do not respect 'their' women, whereas 'we' in 'the West' do. Not to want to preserve this respect is to be inhuman.

She reinscribes the binary between 'East' and 'West', stating that in the United States, 'We respect our mothers, our sisters and daughters', and then holds up the West as liberators: 'Because of our recent military gains in much of Afghanistan, women are no longer imprisoned in their homes [...] The fight against terrorism is also a fight for the rights and dignity of women' (2001: n.p.). Finally, Bush seals the dominant narrative that Western women are liberated while Eastern women are disempowered and she reminds the American listening audience of how lucky they (women) are to be in the United States, for only the United States can ensure the safety of women in the 'East':

> After the events of the last few months, we'll be holding our families even closer. And we will be especially thankful for all the blessings of American life. I hope Americans will join our family in working to ensure that dignity and opportunity will be secured for all the women and children of Afghanistan.

Laura Bush focuses on the brutality 'the terrorists' commit against women's bodies as if it were a new problem that just at that moment the US would need to disrupt. Her reification of the binary between East and West relies on gender and the idea so often deployed at that fraught time: that women in the East lack agency and must find a Western intercessor to initiate the liberation process. Interestingly, up until the morning of 9/11, the Feminist Majority Foundation's pleas to the White House for a discussion of women in Afghanistan had gone unheeded. In *The Terror Dream*, Susan Faludi (2008) reports that suddenly, after 9/11, women's organisations were summoned to the White House to give briefings on an issue about which it cared little before the attacks. The White House even held a conference on Afghan women, and eventually President Bush signed the Afghan Women and Children's Relief Act in December 2001 as part of his 'crusade'. In a moment, women in Afghanistan were the locus of the US administration's interest, which waned once the war on terror began in earnest.

By focusing on the violence perpetrated against women, Laura Bush set up an opportunity to argue that one can only undo this violence with violence; clearly, these people, if they torture their women, cannot be stopped without force. She invokes family life in the US, recently shaken by the attack of 11 September 2001, and uses 'the blessings of life' as the antithesis of women who are denied the right to care for their children. Women in Afghanistan (and soon after the 'axis of evil') are denied their 'natural' life of being mothers and wives; they can do nothing but 'rejoice' at the Coalition of the Willing's efforts to liberate them from their state-imposed chains. Government rhetoric about women in Afghanistan often focused on veiling and the West's reading of the practice as oppressive in every situation. An essential notion of women who veil became embedded in rhetorics of gender and women in connection with war and liberation. Veiling practices were directly connected to women's experiences in the East and were conflated into the same essential idea of the oppressed woman in the East in need of Western military engagement for personal liberation from 'the veil'.[1]

To Americans, the 'veil' became a signifier of all the perceived negative aspects of Islamic culture: patriarchy, lack of freedom of expression, tyranny, and fundamentalism. Much academic work has been done to illustrate this purposeful construction and misreading of veiling. Now we in the West must unpack that powerful signifier and show its complexity – its meanings shaped by nationalist state dictates, governmental laws, women's desires, and anti-nationalist movements – if we are ever going to change the national discourse surrounding women in the East, a topic clearly of interest to Western readers based on the popularity of books like Yousafzai's.

As I remind my students and those attending my lectures, there is, in fact, no one essential 'veil', no singular definition of what it means when a woman places a *hijab, burqa, niqab*, or any other covering on her body.[2] Hence, when discussing this issue, I use the term 'veiling' to dismantle the limiting idea that there is such a single essential entity as 'the veil' and to acknowledge the dynamic nature of this signifier. Said succinctly reminds readers in his preface that 'the worst aspect of this essentializing stuff is that human suffering in all its density and pain is spirited away' (1979: xxi). The focus on veiling in discussions of women in the Islamic world became the cornerstone of the construction of the essential notion of the 'woman' in those regions.

The construction of Eastern women's essential identity in Western readerships' collective imagination

In American popular culture, literature attempting to show the Islamic oppression of women is *de rigueur*. In his talk 'Translating for Bigots', Adam Talib argues that the covers of books from the East, particularly those about women, share a reliance on essentialist discourse in the West. He says (at 7:30 in the video):

> the books that are doing quite well commercially often present themselves to the reader in this way [showing a slide of a variety of covers]. There is still an exotic, orientalizing marketing technique [...] you're tapping into a popular news and political discourse around a part of the world that is going to affect even literary translations.[3]
>
> (2013: n.p.)

Veiling is often deployed as a rhetorical device on the covers of books with female protagonists in the East written for a Western audience. For example, though Marjane Satrapi's main character's extra-diegetic gaze from the centre of her cover could indicate some semblance of agency, the imposing red cover overtakes her small figure. Her look of defiance is there, but small. The rest of the women on popular covers look away; some do not even have faces. The cover of Debbie Rodriguez's *Kabul Beauty School* (2007) advertises that an American woman goes 'behind the veil'. In fact, what she does is go to Kabul to teach hairdressing, but the title intimates that she infiltrated some dark, secret world where Americans never really want, or dare, to go. The author of *Reading Lolita in Tehran*, Azar Nafisi, has even been criticised by fellow Iranian writers for going too far in her depiction of women in Iran and offering an easy target to Republicans who wanted more fuel for their military fire. While she rejects all these accusations, she hasn't been able to shake off the stigma branded upon her by her fellow writers. But even though I argue that her text shows women resisting an oppressive theocracy, the cover gives no inkling of such resistance (Clemens (2013b). The images of women on these covers work towards creating an essential notion of 'the veil', as if all women in some kind of covering are the same and require outside forces to liberate them.

Meyda Yeğenoğlu argues in *Colonial Fantasies* that studying the way in which the West represents 'the veil' teaches more about the construction of Western identity than that of the women who veil:

> By taking the representation of the veil as a test case, I suggest that the presumption of a hidden essence and truth behind the veil is the means by which both the Western/

colonial and the masculine subject constitute their own identity. Moreover, by demonstrating the structural homology between the representations of the Orient, veil, and feminine, I suggest that the discourse of Orientalism is mapped powerfully onto the language of phallocentrism and thereby point to the inextricable link between representations of cultural and sexual difference.

(1998: 11)

Western political action often relies on this mythical 'truth' of the veil: that it is oppressive, demeaning, dangerous, and antithetical to the 'Western' desire for freedom. The 'veil' signifies all that is wrong with the 'Orient', and anglophone narratives are often the first point of contact for a Western audience to engage with this essentialist narrative.

Those in the West who are on a 'crusade' – the language George W. Bush used when discussing the war on terror – often construct themselves as the saviours of women. In *The Terror Dream*, Faludi argues that Americans 'were also enlisted in a symbolic war at home, a war to repair and restore a national myth' (2008: 16). If the myth of America is a place where women are safe and free, there must be another side to the binary in which the women who live under the 'enemy' must be covered and lacking in all freedoms. In these cases, the West uses the trope of 'the veil' as a means of constantly replicating its belief in the dominance of its ideologies, specifically those of freedom and democracy. Yeğenolğu concludes her Introduction with a similar argument:

the desire to unveil women should not be seen simply as an uncovering of their bodies, but as a *re-inscription*, for the discourse of unveiling is no less incorporated in the existential or embodied being of Oriental women than the discourse of veiling.

(1998: 12; emphasis added)

While, in the West, the idea of unveiling is equated with freedom, Yeğenolğu urges caution in simplifying the act. The West has a vested interest in maintaining the idea that women who veil do it under duress and suffer greatly because of it; thereby, in Western discourse, those who work to 'save' those women will be 'greeted as liberators'.

In an interview on National Public Radio in February of 2002, then Secretary of Defence Donald Rumsfeld exploited this essentialist narrative of women in the 'East' and talked about the ways in which the US, in a short time, was able to 'free' Afghani women from the *burqa*:

Women have stopped being repressed. They can actually walk out in the street and not have their entire faces and bodies covered by burkhas [sic]. They can laugh on the street. They can go to a doctor, which they couldn't do. They can go to school, which they couldn't do.

(2002: n.p.)

Historically, we know that many of these victories were short-lived, and women continue to struggle against structural oppression, but of most importance to this chapter's argument is Rumsfeld using women's rights as a sign of improvement in a country, an issue and a population in which his administration had very little interest months before.

Rising from the ashes: the phoenixes Mukhtar and Malala

This notion of liberation, of freeing women, forces readers and scholars to consider a second essentialist character borne out of texts popular in the decades following 11 September 2001: the phoenix. Among an anglophone readership, the phoenix narrative genre came to enjoy success in the academic community and among a public reading audience.

Before Malala, there was Mukhtar. Mai is also from Pakistan, where she lived without access to the same privileges that Malala enjoyed. Mai's 2006 memoir *In the Name of Honor* tells of her desire to die after being gang-raped as retribution for her younger brother flirting with a girl from another tribe. But instead, Mai chooses to fight Pakistan's laws on rape and sues the government. Mai's story would easily have been lost if it were not for the attention paid to it, and to her, by *New York Times* journalist Nicholas Kristoff. In his preface to *In the Name of Honor*, he concludes his introduction of Mai to his readers thus:

> I think you will find a story that is tremendously inspiring rather than one that tells of brutality and despair. By the alchemy of her courage and stubbornness, Mukhtar has taken a sordid tale of gang rape and turned it into something heartwarming and hopeful.
>
> (2006: xvi)

Kristof must make the case to readers that while what they are going to read is in part a 'sordid tale' of structural violence enacted on Mai physically by tribal entities and psychically by national politics, the reader will leave the text feeling hope with a warm heart. Mai's rise out of the ashes, so to speak, inscribes her account with a feeling of do-goodery common in texts telling the stories of women forced into the margins of society by patriarchal family, tribal, cultural, and governmental structures.[4]

The most recent of the books that fall into this genre – and perhaps the one with the most cultural currency – is Malala's story. These two texts contribute to the constructed image of women in the Muslim world. Mai's text is mediated through a Western journalist who found the story of the young girl and wanted it to be heard. This element of assistance gives a clear indication that the audience for Mai's texts is a Western one – and of course the fact that the books were originally written in English illustrates that although both women are Pakistani, their audience is the anglophone world. There is nothing inherently wrong with this, yet these phoenix narratives enjoy a strong currency in the West[5] and are of less interest in the native regions of the authors (Kugelman 2017). These narratives make us Western readers feel better about our own systems, our own treatment of women, and our military engagements pursued in the name of these women.

The covers of these phoenix narratives utilise the veiled woman trope – but in a different way. The phoenix covers play on imagery with which the West has become familiar in the years since 9/11. But in the case of these particular phoenix narratives, we see the actual subject of the text on the cover, not some stock image of Eastern women huddling passively. Also, Mai and Yousafzai engage a more direct gaze on their covers. Mai's cover may be seen as a bridge between the desire for the defeated woman trope, as is evident in the previously discussed book covers, and the emergence of these phoenix narratives from the Muslim world; her look is not direct, but there is a defiance in her face – and readers see her face. Yousafzai looks directly at the viewer, inviting engagement in a partnership between author and reader.

Interestingly, both Mai and Yousafzai were named Woman of the Year by *Glamour* magazine. There is something disconcerting about a magazine dedicated to perpetuating, in the West, the mythology of what a woman should be and using these Pakistani women as their women of the year in 2005 and 2013. Both of these women deserve to be honoured for their work and deserve to be heard – I have no interest in silencing women – yet this chapter's concern is *how* these women and their stories of survival are being deployed for other purposes that conflict with their messages – such as putting Yousafzai in front of a L'Oréal banner or using Mai to sell fashion magazines. When their stories are used for other purposes, readers and consumers must be concerned for these girls and women and hope that they are not being used in the same way 'veiled' women in the Muslim world were used as objects of orientalism instead of being seen as agents of change in need of allies and partners – not in need of saviours.

Phoenix narratives do allow the Western reader some satisfaction. Consider why the story of Yousafzai captured the world's attention: a smart, young, spunky girl who used her mind and her body to fight the most fearsome bogeyman in the US' collective imagination, the Taliban. But is this satisfaction really the end goal of Yousafzai's work? I would argue that Yousafzai does not want us Western readers to feel satisfied and applaud ourselves. Yousafzai argues for action – not satisfaction. As she stated in her Nobel Peace Prize acceptance speech,

> I dedicate the Nobel Peace Prize money to the Malala Fund, to help give girls quality education, everywhere, anywhere in the world and to raise their voices. The first place this funding will go to is where my heart is, to build schools in Pakistan – especially in my home of Swat and Shangla. In my own village, there is still no secondary school for girls. And it is my wish and my commitment, and now my challenge to build one so that my friends and my sisters can go there to school and get quality education and to get this opportunity to fulfil their dreams.
>
> (2014: n.p.)

She is surely looking to create a community of allies in her fight for gender equity instead of creating a phoenix narrative that one may read and then discard as a story that has ended happily, without even remembering the geographic setting. Yousafzai demands action beyond a 'heartwarming' text; hers is a narrative arc that only *begins* on the book's final pages as the reader should turn to association and activism upon completion of the text.

Phoenixes are mythical, not material

In 2014, Texas artist Anat Ronen's mural 'Yes You Can!', depicting Yousafzai in the pose of Rosie the Riveter, shows the conflict between the desire for a 'heartwarming' phoenix narrative and the truth of structural oppression enacted on women's bodies and psyches. Rosie the Riveter was an amalgamation of women – there is no one exact person who was Rosie *per se*. Yousafzai is a person, a young woman recovering from a devastating attack and exiled with her family from the country she loves. Conflating Malala and Rosie signals that the world is asking too much of Yousafzai. To be conflated with an icon of war is too much to ask of an individual – for remember, the goal of this chapter is to undo the essentialism reified by the veil and phoenix narratives. Readers should remember that Rosie the Riveter and the women her image inspired were tossed aside and out of factories as soon as the war was over and the country no longer needed women to work in industry. I do not want to see the same thing done with Yousafzai or her story; she should not be tossed aside when she and her story are no longer serving the West's militaristic or nationalistic needs.

Perhaps it is good that Yousafzai ends the main part of her text in this way: 'When people talk about the way I was shot and what happened, I think it's the story of Malala, 'a girl shot by the Taliban': I don't feel it's a story about me at all' (2013: 301). Mai ends her text with a similar rhetorical move, distancing herself from the ways in which the story went beyond her own experience:

I have become, *in spite of myself*, a symbol for all these women who suffer the violence of patriarchs and tribal chiefs, and if this image of me has spread beyond our borders, it can only be a credit to my country.

(2006: 158; emphasis added)

Part of me cringes and feels great sadness for them not identifying their own selves with their narratives of tragedy and recovery. However, this detachment from their stories may be the strategy that saves them, for if the West is asking too much of their narratives – for them to be mythical phoenixes instead of young women – then maybe they can preserve themselves in the rhetorical process, even if they lose control over the way their readers use their narratives.

Notes

1 For further discussion of the use of unveiling as a liberation trope deployed in rhetorics in the West, see Clemens (2013a).
2 Chandra Talpade Mohanty discusses the ways in which the academy uses (and abuses) 'the veil' to discuss Third-World women: 'it is the analytical leap from the practice of veiling to an assertion of its general significance in controlling women that must be questioned' (1984: 347). She notes that though the coverings may look similar, their disparate cultural meanings cannot be conflated.
3 Readers can see similar images presented during a talk I gave on *I Am Malala* www.youtube.com/watch?v=lZmwM6_rbK0 (at 25:30).
4 Mai has become an agent for girls' education in Pakistan. Mai's Girl's Model School is at the heart of her work through the Mukhtar Mai Women's Organisation.
5 Indicators of their popularity include Simon and Schuster's creation of a reading club guide for Mai's book and the number of Yousafzai's books sold: over a million since October 2013, according to her literary agency Curtis Brown.

Bibliography

Ahmed al-Haj, M.M. (2017) 'Desperate Parents in Yemen are Marrying off their Young Girls for Cash'. *The Independent* [online]. Available from <www.independent.co.uk/news/world/middle-east/yemen-crisis-civil-war-parents-marrying-selling-off-children-girls-cash-a7759981.html> [15 January 2018].

Bush, G.W. (2001) 'George W. Bush: Address before a Joint Session of the Congress on the United States Response to the Terrorist Attacks of September 11'. *The American Presidency Project* [online]. Available from <www.presidency.ucsb.edu/ws/?pid=64731> [15 January 2018].

Bush, L. (2001) 'Laura Bush: The Weekly Address Delivered by the First Lady'. *The American Presidency Project* [online]. Available from: <www.presidency.ucsb.edu/ws/?pid=24992> [15 January 2018].

Clemens, C. (2013a) '"Girl Rising:" What Can We Do To Help Girls? Ask Liam Neeson'. *Bitch Flicks* [online]. Available from <www.btchflcks.com/2013/05/girl-rising-what-can-we-do-to-help-girls-ask-liam-neeson.html> [24 January 2018].

Clemens, C. (2013b) '"Imagine Us in the Act of Reading": A Resistant Reading of *Reading Lolita in Tehran*'. *Journal of Postcolonial Writing* 50(5), 584–595.

Faludi, S. (2008) *The Terror Dream: Myth and Misogyny in an Insecure America*. New York: Picador.

Kugelman, M. (2017) 'Why Pakistan Hates Malala'. *Foreign Policy* [online]. Available from <http://foreignpolicy.com/2017/08/15/why-pakistan-hates-malala/> [18 January 2018].

Mai, M. (2006) *In the Name of Honor: A Memoir*. New York: Simon and Schuster.

Mohanty, C.T. (1984) 'Under Western Eyes: Feminist Scholarship and Colonial Discourses'. *Boundary 2* (12–13), 333–358.

Rumsfeld, D. (2002) 'DefenseLink News Transcript: Secretary Rumsfeld Interview with Bob Edwards, NPR Radio, Morning Edition'. *United States Department of Defence* [online]. Available from <www.defenselink.mil/transcripts/transcript.aspx?transcriptid=2651> [5 January 2009].

Said, E.W. (1979) *Orientalism*. New York: Vintage Books.

Talib, A. (2013) Translating for Bigots [online]. Available from <www.youtube.com/watch?v=aANKpO4zmGA> [15 January 2018].

Warren, R. (2014) 'This Mural of Malala as Feminist Symbol Rosie the Riveter is Wonderful'. *BuzzFeed* [online]. Available from <www.buzzfeed.com/rossalynwarren/this-mural-of-malala-as-feminist-symbol-rosie-the-riveter-is> [15 January 2018].

Yeğenolğu, M. (1998) *Colonial Fantasies: Towards a Feminist Reading of Orientalism*. Cambridge: Cambridge University Press.

Yousafzai, M. (2013) *I Am Malala: The Girl Who Stood up for Education and Was Shot by the Taliban*. New York: Little, Brown.

Yousafzai, M. (2014) 'Malala Yousafzai – Nobel Lecture', Nobelprize.org [online]. Available from <www.nobelprize.org/nobel_prizes/peace/laureates/2014/yousafzai-lecture_en.html> [15 January 2018].

15
WRITING BACK AND/AS ACTIVISM
Refiguring victimhood and remapping the shooting of Malala Yousafzai

Rachel Fox

On 9 October 2012, Malala Yousafzai, a fifteen-year-old girl from the Swat Valley in Pakistan, was shot by the Taliban. It was an event which garnered international attention. This chapter primarily focuses on Yousafzai's memoir, *I am Malala: The Girl Who Stood up for Education and Was Shot by the Taliban* (2013), co-written with British journalist and foreign correspondent, Christina Lamb. Drawing from her memoir, as well as the documentary *He Named Me Malala* (Guggenheim 2015) and her 2014 Nobel Lecture, I discuss the ways in which Yousafzai's various identifiers – activist, spokeswoman, feminist, victim, girl, Muslim, Pakistani – are represented, propagated, and challenged. Before the shooting, and since, Yousafzai has campaigned for girls' right to education and she is now a recognisable feminist icon. Her identifiers of activist and spokeswoman, derived from her role of campaigner, are tied to explicit acts of agency. Although these identifiers might be seen to have diminished against the image of Yousafzai as a victim or – in a more positive frame – a survivor, I argue that the recounting of the shooting as a remediated event by Yousafzai herself unfolds a space for her to establish her own position of agency.

In her 2014 Nobel Lecture, Yousafzai draws attention to multiple facets of her identity. She identifies her position as both a victim and an activist for girls' right to education and also proudly declares that she is 'the first Pashtun, the first Pakistani, and the youngest person to receive this award' (2014: n.p.). These various facets of her identity – victim, activist, female, Pashtun, and Pakistani, alongside the identifiers of Muslim and feminist – are all integral parts of both her public image as it is represented in news and social media, and her self-representation in her memoir and other public speeches and interviews. In this chapter I explore the ways in which the homogenising of some of the individual labels attributed to Yousafzai are challenged, or at least complicated, by her own narrative, and the narrative form of the memoir. I argue that Yousafzai's memoir, as an act of writing back, reframes the events of the shooting in light of her political convictions. She utilises both her victim and activist identities as part of a feminist discourse and her personal narrative galvanises her political campaign for girls' right to education.

A bestselling memoir, a 'veiled bestseller'? Personalising/decentring the political

I am Malala is an international, *bestselling* memoir. Here, I complicate the connection of *I am Malala* to the notion of the 'veiled best-seller' coined by Gillian Whitlock (2007: 88). 'Veiled bestsellers', so-called for the image of veiled women usually featured on their covers, are conceived as biographies of Muslim women which 'can be harnessed by forces of commercialization and consumerism in terms of the exotic appeal of cultural difference. They can also be used to buttress aggressive Western intervention in so-called primitive or dysfunctional national communities' (Whitlock 2007: 55), especially in the context of the War on Terror in the aftermath of the terrorist attacks on the US on 11 September 2001.

The circumstances that Yousafzai describes in *I am Malala*, and the conditions which led to her shooting, are the consequence of a rise in Islamic extremism, especially in rural northern Pakistan, in the political climate of the War on Terror. Aroosa Kanwal connects these political events: 'The post-9/11 situation in Pakistan owes a great deal to [President] Zia [ul-Haq]'s Islamisation policies, which resulted in the rise of Islamic extremism and *Jihadist* culture in Pakistan and Afghanistan' (2015: 15). Arising from these contexts there has been a general shift in focus from the Indo-Pak to the Af-Pak border, which has been reflected in recent Pakistani anglophone literature (Chambers 2011: 125). In the case of *I am Malala*, the Af-Pak border is particularly pronounced given the proximity of the Swat Valley to the northern border of Pakistan, the Taliban activity experienced in the province, and Yousafzai's Pashtun heritage. In *Offence: The Muslim Case* (2009), Kamila Shamsie explains the complicated relationships between Pashtuns in Afghanistan and Pakistan, and Pakistan and the US in the context of the US invasion of Afghanistan in 2001. Shamsie states that although the Pakistani government was ally to the US in its invasion of Afghanistan, 'Pashtuns of the Frontier Province saw it as a war on Pashtuns. The Durand Line, which divides Pakistani Pashtuns from Afghan Pashtuns, had always been viewed as entirely artificial by the Pashtuns themselves' (2009: 69–70). These regional and political contexts, as part of the rhetoric of the War on Terror and alongside Yousafzai's subject matter, which represents the Taliban threat to Muslim women, incorporate *I am Malala* into the literary market of the 'veiled bestseller'.

'Veiled bestsellers', which are marketed on the representation of the oppression of (veiled) Muslim women, are typically read ethnographically or, in related fashion, in ways that enable the metropolitan reader to display 'cosmopolitan tastes, openness, sympathy, political commitment, and benevolent interest in cultural difference' (Whitlock 2007: 55). This cosmopolitan approach to 'veiled bestsellers' is further accentuated by the publicity of Yousafzai's shooting, and therefore her positioning as a clearly recognisable victim of the Taliban. Yousafzai's image as a wounded victim and, in particular, a wounded child, which was expedited by news and social media coverage at the time of the shooting, prompts well-meaning, but almost inevitably un-actioned (or futile) sympathy and 'charitable compassion' (Ahmed 2014: 192). Shenila Khoja-Moolji describes the notion of 'charitable compassion' as an affective response which possesses 'its own politics in that it appropriates the suffering of others for the purpose of empowering the self' (2015: 540). In *I am Malala*, Yousafzai describes some of the gifts, cards, and good wishes she received in the aftermath of her shooting. In one example from her memoir, she describes how 'Beyoncé had written me a card and posted a photo of it on Facebook' (2013: 243–244). This gesture by Beyoncé, a famous feminist icon in her own right, demonstrates the notion of 'charitable compassion': her charitable act is not a private act, but one which is publicised online. Given Beyoncé's popularity, sharing this photograph online may serve to further spread the news of Yousafzai and her cause, but it also receives a metric value of 'likes' and 'shares' which reflects positively on Beyoncé herself.

Khoja-Moolji argues that 'Through acts of charity and consumption, Western audiences assume that they can interrupt the suffering that awaits Muslim girls' (2015: 545). She goes on to add that such 'actions often do not involve understanding the politics, histories, and contexts of Malala's shooting. They depoliticize Malala and can be read as practices of distancing' (2015: 545).

As with the 'veiled bestseller', in which the hugely complex religious, historical, and cultural contexts of the practice of veiling are diminished, instead symbolising oppression, cosmopolitan and charitable responses to Yousafzai's shooting decontextualise the specific regional contexts behind the shooting. In tune with Whitlock's account of the 'veiled bestseller', Jasmin Zine argues that, in the context of Muslim feminist literary production, some 'didactic texts' seeks to 'teach us "truths" about imperilled lives of Muslim women' (2014: 185). Zine argues that 'these kinds of texts construct a "pedagogy of peril" as the central lens through which Muslim women and girls are viewed' (2014: 185), at risk of religious and patriarchal oppression. Yousafzai's memoir, literally marketed off of the shooting that imperilled her life, is at risk of belonging to a market that, as part of a neo-imperial feminist agenda, homogenises, or even demonises, Muslim identity, in spite of the pride with which Yousafzai often speaks about her religion.

This risk is explained by Fatima Bhutto whose own memoir, *Songs of Blood and Sword* (2011), gives a personal account of her family's political history. In an early review (30 October 2013) of Yousafzai's memoir, the niece of the former Pakistani Prime Minister Benazir Bhutto (1993–1996) states that:

> [H]ere in Pakistan anger towards this ambitious young campaigner is as strong as ever. Amid the bile, there is a genuine concern that this extraordinary girl's courageous and articulate message will be colonised by one power or other for its own insidious agendas.
>
> (2013: n.p.)

Indeed, when it was first published, *I am Malala* was banned in many private schools in Pakistan on the grounds of this same concern ('Malala Yousafzai's Book Banned' 2013). *I am Malala*, a bestseller in English-speaking countries, can be appropriated as part of the literary market of 'veiled bestsellers', or 'pedagogies of peril' wherein the cosmopolitan reader who buys the memoir in an act of charitable compassion – or an act of charitable consumption – reads Yousafzai's suffering as representative of the suffering of 'all' girls from Pakistan or, even more broadly, all those who are Muslim and from the Global South (Indo-Pak border) and/or the Middle East (Af-Pak border).

I am Malala is a pedagogical text; a means of 'knowledge production' (Taylor and Zine 2014: 2). However, despite the risk that *I am Malala* could be appropriated as a 'pedagogy of peril', I argue that the written content of the memoir – which, despite her reservations, Bhutto finds 'courageous and articulate' (2013: n.p.) – undermines its paratexts. Yousafzai's self-representation of her personal experiences alongside her political convictions in *I am Malala* challenges homogeneous readings of her identifiers as a Muslim woman and as a victim. Whitlock describes memoir as 'a genre for those who are authorized and who have acquired cultural legitimacy and influence' (2007: 20). Yousafzai proudly identifies with both her national (Pakistani) and her ethnic (Pashtun) identity in her Nobel Lecture and repeatedly in her memoir. Consequently, she situates herself in a position of cultural authority in her discussion of the politics and events that have directly affected her family both before and since her birth.

Yousafzai presents a personal narrative that is explicitly tied to and contemplates within its writing the political, social, cultural, and religious contexts of her recounted life experiences both prior to and since her shooting. Norbert Bugeja describes the genre of the memoir as a remediation of the past:

> By narrating a representational space, the memoir forges the encounter between the claims of unrequited pasts and the present narrative as it interpellates the surviving

traces of those pasts for the world literary stage, hence perpetrating new forms of witness and testimony to their oppression.

(2012: 24)

In memoir, the remediation of past events is inextricably tied to the personal perceptions which are written down retrospectively and subjectively. These past events are remapped through the changing personal, political, and cultural perspectives of the author, who writes back to the events under the influence of experiences that have occurred since. In the case of *I am Malala*, Yousafzai's narratives of historical-political events in Pakistan and the experiences of her parents and herself living and growing up during these events are interpellated through two significant lenses. The first is through Yousafzai's eyes as a Muslim, Pakistani, Pashtun girl, and the reader's perception of these identities; the second lens is the foreknowledge of both the writer and the reader that the earlier events narrated by Yousafzai culminate in her shooting: an experience with huge personal ramifications for Yousazfai, and political ramifications for her campaign for girls' right to education.

The act of writing back as remediation – interpellating the past through both personal and retrospective experience – can be interpreted as a form of border crossing, which I link to Henry A. Giroux's definition of 'border pedagogy' as something that is 'both transformative and emancipatory' (1993: 29). This is established by shifting perspectives in place, time, or media: 'Border pedagogy decenters as it remaps. The terrain of learning becomes inextricably linked to the shifting parameters of place, identity, history, and power' (Giroux 1993: 30). As previously discussed, *I am Malala* has the potential to be appropriated by neo-imperial economic markets and political propaganda, as part of a rhetoric of 'rescue' in support of the War on Terror. However, I argue that in Yousafzai's feminist narrative, which campaigns for girls' right to education in light of both her personal experiences and political convictions, the retrospective nature of writing decentres and remaps such 'Western' neo-imperialist imaginaries.

Female – and feminist – (auto)biographies are typically relational and dialogical. As has been comprehensively argued by numerous critics (see Smith and Watson 1992; Moore-Gilbert 2009), female and postcolonial (auto)biographers aspire, consciously or unconsciously, towards a plural and collective self as opposed to the individuated self that is more commonly recognised in sovereign male autobiography. Supporting this argument, Nawar Al-Hassan Golley asserts that:

> Writing, for women, becomes a way to provide spaces within which women can talk about the complexities and pluralities of their selves. The individualistic model, provided by male writers, especially in the west, becomes inadequate to the lives women lead.
>
> (2003: 69–70)

Thus, (auto)biographies written by women are predicated on the constitution of a plural and dispersed model of self-representation, which forms dialogues socially and locally. As a dispersed model of self-representation, such (auto)biographies enable a space for decentring and remapping female identities, both as they are understood by themselves and by sociopolitical discourses and/or stereotypes. Yousafzai writes within this literary context and her memoir works to establish the complexities and realities of the multiple facets of her identity (e.g. victim, Muslim, woman) which are subject to appropriation and stereotyping by neo-imperial readers and markets.

In the context of black female subjectivity, Mae G. Henderson argues that postcolonial women (auto)biographers speak within two discursive spaces: the space they write about and the space they are writing to; their subject and their market. They 'speak in dialogically racial and gendered voices to the other(s) both within and without' (Henderson 2014: 61). In this sense, their narrative is relational and, publicising the private, 'When a woman writes her own story down on paper or tells it to others, she is asserting her autonomy by ordering her life into a composition and to that extent moving toward feminist consciousness' (Golley 2003: 81). The act of writing or speaking about oneself explicitly builds relational ties with the surrounding world, not only to respond to social, cultural, and political circumstances, but also to establish the writers' own set of politics. In Golley's configuration of the (auto)biographical act, (auto) biography is not merely a form through which the female writer situates herself within a localised or global space. It is also a way of reformulating the way one embodies the space they are writing from or to.

As such, I posit that *I am Malala* is a feminist text wherein Yousafzai publicises her personal experiences as an aspiring student, as an activist for girls' right to education, and, just as significantly, as a survivor. By situating herself in relation to both the identities of activist and victim (of the shooting *and* of Taliban edicts banning girls from school) at the same time, Yousafzai upsets the simplified binary one could imagine between the two roles, and rejects a homogenous identity for herself. By occupying both roles she refigures (or remaps) the way in which her victimhood, or 'oppression', might be understood by a neo-imperial readership, instead using it to galvanise her political roles of activist and spokeswoman.

Yousafzai's role of spokeswoman is also strengthened by her personal connection to the political message she expresses. This is captured in her account of the closing of her school by the Taliban on the 14 January 2009. She tells the documentary makers present at the event: 'They cannot stop me. I will get my education if it's at home, school, or somewhere else' (2013: 135). This bold political statement is immediately followed by her confession that 'When I got home, I cried and cried. I didn't want to stop learning. I was only eleven years old but it felt as though I had lost everything' (2013: 135). Her political message is motivated by her passion for learning and her fear of losing access to her education. Her devastation ('it felt as though I had lost everything') makes her previous statement, 'They cannot stop me', sound not just bold, but also brave. Her account of such personal experiences has the potential to resonate with other women and girls living through similar experiences – relational in a way that politics by itself is not – as the personalised narrative draws attention to, and enhances, her polemical message.

'I am Malala': remapping the shooting of Malala Yousafzai in *I am Malala* and *He Named Me Malala*

Yousafzai does not remember being shot. In the prologue of her biography, she writes that 'I remember that the bus turned right off the main road at the army checkpoint as always and rounded the corner past the deserted cricket ground. I don't remember any more' (2013: 5). Despite her amnesia regarding the event, the shooting is still revisited by both her memoir and the documentary *He Named Me Malala*, twice in each. I argue that in her own recounting of the shooting Yousafzai refigures the identifier of victim/survivor. By 'writing back' to the event of the shooting, Yousafzai charges the political with the personal and unfolds a space to establish her own position of agency within her multifaceted identity. As such, recounting the shooting, in her own words, allows Yousafzai to challenge and decentre neo-imperial and homogenising understandings of 'victimhood' and 'oppression' as it relates to Muslim women's experiences within the context of the War on Terror, by speaking for herself, and for girls' education as part of her own feminist politics.

Writing back and/as activism

Yousafzai's memoir covers an expansive period of her family's life, spanning from her father's activities before she was born and then during her youth; her own experiences as a schoolgirl in Pakistan and her rising involvement in the political scene; and the shooting, her recovery, and her early experiences of living in the UK. These experiences, especially those which occurred prior to Yousafzai's shooting, are written and read with the foreknowledge of the consequences for Yousafzai's and her father's beliefs about education. The narrative anticipates the shooting. This is indicated, first and foremost, in the biography's titular subheading, which casts Yousafzai as 'The Girl Who Stood up for Education and was Shot by the Taliban'. While the order of the statement suggests that she is an education advocate first and foremost, and that the shooting is secondary, the event of the shooting remains embedded in Yousafzai's story: we cannot read her story without it having some kind of impact on our reading of her.

The shooting is also the first point of discussion in a memoir that is otherwise chronological. In the prologue, Yousafzai recounts the shooting in uncensored, graphic detail: 'The first [bullet] went through my left eye socket and out under my left shoulder. I slumped forward onto Moniba, blood coming from my left ear, so the other two bullets hit the girls next to me' (2013: 6). The matter-of-fact sentences that clinically set out the sequence of events of the shooting are shocking to read. At this early, critical stage, the shooting itself is not told sensationally or romantically. It does not pander to faux-interested readers. It warns the reader early on that no matter what else the narrator says, or how it is said, lyrically, fancifully, or otherwise, the events of the shooting are to be treated with horror, disgust, and apprehension.

Lyrical wordplay is used in the prologue of *I am Malala*, which anticipates the shooting, and reminds the reader that, once the narrative proper begins, it will eventually lead back to this point: a shooting of a fifteen-year-old girl. The opening of the prologue reads: 'I come from a country which was created at midnight. When I almost died it was just after midday' (2013: 1). The mirroring of coming/leaving and midnight/midday in these two lines aspires towards a lyrical or poetic expression, but the intrusion of 'just after' discombobulates what would have been an easy symmetry in the depiction of these two moments, alluding to the disruptive reality of the shooting. The following line, 'One year ago I left my home for school and never returned' (2013: 1), is similarly poetic and nostalgic in its expression, ringing like the first line in a fictional story, but again the fatalistic certainty of the words, that the speaker will 'never return', undercuts the illusion that this story is made for children. As we read of her experiences as a child growing up and going to school in the Swat Valley, we read it with this same certainty that one day she will leave home for school and never come back.

The narrative in *I am Malala* thus anticipates the shooting. However, Yousafzai also 'writes back' to it, very explicitly, insofar as her memoir can be read as a direct response to the shooting, and to the shooter. Before choosing his target, the shooter asked, 'Who is Malala?' (2013: 6), to which her declarative title, 'I am Malala', answers. This declarative statement is reiterated at both the opening and close of her book: she ends her prologue and epilogue, respectively, with: 'Who is Malala? I am Malala and this is my story' (2013: 6) and 'I am Malala. My world has changed but I have not' (2013: 265). By bookending her memoir with the self-declarative and oft-repeated phrase 'I am Malala', Yousafzai explicitly emphasises her own position of agency. The framework of her memoir – from its title to the aforementioned bookends, to its manifesto for girls' right to education – as a *response* serves to positively refigure her position as a victim of the Taliban.

Recalling Giroux's definition of border pedagogy as something established through shifting perspectives in place, time, or media, *I am Malala*, as memoir, as a remediation of events, 'decenters as it remaps' (Giroux 1993: 30). Yousafzai writes retrospectively. The foreknowledge, and therefore expectation, that the shooting will occur by both writer and reader codes the events that occurred prior to the shooting with a politics of inevitable injustice and the Taliban threat to Yousafzai's and, by extension, Swat Valley girls' right to be educated. In this way, Yousafzai's personal experiences and recollections about attending school in the Swat Valley become intrinsically political. At the same time, the retrospective nature of *I am Malala*, as an expression of border pedagogy, allows Yousafzai to reframe – or remap – certain events. This is especially notable in her second recounting of the shooting, where she narrates: 'I didn't get a chance to answer their question, "Who is Malala?" or I would have explained to them why they should let us girls go to school as well as their own sisters and daughters' (2013: 203). The retrospective genre of the memoir affords Yousafzai the opportunity to refigure – decentre – the homogenising image of victimhood in this moment. She reframes the events according to her polemical message. Here, the answer to the question 'Who is Malala?' is not an affirmation of her name ('I am Malala') as appears in the title and bookends of her memoir, but an explanation as to why girls should be allowed to go to school. This serves to explicitly tie Yousafzai's identity to education advocacy, and since the shooting she has, in many ways, been both a figurehead and spokeswoman for the campaign for girls' right to education. Aligning her identity with her cause, explaining how she would answer her shooter (and the Taliban) with her manifesto, Yousafzai remaps the event of her shooting, not through the lens of victimhood, but through survival (as she is able to give her answer now) and through her political, feminist vision.

Davis Guggenheim's documentary similarly covers a range of material that is familiar to the memoir, encompassing stories of Yousafzai's family life before and after the shooting and footage of several of her public engagements. The documentary uses an aesthetic and affective conceit in which moments of Yousafzai's narrated past are depicted in animated graphic episodes, often accompanied by composer Thomas Newman's emotively charged music for additional affect. The opening scene depicts the narrative of Yousafzai's namesake, Malalai, which Yousafzai tells in the form of a voiceover.[1] Malalai is dressed in a veil and loose pink clothing, and she resembles, not accidently, the iconic image that Yousafzai has come to be seen as today. Around her are the men who are fighting to defend Afghanistan against the British in the Second Anglo-Afghan War. As Malalai's words encourage Afghanistan's men to fight to defend their lands, Yousafzai's voiceover states that: 'She led the army to a great victory. But she was shot [...] Her name was Malalai' (Guggenheim 2015). As this voiceover is heard, the music, which has been building up to a climax, quietens, and we see a close-up of the flag Malalai had been carrying as it falls from her hand.

The moment which the narration, music, and action onscreen anticipates has occurred, and in the moment of Malalai's death there is only quiet. This is immediately interjected with live-action footage of Yousafzai being carried on a stretcher following her own shooting, her treatment by the doctors, and the vigils being held for her, with archived news reports reporting her shooting. The shift from animated narrative to live-action footage of Yousafzai in the immediate aftermath of the shooting has a jarring effect on the viewer. Ohad Landesman and Roy Bender, writing about the concluding scenes of Ari Folman's *Waltz with Bashir* (2008), which also effectively moves from animated to live-action footage, consider the effect to be:

> an unexpected dénouement, a final chord providing the spectator with an eye-opening, rude awakening. Any layer of shielding distantiation that that may have persisted due to the animated form's beauty [...] is peeled off to disclose the naked, visible evidence.
> (2011: 366)

The shift in cinematographic mode in *He Named Me Malala* results in a rude awakening for the audience at the advent, not the conclusion, of the documentary. The viewer is barely settled when they are confronted with the shocking real-life footage of the shooting. As with the memoir, this first interruption of the shooting's aftermath, using stock live-action footage, serves as a persistent reminder that at the core of this narrative is the violent act of the shooting.

The documentary returns to the events of the shooting some time after its initial recording of it. In this later remediation, the documentary again employs both animated and real-life footage. The animation begins with a remediation of the documentary prologue, showing Yousafzai's namesake Malalai encouraging the men on the battlefield and providing the voiceover, narrated by Yousafzai, that 'When every man was losing courage on the battlefield, a woman raised her voice' (Guggenheim 2015). We are then shown an animation of Yousafzai walking to and attending school, which is spliced with live-action footage of her speaking publicly in Pakistan and audio clips of Radio Mullah. There are also reconstructed scenes which show fragments of moments that immediately led up to the shooting, and which can be recognised from her written account in *I am Malala*: boots walking alongside a bus; the shadow of a gun being raised; two girls holding hands; and a hand held up against a gun being raised, shadowed against the glare of the sunlight. The screen blanks white, the music that has been rising into a crescendo fades abruptly, and then there is silence as the animation returns, showing Malalai's flag from the opening prologue falling to the ground.

There are several layers of remediation at play here: the instant of the shooting is fragmentally reconstructed in live-action cinematography, and draws from elements of Yousafzai's written narrative in her memoir. In particular, Yousafzai writes of a moment in which 'Moniba tells me I squeezed her hand' (2013: 6), which is rendered visually onscreen in the documentary reconstruction. Both the events of the shooting and the death of Yousafzai's namesake Malalai are remediated from when they were recounted in the opening of the documentary, and in this later segment they are remediated alongside one another. The inclusion of the animation with the flag falling to the ground embeds the two stories into one another: both are women who were shot for raising their voices.

The gunshot is signified, paradoxically, by silence. The moment in which the shot occurs is not signified by the sound of a gun firing, but by complete silence as the music abruptly fades and the flag falls. We neither see nor hear the shooting. We see (and hear, via the music) the anticipation, a flurry of movement and noise and voices, and then we hear silence and see still photographs of the aftermath (of the school bus with blood on the seats) which appear onscreen. Given how much the shooting defines Yousafzai's public image onscreen, in writing, and in the news, perhaps the most effective remediation of the event is the one that renders it through absence, omitting it in the form of silence and blank screens. The event of the shooting, which is usually so hyper-present, becomes almost invisible. The audience expects to see it; the onscreen narrative anticipates it. Instead there is only silence and still photographs of the aftermath. And in this audio silence and visual stillness, Yousafzai's voiceover, spoken loud and clear over the top of the reconstruction, is what echoes: 'I will get my education if it is at home, school, or any place. They cannot stop me' (Guggenheim 2015). This statement recalls that which she narrates to the documentary crew in her memoir, which was mentioned earlier. In the space where the audience anticipated a dramatisation of Yousafzai's shooting, there is instead only her voice, declaring her right to be educated. She remains a survivor of a shooting by the Taliban, but at the centre of the narrative of her shooting, and rising above it, is her raised voice, campaigning for her right, and other girls' right, to education.

Writing back and building platforms

Both in emphasising her pride in her Pashtun, Pakistani, and Muslim heritage, and by revisiting (remapping and decentring) the event of her shooting, Yousafzai builds an image, or platform, from which to deliver her politics. Her dual identities of shooting victim and education rights activist, coupled with the remediated events of the shooting, tie her experiences to her continued campaign, and strengthen and substantiate her polemical message. The personal materialises in self-conscious and self-reflective writing, and is politicised not just by the message implied by spoken/written words, but also in Yousafzai's intention to reach the ears of others, to empower others. This is encapsulated in her Nobel Lecture, when she states that 'I tell my story, not because it is unique, but because it is not. It is the story of many girls [...] I am not a lone voice, I am many' (2014: n.p.). In this speech, which continues the polemical message she sets out in her memoir, Yousafzai makes a case for girls' right to education. She does not present herself as exceptional ('unique') in her cause; by aligning herself with other girls, transitioning from 'I am Malala' to 'I am many', Yousafzai testifies on their behalf. This testimony, as with the tenets of postcolonial women's (auto)biography discussed earlier, is relational, not hegemonic. Her 'singularity achieves its identity as an extension of the collective. The singular represents the plural not because it replaces or subsumes the group but because the speaker is a distinguishable part of the whole' (Sommer 1988: 108). Since *I Am Malala* is co-authored with Christina Lamb, there is no certainty as to which words belong to who (although the first-person nature of the memoir means that Yousafzai claims them as her own). In her Nobel Lecture, 'co-authorship' transitions from the British journalist to the other girls', both within and beyond Pakistan, who are unable to gain an education. Yousafzai uses her public platform in order to authoritatively and, as she grows older, increasingly autonomously represent her own and other women's different personal experiences in support of her political, feminist agenda.

This chapter has examined how Yousafzai's ethnicity and gender identities – Pakistani, Muslim, woman – have the potential to be appropriated as part of a neo-imperial project of cosmopolitan interest, sympathy, charity, and 'rescue' within the context of the War on Terror. I have argued that these appropriations are not straightforward, and that Yousafzai's own pride in and presentation of these various identities in *I Am Malala* in regard to both her personal life and her politics serves to challenge the homogenising of these categories. These identifiers, in particular her positioning as a survivor and as an activist, are complex, nuanced, and interconnected, especially in Yousafzai's accounts of the shooting. Yousafzai refigures – or remaps – the events she narrates in her memoir in ways that allow her to return to her position of advocate for education. The strength behind Yousafzai's delivery of her polemical message is partly determined by the interdependence of the two identifiers of survivor and activist. In *I Am Malala*, and in the documentary *He Named Me Malala*, she wields the event of the shooting, and the anticipation of its occurrence, in order to further her agenda for education advocacy. By revisiting the shooting in her own writing and words, by 'writing back', Yousafzai gains control over the narrative, exercising agency and shifting the focus onto *her* politics.

Note

1 Malalai was a Pashtun Afghan girl who encouraged the Afghan army to fight and ultimately defeat the British in 1880 during the Second Anglo-Afghan War, but was killed by enemy fire.

Bibliography

Ahmed, S. (2014) *The Cultural Politics of Emotion*. 2nd edn. Edinburgh: Edinburgh University Press.
Bhutto, F. (2011) *Songs of Blood and Sword: A Daughter's Memoir*. London: Vintage Books.
Bhutto, F. (2013) '*I am Malala* by Malala Yousafzai – Review'. *Guardian* [online]. Available from <www.theguardian.com/books/2013/oct/30/malala-yousafzai-fatima-bhutto-review> [19 January 2018].

Bugeja, N. (2012) *Postcolonial Memoir in the Middle East: Rethinking the Liminal in Mashriqi Writing*. New York: Routledge.
Chambers, C. (2011) 'A Comparative Approach to Pakistani Fiction in English'. *Journal of Postcolonial Writing* 47, 122–134.
Folman, A. (2008) *Waltz with Bashir*. [DVD] New York: Sony Pictures Classics.
Giroux, H.A. (1993) *Border Crossings: Cultural Workers and the Politics of Education*. New York: Routledge.
Golley, N.A. (2003) *Reading Arab Women's Autobiographies: Shahrazad Tells her Story*. Austin: University of Texas Press.
Guggenheim, D. (2015) *He Named Me Malala*. [DVD] Los Angeles: Twentieth Century Fox.
Henderson, M.G. (2014) *Speaking in Tongues and Dancing Diaspora: Black Women Writing and Performing*. New York: Oxford University Press.
Kanwal, A. (2015) *Rethinking Identities in Contemporary Pakistani Fiction: Beyond 9/11*. Basingstoke: Palgrave Macmillan.
Khoja-Moolji, S. (2015) 'Reading Malala: (De)(Re)Territorialization of Muslim Collectives'. *Comparative Studies of South Asia, Africa and the Middle East* 35, 539–559.
Landesman, O. and Bender, R. (2011) 'Animated Recollection and Spectorial Experience in *Waltz with Bashir*'. *Animation: An Interdisciplinary Journal* 6, 353–370.
'Malala Yousafzai's Book Banned in Pakistani Private Schools'. *Guardian* [online]. Available from <www.theguardian.com/world/2013/nov/10/malala-yousafzai-book-banned-pakistan-schools> [19 January 2018].
Moore-Gilbert, B. (2009) *Postcolonial Life-Writing: Culture, Politics and Self-Representation*. London: Routledge.
Shamsie, K. (2009) *Offence: The Muslim Case*. London: Seagull Books.
Smith, S. and Watson, J. (1992) 'Introduction: De/Colonization and the Politics of Discourse in Women's Autobiographical Practices'. In *De/Colonizing the Subject: The Politics of Gender in Women's Autobiography*. Ed. by Smith, S. and Watson, J. Minneapolis: University of Minnesota Press, xiii–xxxi.
Sommer, D. (1988) '"Not Just a Personal Story": Women's *Testimonios* and the Plural Self'. In *Life/Lines: Theorizing Women's Autobiography*. Ed. by Brodzki, B. and Schenck, C. Ithaca: Cornell University Press, 107–130.
Whitlock, G. (2007) *Soft Weapons: Autobiography in Transit*. Chicago: The University of Chicago Press.
Yousafzai, M. (2013) *I Am Malala: The Girl Who Stood up for Education and was Shot by the Taliban*. London: Phoenix.
Yousafzai, M. (2014) *Malala Yousafzai Nobel Peace Prize Speech* [online]. Available from <www.youtube.com/watch?v=MOqIotJrFVM> [30 September 2016].
Zine, J. (2014) 'Cartographies of Difference and Pedagogies of Peril: Muslim Girls and Women in Western Young Adult Fiction Novels'. In *Muslim Women, Transnational Feminism and the Ethics of Pedagogy*. Ed. by Zine, J. and Taylor, L.K. New York: Routledge, 175–197.
Zine, J. and Taylor, L.K. (2014) 'Introduction: The Contested Imaginaries of Reading Muslim Women and Muslim Women Reading Back'. In *Muslim Women, Transnational Feminism and the Ethics of Pedagogy*. Ed. by Zine, J. and Taylor, L.K. New York: Routledge, 1–24.

PART IV

Identities in question
Shifting perspectives on gender

16
DOING HISTORY RIGHT
Challenging masculinist postcolonialism in Pakistani anglophone literature

Fawzia Afzal-Khan

According to Walter Benjamin's Angel of History, a figure based on Paul Klee's painting of the *Angelus Novus*, History is not an accident (1942: Thesis IX). Indeed, we must move away from an attachment to what he calls 'erotic historicism' – or the impulse to see history through the eyes of mysticism – into the phase of historical materialism, in order to grow up and do history 'right'. That is, be able to connect present to past and past to present so as to move to a futurity that may be more hopeful than what has gone before. Adding a feminist lens to this Angel of History suggests that one can learn to read/uncover the buried remains in the gaps and fissures of official narratives that constitute History with a capital H – thus giving voice to the marginalised and the forgotten (who are often women, and the dark 'others' of History).

In this chapter I would like to proffer a symptomatic reading of a handful of novels by some prominent contemporary Pakistani and Pakistani-American male novelists, to assess the degree to which they do 'history right' in the ways I deem important – nay urgent – in these challenging times we live in, as I have outlined above. Contemporary women writers of Pakistani origin writing and receiving recognition today, such as Kamila Shamsie, Uzma Aslam Khan, of course our literary godmother Bapsi Sidhwa and a host of others, are, in my opinion, already are/have been 'doing history right'. They are courageous feminist humanists (mostly of the liberal variety, it is true) – connecting past and present in service of delineating more hopeful future possibilities for Pakistan and the world. The men, on the other hand, who are – as is usually the case – receiving far more attention and accolades (in the latest Booker Award news, Mohsin Hamid's novel *Exit West* has been shortlisted, while Shamsie's *Home Fire* has not) – need closer attention for my unabashedly polemical study. In order to arrive at an answer to my question, I would like to begin connecting the past-present continuum by referring to a fairly recent event in the shared history of the world we inhabit, which I refer to as 'the *Charlie Hebdo* affair', and point out its relevance to connecting our global imperialist present to a past colonialist one via a brief reading of Sudanese novelist Tayeb Salih's *Season of Migration to the North* (1966). The term 'postcolonial' seems apt, in this context, in signalling the continuities of oppression in the Global South, unleashed by Western colonialist and imperialist History, but then also propelled by a self-hating mechanism on the part of the postcolonial subjects of that History (Fanon 2008: 16), into a futurity that is a dead end, rather than an opening-out. When the voices of the marginalised remain trapped in masculinist ideologies, the future remains a captive of the past. I refer to Salih's novel as a foundational text that informs the repetition of self-hating tropes found in the work of Hamid, Ali Eteraz, and Ayad Akhtar in ways which suggest that they remain trapped in the past, unlike the narrator of Salih's novel, who at least tries to swim ashore to a different land and take responsibility for creating a better future. *Exit West* (2017), Hamid's latest work of fiction, comes closest to breaking out of the prison house of masculinist (self-hating) melancholia.

The *Charlie Hebdo* affair and postcolonial male melancholia

In the wake of the *Charlie Hebdo* affair, we have been thrust into a world of postcolonial claims that belie the Keatsian dictum 'beauty is truth, truth beauty; that is all you know, and all that you need to know' – or at least complicate it ('Ode to a Grecian Urn'). Thus, at the very least, we have been forced to ask, whose truth is beautiful? Whose definition of the beautiful (*viz.* satire in this context) gets to represent 'the truth'? Surely value judgements are being made and this value system which is always specific and local to its political and cultural context, though it masquerades as universal and absolute (freedom of speech!), is what ideological critique exposes, as it unmasks the contradictions that systems of power seek to conceal through what French Marxist thinker Louis Althusser dubbed 'ideological state apparatuses' (1971). Newspapers, magazines, books and other media, places of worship, educational institutions, etc. are all part of the ideological state apparatuses through which state power consolidates itself to produce a docile citizenry, or what the Italian Marxist theorist Antonio Gramsci called 'the consent of the governed': where state repression ends, ideological hegemony begins.

However, as we all know, the work of ideology is never finished – it must constantly reproduce itself to ensure compliance; and, of course, compliance is never guaranteed – because power can be questioned, subjects of power can be radicalised and speak their truth to power. As Paul-Michel Foucault reminded us, power is never unidirectional, victims can have agency (1991). Thus, while those waving 'Je Suis Charlie' banners and placards could be read in this interpretive scheme as those who allowed themselves to be interpellated by the French (read Western/liberal/secular) hegemonic discourse of History with a capital 'H', the killers were counter-interpellating the ideological state apparatus represented by *Charlie Hebdo* (an ironic turnaround for a magazine that started out occupying a counter-hegemonic space in France!) – and thus giving 'voice' to the marginalised.

Many have written about the economic marginality of the Kouachi brothers being representative of the majority of citizens in France of Muslim Algerian descent and, as such, a major contributing factor to their radicalisation in the face of their continued precarity. Such disenfranchisement under neoliberal regimes of power, coupled with Western wars on Muslim lands in the present and the not-so-distant past (especially as far as France's occupation of Algeria is concerned), has been cited as an obvious cause leading to events such as the murder of the *Charlie Hebdo* journalists (see Sharma 2015).

I would like to add a third component to this narrative of marginalised voices: that of the psychic alienation which uprootedness from one's cultural background produces (though leading to different results and possibilities, as I will argue a bit later on). Religion is only one facet of this cultural baggage we all carry. Indeed, as the Sudanese writer Salih's eerily prescient novel *Season of Migration to the North* sets out for us as early as 1966, when it was first published in Arabic, in the aftermath of British colonialism's physical and cultural imperialism in the Sudan, even gifted and brilliant young men who have no affinity to their Muslimness, like the secular protagonist Mustafa Saeed, can become murderers of their oppressors; even when those oppressors become supposed benefactors, welcoming the likes of Mustafa into their countries, their educational institutions, their homes, and lives. This is precisely the plot line of Hamid's post-9/11 novel, *The Reluctant Fundamentalist* (2007), which so brilliantly traces the interconnected histories of past and present, West/East, giving voice to the marginalised 'other' of US History, the novel's Pakistani-American protagonist, Changez. On the one hand, the description of the 'other' – in this case the city of Lahore – can be read as an ironising tactic to crack open Western orientalist tropes, as Anna Hartnell argues:

> Hamid provocatively paints a forbidding picture of Lahore, the frame-story's immediate setting, which evokes what Hamid describes elsewhere as Pakistan's 'recurring role as a villain' ('It had to be a sign'). Though the narrator makes much of the city's rich cuisine, its decidedly bloody nature along with the 'shadowy' figures and places that characterize Hamid's Lahore underscore the fact that the novel deliberately filters the city through Orientalist stereotypes, demonstrating its status as a menace in the imagination of the western reader.
>
> (2010: 337)

Yet, one can also argue, as I will later on, that this Pakistani-American novel fails to live up to the Angel of History's dictum for moving beyond an 'erotic history' (the orientalist framing of Lahore in this case) – and into a more mature, more materialistic conception of history that could point to a more hopeful (feminist) futurity, whereas Salih's much earlier novel – despite having a protagonist whose journey to Europe and back home to the Sudan mirrors that of Hamid's narrator Changez – succeeds in this endeavour because of its materialist rather than romantic embrace of history.

Why and how does Salih's *Season of Migration* succeed in puncturing the repugnant present and past of colonialism, to gesture to a more hopeful future rooted in reality and a pragmatic embrace of such reality (without sacrificing principle)? This is a difficult question to answer, especially for my students, who can only deal with Mustafa Saeed as long as they can see/ understand him as pathologically disturbed, a crazy man, rather than as a symbolic avenger of the British colonial rule inflicted on his country through his 'conquest' of British women via elaborate sexual games he plays with them, turning them mad and suicidal over time. The only English woman who sees through and resists his counter-orientalist, counter-interpellative but deeply misogynistic moves is Jean Morris, whom he marries; and when he still can't 'conquer' her, he kills her (she invites him to, but only if he also kills himself, which he doesn't do). At his trial, he is exonerated thanks to his defence lawyer, a former professor of his at Oxford – who argues that Saeed was undone by his own brilliance, which these English women whom he bedded simply couldn't comprehend, given their own (em)beddedness in colonialist ideology. According to his English lawyer, Saeed had become Othello, the Moor, one who can never be accepted by the West, and this was the cause of his mental and psychic breakdown, which led to the awful denouement of the murder of Jean Morris, a modern-day Desdemona. In the last scene of this farcical trial, at the end of which Saeed is released and returns to Sudan, he wants to yell out to the courtroom that he is no Othello, that Othello is a Lie, a figment of the West's imagination. It is this Lie, which has haunted his entire existence up until this point, that Saeed has wished to kill; with his exoneration, which he pleads against, the Lie unfortunately lives on, just as his inability to kill himself as he plunges the knife into Jean Morris' heart leads to the continuation of the cycle of history, and the 'other' and 'self-' hatred unleashed by such a history.

What is this 'Lie', and how does it bring this twentieth-century novel and its protagonist into conversation with the *Charlie Hebdo* affair that unfolded in the heart of twenty-first-century Western civilisation, about which Gandhi once famously quipped, 'it would be a good idea'?

Could it be the Lie the West needs to tell itself, about how its actions are solely responsible for the moment we are living in today? Could it be that the Lie of Western civilisation is the insistence on understanding/explaining the murderous behaviour of Othello through the prism/lens that frames him as an 'other', an 'outsider' to norms of emotional control that are supposedly the hallmark of the civilised Western (white) man? As a transplanted 'subject' of Empire, surely (according to the orientalist discourse within which he is located) it is perfectly understandable that Othello falls back on his atavistic urges of uncontrolled jealousy and irrational rage when confronted with his wife's supposed infidelity?

On the one hand, it might be argued that *Season of Migration* simply fuels anti-Muslim prejudices, extending the sphere of Muslim killers to all Muslims, even those who are not *jihadists*, and maybe not even real believers, like Saeed. By extension, anyone – whether a liberal Westerner or a sympathetic fellow Muslim – who brings colonial legacies as an explicating factor into the discussion at hand becomes suspect, an 'apologist' for the vilest extremism, for the killing of innocent women, for Islamist reasons or otherwise. The Lie, then, that Mustafa himself wants to see killed, and thus be liberated from, could be the lie of Blaming the West, the Lie that blames colonialism for all of the ills faced by Muslim nations (and Muslim immigrants to Europe today) – the Lie that Saeed has bought into as an excuse for his own horribly misogynistic behaviour towards the 'prized possessions' of his enemy – 'his' women. On the other hand, if Othello is indeed a creation of the West (much as Saeed proves by telling elaborate lies to the white women he seduces in London regarding the lions and tigers and crocodiles that roam around in his backyard in Cairo!), then later – by becoming the West's object of pity because he has been 'misjudged' and 'victimised' like Othello by his colonial masters (and mistresses) – the Lie could also be one that the West has created, that of the 'poor oppressed Muslim subject' who must be 'saved' through exposure to the superior (and forgiving) civilisation of the West. Both Saeed and Changez – who appears as the protagonist in Hamid's novel half a century after Salih's novel – refuse this objectification by their Western paymasters, and suffer accordingly, trapped in the roles of victims-turned-victimisers, much like the Kouachi brothers and their ilk.

Saeed, the Kouachi brothers, and Changez – and most of the heroes and villains in this continuing saga of colonial history redux – are caught, therefore, in a trap. It's a trap in which the only heuristic model is that of the West and the Rest (Rest = Muslims). And the Rest can be either saved or not, understood or not, accommodated or not, only by the West (or North), which continues to be the point of reference for everything, good, bad, or ugly, in our world.

In such a view of the world, the subaltern truly cannot speak, because the discursive parameters within which subjectivities are shaped and understood are always already in place. It matters not whether the subaltern is poor, ill-educated, living in precarious conditions in the *banlieues* of Paris, like the Kouachi brothers, or an elite-educated professor of economics at Oxford University, like the protagonist of Salih's novel or, more recently, a Princeton-educated Pakistani man like Changez in the *Reluctant Fundamentalist*. The faulty vision of these subalterns who have bought into their own 'otherness' as defined by the dominant discourse – the fact that they can see only with one eye/only in terms of Black and White, Us and Them, the West and Islam, Male/Female, Victim/Oppressor – is matched by the equally exaggerated binaristic visions and discourse of those on the Western/Northern side – such as the discourse of the liberal-left variety, who can only see these 'others' as poor, victimised Muslims to be 'saved'. The unsuspecting white women whom Saeed manipulates can be said to belong to this category, as does Erica in *The Reluctant Fundamentalist*, and they make odd bedfellows with the right-wingers like Marine le Pen (for whom the Muslim 'others' in their midst are nothing more than savages to be obliterated). Perhaps Jean Morris of *Season of Migration*, the only white English woman who challenges Saeed and is murdered by him in turn, fits this latter category too? An exaggerated hate for the Other may not be that different from an exaggerated Love for the othered 'object'? – something Hamid's protagonist realises about the way Erica treats him, in the movie version of the novel, which prompts his final irrevocable rejection of the West (in this instance, the imperial USA) – and return 'home' to Lahore to become the 'reluctant fundamentalist' of the novel's title. In the novel itself, Erica is more akin to Jean Morris (though without the latter's murderous rage towards her 'other' object of affection) – in that she withdraws slowly, but surely, from Changez into her own world, which has room only for her 'true' lost love, Christian, symbol of the white Christian America that she is losing, the Am/Erica she truly wants to hold on to (dalliances with brown Muslim men aside). Can Trump's Am/Erica be far behind?

However, what differentiates *Season of Migration* from *Reluctant Fundamentalist*, and from the novels and plays of Pakistani-American writers like Akhtar and Eteraz for instance, is the presence of the protagonist Saeed's doppelganger. This nameless narrator of *Season* is a product of the *same* history as Saeed, yet points to a different possible future, his thinking/actions exhibiting a materialist conception of history in contrast to Saeed's – and Changez's, or that of Akhtar's Amir in his play *Disgraced*, or of Eteraz's protagonist in his novel *Native Believer* (2006) – more *erotic* fixations on the White woman who, as symbolic avatar of the West, is the prize that must be obtained for the colonised man's injured masculinity to be set right. Truly, these male writers' sensibilities are more romantic/mythic than realist/materialist, more Northrop Frye than George Lukacs!

This desire for the White woman, mingled with a concomitant fear of her sexual prowess that mocks the colonised/conquered man's feminisation – has been accepted as the neurotic symptom par excellence of the Black (or Brown) man in a colonised world. Both the trope and its analysis, by postcolonial theorist and psychiatrist Frantz Fanon, seem to apply rather well to the situation of the Brown Muslim man in our neocolonial, imperial times.

Certainly, parts of Fanon's *Black Skin, White Masks* are highly apropos in this context, specifically the chapter on 'The Man of Color and the White Woman', which thematises Fanonian insights into the Black Man as Salih's *Season of Migration* does through Mustafa Saeed's obsession with 'conquering' white English women as a mode of 'revenge' against the colonial 'master' who came and took over the Black man's lands, rendering him as powerless as a wo/man, a no/man.

Season's thematisation of the Black man's psychosexual 'split' – his simultaneous desire for the White Man's world (including 'his' prized women), and his inevitable fear and hatred of them and of himself for following the hackneyed path of erotic revenge and other extremist behaviours – acknowledges that split by giving us two different characters who each provides different possible revisionings of the tragedy of colonialism. However, Hamid's *Reluctant Fundamentalist* falls into a dead end of history doomed to repeat the worst, most extremist of its tropes. As indeed do the male protagonists of Akhtar's *Disgraced*, and Eteraz's protagonist in *Native Believer*. These 'heroes' simply become, again in Fanon's terms, 'reactional' and 'negational' (2008: 90). Clearly there are 'actional' and 'affirmative' responses to the situation in which Muslims find themselves today in the West (and elsewhere), circumstances not too different from those of the Antillean Black man (and woman, though her set of neuroses is under-theorised), of the era of colonisation which Fanon analyses. It is the 'actional' responses that Fanon seeks to validate so that we (Blacks, Browns/Others/Muslims) can see that another solution is possible through a restructuring of the world, a way set forth by challenging the backward glance of Walter Benjamin's Angel of History (Marker 2012: n.p.).

Such an 'actional' response requires, I suggest, the desire to discover an alternative path to extremist thinking (West or East, North or South). As the nameless narrator of Salih's novel (who is himself dealing with psychic alienation as a Sudanese returned from England with a

PhD in English literature, and mocked for this by Saeed, who has become a 'nativist' leader in his own village), soliloquises at one point, 'where lies the middle'? In the end, Saeed does come to realise the futility of his actions, which are a result of his own capitulation to extremist modes of thinking and behaviour. But it is the wishy-washy narrator – who has, over the course of the novel, become obsessed with Saeed's symbolic acts of vengeance against the big bad West, and has cast him idealistically as a man of action, seeing himself by contrast as weak because he is unable to pick sides – who actually comes of age in the novel; as such, he points to a different resolution of the psychic alienation unleashed by the ills of colonialism. Finding himself drowning in a river that connects South to North (or East to West), he decides to swim with the current, rather than fight against it, and to swim to the shore, wherever that might land him, whether South or North. In doing so, he makes a choice to fight for life, rather than death. By choosing life, he takes responsibility at long last for his own actions – rather than basking in the destructive glory of the phantasm that Saeed has symbolised. He rejects a Saeedian one-eyed view of the world that can only result in binaristic simplifications, and embraces instead a *jouissance* that moves away from a singular and dualistic vision into a world of multiple visions, allowing for the possibility of several points to land safely, to connect with others, to breathe, to live. Perhaps this is a welcoming vision that can only be promised by a borderless world, where South and North can no longer be distinguished.

This nameless narrator's more historical materialist vision (though stuck within a liberal humanism rather than bespeaking a radical progressive vision) may very well be the one that is presented to us in Hamid's latest novel, *Exit West* – though in *The Reluctant Fundamentalist*, Saeed's ghost seems to be the guiding spirit for protagonist Changez. Before concluding with a few remarks about *Exit West*, I would like to turn briefly to a discussion of Amir in Akhtar's play *Disgraced* (2013), and of the nameless protagonist of Eteraz's novel *Native Believer*.

Native Believer's protagonist tells us in his opening salvo that 'In America, those who want something have to dress like those who already have everything' (2006: 7). Like Amir in Akhtar's *Disgraced*, the first-generation Pakistani-American Muslim male in Eteraz's novel – who is defined only as the white Anglo-Saxon blue-blooded Marie-Anne's husband – is someone who is desperate to 'make it' in America, success being measured by how quickly one can ascend the corporate hierarchy and by the fancy clothes, cars, houses, and 'trophy wife' one acquires. The trope of the 'white woman as symbol of success', nay even 'conquest', over those (men) who once ruled the brown or black country whence came these once-colonised men/their forbears, is present front and centre in both these works (as in Hamid's *Reluctant Fundamentalist* and Salih's *Season of Migration* before them). But rather than ironise the trope as Salih does – to reveal its fatuousness and expose the cupidity and self-hatred of the postcolonial male who adopts it (mis-takenly) as a mark of success – both Eteraz and Akhtar create protagonists who, like Hamid's Changez, are undone not so much by their own foolish belief in such avatars of success, but by the fact that these white women are truly out of their reach, are uncaring, cold, or simply (as in Eteraz's novel) diseased and morbid (universalist misogyny, anyone?) – and of course, truly out of reach for men who believe themselves to be 'below' them. Eteraz's eponymous protagonist reveals as much when thinking about his wife Marie-Anne:

> We were so different, situated in distinct levels of the American caste-system. She came from the priestly class, from those who were presumed to be born with access to divinity. I was from something far lower. Perhaps even an untouchable place. My one hope had been to merge my dirty blood with her pure blood and dilute myself in a new generation. Even that hadn't worked out.
>
> (2016: 178)

Turning his profound self-loathing and attendant melancholia at his 'failed manhood' into a virulent misogyny becomes the *modus operandi* of our erstwhile hero. Thus, his wife Marie-Anne is described as a woman who has grown huge, thanks to some bodily disorder, but even without the extra weight she has always been larger and taller than him, standing 'six-foot-one' over his 'five-foot-eight'; and he tells us that when she 'wore heeled riding boots, […] I had to look up at her even more than usual' (2016: 8, 9). She walks 'bow-legged' and during sex she likes to play dominatrix games in which she becomes a racist lesbian vampire, making the protagonist a slave to her sexual appetite that is as exhausting as it is unattractive and humiliating, and yet it is a scenario he participates in willingly. Here is a bedroom scene in which the fetishised object for Marie-Anne is a small black co-worker they'd invited to the dinner party that sets the Islamophobic events of the novel in motion, which end up making the protagonist a Kouachi brothers-type of 'native believer' by the apocalyptic end. The black girl who becomes the object of the sexual fantasy game and whom Marie Anne requires to reach her orgasm, might be seen to represent the emasculation of the brown Muslim male at the hands of the all-powerful white woman who, despite being his wife, is never someone he feels he can claim to be equal to; the black woman becomes the 'doll' – like him – to be 'played with'. Self-hatingly, it is the protagonist who serves the role of the 'house slave':

> 'Yes,' I licked her nipple, 'you tell her she's tiny. A toy.'
> 'She's a doll.'
> I licked harder. 'You know what to do with dolls.'
> Marie-Anne nodded and increased her pace. 'I know what to do with dolls. They are to be played with.'
> 'Do you play with her?'
> 'I take her home. I play with her. All the people see me leave with her. All the men. All the men were staring at her. All the black men and all the white men. They all want her. All the big swinging dicks. But I take her.'
>
> (2016: 28–29)

Not only is the white woman in this scenario a stand-in for white men's desires and power over black and brown men and women, she is also a white mistress with power over the black man's 'woman' and, in taking her, she strikes a deadly blow to seal the colonised man's emasculation.

The protagonist continues in his abjection to his white mistress, and the sex scene becomes a satire not to expose or comment on the black (brown) man's self-hatred as much as an easy misogyny directed at the white woman barking sex commands to her slave:

> 'Mistress!' Marie-Anne screamed her trigger word. Whenever she uttered it I knew my job was to start licking her nipple even harder […] Her mouth opened. She was in that imaginary bed with Candace [the black co-worker], where Marie-Anne was the owner, where Marie-Anne was the empress. I licked. My mouth grew tired. Still I licked. My tongue dried up, still I licked. My jaw hurt, still I licked. It wouldn't be long now. Within her vision Marie-Anne would soon reach her desired apogee. The moment when her authority over Candace would be so immense that it would make her explode […] And then she was still. She'd consumed Candace, chewed her up, turned her into wetness.
>
> (2016: 29–30)

The brown counterparts to these white, emasculating women (like Amir's anti-Semitic mother in *Disgraced*, or the Pakistani-American Muslim woman with whom Eteraz's protagonist has sexual relations while married to Marie-Anne, like Candace, or even his own loving but uncomprehending mother whose placement of the tiny Qur'an in his living room is the catalyst for his downfall in white America) are portrayed as similarly un-sympatico, major contributors to the psychic alienation their sons and lovers experience in white capitalist America. Muslim misogyny thus becomes a facet of a complex self-orientalising gaze.

(Self-)orientalism reiterated in our times

And this brings us to the final example of orientalism reiterated, the Pulitzer-winning play *Disgraced* by Pakistani-American Akhtar. If we grant, with Michel Thévoz, that 'exotic representation [is] a constant negotiation between the modalities of ethnographic documentation on the one hand, and fantasy on the other' (qtd. in Kuehl 2011: 33), then certainly Akhtar's play and its reception, both by some of the main actors (whom I interviewed informally after a performance on 8 December 2012) as well as a handful of audience members whom I questioned similarly, would suggest the combative terrain of the play itself as a useful site for the citing and re-citing of orientalist tropes with a difference. These comments ranged from several of the actors stating that they thought the play exposed all of the characters equally as 'tribal-minded' in the final analysis, to a group of South Asian audience members (male and female) saying they saw the main theme as a 'self-loathing that bubbles beneath the surface of the most cosmopolitan of liberal Muslims', which bothered a few of them, though it also felt 'true' to them, to a couple of liberal white women from Dartmouth who felt the play catered to stereotypes of Muslims. Thus, the liminal or border space opened up between the ethnographic impulse for 'authentic' documentation of a multiracial and multi- as well as anti-religious post-9/11 American 'reality' rubs up uncomfortably against not just the fantasy of the white and black Christian/Jewish/atheist/secular characters of the play towards the Muslim(s) in their midst but, more importantly perhaps, against the self-orientalising fantasy to which the main character, a Muslim who has changed his name to the Indian/Hindu moniker Amir Kapoor, succumbs with tragic effect. I would say that this character's final comeuppance (or downfall) ultimately reiterates, and in the process reifies, a white, Western, Judeo-Christian fantasy: the iconic image of the Moorish slave, a *morisco* named Juan de Pareja, who was painted by his master Diego Velásquez in the mid-sixteenth century. Kapoor's wife, an upper-class 'liberal' white woman who is an ambitious artist, is painting a portrait of him based on Velásquez's portrait of his slave – but with a difference: her husband is a well-clad, well-heeled lawyer on the make in a New York law firm specialising in – what else – mergers and acquisitions. Unlike the modest (but clean) lace-front shirt of the slave Juan de Pareja as seen in Velásquez's portrait, Amir's shirts are 'Charvets', high cotton count and costing upwards of $600 apiece (Akhtar 2013: 38), indicating his status as a supposed master of his destiny. Yet something binds him to the Muslim slave of the earlier portrait. Scholars Thomas Freller and Stephan Herget remind us of the historical context that brought forth the performative of the *morisco* (the Muslim Moor of Spain after the Reconquista) as a 'suspicious subject' of Spain:

> under the reign of Philip II, the situation of the Moriscos, as the newly Christianized Muslims living in Spain became known, created conflicts and tension. This in turn gave way to a period fraught with psychological undertones, fear and enmity. As several recent studies have made clear, a person recognized as 'Morisco' at the height of this obsession with *limpieza di sangre* [sic] ('purity of blood'), during the second half of the sixteenth and the beginning of the seventeenth century [the time of Velásquez and of kings Philip III and IV], meant their exclusion from all military and many of

> the religious orders, from the prime positions within the state bureaucracy and from all university colleges.
>
> (Freller and Hegret 1999: 110)

Like the orientalist painters whom scholars like Kuehl would have us refer to as painters of the 'Exotic', Velásquez became famous for his 'realism', especially after painting this portrait, whose details of physiognomy and clean but battered clothing (befitting a servant/slave's station) were praised by the most important European painters of the day as 'exhibiting an impressive economy of brushwork' ('Velázquez' 2014: n.p.).

One might argue that Velásquez's famous portrait of Juan de Pareja oscillates between the realistic exterior of a man (a Moorish slave to be precise) depicted in a dignified manner by his master and thus, at one level, serving to destabilise the fantasy stereotypes of unkempt, dirty, and untrustworthy Moors – and the 'covered up' reality of his Moorish slave heritage, which reactivates another level of 'truth': the one that animates a white, Western Christian power fantasy of Empire. A similar fantasy operates in the performative register of *Disgraced*, wherein Amir Kapoor's Charvet shirts do not succeed in liberating him from a slave-like status in the Judeo-Christian painterly and economic realms of which his wife, and her Jewish former lover Isaac, are the obvious rulers. Just as the iterative traces of a previous phantasmagorical painting Velásquez created in 1627 showing the *moriscos* (like Pareja) being driven out of Spain cannot be erased from this latter 'realist' portrait, so too this same oscillating world view, a feeling of being caught between competing ideologies and that in-between space of an orientalist exoticism, permeates *Disgraced* and causes at least two different kinds of reviewer response. On the one hand, according to a review in *Variety*, 'Playwright Ayad Akhtar really sticks it to upper-class liberals in *Disgraced*, his blistering social drama about the racial prejudices that secretly persist in progressive cultural circles' (Stasio 2012: n.p.). On the other, Charles Isherwood writing for the *New York Times* notes:

> In dialogue that bristles with wit and intelligence, Mr. Akhtar, a novelist and screenwriter, puts contemporary attitudes toward religion under a microscope, *revealing how tenuous self-image can be for people born into one way of being who have embraced another* […] and what will ultimately tear apart at least one of the relationships in the play is who they really are and what they stand for, once the veneer of civilized achievement has been scraped away to reveal more atavistic urges.
>
> (2012: n.p.; emphasis added)

Thus, Stasio's review for *Variety* reads the play – and playwright – in a realist mode as 'sticking it to upper class liberals' (2012: n.p.) – in which circle he presumably does not include the Johnny-come-lately Amir Kapoor or his nephew-turned-fundo, but focuses rather (and sees the play as focusing its ire) on the other three characters, *viz*. Kapoor's white upper-class artist wife, Emily; a snooty Jewish art curator named Isaac; and his African-American 'boogie' wife, a competitive colleague at Amir's swanky Manhattan law firm. Isherwood, on the other hand, sees the play's animus as directed against the Muslim male at the centre of the quadrangle. The 'one relationship' that Isherwood sees as 'torn asunder' most obviously is that between Amir and his waspy wife Emily, and when Isherwood states the cause as the 'scraping away' of a 'veneer of civilized achievement' which 'reveal[s …] atavistic urges' (Isherwood 2012: n.p.), one is put in mind immediately of Joseph Conrad's imperialist fantasy novel, *Heart of Darkness*, where all of the achievements of Western civilisation are shown as facing continuing threat of extinction from the forces of darkness, those savage urges of primal man located in the black jungles of Africa and its supposedly primitive peoples. Clearly, the most obvious example in *Disgraced* of someone whose 'self-image' is tenuous because he was 'born into one way of being' – that of the brown Muslim man from Pakistan – and who has embraced another mode of being, one where he is hell-bent on distancing himself from his 'atavistic' past and entering the rarefied and aspirational realms of white, upper-class, 'civilised' America – is Amir. The play reverses the nineteenth-century Conradian journey of the civilised white man into the jungles of Africa – where he turns into the worst of the savages he encounters whilst taking a black woman as his mistress – to a contemporary fable where the Black (or Brown) man comes to the Heart of Civilisation in the twentieth century – New York City – to achieve the glories of a well-heeled 'civilised' life in the West, acquiring his white 'trophy' wife to cement his virile success. In the process, it isn't he who turns into a likeness of those he aspires to – rather, he exposes the darkness lurking in their hearts – but ultimately, this being the USA and not the Congo (or Pakistan), civilised norms prevail for the three 'natives' (white/black/Christian/Jewish) who were 'born' (or at least 'bred' from an early age) into their proper 'classed' roles which subsume/ smooth over presumed differences of race, gender, ethnicity, and religion, whereas poor Amir regresses back into the savage he always/already was.

And, of course, the savagery has a gendered/sexual dimension, for otherwise the orientalist trope would not be complete. Upon learning that his wife has had an affair with Isaac, he exhibits the Moor's innate and uncontrollable jealousy (think *Othello*), and all the lovey-dovey cooing and gentle bickering with his wife earlier in the play gives way to rage expressed in a symbolic slap across Emily's face, followed by some vicious kicking thrown in for extra measure as she writhes on the floor of their sophisticated living room. This being twenty-first-century Manhattan – rather than sixteenth-century Venice or, which amounts to the same thing in the play, twenty-first-century Pakistan – and Emily a modern twenty-first-century woman with means of her own, she leaves rather than waiting to be disfigured or killed by the jealous Muslim male now giving full reign to his long-repressed savage instincts that, as he himself earlier reminded his wife and dinner guests, are sanctioned by the Qur'an. In this interpretation of an (in)famous Quranic verse, he had ironically been challenged by the same wife who is now the victim of his abuse. The scene where the play enacts the thin and essentially non-negotiable difference between the exotic and the orientalist is the final one which collapses into the sameness of a recognisable iterative performativity: that of the slave/Moor/Muslim gazing forlornly as his white mistress/wife slips, like the civilisation she represents, always and already beyond his grasp. As he is packing up his belongings to move out of the apartment they had once shared – and listening to the story of FBI harassment by his nephew who had changed his name from Hussein Malik to Abe Jensen to 'fit in' at the play's beginning, and has now has re-embraced his Muslim identity by changing his name back and donning a *kufi* (skull) cap – Amir's ex-wife shows up. She is there to hand him the portrait she had been painting of him in the opening scene of the play. What exactly is she 'returning' to Amir here?

At the conclusion of the ill-fated dinner scene, when all civilisational masks had fallen off, and everyone's prejudices and uglinesses had been revealed, the ugliest and most atavistic of all interior spaces to be denuded was most clearly Amir's. Echoing the sentiments of Hamid's protagonist in *The Reluctant Fundamentalist*, Amir at that turning point in the play had triumphantly admitted to feeling a sense of 'pride' with other co-religionists on 9/11 when the Twin Towers were hit. After such an admission – no matter that he immediately says he felt horrified by feeling this way – there is no redemptive possibility for Amir. When he leaves the party to get a bottle of wine with Jory (his African-American colleague and wife of art curator Isaac) to celebrate the news that his own wife has made it into Isaac's show at the Whitney (after Emily has taken him into the kitchen apparently to admonish him for his bad behaviour thus far), Isaac, left alone with Emily, reminds her of their affair in London, which she then proceeds to insist was a mistake. Isaac's response is that it is her marriage to Amir that is a mistake. After telling Emily that her husband 'doesn't understand you', Isaac claims that it is clear from his expression in her portrait of him that Amir 'is looking at you [with an] expression [of] shame, anger, pride: the slave finally has the master's wife'. When Emily protests weakly at this interpretation of her portrait and Amir's gaze in it, Isaac continues: 'A man like that [...] you will cheat on him again [...] and then you will leave him' (Akhtar 2013: 61, 62).

Arguably then what Emily is 'returning' to Amir in the sad final scene – after the dinner party has ended in catastrophe, in the apartment where he now stands alone, humiliated and shorn of all of his 'civilisational' achievements and aspirations, pleading with her, 'I just want you to be proud [...] proud that you were with me' (Akhtar 2013: 76) – is that 'gaze' which Isaac had described as a slave's gaze combining shame, anger, and pride at finally 'owning' the master's wife. If Malek Alloula claimed in his *Colonial Harem* (1987) that the work of postcolonial critics like himself, following Said, was a belated 'returning' of the colonial photographers' orientalist 'gaze' to the colonisers who tried to appropriate the lands and the women of the Muslim lands they conquered through their phantasmic portraits of native women (Algerian women in Alloula's case), then Emily, in a classic double-reversal of the postcolonial returning of the master's gaze (much like Jean Morris in Salih's novel), is re-turning the imperial gaze back on its 'subject', and thus reiterating the orientalist performative: You, O Slave, will never 'own' me, so take back that look of pride, anger, resentment with which you foolishly thought you could lay claim to my domain. Unlike Jean, who kills herself in a symbolic gesture that acknowledges white imperial culpability in the cycle of violence, Emily – in a play written by a brown Muslim man half a century after *Season of Migration* tried to suggest a path out of orientalism's morass – ends up signifying its return, bigger and badder than ever.

Suffice it to say that in Eteraz's novel too, as recently as 2016, we are presented with a series of tropes that mimic Akhtar's reiterative orientalism. Pauls Toutonghi, reviewing *Native Believer* for the *New York Times Book Review*, asks an important question about the tripling of hate crimes in the US against Muslims in 2016, a question that is central to my own argument in this chapter:

> How much is our cultural marketplace to blame – where the narratives that sell most widely are ones that, arguably, do little to advance understanding, or even dialogue, across difference?
>
> (2016: 17)

My thesis has been that most of the Pakistani/Pakistani-origin male writers who have been or are being lionised by the West have produced works that reiterate orientalist clichés about Islam, Muslims, and Brown 'others' as essentially 'exotic', unknowable, given to atavistic urges that confirm the savagery lurking beneath supposedly civilised exteriors; repeating the trope of the Muslim male as always-already an Othello, his obsessive lust for, combined with his jealous mistrust of, a white woman, the reigning trope of his desire to be seen as a Man, an impossibility given his inferiority complex *vis-à-vis* the white master who colonised his lands; especially when the white woman he painfully 'acquires' (Jean Morris, Marie-Anne, Erica, Emily) as a possible symbol of his counter-conquest turns out to be yet another emasculator, in league with her 'own' race. 'What a history', to quote Sara Ahmed (2014: 203). It is one that persists in our times, but requires of us different moves if we wish for new and better futures; to move away from erotic historicism to a materialist conception of history; away from misogyny and self-hatred spun as dreams of conquest, into 'wilful arms' that, as part of a collective historical struggle, can actually bring down the walls of a history that has become concrete and tiresome in its clichés. The 'persistence of protest' can help prevent 'every hand' played by the

Black/Brown/Muslim man from becoming a 'losing hand', such as to liberate the arms of the Other from their 'otherness', smashing the Hegelian dialectic in the process, and thus realising Frantz Fanon's 'decolonizing humanist project', however belatedly (Ahmed 2014: 203).

None of the male Pakistani/Pakistani-American writers I have discussed in this chapter inhabit such a decolonising humanist project, though each does hint at the need to move away from a nihilistic despair and regurgitation of old clichés towards some new vision, even if expressed negatively. Part of the problem each of these writers faces is their inability (unwillingness?) to tell a story in which their protagonists see themselves as part of a collective historical struggle, which is what saves the narrator of Salih's *Season of Migration* from succumbing to nihilistic despair and, instead, has him commit at the end to a desire to land on the shore, to build connections between South and North; unlike Saeed, who warned of the danger of 'seeing only with one eye', Salih's narrator keeps both eyes open and on the horizon of change. Changez does return to inhabit a collective struggle back in his homeland of Pakistan, but his larger struggle is subservient to the demands of fictional strategy – the author's need to tell a gripping tale in which the reader is kept guessing until the end whether or not Changez's struggle is a worthy one or negatively in thrall to the demands of 'terrorists'. Akhtar faces a similar dilemma in his portrayal of Amir, who stands against the twin demands of Islamophobia and Islamism, which are essentially communitarian ideological visions. In order to take a stand against both ideologies, Akhtar creates a protagonist who remains an isolated individual, unable to connect to any sense of a community or to a larger struggle for justice for Muslims, or Palestinians, or for other people of colour such as Jory. It is his individual plight that the play focuses on, which is doomed to failure given its tethering to a romanticist, erotic historicity rather than a dialectical materialist one. Similarly, Eteraz's nameless protagonist does not see himself as part of a collective historical struggle, even when he is rejected and cast aside as an employee because of his boss' Islamophobia. His professionally successful wife's ballooning size, while he starves metaphorically in the workplace without a job, could be read as the diminishment of his individual masculine ego, while America's imperial might balloons unchecked. The 'Commie Muzzies' he begins to hang out with are presented as a joke, rather than as an example of a truly progressive collective struggle for justice that might help recast the terms of the historical impasse of our current *poco* moment in favour of a decolonising futurity. Unfortunately, the work discussed here is mired in a present in which an individualist ethos in thrall to global capitalism reigns supreme, whether of the imperialist or the Islamist variety, no exit in sight …

Exit West – and East?

Unless we exit West. That, in a nutshell, is the vision adumbrated in Hamid's latest novel, an interesting stylistic and thematic cross between J.K. Rowling's *Harry Potter* and Jean-Paul Sartre's *No Exit*. Where, in Sartre's play, 'L'enfer, c'est les autres' or 'Hell is other people', Hamid's novel moves from such a pessimistic Sartrean existentialism to a more joyous sense of community that is the heart of the Potter universe and saves its inhabitants from the tyranny of rule by one supreme power, a He who cannot be named. Hamid's Pakistani protagonists, who start out as the young lovers Nadia and Saeed, flee through mysterious trapdoors, once the decimation of their country by Islamist gangs begins, into different countries of Europe which they keep exiting, from Greece, into England, ending up by the end of the novel at the furthest end of America, in Marin county, where:

> there was nonetheless a spirit of at least intermittent optimism that refused entirely to die [...] perhaps because Marin was less violent than most of the places its residents

had fled, or because of the view, its position on the edge of a continent, overlooking the world's widest ocean, or because of the mix of its people.

(2017: 192–193)

This mix of people in Marin includes very few 'Natives' who, we are told, had either 'died out or been exterminated long ago' but whose surviving elders, when they appeared, told 'tales [...] that people from all over now gathered to hear, for the tales of these natives felt appropriate to this time of migration, and gave listeners much-needed sustenance' (2017: 196).

This present time is rendered within a materialist dialectic that brings together the experiences of descendants of African slaves brought forcefully from their homes to the shores of the American continent three centuries ago, with those of the 'other' natives – those who trace their 'nativeness' to the white colonists from Britain. Yet, in this latter time of mass migration brought on by the depredations of a coloniser-capitalist-imperialist-patriarchal class system culminating in a violent globalisation that has left no one untouched, Hamid paints a picture of a post-apocalyptic world where we have all become refugees, including the white folk who are now also experiencing things falling apart:

It seemed to Saeed that the people [...] who claimed the rights of nativeness most forcefully, tended to be drawn from the ranks of those with light skin who looked most like the natives of Britain – and as had been the case with many of the natives of Britain, many of these people seemed stunned by what was happening to their homeland [...] and some seemed angry as well.

(2017: 196)

For Saeed, it is the African-American descendants of slaves who provide the greatest source of comfort in a world whose history demands to be remade if humanity is to survive and perhaps thrive once again:

A third layer of nativeness was composed of those who [...] had been brought from Africa to this continent centuries ago as slaves [...] this layer [...] had vast importance, for society had been shaped in reaction to it, and unspeakable violence had occurred in relation to it, and yet it endured, fertile, a stratum of soil that perhaps made possible all future transplanted soils, and to which Saeed in particular was attracted, since at a place of worship where he had gone one Friday the communal prayer was led by a man from this tradition [...] and Saeed had found [...] this man's words to be full of soul-soothing wisdom.

(2017: 197)

We can see that Saeed's attachment to the ritual of Muslim prayer becomes a conduit for remembering his parents, for what was past, but also for developing attachment to other traditions of prayer, such as that represented by this African-American preacher. Through participating in this communal activity, he finds love anew with the preacher's daughter, but only after both he and Nadia separate in a peaceful and loving way, and Nadia embraces her desire for communion through same-sex love for a woman with blue eyes, a cook in their community of migrants.

Exit West embraces the art of collective survival, and all the different types of border crossings that it demands of us, including a leap of faith across the gender, religious, class, and race divisions that keep us trapped in a world without exit. Whilst the narrator of *Season of Migration to the*

North finally accepts life and the need to negotiate its demands for justice without succumbing to nihilistic violence despite the unfairness of history for its victims – just as, half a century later, the protagonists of *Exit West* attempt do the same in the imperial centres that continue to victimise them – the real question now is: will the North/West similarly show itself capable of absorbing these 'other' narrators of his/her/story? Will the (waning) West allow its power a safe exit, so that the horrors of hell, where all protagonists and antagonists remain tethered to otherness, can be avoided? Will the East jettison its self-orientalising habits? Or, to circle back to Benjamin (via Chris Marker), can we turn the Messianic impulse so prevalent in our present moment into 'a secular acknowledgement of the possibilities of creating Heaven on Earth, interpreted as the *potential* in each moment for the radical change of everyday conditions'? According to Marker, '*this* is the service of theology that Benjamin wished to enlist. Not the promise of a redemptive afterlife, but the political charging of each and every moment of experience' so as to create 'Heaven on Earth' (2012: n.p.; emphasis added). Surely, by locating the theological impulse within a secularist mode of class, race, and gender struggles for equity, a new kind of Angel will come forth, consigning its white wings to a debunked history in favour of another world of multicoloured herstories. This 'other' world is not only possible, it is already here.

Bibliography

Afzal-Khan, F. (2014) 'Re-Orienting Orientalism'. *Arab Stages* [online]. Available from <http://arabstages.org/2014/12/re-orienting-orientalism-from-shafik-gabrs-what-orientalist-painters-can-teach-us-about-the-art-of-east-west-dialogue-to-ayad-akhtars-disgraced/> [22 October 2017].

Afzal-Khan, F. (2015) '*Charlie Hebdo* and the Return of the Postcolonial'. *Counterpunch* [online]. Available from <www.counterpunch.org/2015/01/21/charlie-hebdo-and-the-return-of-the-postcolonial/> [22 October 2017].

Afzal-Khan, F., Bose, N., and Khoury, J. (2016) 'The Dramaturgy of Political Violence: Muslims Americans on American Stages'. *Performing Islam* 5(1–2), 29–41.

Ahmed, S. (2014) *Willful Subjects*. Durham: Duke University Press.

Akhtar, A. (2013) *Disgraced*. London: Bloomsbury.

Alloula, M. (1987) *The Colonial Harem*. Manchester: Manchester University Press.

Althusser, L. (1971) *Lenin and Philosophy and Other Essays*. New York: Monthly Review Press.

Benjamin, W. (1942) 'Theses on the Philosophy of History'. Book 1X [online]. Available from <www.sfu.ca/~andrewf/CONCEPT2.html> [24 October 2017].

Conrad, J. (1990) *The Heart of Darkness*. Mineola: Dover Thrift.

'Diego Velázquez'. NNDB [online]. Available from <www.nndb.com/people/913/000071700/> [20 June 2013].

'East-West: Art of Dialogue Symposium'. *New York Times*. 30 November 2012. sec. A, 18.

Eteraz, A. (2016) *Native Believer*. Brooklyn: Akashic Books.

Fanon, F. (2008) *Black Skin, White Masks*. New York: Grove Press.

Foucault, M. (1991) *Discipline and Punish: The Birth of a Prison*. London: Penguin.

Freller, T. and Herget, S. (1999) 'The Morisco and Hispano-Arabic Culture and Malta: Some Highlights on Late Medieval and Early Modern Links'. *MEAH, Sección Árabe-Islam* 48, 105–120 [online]. Available from <https://azslide.com/the-morisco-and-hispano-arabic-culture-and-malta-some-highlights-on-late-medieva_5a3686761723ddbe85f195c8.html> [30 December 2017].

Frye, N. (1970) *Anatomy of Criticism: Four Essays*. New York: Atheneum Press.

Gramsci, A. (1971) *The Prison Notebook*. In *Selections from the Prison Notebooks of Antonio Gramsci*. Ed. and trans. by Hoare, Q. and Smith, G.N. New York: International Publishers.

Hamid, M. (2007) *The Reluctant Fundamentalist*. Oxford: Oxford University Press.

Hamid, M. (2017) *Exit West*. London: Penguin Random House.

Hartnell, A. (2010) 'Moving through America: Race, Place and Resistance in Mohsin Hamid's *The Reluctant Fundamentalist*'. *Journal of Postcolonial Writing* 46(3–4), 336–348.

Hoeveler, D. and Cass, J. (eds.) (2006) *Interrogating Orientalism: Contextual Practices and Pedagogical Approaches*. Columbus: Ohio State University Press.

Isherwood, C. (2012) 'Beware Dinner Talk on Identity and Islam: "Disgraced," by Ayad Akhtar, with Aasif Mandvi'. *New York Times* [online]. Available from <www.nytimes.com/2012/10/23/theater/reviews/disgraced-by-ayad-akhtar-with-aasif-mandvi.html?_r=0> [2 February 2013].

Johnson, B. (2013) 'Diego Rodriguez de Silva Velazquez' [online]. Available from <http://hoocher.com/Diego_Velazquez/Diego_Velazquez.htm> [24 June 2013].

Kuehl, J. (2011) 'Exotic Harem Paintings: Gender, Documentation, and Imagination'. *Frontiers: A Journal of Women Studies* 32(2), 31–63.

Lukacs, G. (1964) *Realism in Our Time: Literature and the Class Struggle*. New York: Harper and Row.

Marker, C. (2012) 'Walter Benjamin and Architecture: An Exploration of Porosity and Ruin' [online]. Available from <https://allfordeadtime.wordpress.com/2012/07/16/walter-benjamin-and-architecture-an-exploration-of-porosity-and-ruin/> [20 December 2017].

Salih, T. (1966) *Season of Migration to the North*. Trans. by Johnson-Davies, D. Oxford: Heinemann.

Shakespeare, W. (2001) *Othello*. New York: Penguin Putnam.

Sharma, P. (2015) 'Tariq Ali: France Tries to Mask its Islamophobia behind Secular Values'. *Tikkun* [online]. Available from <www.tikkun.org/nextgen/tariq-ali-france-tries-to-hide-its-islamophobia-behind-secular-values> [4 June 2015].

Stasio, M. (2012) 'Broadway Review: "Disgraced"'. *Variety* [online]. Available from <http://variety.com/2012/legit/reviews/disgraced-1117948621/> [1 July 2013].

Toutonghi, P. (2016) 'In an New Novel, a Secular Muslim American Rejects the Burden of Labels'. *New York Times Book Review* [online]. Available from <www.nytimes.com/2016/06/26/books/review/in-a-new-novel-a-secular-muslim-american-rejects-the-burden-of-labels.html> [24 June 2016].

Trueman, M. (2013) 'Pulitzer Prize for 2013 Won by Ayad Akhtar's *Disgraced*'. *Guardian* [online]. Available from <www.guardian.co.uk/stage/2013/apr/16/pulitzer-prize-drama-2013-disgraced> [2 July 2013].

17
LOVE, SEX, AND DESIRE VS ISLAM IN BRITISH MUSLIM LITERATURE

Kavita Bhanot

At the 2015 Jaipur Literature Festival, in a discussion on sex and writing, Hanif Kureishi declared sex and writing about it to be acts of political resistance against 'Muslim fascism'. 'It's important to write about sex', he said:

> because we are desiring creatures. Particularly in the Muslim world, it's distorted and forbidden [...] In the present context the love of sensuality, love of desire, our sexual love of one another seems to have become a political act. Remember that, every time you're f******, you're defying political Islam. One of the things radical Islam thinks about is pleasure, all the time, in the negative [...] Islam is a death cult of extreme fascism – we also have to have a resistance from the side of pleasure. It's partly our duty to keep pleasure alive.
>
> (quoted in Nelson 2015: n.p.)

This pitching of love, sex, desire, and pleasure in opposition to Islam has been central to Kureishi's fiction, in particular his novel *The Black Album* (1995), about the Rushdie Affair.

The aftermath to the publication of *The Satanic Verses* signified the emergence and development of a perceived British Muslim identity, while subsequent events, such as 9/11, 7/7, the Bradford riots, and state media responses to these continued to contribute to a process of creating and fixing a British Muslim subject. A number of critics (Mondal 2015; Ahmed 2017; Nash 2012; Yaqin 2012; Morey 2012; Upstone 2010) have articulated the role that British literature has played in reflecting and contributing to the idea of a threatening Muslim 'other'. Apart from novels by writers such as Ian McEwan and John Updike, a number of texts by Muslim/South Asian writers have grappled, overtly or implicitly, with the Rushdie Affair, as well as ensuing events, such as 9/11 and 7/7, that have formed pressure points for British Muslims. Above all, while seeming to give a voice to the British Muslim perspective, they have reflected and confirmed mainstream representations and suspicions of British Muslims; young British Muslim believers are caricatured in this literature as radical, rigid, unreasonable, fundamentalists.

These literary representations can be traced to *The Black Album*, published in 1995. The novel charts the main character/narrator Shahid's simultaneous attraction to what are presented as dichotomous ways of living: the liberal pleasure-seeking hedonism of his teacher, Deedee

Osgood, and the revivalist, politicised religiosity of the Muslim students at his college. These students are presented in sinister and caricatured tones, and it is therefore inevitable, as the plot hurtles towards its climax, in which a book (unnamed but analogous to *The Satanic Verses*) is burnt by these students, that Shahid will ultimately choose the pleasure-seeking liberalism signified by his teacher/lover. According to Anshuman Mondal, this paradigm in *The Black Album*, along with the accompanying representation of young British Muslims, has become an archetype or resource that has been recreated in a number of literary works that followed Kureishi's novel – including Kureishi's own short story 'My Son the Fanatic', Monica Ali's *Brick Lane*, and Zadie Smith's *White Teeth* (Mondal 2015: 34–35).

This chapter focuses on love, sex, and desire as a central aspect of this dichotomy, in three texts that form a central thread through the category of 'British Muslim' literature: Kureishi's *The Black Album*, Nadeem Aslam's *Maps for Lost Lovers* (2004), and Sarfraz Manzoor's memoir *Greetings from Bury Park* (2007). All of these texts grapple with love, desire, and sexuality (as aspects of Western liberalism, entangled with abstract notions of music, literature, creativity, imagination, beauty, and freedom) in relation to Islam, which is seen to repress and forbid them. Whilst the binary is stark in *The Black Album* and *Greetings from Bury Park*, with a clear association with whiteness (e.g. love and sexual pleasure are associated with a white lover), this dynamic is more complicated and somewhat obscured in Aslam's novel due to the articulation of what Sadia Abbas refers to as a 'Sufi aesthetic' (2014: 193) that is rooted in the subcontinent, and entangled with Islam.

The Black Album

At the heart of *The Black Album* is a dichotomy between Islam and literature (along with everything that the narrator Shahid associates with literature: intelligence, love, imagination and creativity). Islam's rejection of these is captured in the novel's representation of the Rushdie Affair. The novel appears to present different critical arguments via characters such as Riaz and Chad (Shahid's Muslim friends) and the socialist Brownlaw, who questions Shahid's elevation of literature and intellectuals, his assumption that literature represents a neutral perspective, and the 'good intentions' of liberals. Shahid is shown at times to have been swayed by the arguments of his new friends; however, the moment when the book is burned in the college is a turning point. It becomes clear to Shahid at that moment which side he is on: 'He never wanted his face to show such ecstatic rigidity! The stupidity of the demonstration appalled him. How narrow they were, how unintelligent, how […] embarrassing it all was!' (Kureishi 1995: 225). Characters who represent alternative perspectives ultimately slip into caricature or carry a sinister edge, undermining their arguments, ratifying the liberal perspective of the novel. What Shahid finally chooses, over what is presented as the certainty, narrowness, and rigidity of young Muslims, is to embrace fluidity, openness, freedom: 'There was no fixed self; surely our several selves melted and mutated daily? There had to be innumerable ways of being in the world. He would spread himself out, in his work and in love, following his curiosity' (Kureishi 1995: 274). In this way, the specific perspective which Shahid/the novel represents assumes a neutrality, objectivity, and universality, with love and pleasure as aspects of this apparently free, fluid, and creative path. Shahid's Muslim friends are shown to deny themselves this pleasure. For example, Shahid describes the repressed sexual energies between Nina and Sadiq: 'Forbidden to kiss or touch, they liked to fight: Sadiq had pinched her and now Nina was poised for the chance to pinch him back' (Kureishi 1995: 126).

'Pleasure and self-absorption isn't everything', Chad explains to Shahid (in whose mind a 'terrible torment' is 'working itself up') 'One pleasure […] can only lead to another […] A man is more advanced, surely, if he conquers himself, rather than submits to every desire?' (Kureishi 1995: 128–129). Around these Muslim friends, Shahid is filled with guilt about the parallel life of pleasure, sex, drugs, raves, and alcohol that he is leading with his teacher, Deedee. He repeatedly uses imagery of water, of drowning, of being carried by a current, almost against his will. He has 'plunged', he thinks as he watches the men pray, 'into a river of desire and excitement' (Kureishi 1995: 132). Out of guilt, he tries to expunge thoughts of Deedee from his mind while with his new friends: 'Instead of bathing in the warm memory of the love they'd made and the pleasures she'd introduced him to […] he became aware of a bitter, disillusioned feeling. How he'd been drowning in his senses in the past hours!' (Kureishi 1995: 130). At one point, he feels himself 'empty of passion and somewhat delivered and cleansed' while praying (Kureishi 1995: 131). By the end of the novel, Shahid frees himself of the influence of these friends, and therefore of any guilt, in order to succumb to all the joys that life has to offer. He and Deedee commit themselves, finally, to their latest adventure, 'until it stops being fun' (Kureishi 1995: 276).

The novel is an ode to hedonism, pleasure, playfulness. This is what constitutes the sacred for Shahid; feeling unsure of what he is supposed to think during prayer,

> on his knees, he celebrated […] the inexplicable phenomenon of life, art, humour and love itself – in murmured language, itself another sacred miracle. He accompanied this awe and wonder with suitable music, the 'Ode to Joy' from Beethoven's Ninth […] which he hummed inaudibly.
>
> (Kureishi 1995: 92)

Sexual pleasure and love become intertwined with, and analogous to, forms of art such as literature and music. Thinking of Deedee, for Shahid, is 'like listening to his favourite music; she was a tune he liked to play' (Kureishi 1995: 130). And at another point, as he is writing, Shahid's 'typing fingers, sensing Deedee's body beneath them, danced on the keys too euphorically for the subject matter […] He pulled himself together, but got an erection which just wouldn't go away' (Kureishi 1995: 76). Shahid is here typing up Riaz's work on religion and, as an act of mischief and what is shown to be innocent joy in his relationship, and therefore almost accidental, he brings sex and innuendo into Riaz's writing. It was a celebration of passion (Kureishi 1995: 234), he later tells Hat, one of his Muslim friends. This act of blasphemy, or of rebellion, becomes a small feat of heroism in the novel (and also a comment on the Rushdie Affair). We see Shahid perpetually writing or imagining writing stories about sex, weaving in religious imagery: 'He began composing an erotic story for Deedee, "the Prayer-mat of the Flesh"' (Kureishi 1995: 134). Later, 'he embarked on a story which he wanted to call "The Flesh, the Flesh"' (Kureishi 1995: 166). The implication is that it is the job of the writer to offend religious sentiment. As he is quoted as saying at the beginning of this chapter, for Kureishi, writing about sexual pleasure is a form of resistance to Muslim fascism.

The idea of love is evoked throughout the novel: 'He would spread himself out, in his work, and in love' (Kureishi 1995: 274), Shahid decides in the final pages of the novel. He does question, at one point, whether his relationship with Deedee is love, reflecting on Riaz's assertions that:

> Without a framework in which love [can] flourish […] love [is] impossible […] people merely rented one another for a period. In this faithless interlude they hoped to obtain pleasure and distraction; they even hoped to discover something which would complete them. And if they didn't soon receive it, they threw the person over and moved on. […] In such circumstances what permanence or deep knowing could there be?
>
> (Kureishi 1995: 240)

Shahid wonders if his relationship with Deedee is an instance of this, whether they

> had plunged into a compelling familiarity. They'd gone out a few times, confessed, and shared the most uninhibited passions people could participate in. Surely though, their lovemaking was merely an exchange of skills and performances? How much did they know one another? They had been tourists in one another's lives.
> (Kureishi 1995: 240)

However, such questioning, attributed to his Muslim friends' influence, becomes another instance in the novel of a counter-perspective being offered, but not taken up.

The implication by the end is that Shahid has chosen the path of love. Apart from a lack of depth and emotion in the depiction of love in the novel, there is also a lack of complexity and politics. Instead, love, as well as creativity, beauty, music, art, and imagination, are ultimately idealised and abstracted. Although we see hints of the inequalities between Deedee and Shahid, these are brushed under the carpet, absolved of significance. We don't get a sense that power dynamics are addressed or overcome in order for their love to flourish. For example, at one point, Shahid reflects on his relationship with Deedee, the fact that she is an older white woman, and his teacher. 'What prevented her taking other Asian or black lovers?' he wonders. 'Perhaps she took a different lover each year, using men as [Shahid's brother] Chili had used women' (Kureishi 1995: 240). Shahid is echoing here what Sadiq has suggested to him: 'Osgood is taking lovers among the Afro-Caribbean and Asian students [...] For political reasons she selects only black or Asian lovers now'. Tahira echoes this: 'Our people have always been sexual objects for whites' (Kureishi 1995: 228). This is another example of a counter-perspective in the novel, but in the logic of the narrative, such questions simply remain as paranoia or petty vilifying, not truly considered.

Abstract ideas of love and sex are emptied of complexity and power relations. However, the fetishisation of young black/brown male bodies is an obstacle to the possibility of love, in the same way that men's objectification of women is. At one point, during one of their liaisons, Shahid says: '"You're looking at me as if I were a piece of cake. What are you thinking?' 'I deserve you"', Deedee replies. 'I'm going to like eating you' (Kureishi 1995: 117). Fetishising Shahid's skin colour from a location of power, Deedee tells him to undo his shirt. 'I love that café-au-lait skin', she says (Kureishi 1995: 210). Perhaps this power dynamic is all the starker because it tends to be normalised when the female is being objectified by a man. It is perhaps a decolonial counter-reading of the novel that leads us to think about Deedee's whiteness in the relationship. Meanwhile, it also remains the case that the novel inhabits a male gaze in its representation of love and desire. This is how Shahid recalls his first meeting with Deedee:

> She crossed her legs and tugged her skirt down. He had, so far, successfully kept his eyes averted from her breasts and legs. But the whole eloquent movement – what amounted in that room to an erotic landslide of rustling and hissing – was so sensational and almost provided the total effect of a Prince concert that his mind took off into a scenario about how he might be able to tape-record the whisper of her legs, copy it, add a backbeat and play it through his headphones.
> (Kureishi 1995: 25)

This description (again bringing together music and desire), from Shahid's point of view as the narrator, is normalised as the perspective of the novel. It is not problematised or separated as the perspective of the main character or narrator. Although we see glimpses of Deedee's insecurity in the novel, the relationship between her and Shahid seems to rest on her self-alienation, a disconnection from her own vulnerability. In this way, Deedee, as a sexually liberated, assertive female teacher, appears as a male fantasy. She talks to Shahid about 'The Story of O' – which is about female submission; the female protagonist is prepared to be a slave. She is whipped and says, 'I'll be whatever you want me to be' (Kureishi 1995: 118). Deedee says, 'I'm thinking of preparing a literary wank list for my students'. And Shahid says, 'How do you turn the pages?' (Kureishi 1995: 118). It is clear in his comment that he assumes it to be men who are the recipients of this 'literary wank list'. As Deedee masturbates before him, he thinks 'without losing her soul she was turning herself into pornography' (Kureishi 1995: 119). From a male perspective, this is perhaps ideal: a woman willingly objectifying herself. The dynamic between Deedee and Shahid, the expression of their desire and sexuality, is specific to a particular context, history, and cultural expression, and perhaps, through these cracks in (or in the illusion of) abstraction, the specificity or parochialism of the Western liberalism which the book embraces is revealed.

Greetings from Bury Park

While Manzoor's memoir *Greetings from Bury Park* is chronologically the latter of the texts I am discussing, it is a clearer articulation, in continuity with Kureishi's novel, of the binary of a liberal, Western framework contrasted with Islam. It all the more clearly occupies a position that is simultaneously 'post-ethnic' and proudly British. An inheritor of Kureishi's ideological framework, Manzoor's memoir clearly reveals its implications to us.

Greetings from Bury Park is a commercial response to 7/7. It is also located in the post-9/11 and post-2001 Bradford riots context, wherein former *Prospect* editor David Goodhart recommended 'earned citizenship' (citizenship granted only to the most assimilated subjects). This has been the face of aggressive British government policy since 2002, when multiculturalism and the allowing of 'difference' to flourish was blamed for the growing 'segregation' behind the Bradford riots. In the background, dating back to the Rushdie Affair, exacerbated and overt since 9/11 and 7/7, has been the demonisation of Muslims as the embodiment of the uncivilised 'other'.

Post-9/11 and 7/7, there has been a political and commercial imperative to present 'authentic' Muslim voices – but also for writers to illustrate, through their work, that they are 'good', integrated, 'normal' Muslims with a shared understanding with the white middle-class reader towards whom a text such as Manzoor's is directed, of what it is to be normal. This is one of the key functions of Manzoor's text – it is overt in its celebration of Britishness, declaring by the end that 'every opportunity, every job, and every chance to pursue my dreams has been offered by this country [...] Britain [...] is my land of hope and dreams' (2007: 268–269).

At the centre of the memoir is a celebration of Bruce Springsteen's music, which becomes a signifier in the memoir of integration/assimilation into the West. The subtitle for the book is *Race. Religion. Rock 'n' Roll*, and the blurb talks about the book as a tribute to the 'power of music to transcend race and religion'. Blurring the specificity of the music that Manzoor's book is celebrating and the accompanying liberal ideology, music is assumed to be a pure, universal realm that brings people together: 'It was this shared love of music that quickly helped me see Kenny and Al as friends first and Americans second' (2007: 142).

An aspect of the dichotomy (West vs East/Islam) at the centre of Manzoor's work is the idea of romantic love and sexual pleasure. It is from Western music that Manzoor has acquired a sense of the importance, even the concept, of falling in love: 'I didn't know what love felt like, but according to the songs I was listening to when I was fourteen, it was overpowering, and its power overwhelming' (2007: 186). Elsewhere, he tells us that 'listening to Bruce had ruined my love life. All those songs about love had affected my expectation' (2007: 204).

Being a 'true fan' of Springsteen, 'absorb[ing] the wisdom in his songs', seeing him as 'a role model, someone who had married a woman he loved and did a job he enjoyed, surrounded by some of his best friends' (2007: 203), involves a responsibility to follow the same path. Islam is presented as being an obstacle since it is shown to be fundamentally opposed to individual freedom, pleasure, sensuality. The only way to be Muslim, he had thought, 'was to be obedient, deferential and unquestioning, it was to reject pleasure and embrace duty, to renounce sensuality and to never ever ask why' (2007: 238). His parents' faith torments him as he apprehends the forbidden possibility of falling in love, which

> would have been deeply inconvenient as it would have involved my parents disowning me and throwing me out of their home [...] My father treated the concept of love with a withering mixture of contempt and pity. 'What is love, anyway?' he would ask. Love is childish, anyone can fall in love. [...] Naïve individuals fell in love, good sons got married.
>
> (2007: 186–187)

A dichotomy is created between love and marriage; while the West signifies love, Muslims and Pakistanis are concerned with the practicalities of marriage, including its cynical use/abuse for visa purposes. 'That was one of the problems with arranged marriages and importing husbands and wives from Pakistan', Manzoor writes at one point, 'they thought marriage was a free ticket to an easy life' (2007: 68). In this way, the text becomes almost a form of propaganda for state policies which argued – in the name of community cohesion after the 2002 Bradford riots – for 'integrationism as the new framework for race, immigration policies' (Kundnani 2007: 131), and recommended to this end a clampdown on arranged marriages with foreign spouses.

Manzoor writes about the unlikelihood of meeting a Pakistani girl he can fall in love with – a girl who listens to Springsteen; 'my ideal girl would be someone to whom I could play "Born to Run", "Backstreets" and "Racing in the Street" and who would get it. There wasn't a chance I was going to find that amongst any Pakistani girls' (2007: 204).

Love, sex, and desire are entangled in Manzoor's memoir, along with whiteness – all the more overtly since there is no girlfriend/lover, real or fictional. But the assumption is that any girlfriend Manzoor might have is likely to be white; the assumed inevitability of this feeds Manzoor's angst in the memoir. Looking through the local newspaper, Manzoor says that he has never seen 'an Asian man with a white bride' (2007: 179). Reminiscent of Frantz Fanon's writing about the black man's attraction to the white woman (2008), Manzoor writes: 'I sometimes wondered if perhaps the price of having gone to school and grown up with whites was that it was only going to be white girls to whom I would be attracted and who would like me' (2007: 198).

This supposition that the woman with whom he will fall in love will be white belies the apparent freedom that the 'West' is supposed to signify, in opposition to the rigidity of arranged marriage. It suggests a certain conformity or ideology in the cultural expressions that Manzoor is celebrating, which renders only white women attractive, and also instils in Manzoor a sense of inferiority. Indeed, Manzoor repeatedly articulates an adolescent self-loathing connected to not being white – a feeling that he is not attractive to women (2007: 185–186).

When he is asked by his friend's mother if it would matter if he fell in love with a white girl, and when his friend responds that Sarfraz would never have an arranged marriage – that he is 'English like me', Manzoor's response is 'he was right of course' (2007: 193). There is no bristling at his friend's mother's patronising question, or his friend's declaration. Implicit in this recounted scene is the assumption that if he doesn't have an arranged marriage, Manzoor will inevitably fall in love with/marry a white woman.

All this suggests a need to interrogate the 'abstract' pure idea of love that Manzoor asserts he has inherited through Western culture, which is contrasted with oppressive Islam. There is also no critical engagement with the power dynamic between men and women in this articulation of love and sex, of the male gaze, of the exploitation and objectification of women. As a boy, Manzoor would look at pages from pornographic magazines, with a 'delectable cover girl [...] displayed in all her naked glory', and would feel 'a surge of electric pleasure' (2007: 184). He talks about blue movies, about secretly looking at the photographs of naked women in back copies of *The Sun* in his father's friend's home. Pornography is simply a part of the sphere of pleasure, sex, and desire which Islam is shown to suppress, and Manzoor articulates his torment due to the guilt induced by his religion and family:

> While I spent my afternoons poring over discarded porn magazines or browsing the videos on the top shelf of the video store [...] I spent my evenings reading the Koran. [...] I [...] hoped that my teenage curiosity did not make me a bad Muslim. Was I going to suffer in Hell because I had lingered too long on the underwear models in the catalogue?
>
> (2007: 184)

This angst is reminiscent of the guilt that Shahid goes through in *The Black Album*, which carries a similar dichotomy or dilemma. These magazines and videos are shown to represent healthy desire, 'teenage curiosity'. Meanwhile, it is not only Islam that is opposed to the 'freedom' of the West to 'love'. 'Fact is', says his friend Amalok, who is shown to 'endure' wearing a turban due to parental pressure, 'there's no way I'm getting any pussy with this on my head' (Manzoor 2007: 100). 'Getting pussy' is normalised as an aspect of the freedom, the love, sex, and desire, that is being oppressed by the young boys' prospective cultures and religions.

Maps for Lost Lovers

Both *The Black Album* and *Greetings from Bury Park* are responses to pivotal moments for Muslims in Britain, where pressure was exerted upon them to assert their allegiance to Britishness. The writing and publication of these texts have also been intertwined with a commercial and political imperative. In this way, the political agendas and positions in these works are overt. This dichotomy appears to be more complicated in Aslam's novel, which was written over eleven years. This is largely because *Maps for Lost Lovers* is more deeply immersed in the details and lived lives of the South Asian/Pakistani community in a fictional northern British town. Rather than setting up an East vs West dichotomy in which a normative white Britishness is contrasted with a traditional South Asian identity, the context of the novel appears to be a more specifically British-Pakistani identity.

This specificity exposes, perhaps inadvertently, the false universalism assigned to love, beauty, art, music, and literature in the work of Kureishi and Manzoor. Whilst *Maps for Lost Lovers* also articulates such apparently universal values, it is primarily through a specific Punjabi/Urdu Sufi perspective and context, revealing the narrow frame through which Kureishi and Manzoor articulate these values. For example, unlike Kureishi's novel and Manzoor's memoir, and most British-Asian literature (where the possibility or idea of love is usually entangled with whiteness), the beloved in *Maps for Lost Lovers* is not necessarily white. The only white character in the novel is Stella, the ex-wife of Charag, Shamas and Kaukab's son. Similarly, while both

Manzoor and Kureishi celebrate an abstract idea of music, their references are almost entirely Western: singers such as Springsteen (Manzoor's memoir) and Prince (Kureishi's novel), along with the specific ideologies intertwined with these forms of music. It is this music that is seen to signify love in opposition to Islam. However, even in these works, Sufism is hinted at as an exception. In both *The Black Album* and *Greetings from Bury Park*, references are made, albeit in passing, to the Sufi music of Nusrat Fateh Ali Khan and his nephew, Rahat Fateh Ali Khan; their music seems to have transcended cultural boundaries into the Western sphere (Manzoor 2007: 226, 237; Kureishi 1995: 45). Sufism and Sufi music and poetry alone have come to signify an acceptable aspect of Islam – often adopted or appropriated by secular left liberal elites in the subcontinent or by the West.

Sufi music and literature are also exceptionalised, indeed centred, in Aslam's novel as signifying the idea of love; the novel is entangled in what Sadia Abbas refers to as Sufi aesthetics (2014: 193). This engagement frames the novel's articulations of love, sex, and desire through a specific context and history. In particular, we see references throughout Aslam's novel to Nusrat Fateh Ali Khan, who sings Sufi *qawwalis*. It is no coincidence that it is at a concert by him that Suraya and Shamas, who will have a short-lived affair, meet. Nusrat's *qawwalis* represent freedom, sensuality, disorder, and defiance in the novel. Their performance, as articulated in Virinder Kalra's work, in some contexts (e.g. in an all-night *urs* in Pakistan) become 'demotic and carnivalesque' (2014: 5). We see a glimpse of the transgressive aspects of these performances in Aslam's novel, where Nusrat comes to perform in the fictional town:

> People are jubilantly throwing double handfuls of banknotes at Nusrat as he sings. A young woman gets up and, dancing there and back, goes to place a rose in Nusrat's lap; her open movements of pleasure are seen by some as a lack of womanly restraint and they win disapproving looks from a number of people in the audience, male and female.
>
> (2004: 190–191)

Sufi *qawwalis* are closely associated with the *qissa* or 'fable' tradition. Throughout *Maps for Lost Lovers*, references to the *qissa* of Heer are contrasted with the terrifying Islam that pervades the closed community. Heer becomes the defiant female figure who devotes herself to love. Forced to marry into another family, she refuses to consummate the marriage and continues to pine for her lover. Nusrat sings from Heer's perspective in the novel:

> Nusrat's voice has now become the fabled Heer [...] *Don't anybody call me Heer*, says Nusrat-Heer in a pining tone, *call me Ranjha, for I have spoken his name so many times during this separation that I am become him.*
>
> (Aslam 2004: 191)

This is a specific kind of love, in which the female and the male merge, through submission to love. The male lover represents the *murshid* or guru, who also embodies love and leads the devotee (signified by the female) to God. Love exists on these two levels, the mystical and the worldly – perhaps the worldly is a metaphor for the mystical, perhaps there is no distinction. An abstract God is signified by the human figure of the *murshid*/guru, while romantic love is intertwined with the material, with sexuality, desire, lust. And so, in stories such as that of Heer, the merging of the bodies is central to the idea of losing oneself in love.

The novel's emphasis on 'the worldliness of love' (Abbas 2014: 193) is tied to a certain interpretation of Sufi *qissas* that elides, perhaps, the spiritual dimension. As Sadia Abbas argues, the novel is concerned with the idea that 'the body is all that humans have [...] If everything ends with the grave, there is no reward to be gained by deferring the body's pleasure [...] the idea of resurrection is a cheat, not a promise' (2014: 193). The novel is therefore a counter to the denial or postponement by orthodox Muslims (or indeed, in Aslam's novel, all believing Muslims) of pleasure and desire, echoing Kureshi's articulation quoted at the opening of this essay. For Shamas (the character closest to the novel's perspective),

> there was hardly anything more beautiful than [...] young people, fumbling their way through life, full of new doubts and certainties, finding comfort in their own and others' bodies:
> And more wonderful still the single sheet
> over two lovers on a bed.
>
> (Aslam 2004: 144)

Worldly, physical love is given importance in *Maps for Lost Lovers*. Chanda and Jugnu are killed for living together outside of marriage. The last we see of them, towards the end of the novel, is an elegy of sorts to their lovemaking:

> They – Chanda and Jugnu – would lie in the various rooms of this house on secret trysts, the windows curtained and the clocks daringly put away the way they are in casinos – but they wouldn't know in enough time that they were gambling with their lives. They contrived to meet for sensual dalliance in other places too, in the age-old manner of lovers.
>
> (Aslam 2004: 362)

This reminds us of Heer Ranjha, who also met for secret trysts over twelve years (this number could be metaphorical rather than literal). Aslam's novel refers repeatedly to Heer, who has been depicted in Sufi literature, poetry, and music as a fearless woman going against her family and society, and, above all, taking on her religion and its clergy, for love (2004: 191). The Sufi saints, and the poetry they wrote, which Nusrat sings, celebrate Heer's rebellion and resistance to the hegemony of her time: her family, the community, orthodox clerics. Similarly, Chanda is shown to display agency and defiance, going against her family and community, loving Jugnu openly. She is perhaps the only Muslim woman in the novel who shows the strength and courage to do this and, like Heer, dies for her rebellion, killed by her brothers in the name of honour:

> Always it was the vulnerability of women that was used by the poet-saints to portray the intolerance and oppression of their times: in their verses, the women rebel and try bravely to face all opposition [...] And, in every poem and every story, they fail. But by striving they become part of the universal story of human hope.
>
> (2004: 191–192)

It is this idea of universality (tying in with the assumed universality of Kureishi's *The Black Album* and Manzoor's *Greetings from Bury Park*) that becomes problematic in Aslam's novel. For the form that love/resistance takes in the different contexts represented in these novels is not universal, and neither is the form that power takes.

For example, the idea of love/desire, freedom, and agency in the Sufi context, as a kind of submission to love, a willingness even to face death for love, does not resemble the conception of love in Kureishi's and Manzoor's works, it is not analogous, for example, to the hedonism of

The Black Album. Instead, it is closer to the idea of agency through submission that is articulated in the work of Talal Asad (1993, 2003) and Saba Mahmood (2011), as they complicate the idea of agency.

Meanwhile, the form that power takes is also not universal. Aslam's novel draws on eighteenth-century Sufi *qissa*s which articulate forms of resistance, through love, to Muslim orthodoxy combined with institutions such as the family and the state. This is applied to the present in a way that becomes disingenuous, even duplicitous. Referring to stories of resistance to power in an earlier period, and applying these, as if there were a line of continuity, to the contemporary moment, to oppression by a community that is amongst the most oppressed today, thus contributing to an endemic Islamophobia, is a distortion of the political and philosophical foundations of such traditions which fail to take account of power dynamics in the world today.

The oppression enacted by Muslims depicted in the novel is relentless. There is an honour killing at the centre, that of Chanda and Jugnu. Chanda's brothers, who have killed the couple, are shown as violent, hypocritical, monstrous; they kill Chanda and Jugnu for living together without being married. Meanwhile, the couple were unable to get married, because of religion (Chanda's husband had to divorce her first and refused to): 'Chanda too could not marry Jugnu due to the laws about Islamic divorce and women' (Aslam 2004: 201). Suraya, with whom Shamas has a brief relationship, is similarly shown to be in a difficult situation due to Islam – her violent husband says *talaq* three times when drunk one night. In the morning, he regrets having accidentally divorced his wife – who now, according to Islamic law, must find another man to marry and then divorce her so that she can remarry her first husband, with whom she has a child.

This is not to suggest that religion, especially in its orthodox form, is not experienced as oppressive in certain contexts, by women in particular. However, the relentless articulation in the novel of all that is wrong with Islam, and all believing Muslims, suggests another agenda in Aslam's work. There is only occasional mention of racism, including Islamophobia, in local, national, and global contexts. The primary oppression for the inhabitants of Dasht-e-Tanhaii, particularly those who pursue love and desire, is the relentless violence of Islam. Virtually every Muslim man in the novel is shown to be dangerous and abusive, while the entire town, predominantly Pakistani Muslim, is shown to be inward-looking, claustrophobic, a place of sheer terror; murders happen regularly, everybody is under constant surveillance by the community. The words 'terror' or 'danger' are used repeatedly. As Shamas thinks about Suraya, there is 'fear that someone had seen her talking to him and that she is even now – somewhere – being harmed for it. This terror has been hurtling around inside him like a grenade with the pin pulled out' (Aslam 2004: 162). As he waits for Suraya, 'a part of him hopes she doesn't come [...] he is too aware of the dangers' (2004: 163).

Meanwhile, female characters such as Kaukab and Suraya are depicted as simultaneously oppressed and oppressive, reproducing patriarchy as much, if not more than, the men, shown to be hardly aware of the ways in which the religion they follow oppresses them. Mah-Jabin reflects on Kaukab: 'Trapped within the cage of permitted thinking, this woman – her mother – is the most dangerous animal she'll ever have to confront' (Aslam 2004: 110). Kaukab's religiosity is shown to contribute to the breakdown of her relationship with her husband – the discovery that she is making their youngest son, a baby at the time, fast for Ramadan leads Shamas to hit Kaukab for the first and only time in their married life (feeling his frustration, the reader does not judge him harshly for it) and he temporarily leaves her. She is shown not to satisfy Shamas' emotional and physical needs, due to her faith, so the reader is sympathetic when he seeks a relationship with Suraya. We see, in this way, the patriarchy or maleness inherent in the novel's perspective.

Shamas (along with his murdered brother Jugnu) is a reasonable character – kind, compassionate, in touch with nature, beauty, art, and literature. He is an atheist who loves Sufism. Beauty, art, and literature are shown to be the connection between him and Suraya – she represents, for him, all the things that he values; they meet at the Nusrat concert, they often meet at the Safeena bookshop and discuss literature. She tells him of going, as a girl, to a poetry performance by the poet Wamaq Saleem which, as it happens, Shamas co-organised, and she talks of presenting a shawl to the poet. Shamas 'realises he's smiling, feeling light if not lightheaded. She seems to be one of those people to meet whom is to meet oneself' (Aslam 2004: 155). Suraya encourages Shamas to start writing poetry again. All this is part of what Rehana Ahmed refers to as the 'fetishization of creativity' in the novel (2017: 214).

These associations signify the sanctity of Shamas' love for Suraya. On one occasion, after they have made love, 'he slid his hand out from under her head and gave her a book of henna patterns to rest her head on: "Quite appropriate. Pillows filled with henna blossom are used to induce restful sleep"' (Aslam 2004: 201). Nature, beauty, and art are in this way intertwined with love, sexuality, and pleasure. Shamas is shown to be a gentle, generous lover, unlike virtually every other man in the book, including the abusive husband whom Suraya believes that she loves and wants to return to, even if it is primarily to be with her son. She ends up with another man who exploits her, marrying her because he wants a child. It is due to Suraya's attachment to her religion, her inability to shed the conventions of religiosity and internalised patriarchy, that she is shown as unable to fully embrace Shamas' love.

This mystification of love and desire in *Maps for Lost Lovers*, entangled with Sufism, must be questioned. There is little engagement with its politics, for instance with the power dynamic in the relationship between Shamas and Suraya, who is a woman in her late thirties, while Shamas is an important community figure, married, in his sixties. There is inequality and a degree of exploitation in such a relationship, all the more due to Suraya's vulnerability, her situation. But the novel leads us to dwell instead on Suraya's duplicity, as she tries to 'trap' Shamas into marrying her. This is contrasted with Shamas' earnest, boyish enthusiasm as he falls for Suraya – fantasising about her, forming an obsession that could be seen as sinister and disturbing. Similarly, the relationship that is central to the novel, although it takes place in its margins, that between Jugnu and Chanda, is also more complicated than the beautiful rebellion it is depicted as. For Jugnu is also three decades older than Chanda – he has travelled the world, is worldly and educated, while Chanda has always lived in Dast-e-Tanhaii. There is no exploration of the politics/layers in such a relationship. Instead, an abstract idea of love/desire, with an assumption of its radical potential for resistance, is suggested to be equalising. Chanda's (and Heer's) efforts to negotiate patriarchy, the celebration of their devotion to men, at the cost of both their deaths, and the reading of this as female agency, can also be connected to the male gaze. Meanwhile, this almost metaphorical idea of love, entangled in Sufism, is conflated in the novel with a Western liberal idea of individual freedom – which Britain/British laws are seen to protect.

According to Abbas, Aslam's novel is an example, like 'Pakistan's most popular band, Junoon, which calls its music Sufi-rock', of Sufi forms and themes being adopted as forms of 'counter-cultural assertion [...] fight[ing] the neo-orthodox revival that the Islamists prefer and reject(ing) Western imperialism' (2014: 195). However, this understanding doesn't account for the power, class, and location of those such as the Sufi-rock band Junoon and writers such as Aslam. Abbas and the novel conflate Sufism, which is entangled with the lived religiosity of ordinary people's lives, with resistance or resilience 'from below', with an elite secular perspective that is threatened by the form of religiosity constituted by Islam. This is another instance of Sufism being used in the service of Islamophobia – in the West, such differentiation between good

Islam (Sufism) and bad Islam has been a common practice of proponents of global imperialism. 'The secular elites' writes Geoffery Nash:

> have frequently adopted anti-religious positions, attacking the Islamic beliefs, practices and cultures of the lands to which they notionally belong [...] Sometimes non-authoritarian forms of Muslim culture such as Sufism or local traditional Islams are appropriated to attack revivalist Islam.
>
> (2012: 36)

In *Maps for Lost Lovers*, it is not Sufism but a hammering anti-Islam sentiment that pervades the novel. It is therefore questionable whether, as Abbas asserts, by using Sufi poetics, Aslam 'deAnglicises' the novel, 'hook[ing] it firmly to a South Asian literary genealogy, and through that process, claim[ing] English literature for Britain's most despised immigrants' (2014: 192). Rather, Aslam seems to have set out to vilify Muslims, Britain's 'most despised immigrants', primarily for white readers – confirming their worst fears. This ties in well with British foreign and domestic policy (which emphasises integration as assimilation); demonising Muslims has eased the attacks on and invasion of Muslim countries. As Ahmed argues of Sufism 'in its modern form', 'It is no coincidence that the only acceptable form of Islam is a politically quietist individualised understanding of faith and culture' (2017: 219).

Sufism, allied with the West/Britain, is presented as the only positive aspect of Muslim/South Asian culture. For while, on the one hand, Pakistani Muslims are shown as creating their own mini-Pakistan in a corner of Britain, Pakistan is shown to be much worse, particularly in how it treats its women. It is there that Mah-Jabin endures her Pakistani husband's violence, as does Suraya, along with the violence of other men in her husband's family. Shamas, the voice of conscience in the novel, says, 'Pakistan is not just a wife-beating country, it's a wife-murdering one' (Aslam 2004: 226). Towards the end of the novel, we are told that killings such as that of Chanda and Jugnu 'are not uncommon in Pakistan, but the killers usually killed openly and were proud of their deed' (2004: 347).

England is therefore shown to be a safe haven compared to Pakistan. The inhabitants of Dasht-e-Tanhaii, especially women, are protected somewhat by British laws. We are told that Suraya's husband won't send their son to visit her in England, saying that 'the laws in the West are favourable to women: the authorities will side with you and I won't be able to do anything' (Aslam 2004: 199). It is thanks to the British legal system that Chanda's and Jugnu's killers (Chanda's brothers) are rightfully convicted and punished. We are told that:

> they knew the law of this country would not view their crimes indulgently. They boasted of having killed her and Jugnu – but only in Pakistan, where the laws and religion and the customs reinforced their sense of having acted properly, legitimately, correctly.
>
> (2004: 348)

The message at the heart of the novel seems to be, like that in *The Black Album* and *Greetings from Bury Park*, the need to integrate. Shamas' children are all shown to have escaped the town of their birth, they are secular and integrated into white Britain. Shamas' ultimate tragedy in the novel is that, due to his good intentions and politics, because he wanted to help the community, he never left. In this way, the articulation of love, sex, and desire in all three texts discussed here is tied up with Britishness – the suggestion is that it is only in inhabiting a conditional

Britishness (integrating into the mainstream) that love and desire can be expressed, fitting well into dominant ideologies and propaganda of the British state and media.

Bibliography

Abbas, S. (2014) *At Freedom's Limit: Islam and the Postcolonial Predicament*. New York: Fordham University Press.

Ahmed, R. (2017) *Writing British Muslims: Religion, Class and Multiculturalism*. Manchester: Manchester University Press.

Ahmed, R., Morey, P., and Yaqin, A. (eds.) (2012) *Culture, Diaspora, and Modernity in Muslim Writing*. New York: Routledge.

Asad, T. (1993) *Genealogies of Religion: Discipline and Reasons of Power in Christianity and Islam*. Baltimore: Johns Hopkins University Press.

Asad, T. (2003) *Formations of the Secular: Christianity, Islam, Modernity*. California: Stanford University Press.

Aslam, N. (2004) *Maps for Lost Lovers*. London: Faber and Faber.

Fanon, F. (2008) *Black Skin, White Masks*. Trans. Markmann, C.L. London: Pluto Press.

Goldberg, D.T. (2002) *The Racial State*. Malden: Blackwell Publishing.

Kalra, V.S. (2014) 'Punjabiyat and the Music of Nusrat Fateh Ali Khan'. *South Asian Diaspora* 6(2), 179–192.

Kundnani, A. (2007) *Racism in 21st Century Britain*. London: Pluto Press.

Kureishi, H. (1995) *The Black Album*. London: Faber and Faber.

Mahmood, S. (2011) *Politics of Piety: The Islamic Revival and the Feminist Subject*. Princeton: Princeton University Press.

Manzoor, S. (2007) *Greetings from Bury Park: Race, Religion and Rock 'n' Roll*. London: Bloomsbury.

Mondal, A. (2015) 'Representations of Young Muslims in Contemporary British South Asian Fiction'. In *Imagining Muslims in South Asia and the Diaspora: Secularism, Religion, Representations*. Ed. by Chambers, C. and Herbert, C. New York: Routledge, 30–41.

Morey, P. (2012) 'Mourning Becomes Kashmira: Islam, Melancholia and the Evacuation of Politics in Salman Rushdie's *Shalimar the Clown*'. In *Culture, Diaspora, and Modernity in Muslim Writing*. Ed. by Ahmed, R., Morey, P., and Yaqin, A. New York: Routledge, 215–230.

Nash, G. (2012) *Writing Muslim Identity*. London: Continuum.

Nelson, D. (2015) 'Hanif Kureishi: Writers Must Continue to Write about Sex to Defy Islamic Fascism'. *The Telegraph* [online]. Available from <www.telegraph.co.uk/news/worldnews/asia/india/11365844/Hanif-Kureishi-Writers-must-continue-to-write-about-sex-to-defy-Islamic-fascism.html> [18 December 2017].

Stein, M. (2004) *Black British Literature: Novels of Transformation*. Columbus: Ohio State University Press.

Upstone, S. (2010) *British Asian Fiction: Twenty-First-Century Voices*. Manchester: Manchester University Press.

Yaqin, A. (2012) 'Muslims as Multicultural Misfits in Nadeem Aslam's *Maps for Lost Lovers*'. In *Culture, Diaspora, and Modernity in Muslim Writing*. Ed. by Ahmed, R., Morey, P., and Yaqin, A. New York: Routledge, 101–116.

18
TRANSGRESSIVE DESIRE, EVERYDAY LIFE, AND THE PRODUCTION OF 'MODERNITY' IN PAKISTANI ANGLOPHONE FICTION

Mosarrap Hossain Khan

On 27 May 2014, a twenty-something Pakistani woman, Farzana, was killed outside the Lahore High Court by members of her own family, who included her father, brother, a cousin, and possibly a female relative, for falling in love with an elderly married man, Muhammad Iqbal, and marrying him. Erum Haider reported that she was killed because 'Many conservative families consider it shameful for a woman to fall in love and choose her own husband' (2014: n.p.). Haider very perceptively points out that love is something that women cannot experience in conservative societies. It is something done to them. The agency of loving is ascribed to men because women are merely 'loved'. This narrative framing of the incident renders the voice of the woman silent, as she is killed while men live to tell the tale. I start with this incident of 'honour killing'[1] because this essay will explore, through a reading of Mohsin Hamid's *Moth Smoke* (2000) and Nadeem Aslam's *Maps for Lost Lovers* (2004), the question of 'deviant' sexual desire in everyday life and the production of what I term a 'worldly subjectivity'.

The events of 9/11 have enabled the emergence of new texts and connections that may be termed 'Muslim writing' (Chambers 2011: 125). This corpus – 'Muslim writing' – represents, in general, 'the culture and civilization of Islam from within' (Malak 2005: 2), as opposed to earlier writings, especially in the context of Pakistani anglophone fiction, which focused, according to Cara Cilano, on issues of migration and diaspora (2009). In contemporary Pakistani writing, there is a corpus of novels in which romantic/illicit love takes centre stage: Hamid's *Moth Smoke*, Aslam's *Maps for Lost Lovers*, Moni Mohsin's *The End of Innocence* (2006), Musharraf Ali Farooqi's *The Story of a Widow* (2008), etc. Through a reading of *Moth Smoke* and *Maps for Lost Lovers*, this chapter will argue that individual subjects seek to defamiliarise their ordinary life, suffused with extreme religiosity, by engaging in romantic/illicit love, which becomes a site for the production of an incipient 'modern' Muslim subjectivity. According to Henri Lefebvre (2008), 'defamiliarization' denotes utopian moments of transformation, which surmount the dreary routine of everyday life. Here I argue that transgressive desire becomes utopian, transformative in the way it de-alienates the lives of individual characters in Hamid's and Aslam's novels.

Since these novels deal with the supposedly controversial themes of Muslim sexuality and violence, their popularity is thought to be a consequence of a stereotypical representation of Pakistani society. While some critics have attributed the creative vigour of Pakistani anglophone fiction after 9/11 to political turbulence at home,[2] some others (*Hindustan Times* 2010; Rehman 2014) have argued that these novels are popular in the West and in India – a major publishing site for much of this fiction – because of their handling of sensational themes of oppression, violence, terrorism, and Islamisation, all of which generate interest in Pakistani fiction by reducing a complex country to a simplistic duality. Cilano, however, offers a different perspective on the inward turn in contemporary Pakistani anglophone fiction (2009). While commenting on the marketability of fiction from Pakistan, she highlights the difficulty of selling fiction produced by indigenous Pakistani publishers (e.g. Alhamra) in the West, because this fiction does not fit the frame of expectation of international publishers, distributors, and readers.

Tension between transgressive desire and social order

Set in Lahore against the backdrop of the nuclear tests by India and Pakistan in 1998, Hamid's *Moth Smoke* sets up a tension between individual choice and social order through a depiction of the transgressive sexual desire of Darashikoh Shezad, or Daru, and Mumtaz. Hamid metafictionally comments on his own intention to write about the surface that lies beneath what realism can achieve (i.e. his writing is not about social ills that can be straightened out but about the unseemly side of Lahore). Hamid evokes the figure of Saadat Hasan Manto,[3] who also wrote about elements that many of his contemporaries in the Progressive Writers' Movement castigated. Hamid's novel employs modernist techniques of multiple narrative voices, deliberate rupturing of causal time, and the protagonists' alienation from both tradition and consumer capitalism. The novel is structured around three layers of time: historical time, which frames the novel by taking it back to the Mughal past and the brutal battle of succession between Shahjahan's two sons, Darashikoh and Aurangzeb, the latter of whom emerges victorious; film time, which frames most of the court scenes, as if Darashikoh's trial and judgement are performances and not real; and chronometric time, which undergirds Darashikoh's mundane life in the novel. While Hamid inverts the historical narrative of Shah Jahan and the Mughal Empire, the mode of representation is ironic and yet resonant of a deep similarity between the two historical moments. In an interview with the *Guardian*, Hamid claims that he considers himself to be part of the 'post-post-colonial generation' in Pakistan that has no direct knowledge of colonial rule (Khalili 2013: n.p.). Kamila Shamsie makes a similar point in an interview with Cilano (2007). The use of Mughal allegory is meant to bypass the colonial experience, which is a staple in much contemporary anglophone fiction from the subcontinent. Along with time, *Moth Smoke* experiments, in modernist vein, with multiple narrative voices which, as Paul Jay writes, 'call into question the truthfulness of all the characters' (2005: 53). The narrative of ordinary life is defamiliarised by these rupturing techniques, demonstrating the difficulty of narrating the contingency and fluidity of everyday life without deflecting it through other narrative voices and times.

Aslam's *Maps for Lost Lovers* is set in the fictional town of Dasht-e-Tanhaii ('Desert of Loneliness') in the north of England, populated by an impoverished immigrant Pakistani population from the Indian subcontinent.[4] Following the seasonal patterns in England, the novel revolves through winter, spring, summer, and autumn, the absence of monsoon, a prominent season in Pakistan, denoting loss because of exile and banishment. This sense of loss is accentuated by the murder of two lovers, Jugnu and Chanda, who are allegedly killed for defying traditional religious norms and living together. As the immigrant Muslim community copes with alienation in a host country, Shamas and Kaukab, the main protagonists in the novel, reflect on their individual losses: Kaukab's children are lost to her because they have taken up British liberal values; for Shamas, his brother, Jugnu's disappearance is a result of the rigid cultural/religious norms of the immigrant population. However, intergenerational conflict between first- and second-generation Pakistani immigrants is undercut by male characters such as Shamas and Jugnu, who transgress traditional cultural and community norms, and also by female characters such as Mah-Jabin, Kiran, and Chanda, who rebel against patriarchal norms imported from their home countries in the subcontinent. The novel weaves together multiple 'uneasy intersections of ethnicity, religion, gender and class in the margins of social space' (Moore 2009: n.p.) – these loose strands are reminiscent of the traditional *dastaan* (romance) genre in Urdu literature. As Lindsey Moore points out, the key symbols in the novel – butterflies, moths, and peacocks, foregrounding sexual transgression as in Hamid's novel – and the rejection of Islam by Shamas and Jugnu in favour of some other object of erotic devotion draw on the genres of *dastaan* and *ghazal*. Speaking of Islamic cultural influence on the novel, Aslam says: 'The book in many ways is about the classic theme of Islamic literature: the quest for the beloved. The book wouldn't be what it is without *1001 Nights*, the Koran, *Bihzad*' (O'Connor 2005: n.p.). The conflict between individual freedom and social order is encoded as one of sexual transgression between first- and second-generation British-Pakistani Muslims. As Nadia Butt writes, the strife between an orthodox, dogmatic version of Islam and modernity, undergirded by British secular values, manifests as a tension between individuals and families or community (2008: 154), leading to practices such as 'honour killing' and 'forced marriage'.

In 'Modernism and Postmodernism in African Literature', Ato Quayson (2008) writes about the historical strain that constitutes modernism in the West: a crisis of the self and the techniques of introspection, stream-of-consciousness, and a limited point of view. Since African writers constantly struggle to navigate between individualism and communal sensibility in their writing, alienation, the mainstay of modernist writing, is often viewed suspiciously in African literature. Early Indian anglophone writers, such as Mulk Raj Anand (1986) and Ahmed Ali (1984), inaugurated this moment of disjunction between social cohesion and individual alienation in their writing in a realistic mode. Since both these writers were part of the Progressive Writers' Movement, they were committed to the narrative mode of social realism, despite the modernist impetus to represent a crisis of the self under colonialism, nationalism, colonial modernity, and religious reform movements. While alienation and a crisis in knowledge of the self seem to be the focus of Hamid's and Aslam's novels, their narrative modes depict multiple worlds within a single fictional space. In Hamid's novel, Daru and Mumtaz inhabit a globalised, cosmopolitan milieu in which transgressive desire is a marker of secular and 'modern' identity, as is the case with Jugnu and Chanda in Aslam's novel. In contrast, the 'fundos' in Hamid's novel represents a traditional, non-modern, religious sensibility, as embodied by Kaukab in Aslam's novel. To recreate these differing worlds in their fiction, Hamid and Aslam draw on the indigenous traditions of *masnavi* (romance), *ghazals*, and Mughal history, narrativised through a fragmentary technique with a limited omniscient narrator.

Where, in *Moth Smoke*, the tension between individual choice and social order is foregrounded through the alienation and transgressive desire of its protagonists, Daru and Mumtaz, *Maps for Lost Lovers* depicts this tension more directly in Jugnu and Chanda's decision to live together and in Shamas' love for Suraya. Although the depiction of transgressive love in literature in general and in the novel in particular is certainly not a consequence of colonial modernity, cultural transactions during the colonial period introduced a new notion of conjugality in the fictional space.[5] Unlike many of the Sanskritic *shringara* aesthetics and the Perso-Arabic aesthetics of *ishq* and *muhabbat*, lovers in modern literature can consummate their love in the fictional space. And the new ethic of romantic love is intimately connected with the new aesthetic mode of realism, where the idea of conjugality is imported from Victorian novels.[6] Citing the example of Chandu Menon's Malayalam novel, *Indulekha* (1889), which narrativises romantic love premised on individual choices and aspirations, Meenakshi Mukherjee (1985) writes that the challenge for Indian novelists in the late nineteenth century was to make the action more exciting in a setting where there was no notion of individualism. Mukherjee further argues that in the late nineteenth century, rigid social norms in India made only two kinds of romantic love fictionally depictable – illicit love for a widow or a courtesan – because 'these two categories of women were without legal "proprietors" and thus seemed to embody a certain amount of unharnessed sexual energy' (1985: 70). However, love of this kind was doomed from the very beginning, because these women were outside of structured society. In Pakistani anglophone novels, this tension between transgressive desire and preservation of the social order becomes a persistent trope, much like what Mukherjee (1985) explores in Bankimchandra Chatterjee's novels or Sudipta Kaviraj (2006) finds in Rabindranath Tagore's writing. In Hamid's *Moth Smoke* and Aslam's *Maps for Lost Lovers*, illicit love and the transgression of social conventions form the pegs on which hang the plots of the novels, finally leading to censure and punishment for preservation of the social order. In the banality and boredom of everyday life, illicit love functions as an ideal or as a means of defamiliarising routine, ordinary life, thereby making everyday life and romantic ideals appear to be at odds with each other.

Transgressive desire and the defamiliarisation of everyday life

In rigid, formalised everyday life in *Moth Smoke*, Daru and Mumtaz's illicit sex and drug use become residues of transgressive desire beneath the surface of the ordinary. In *The Psychopathology of Everyday Life* (2002), Sigmund Freud analyses such disorderliness beneath the supposed routine order and structure of everyday life, which he terms 'parapraxes': for example, forgetting proper names, foreign words, and certain childhood memories. The stable structure of orderliness is vulnerable to our unconscious ('id') desires and fears, as in the case of hysteria, where the normal is suspended. Freud's notion of 'parapraxes' is located in the everyday traces of a temporality other than the one we see in everyday life, and this notion of simultaneous temporality enables resistance and a creative circumventing of the immutable temporality of religious tradition. Besides Daru and Mumtaz, there are other instances of transgressive, residual desire in the novel: Mumtaz shows Daru a newspaper report about a young missing girl whose family is suspected of having killed her because she had a lover (Hamid 2000: 14). This instance already demonstrates how everyday life is highly regulated and how transgressive desire is particularly disciplined and policed in the name of family honour. Paradoxically, there are places like Heera Mandi (the 'Diamond Market'), Lahore's infamous pleasure district where men satisfy their transgressive sexual desires. One way to understand the existence of such a place is to see it as a space of fluid, subversive desire that existed before such illicit sexual practices were critiqued and disciplined by the colonial regime and the religious reform movements, both of which discouraged decadent Indian sexuality and encouraged conjugal love (Kaviraj 2006; Minault 1998) towards the second half of the nineteenth century. In the case of Pakistan, this fluid notion of sexuality was further regulated after Zia-ul-Haq rose to power in 1978 and declared Pakistan an Islamic state. Another way to understand the presence of Heera Mandi is to see it as a space of masculine transgressive desire, similar to the *kotha*s (residences of courtesans) in nineteenth-century North India, which were frequented by men.

Despite the covert acceptance of subversive desire, religion and its attendant traditions – equated, for the most part, with growing religious fundamentalism – loom menacingly as a spectre that regulates, controls, and polices everyday life in *Moth Smoke*. Since the everyday is strictly regimented by tradition and religion, transgressive sexual encounters become one of the sites for defamiliarising everyday life. There are multiple layers of desire in the novel: those of the lower classes at Heera Mandi and those of the educated upper and middle classes, who engage in covert affairs. Mumtaz confesses that covert sexual relations are 'the most popular form of entertainment around. And I know why. My affair with Daru was, at first at least, the most liberating experience I have ever had. I felt bad, of course. Selfish. But I also felt good' (Hamid 2000: 158). Despite class differences, subversive desire seems to seep into every stratum of society and rupture the rhythm of daily life. Daru and Mumtaz's transgressive sexual liaison is framed through two conventions: the violent and unconsummated love between lovers and the passive, selfless love of the lover for the beloved. The first kind, violent, unconsummated love, is typified in a nuclear explosion, which is metaphorically described as a sexual act with 'a huge gasp, smothered unsatisfied' (Hamid 2000: 100), making it appear almost prosaic. In contrast, the trope of passive, selfless love, embodied in the moths visiting Daru's house, is drawn from the conventions of *ghazal*:

> But she keeps coming, like a moth to my candle, staying longer than she should, leaving for dinners and birthday parties, singeing her wings [...] And I, the moth circling her candle, realize that she's not just a candle. She's a moth as well, circling me. I look at her and see myself reflected, my feelings, my desires. And she, looking at me, must see herself. And which of us is moth and which is candle hardly seems to matter. We're both the same.
>
> (Hamid 2000: 204)

In Hamid's aesthetic, the moth's attraction to the candle is equated with the attraction of a lover to their beloved, following the traditions of Sufi poetry,[7] in which love for God is couched as love for one's Beloved. In Hamid's reworking of the trope, lover and beloved become interchangeable in a selfless union, foregrounding utopic transformative possibilities in everyday life.

In Aslam's *Maps for Lost Lovers*, the rigid tradition-bound everyday life in which laws and codes have been dragged into England from Pakistan like shit on shoes (2004: 163) is defamiliarised through the tragic transgressive love of Shamas for Suraya, of Jugnu and Chanda, of the murdered Muslim girl for her Hindu lover. In each of these cases, transgressive love is gendered in the way men have access to spaces such as Heera Mandi in Lahore and the white prostitute at Dasht, while women are punished, as in the cases of the unnamed girls in both novels. In this context, Kaukab's stream-of-consciousness on the Islamic idea of love, as one felt for all creatures within the laws of permissibility, foregrounds the asymmetrical nature of power inherent in transgression:

> Love. Islam said that in order not to be unworthy of being, only one thing was required: love. And, said the True Faith, it did not even begin with humans and animals: even the trees were in love. The very stones sang of love. Allah Himself was a being in love with His own creations.
>
> (Aslam 2004: 91)

This notion of a higher love is reiterated during Nusrat Fateh Ali Khan's concert at Dasht, when 'he points to the sky with his index finger to indicate and include Allah in the love being felt and celebrated – a lover looking for the beloved represents the human soul looking for salvation' (2004: 270). While incompatible with her more stringent faith, Kaukab reflects on the pervasiveness of love in people's lives, more particularly in the context of people in Dasht, who might have loved someone or other at some point in their lives. And, yet, for Kaukab, the idea of transgression can only go so far, because she finds sublimation in prayers, in her unflinching faith in Allah.

Like Heera Mandi in Hamid's novel, Dasht does have a space for the fulfilment of transgressive male sexual desire: the house of the white prostitute whose presence falls outside the permissible boundaries of purity and honour: 'had she been Indian or Pakistani, she would have been assaulted and driven out of the area within days of moving in for bringing shame upon her people' (2004: 14). Aslam refers to Heera Mandi (the 'Diamond Market') in Lahore as a transgressive space of sexual awakening for Shamas:

> An unmarried young man's sexual life, in those days and in a segregated country like Pakistan, began late, and so they were also years of his sexual initiation, exploration, and gratification – in the 'Diamond Market' district of prostitutes in Lahore.
>
> (Aslam 2004: 113)

Shamas' initial foray into transgressive sexuality in Dasht is limited to his desire to visit the white prostitute, thereby replicating his sexual initiation in Heera Mandi. This traversing of borders between Pakistan and England is symptomatic of Aslam's attempt to illustrate how transgressive desire defamiliarises everyday life transnationally across cultures. And yet, as already mentioned in the previous paragraph, the transformative possibilities of transgressive love are gendered, rendering invisible even those women who participate in the sex trade at Heera Mandi.

Shamas' love for Suraya and their secret rendezvous at the bookshop are undergirded by two different sets of motives, both worldly. For Shamas, his love for Suraya is a way of defamiliarising the ossified ordinary, as is evident when he meets her for the first time: 'Like a matchstick struck on the inside of his skull, spilling sparks, the ecstatic torpor of adolescent summers comes to him in a brief warm illumination, and he experiences a thrill which is very close to happiness' (Aslam 2004: 195). He searches for a love that will regenerate him, releasing from his atrophied everyday life with the help of Suraya's 'youth, the life in her […] her living breath on his face' (2004: 278). For Suraya, transgressive love is tempered by the mundane consideration of finding a temporary husband who will help her reunite with her husband in Pakistan, who divorced her in a drunken state. Despite staying close to the Islamic ideal of marriage, she falls in love with Shamas, his poetry, and his gentleness:

> Suraya has started to pay attention to her physical appearance. And, yes, it must be admitted that there are times when she enjoys his compliments concerning her beauty, a sense of well-being spreading over for a while, before she is reminded of her adversity, of her husband, her son, her Allah.
>
> (2004: 301)

Her practical necessities make Suraya negotiate 'the dinful strife of faith and disbelief' (2004: 279), knowing full well that sex outside marriage is one of the greatest sins in Islam. In Jugnu and Chanda's case, their live-in relationship works as a motif of life in the midst of death that surrounds them in Dasht. Jugnu's love for butterflies is in consonance with the reputation of his family, who did not wish 'to be bound by any tradition and custom' (2004: 514). His house is a museum of dead objects: 'pinned butterflies in glass frames' (2004: 513). When Chanda comes to his house for the first time to deliver food for the butterflies, she accidentally rouses the Bhutan glories, which he had put into ice-induced sleep. Jugnu and Chanda's transgressive love metaphorically defamiliarises their tradition-bound oppressive everyday life, rousing them from a 'somnolent state' (2004: 515). Aslam's deployment of the myth of Krishna and his companions' love for their beloveds on opposite shores of the Jamuna River illustrates how the fulfilment of transgressive desire circumvents 'the disapproving world' (2004: 516), the reified mundane life in a rigid tradition-bound society.

At the end of *Moth Smoke*, the prosecution argues that the illicit sexual relation between Mumtaz and Daru is a breach of the sacred institution of marriage and the court judgement upholds the sanctity of tradition, endorsed through everyday norms, by punishing transgressive desire that ruptures this norm. In *Maps for Lost Lovers*, too, transgressive love is punished and Shamas, Jugnu, Chanda, and the unnamed Muslim girl pay with their lives. The mundane social order is restored at the end by returning to the community of fellow humans, as the illegal immigrant ponders: 'at dawn today he had told himself to go out into the world again. If calamity is coming then where else would he rather be than with his fellow humans? What else is there but them?' (Aslam 2004: 525). In the Indian context, Mukherjee (1985) claims that the representation of such illicit sexual relations in fiction is doomed from the very beginning, because it is at variance with the traditional social reality, which demands that the social order be upheld at the end. While *Moth Smoke* and *Maps for Lost Lovers* depart from the conventions of realism – in their choices of subject matter, which are more suited to the conventions of naturalism, and a narrative technique which closely resembles that of modernist fiction – the protagonists in Hamid's and Aslam's novels fail to disrupt the ossified tradition, despite their momentary defamiliarisation of norm-bound everyday practices, reiterating the conventions of *masnavi* romances, which set up a contest between individual love and obligation towards traditional norms of honour.[8]

In Hamid's *Moth Smoke* and Aslam's *Maps for Lost Lovers*, Mumtaz, Daru, Shamas, Suraya, Jugnu, and Chanda transgress moral codes engendered by traditional religious values. While transgressive desire in these novels encapsulates transformative possibilities in the form of defamiliarisation of the ordinary, such transgressions contain within them despair at non-fulfilment, as enunciated in the death or punishment of those who transgress. And yet, Hamid's and Aslam's fictional aesthetics produce a contingent Muslim modernity, despite the gendered nature of transgressions in which women are rendered invisible and punished. The motivations for transgression and engagement with the 'worldly' come from encounters with consumer capitalism, Western secular values, new consumption patterns and lifestyles.[9] Pakistani anglophone writers, however, seem to encounter a challenge because social ethics and literary aesthetics are in conflict here. Recent religious resurgence, which reinforces and reinvents tradition in Pakistani society, makes difficult the emergence of an individual self, that is able to determine her own course of action, independent of the social structure (Iqtidar 2011). In other words, the project of self-fashioning through transgressive love in Pakistani fiction is almost doomed from the very beginning because writers' aesthetic inclinations and social ethics clash.

Notes

1 This chapter does not engage directly with the question of 'honour killing', a violent act most often perpetrated against women in many conservative societies, including Pakistan, for defiling the honour of the family/community through romantic and sexual acts outside marriage. Amir Jafri (2008) contends that 'honour killing' is at once a male performative act demarcating social boundaries and a public

spectacle. Aroosa Kanwal (2015) asserts that 'honour killing' is actually a pre-Islamic, tribal act which has been maintained, incorporated into practices in Islamic countries. In this chapter, I engage with acts of transgressive desire in everyday life, instead of exploring the place of 'honour killing' in Pakistani society.
2 See William Dalrymple's 'Moonlight's Children: Pakistani fiction, long eclipsed by India's, is now emerging from the shadows' (2008), an assessment of Pakistani anglophone fiction which he later followed up in his review of Daniyal Mueenuddin's short story collection *Other Rooms* in the *Financial Times* (2009).
3 Hamid talks about Manto's influence on his writing in an interview with the Duke University newspaper, *The Chronicle*, 18 February 2000.
4 While Aslam's novel engages with British multicultural discourse, it does so by rendering White England absent from the novel and focusing its attention on the micro violence within the Pakistani immigrant community. See O'Connor (2005).
5 However, romantic love in European fiction, including British fiction, which Indians were reading in the nineteenth and twentieth centuries, was never without a conflict between romance and social realities. What Indians inherited was a fantasy of romantic love and conjugality from such fiction because of the impossibility of romantic fulfilment in a tradition-bound Indian society.
6 The idea of romantic love travelled to India from the West as a fantasy, which in European fiction was more a conflictual desire in which the protagonists, especially women, often followed the head rather than the heart. Yet this idea of companionate marriage and love exerted tremendous influence on Indian fiction writers.
7 See, 'Mohsin Hamid', *The Chronicle*, 18 February 2000, in which Hamid elaborates on the influence of Sufi poetry in his novel.
8 In this context, it is apt to remember that the Urdu fiction serialised in Pakistan in the 1970s, which had a predominantly female readership, presents another aesthetic model where rebellious and independent women creatively negotiate with tradition, and often dealt with taboo topics, such as gay sex, illicit desire, etc. As Adam B. Ellick (2010) writes, such risqué writing was extremely popular in the 1970s but banned in the 1980s under Zia-ul-Haq's regime.
9 For recent studies on the impact of consumer culture on Muslims, especially youth, see, Hossein Godazgar (2011) and Mona Abaza (2001).

Bibliography

Abaza, M. (2001) 'Shopping Malls, Consumer Culture, and the Reshaping of Public Space in Egypt'. *Theory, Culture, and Society* 18(5), 97–122.
Ali, A. (1984) *Twilight in Delhi*. Karachi: Oxford University Press.
Anand, M.R. (1986) *Untouchables*. New York: Penguin.
Aslam, N. (2004) *Maps for Lost Lovers*. New Delhi: Random House.
Butt, N. (2008) 'Between Orthodoxy and Modernity: Mapping the Transcultural Predicaments of Pakistani Immigrants in Multi-Ethnic Britain in Nadeem Aslam's *Maps for Lost Lovers* (2004)'. In *Multi-Ethnic Britain 2000+: New Perspectives in Literature, Film and the Arts*. Ed. by Eckstein, L. et al. New York: Rodopi, 153–169.
Chambers, C. (2011) 'A Comparative Approach to Pakistani Fiction in English'. *Journal of Postcolonial Writing* 47(2), 122–134.
Cilano, C. (2007) '"In a World of Consequences": An Interview with Kamila Shamsie'. *Kunapipi: Journal of Postcolonial Writing and Culture* 39(1), 150–162.
Cilano, C. (2009) '"Writing from Extreme Edges": Pakistani English-Language Fiction'. *ARIEL: A Review of International English Literature* 40(2–3), 183–201.
Dalrymple, W. (2008) 'Moonlight's Children: Pakistani Fiction, Long Eclipsed by India's, is Now Emerging from the Shadows'. *Financial Times* [online]. Available from <www.ft.com/content/76a9c204-9662-11dd-9dce-000077b07658> [20 October 2017].
Dalrymple, W. (2009) 'In Other Rooms, Other Wonders'. *Financial Times* [online]. Available from <www.ft.com/content/8f26a696-09dd-11de-add8-0000779fd2ac> [20 October 2017].
Ellick, A.B. (2010) 'Risqué Writing in Pakistan'. *New York Times* [online]. Available from <https://atwar.blogs.nytimes.com/2010/11/24/risque-writing-in-pakistan/> [20 October 2017].
Farooqi, M.A. (2009) *The Story of a Widow*. New Delhi: Picador.
Freud, S. (1901) *The Psychopathology of Everyday Life*. New York: Penguin Books.

Godazgar, H. (2011) 'Islam in the Globalized World: Consumerism and Environmental Ethics'. In *Religion, Consumerism and Sustainability: Paradise Lost?* Ed. by Lyn, T. New York: Palgrave Macmillan, 115–136.

Haider, E. (2014) 'The Love Affairs of Muhammad Iqbal'. *Tanqeed* [online]. Available from <www.tanqeed.org/2014/06/the-love-affairs-of-muhammad-iqbal/> [21 October 2017].

Hamid, M. (2000) *Moth Smoke*. New York: Picador.

Hindustan Times. (2010) 'New Genre of Pakistani Fiction a Hit in India' [online]. Available from <www.hindustantimes.com/delhi/new-genre-of-pakistani-fiction-a-hit-in-india/story-YT9yZ3rrCtRTaVybvwh8PL.html> [21 October 2017].

Iqtidar, H. (2011) *Secularizing Islamists? Jama'at-e-Islami and Jama'at-ud-Da'wa in Urban Pakistan*. Chicago: The University of Chicago Press.

Jafri, A.H. (2008) *Honour Killing: Dilemma, Ritual, Understanding*. Oxford: Oxford University Press.

Jay, P. (2005) 'The Post-Post Colonial Condition: Globalization and Historical Allegory in Mohsin Hamid's *Moth Smoke*'. *Ariel: A Review of International English Literature* 36(1–2), 51–71.

Kanwal, A. (2015) *Rethinking Identities in Contemporary Pakistani Fiction: Beyond 9/11*. New York: Palgrave Macmillan.

Kaviraj, S. (2006) 'Tagore and Transformations in the Ideals of Love'. In *Love in South Asia: A Cultural History*. Ed. by Orsini, F. Cambridge: Cambridge University Press, 161–182.

Khalili, H. (2013) 'Hamid Mohsin: Pakistan and India are Incredibly Similar'. *Guardian* [online]. Available from www.theguardian.com/books/2013/mar/26/mohsin-hamid-pakistan-india-similar [20 October 2017].

Lefebvre, H. (2008) *Critique of Everyday Life, Vol. 1*. Trans. by Moore, J. London: Verso.

Mahmood, S. (2005) *Politics of Piety: Islamic Revival and the Feminist Subject*. Princeton: Princeton University Press.

Malak, A. (2005) *Muslim Narratives and the Discourse of English*. Albany: SUNY University Press.

Minault, G. (1998) *Secluded Scholars: Women's Education and Muslim Social Reform in Colonial India*. Delhi: Oxford University Press.

Mohsin, M. (2006) *The End of Innocence*. London: Penguin Books.

Moore, L. (2009) 'British Muslim Identities and Spectres of Terror in Nadeem Aslam's *Maps for Lost Lovers*'. *Postcolonial Text* 5(2) [online]. Available from <http://postcolonial.org/index.php/pct/article/view/1017/946> [30 January 2018].

Mukherjee, M. (1985) *Realism and Reality: The Novel and Society in India*. Delhi: Oxford University Press.

O'Connor, M. (2005) 'Writing against Terror – Nadeem Aslam'. *Three Monkeys* [online]. Available from <www.threemonkeysonline.com/writing-against-terror-nadeem-aslam/> [20 October 2017].

Quayson, A. (2008) 'Modernism and Postmodernism in African Literature'. In *The Cambridge History of African and Caribbean Literature, Vol. 2*. Ed. by Irele, F.A. and Gikandi, S. Cambridge: Cambridge University Press, 824–852.

Rehman, S. (2014) 'Pakistani Authors Find a Market in India'. *The Diplomat* [online]. Available from <http://thediplomat.com/2014/07/pakistani-authors-find-a-market-in-india/> [20 October 2017].

PART V

Spaces of female subjectivity
Identity, difference, agency

19
AGENCY, GENDER, NATIONALISM, AND THE ROMANTIC IMAGINARY IN PAKISTAN

Abu-Bakar Ali

This chapter will explore Qaisra Shahraz's novel *The Holy Woman* (2001), which, beside selected material from author-activist Fahmida Riaz and a consideration of contemporary anglophone writers Shaila Abdullah and Kamila Shamsie, will form the basis for an engagement with the romance genre in the writing of Pakistani women. The development of mass media in the nascent Pakistani nation is characterised by the emergence of one particular generic form that continues to be, by far, the most popular. The romance narrative, whether in its classic or family guise, dominates Pakistani television in epic, panoramic dramas and is, more significantly, voraciously consumed when it appears in its most ubiquitous literary form, serialised in newspapers and magazines targeted at women.[1] *The Holy Woman* retrospectively reimagines the period against which the burgeoning popularity of the romance will be contextualised; a period in which Riaz also makes political inscriptions. The copious pseudo-novels which were serialised during the especially significant Zia period were published in Urdu and, given Pakistan's fragile archival resources, are notoriously difficult to obtain. Writers such as Shahraz, Shamsie, and Abdullah refashion the genre with sufficient nostalgia, referentiality, and, in the case of Riaz, epistemological and political consciousness, to shine a light on the way the relationship between 'national culture', feminism, and romance literature can be read against the wider backdrop of Pakistan's fractious history. There are several interesting issues to consider here. Rather than focus on whether agency is ever possible in the discourses of Pakistani romance novels, it is more fruitful to look at why the recurring tropes of the popular romance genre, which appear in Shahraz's work and in the diasporic fiction of Abdullah and Shamsie, are as widely successful as they have been.

It may appear peculiar to employ the generic discourse of romance literature as a repository in feminist debates on nationalism and the effect of nationalist ideologies on gendered expressions of sexuality, class, and (most significantly) agency, in a Pakistani context. Romance narratives do seem to have something of an image problem in this sense. As Janice Radaway explains in her seminal study on romance literature, 'Elaborate female fantasies' notwithstanding, readers are 'in effect, instructed about the nature of patriarchy and its meanings for them as women' (1991: 149). Ominously, the ideologies that pervade the text's easily identifiable generic conventions 'evoke the material consequences of refusal to mould oneself in the image of femininity prescribed by the culture but also displays the remarkable benefits of conformity' (Radaway 1991: 149). And, presumably, these 'benefits' can be found in the pleasures that accrue from reading such a text and sharing in the 'female fantasy' where 'the heroine is gathered into the arms of the hero' (Radaway 1991: 149). These pleasures thus paradoxically bring the female reader back into the patriarchal fold, expressing her hopes and dreams, her agency, through the very ideological framework that would curtail such aspirations. Needless to say, the kind of readership relevant to this chapter has a very different history and epistemology to the bored, suburban white middle-class housewife of middle America. Very little research has been conducted on the way popular romance is played out across both literary and theoretical postcolonial discourses, let alone a further consideration of postcolonial feminisms. The question is not one of cultural relativity, but how representations of feminist agency within Pakistani romance texts provide continuity with the country's past, a past nationalist in hue, tainted by the violence inflicted on scores of women.

The narrative of romance appears to pan out in the following way: a strong-willed and assertive woman vows that she can exist without (heterosexual) love; she meets an equally stubborn man who apparently does not know how to love; he exhibits crude, even violent behaviour towards the heroine and, as they both struggle with various obstacles that include their own insecurities, the hero realises that said heroine is the one he 'loves', climaxing in her being 'gathered' into his now more than welcome embrace (Chaney 1979). As far as agency is concerned, it is a case of 'now you see it, now you don't'. The text performs its own Foucauldian manoeuvre, producing ideological opposition to its patriarchal discourse in the form of a vaguely feminist heroine, and then consuming the subversion it has created in those all-enveloping 'arms'. 'Love' is expressed in that familiar discourse of 'chivalry', a representational device that effaces the female epistemology once again. Agency becomes a kind of strained, lost fantasy, effaced between violence and 'protection'. In 1984, Janice Radaway published her theoretical observations in a groundbreaking ethnographic research project she had undertaken. Basing herself in the small but affluent city of Smithton, North Carolina, Radaway meticulously recorded the reading habits and practices of a group of women who were self-confessed romance novel aficionados. She discusses their preferences for the types of romance, genre characteristics that they like or dislike, and probes their responses, attempting to situate these, and the novels themselves, in a theoretical and ideological context. There are the obvious questions of how relevant a framework exploring Western romances and their effect on a small selection of women in the mid-West is to this task. As Radaway emphasises, the narrative trajectory of the type of texts the Smithton women consume is ideologically reflective of their interpellation. They accede to the politics at play but only because they recognise 'the remarkable benefits of' this 'conformity' (1991: 149). The perks of middle-class suburbia may not be the same as those available to the working-class Pakistani women who read romances, or even to those from the higher classes.

Romance at the limits: the strained interventions of Fahmida Raiz

The immediate task here is to interrogate exactly what sort of intervention romance literature represents in this young country's gendered history. Hence it is interesting to explore the position of romance tropes in the work of a prominent author and poet whose most influential pieces were produced within the very historical moment with which this chapter is concerned. The notorious period of General Zia's martial rule in Pakistan, swiftly followed after his death by democratic elections and the appointment of the country's first woman prime minister, saw an exponential rise in the amount of popular romances being consumed and written on the

Pakistani literary scene. The poems, political essays, and short stories of Riaz provide a unique counterpoint to the popular generic discourse of her time, as well as a lens through which Pakistani romance fiction's own intervention can be read both historically and in feminist terms. In the foreword to *Four Walls and Black Veils* (2005), Aamer Hussein describes the author and her literature in the following terms:

> From the outset she refused to be typecast as a woman poet and conform to what are generally regarded as the confines of 'proper' literary and creative traditions of feminine poetry […] she broke out of the inhibitions imposed on her gender.
>
> (Riaz 2005a: 6)

Her writings were oppositional in every sense of the word. Riaz's politically charged repudiations of 'the inhibitions imposed on her gender' (2005a: 6) were not simply to be found in the political unconscious of allegorical fictions, they were dangerously critical of state and society. She was not only a poet and a writer but an activist, and the regime of the period in which she developed a political consciousness provided a target against which her intellectual sensibilities could be directed.

Initially, Riaz was influenced by her exposure to the Marxist political scene in London during the rise of Thatcherism in the late '70s. She became part of a growing middle-class intelligentsia who were mobilised by Zia's plans to hang the democratically elected Prime Minister Zulfikhar Ali Bhutto and seize power. This was a watershed in Riaz's life. She and her husband were imprisoned for inciting civil unrest and anarchy. Riaz was bailed by an admirer of her work and then chose to go into exile to India, under threat of house arrest. From the relative safety of her adopted home, her awareness as a feminist took shape, undoubtedly as a direct result of the stories of injustice and violence against women that were reaching her from across the border (Rahman 1991). General Zia had engaged familiar ideological tropes in a politics that associated all that was pure, and also by association impure in the parlous Pakistani state, with the symbolic and real female body.

Riaz's annexation of class and gender concerns raises some interesting complexities in her work. These are apparent in the short story 'Some Misaddressed Letters', written in exile. It narrates a story of displacement similar to her own, in which Amina, a female activist, and Murad, her male colleague, are sent to India but return to a politically chaotic and unstable Pakistan (Riaz 2005b). As Amina works through her memories, she finds that as a woman representing working-class causes she is the site of a curious double colonisation:

> Amina was beginning to feel exhausted. She looked at the room, the flowers, the photograph of the Founding Father on the wall. She knew how he felt, knew that despite his affected mannerisms, he was really feeling sick at heart. […] He was not frightened like Amina.
>
> (Riaz 2005b: 98)

The site of this epiphany is the 'host country' of India, where Amina finds herself intellectually neutered, her offerings dismissed by the male intelligentsia as 'sincere attempts' (Riaz 2005b: 99). The author's gender here has problematised any routes to agency she may have attempted to fashion through a working-class position. But it is what happens next in the narrative that is most interesting from the perspective of romance conventions. Amina tackles the irreconcilability she is confronted with by nostalgically conjuring up an Indian man who could have been her lover, the subject of 'misaddressed letters' that she had composed and sent some years ago: 'her love for this young man was like the legendry flame in the faraway place on which the washerman fixed his gaze' (Riaz 2005b: 97). And at this point the romance threatens to become a parody of itself, as this man emerges in a similar memory of Murad, in the form of the husband of a peasant woman he is about to make love to. Riaz employs romance conventions cleverly to traverse a multitude of points in Pakistani history where class and gender are far from frameworks that share common political ground. Feminist concerns and agency are produced as silence at each of these sites.

The period of the late 1970s to the cusp of the '80s provides the backdrop for this silencing and has been commonly historicised as one of the darker periods in Pakistan's already bloody history, shaped by ideologically marked discourses of gender. In 1977, General Zia-ul-Haq seized power from the democratically elected incumbent, Zulfikar Ali Bhutto, in a bloodless military coup. The subsequent recriminations were unprecedented and saw a change in the cultural, social, and political terrains, as Sadia Toor articulates so well (2011: 161). After sanctioning the hanging of his political rival, Zia turned his attention to what was to be the bedrock of his political *modus operandi*: the reconstruction of the country's national identity. Ostensibly, the way the country's women were marginalised in such a refashioning does not appear surprising and simply seems to be a continuation of a common theme in nationalist politics: 'Zia attempted to secure his power through the propagation of an explicitly misogynist ideology and by proclaiming a mission to revitalise society by correcting the immorality of women' (Toor 2011: 160). Zia's state assumed the role of 'correcting' mechanism and this is where Islam entered the equation. Zia required a framework through which his discourse could unquestionably be essentialised and there was none better than the *raison d'être* of Pakistan itself. For Zia, the cleansing process had to begin in an area which Bhutto had dangerously neglected. The binaries for the establishment of this ideology changed subtly. National identity was mediated not against the 'morally bankrupt' West, but the Pakistani woman.

In her novel *An American Brat* (1993), Bapsi Sidhwa reflects on the zeitgeist of the Zia years in typically incisive yet emotive fashion. The impact of the Hudood ordinances on the gendered landscape of the Pakistani woman is expressed through an extended metaphor:

> The new mischief in their midst had sneaked up on them unawares and surprised them one day when they read about the Famida and Allah Baksh case. The couple, who had eloped to get married, had been accused of committing adultery, or *zina*, by the girl's father. They were sentenced to death by stoning.
>
> (Sidhwa 1993: 246)

Zia's refashioning of the state's role in the private and public spaces may well have been Machiavellian, with the newly configured nationalist ideology acting as the moral regulator of bodies and minds. But his 'mischief' also carried a painful sting, with the threat of violence often culminating in the *deux ex machina* which the new, male-centric national character of Pakistan dictated.[2]

It appears tempting, in light of the historical discourse concerning the period, to view the Zia era as a grim corollary of the country's dark past, in terms of the way the question of gender has been negotiated violently by its successive nationalisms. However, from the late '70s onwards, in the lead up to the General's coup d'état and his subsequent changes to the constitution within the *Chaadar aur Char Diwari* framework of Islamisation, Pakistan certainly experienced its most substantial and significant period of feminist intervention and activism.[3] These contributions played an equally pertinent role in shaping what was fast becoming a gendered nationalist consciousness. The violence that characterised the Zia years and the many victims it claimed still reverberate powerfully when the past is revisited. But alongside this legacy of pain stands a compelling narrative of resistance, which tends to be sidelined if not subsumed by the totemic image of the Pakistani woman as historic victim ever since the country's fractious inception.

Postmodernity and the (trans)national Pakistani romance

Whilst the fiction of Shahraz makes subversive interventions from within the limits of the patriarchal discursive framework which underpins the romantic imaginary, her anglophone contemporaries have predictably realigned their focus. Both Shamsie and Abdullah concentrate on the politics and poetics of a postcoloniality which is expressed through the pleasures and pain of diasporic migration and displacement. Of course, the transnational turn is not unique in the tenuous canon of 'Pakistani' literature. What primarily interests me in this instance is the way these authors make their diasporic inscriptions within the conventions of a genre that can still be identified as belonging to the romance tradition. The Pakistani romantic imaginary therefore becomes an intertext which can be reconfigured and reshaped in a dissonant migratory space. The discourse of romance is destabilised and refashioned from within the limits of diasporic movement, a movement which shapes a potential feminist agency.

As a practitioner of this genre, Abdullah's most intriguing work is *Beyond the Cayenne Wall* (2005), which is a collection of short stories focusing around the twin spaces of the 'Home' and 'World'. 'Crimson Calling' is an example of one of these narratives, which employs the romance trope at the same time as it seeks to reimagine it through the postmodern identity politics of diaspora. The binaries are familiar here as the story concerns Minnah, a woman who has returned to the 'constricted' city of Karachi from 'the biggest University in Texas', where 'she felt she had it all' (2005: 32). The regenerative migratory spaces have been curtailed for Minnah, however, by the end of an affair which she was involved in with her University professor, who failed to disclose that he had a young family. It is in the return to Karachi that the trope of romance is most apparent. As she 'gazed into the eyes of her husband of only a few minutes and smiled' (2005: 43), the play of ambivalence underpins the ostensible mimesis of romance in the homeland. Minnah is either wholly invested in this or, perhaps more plausibly, she retains hope of reconfiguring the patriarchal landscape with the shifting, fluid transnational expression of identity that is the corollary of her migration to the 'World' of America. The real epistemological crisis lies at the border of these inscriptions, however, as Minnah explores the idea of revealing her affair to her new husband. This may be a manoeuvre that is full of wishful thinking, at best, emphasising a reductive outlook in which the conservative space of 'Home' is transformed and 'liberated' by the diasporic migrant returning. Moreover, Abdullah is perhaps also aware of the corporeal risk that such an intervention necessarily involves, again highlighting the spectre of violence and erasure.

The romance trope therefore appears at the site of a curious double bind in Abdullah's story, which telegraphs an alternative gendered historiography; a historiography underpinned by the enabling narrative of transnational movement. As Meenah returns home, her 'love' is both 'fluid-like and fragile' (2005: 43); her 'Ma had no idea how independent her little daughter had become' (2005: 42). She exhibits this confidence by taking a romance discourse at whose limits she had strained as a diasporic woman, and superimposing it textually onto its diametric opposite – the arranged marriage. It is an unsettling hybridity which raises questions about the many Pakistani women who cannot refashion patriarchy. In the end, the spectres of cultural memory threaten to destabilise Minnah's romantic imaginary.

There is therefore a caveat to such an attenuated postmodern postcoloniality and it is conspicuous in Shamsie's novel *Kartography* (2002). The main thematic and contextual dialogue

Shamsie employs to mediate both the romance narrative and the wider politics of her novel lies in the conflicting, oppositional views of the two lovers, Raheen and Karim, on maps and mapping, specifically the cartography of Karachi. Raheen's perspective is evident in the opening pages of the text:

> The globe spins. Mountain ranges skim my fingers; there is static above the Arabian Sea. Pakistan is split in two, but undivided. This world is out of date. [...] I close my eyes, and wrap my fingers around a diamond-shaped bone. I still hear the world spinning. I spin with it, spin into a garden. At dusk. And yes, those are shoulder pads stitched into my shirt.
>
> (Shamsie 2002: 1)

There is more at stake in this cartographical project than the metaphorical, in terms of the romance conventions that evidently underpin the text. The valorisation of Raheen's alternative, romanticised landscape is unsettling. It must be remembered that her fluid and flexible conception of Karachi's spatial markings, where movement is entirely predicated on the liberal scope of imagination and memory, also produces an essentialist map of its own. The very real violence and 'crisis' that shape the trauma etched in Karachi's cultural memory and landscape, are eschewed by Raheen's desire to map space in a certain way. These particular postcolonial sensibilities are rooted in a diasporic migration away from, and the subsequent return to, the postcolonial homeland. Raheen's and Karim's migratory experiences represent the seamless movement through transnational space of the diasporic subject who is clearly comfortable in their own globalised skin. The inscriptions which Shamsie's characters make eschew other dissenting identities from their ostensibly apolitical framework. And, significantly, it is only the diasporic *flâneur* – from a specific class and enlightened by their journey across specific transnational flows – who has the privilege to make such fluid markings on their refashioned map of Karachi.

'She has discovered a new lease of life': cultural memory, contingency, and the play of imagination in the romance of Qaisra Shahraz

The geopolitical position of Shahraz perhaps mirrors those contemporary postcolonial voices purporting to vocalise the concerns of the country from which they have been exiled, either by birth or circumstance. Yet her work does not possess a Rushdie-esque postmodern expression of postcoloniality, nor does it establish continuity with the diasporic traditions of her immediate contemporaries such as Shamsie or Abdullah. *The Holy Woman* undoubtedly makes references to, and effectively is, a romance novel in many of the ways Radaway identifies. The copies of the novel being circulated in Pakistan are not imported either, so that with an altogether different readership and a unique nationalist and historical backdrop against which feminist interventions have been played out, it appears significant to question whether a more nuanced approach to reading the Pakistani romance is required. In terms of locating Shahraz's work against Abudullah's and especially Shamsie's, the important question is how the liminal, female Pakistani voice is mapped and imagined. In this sense, Shahraz does not situate agency through performative politics that have been appropriated by diasporic postcoloniality. Her representation of performativity emerges from a mimesis of the romance genre that necessarily collapses under the weight of its contingencies, the most glaring of which is the erasure of the female body. Agency, therefore, is always fashioned with a recognition of absence, a recognition which the texts of the other authors and their migratory inscriptions do not accommodate.

What is immediately evident for readers of *The Holy Woman*, then, is the way the representation of a gendered, feminist agency is foregrounded. It is an agency forged from within the limits of its own tenuous literary conventions, which the evocation of romance struggles to transcend. These representational limits stem from the pressures of a nationalist history whose ideological presence proves at once unsettling and enabling. Shahraz's romance, far from performing a Radaway-style containment of agency, continuously stimulates its readers' interests by suggesting how the former could possibly be achieved without necessarily being subsumed by the very cultural and nationalist patriarchies it is challenging, a reality her audience would be all too familiar with. Agency exists as a dynamic question, constantly changing and always locked in conflict, rather than a static, stage-managed corollary both produced and appropriated by the ideological work of successive romance fictions.

Shahraz's novel in this sense is a veritable patchwork quilt of different social, cultural, and literary representational material. More than resonating on a textual level, to any reader familiar with the author's work in the genre of Pakistani television drama, or examples of these generally, *The Holy Woman* reads like a novelisation of such sprawling serials, epic family melodramas that are typically broadcast across six to eight months of screen time. The melodrama in Shahraz's epic has a decidedly visual quality, with other literary devices subordinated to reams of dialogue between protagonists or healthy doses of knowingly clichéd, free indirect discourse. So far, so romance novelesque. Indeed, part of the front cover, beneath some orientalist artwork, consists of a quotation by newspaper critic Michele Roberts, enthusiastically proclaiming the novel to be 'a dramatic story of family intrigue, religious passions and riproaring romance'. And an initial overview of the narrative apparently reinforces such an appreciation, which speaks to the stock conventions that shape the genre as described by Radaway.

The eponymous holy woman is the heroine of the piece, Zarri Bano. She is the eldest daughter of Habib Khan, son of Siraj Din and overlord of his landed wealth, presided over by both men in the rural district of Sindh. Invoking Sindhi rural tradition, Habib weds Zarri Bano to the Qur'an, despite the vehement protestations of both daughter and wife. It is essentially a *sponsa Christi*, with a difference, being a complete anathema to the religion it is allegedly a ritual of. Habib's daughter is to be shrouded in a black veil at all times when she leaves her home, and in adopting the title of 'the holy woman' in the village, she renounces the possibility of marriage. Her new role entails devotion to the religion and its rigorous study. More significantly, however, in remaining a virgin and thus unmarried, she has also protected Habib's estate as the ritual also crucially necessitates that the inheritance in its entirety be passed onto her. The opening quotation in this chapter relates to this point in the narrative where the same forces that attempted to convince the novel's heroine of the worthiness of her new position now wish to extricate her from that very role. Amidst much reluctance and recrimination, Zarri Bano agrees to marry her former suitor Sikander on her conditions, which make abundantly clear that the reason for her surrender to the pressure imposed on her is the welfare of her nephew, Haris. The nuclear family is reformed then, but is also pervaded by an unease and anxiety, as the reader is left to imagine the consummation of a romance that may never occur.

Even in the somewhat compressed overview given, the stresses and strains within the narrative framework are apparent. And these are produced at the site where gendered agency is enunciated through the ideological work of a patriarchal literary discourse. Two conflicting, irreconcilable discursive frameworks are superimposed in *The Holy Woman*. The expression of feminist agency is qualified by an appreciation of the violent gaps and silences characterising the relationship Pakistani women have with their country's history. But, at the same time, such an enunciation from within the confines of time-honoured patriarchal conventions is confidently asserted against the backdrop of the significant feminist interventions made historically at a time when state-driven, religiously defined nationalism was presenting another oppressive challenge to Pakistani women. Retrospectively or otherwise, the legacy of the Zia regime reverberates throughout Shahraz's novel, so that agency is the product of both the glaring contingencies that continue to mark its legacy and the tenuous possibilities the historical, feminist response to it may have provided for the expression of the former.

The marriage of Zarri Bano to the Qur'an is the stage where such a potentially enabling refashioning is enacted and also the symbolic site at which localised rural patriarchies both enunciate themselves and unravel. Once it becomes patently obvious that the heroine's sacrificial gesture signifies nothing beyond the preservation of land, the ritual struggles to reify itself ideologically. At this point, gendered identity across various spectrums, not just the religiously cultivated, becomes vulnerable to questioning, threatening to collapse under the weight of its own contingencies. Zarri Bano's ceremonial veiling therefore *unveils* the material conditions underpinning the interpellation of identity and subjectivity for women such as herself. This is apparent in her impassioned response as her father dictates her fate to her for the first time:

> I want to be a normal woman, Father, and live a normal life! I want to get married. I am not a very religious person, as you know. I am a twentieth-century, modern, educated woman. I am not living in the Mughal period – a pawn in a game of male chess. Don't you see, Father, I have hardly ever prayed in my life nor opened the Holy Quran on a regular basis.
>
> (Shahraz 2001: 90)

Yet even as she reasons forlornly, the implications of her words appear to unravel before her. Her father's actions have suddenly brought into sharp focus the whole concept of 'normality' as far as women and their socially constituted roles are concerned. A contradiction begins to emerge in what Zarri Bano is saying here. Being a 'normal woman' and leading 'a normal life', rather than offering a magical passport to enfranchisement, itself entails being 'a pawn in a male game of chess'. The central protagonist's 'twentieth-century, modern' education, far from safeguarding her entry into such a world, acts as a facilitator in a very ideologically specific construction of the 'normal woman'. She may be 'educated' and dress in a manner that is less conservative than her female peers in the village, but her identity, 'the essence of her womanhood', is still defined by her place in the patriarchal hierarchy which involves heterosexual love, marriage, and children (Shahraz 2001: 92). This is the type of 'normality' that a cherished union with Sikander would have provided her with. Very quickly, however, Zarri Bano becomes aware of the precarious foundations undergirding the 'choices' available to her:

> The Holy Woman. The woman he [Habib] created by killing me. Did you not know that men are the true creators in our culture, Mother? They mould our lives and destinies according to their whims and desires. The irony of all ironies, for which I can never forgive myself, is that it has happened to me – a feminist, a defender of women's rights. I have been living in a glass house of make-believe.
>
> (Shahraz 2001: 94)

Therefore, whether she opts for a ceremonial marriage to the Qur'an and a life shaped by apparent enclosure and devotion to her religion, or marriage to Sikander, the hero, and the promise of a 'freedom' that is very much ideologically circumscribed, Zarri Bano's agency, her identity, will always be the product of epistemic violence, conspicuous only by its absence on the margins of competing essentialisms.

In this rather bleak landscape, it is logical to question what is actually enabling about the veiled identity which the heroine of the novel assumes. It is important to tread carefully here as it would be inaccurate to suggest that Zarri Bano's shrouded appearance offers some kind of transformative potential. Yet if her imposed role is not a starting point for the conscious performance of various identities whose material parameters have now become transparent, there is little doubt that the holy woman of the title is the springboard for a visible (re)configuration. From behind her religious garb and the authority it gives her, Zarri Bano feels empowered enough to expose how the 'identity' of the Pakistani woman cannot transcend its own materiality. The role she occupies is a corporeal testament to this, where the previously mythical, essentialist significance of religion is reduced to the symbolic, unable to escape that for which it is a mere patina – which is ultimately the preservation of land and wealth through the enclosure of the female body. And it is with the body that Zarri Bano begins to explore the enabling possibilities of her position:

> The cloak hid the shape of her body totally. 'I could be fifteen stones in weight and obese, but nobody would know the difference', Zarri Bano mused. In effect nobody would ever guess that apart from a silky slip and other pieces of lingerie, she wore nothing else.
>
> (Shahraz 2001: 162)

Zarri Bano's newly veiled persona provides her with a position from which she can interrogate the way her body was figured and represented in her previous, 'liberated' existence. Far from rendering her invisible, the covered position becomes an enlightening one in that it illuminates, for her, how the 'norm' that she once craved was one in which her corporeal appearance was shaped by the politics of various benign patriarchies. The way her body was figured changed accordingly as she was exchanged between the spaces of these subtly distinct frameworks. 'Propriety' in this sense would necessitate that she appears differently in front of her father from the 'fashionable' sartorial elegance that her meetings with Sikander or a trip to the village fete would demand. But the end game remained the same, with the control of the female body by either the paternalistic or sexually charged patriarchal gaze marking the stable 'norm' of the 'ordinary woman' Zarri Bano assumed she always was (Shahraz 2001: 159). Her identity at this point becomes an entirely contingent, ideological construction.

It must be reiterated here that Shahraz's epic romance text is a simulacra of the discourses through which, in many ways, she nostalgically reimagines the Sindhi landscape of her past. Yet the type of destabilising feminist intervention that emerges in the shape of her holy woman does not become enclosed in its own hyperreality. The risk with this type of representational politics is that it threatens to become hegemonic in its own right, where any alternative discursive or political intervention is repudiated because a preoccupation with the material is not its defining principle. This is avoided in Shahraz's text, even though it appears in every way to be vulnerable to such criticism. The pleasures her novel speaks to, both in a contemporary sense and those it seeks to recapture from the past, are energised by very specific historical processes shaping the ongoing conflict between gender and nation in Pakistan. Zarri Bano's reclamation of her body within the ideological frameworks of the various local and national patriarchies that would seek to possess and enclose it, never becomes lost in its own representation or materiality. Instead, such a gendered politics of the body actually stems from an awareness of what is lost, what is perpetually on the margins. What is empowering, therefore, for the heroine of Shahraz's romance is not the forming of her own illusory opposition, in which she is either sustaining patriarchy, or marginalising other Pakistani women from different classes and ethnicities, but instead always remaining in that space which is between even the in-between, revealing what is alienated and marginalised from behind the patina of ideological legitimacy.

At a time when Pakistan was seeing an unprecedented rise in feminist opposition to the institutionalised gendered violence of the Zia regime, the guerrilla resistance of a Zarri Bano would undoubtedly have resonated with Pakistani women across the spectrums of class and ethnicity. Localised patriarchal practices such as the wedding of the bride to the holy book were ones that Zia had ironically attempted to eradicate and bring under the banner of his own nationally marked, gendered ideology. He initially had to support powerful feudal regions such as the Sindh as a precursor to gaining political power, and this came with a tacit understanding that traditions such as those depicted in Shahraz's novel would inevitably continue (Mahmud 1995). Nostalgic romances such as *The Holy Woman* therefore suggest that whilst opposition to Zia's policies continued to be orchestrated on a national level, the most significant subversion was being expressed by women, across the discrete, localised spaces of Pakistan, and within the pleasures they derived from their reading practices.

The purpose of this chapter has been to demonstrate the unique trajectory taken by the development of writing by Pakistani women in the form of the popular romance, especially during the period of General Zia's rule. The adoption of such a globalised generic form inevitably provokes the immediate queries of what exactly the romance – in terms of its enduring, conventional narrativity, ideological work, and textual pleasures – has to offer writing that is taking place in a radically different context. What I have concluded is that examples of the rise in romance literature during the period in question must be theorised against the historical context of contemporary Pakistan and, significantly, the legacy of the relationship which feminist interventions of the past have had with the country's previous nationalism and their discourses. The work of Riaz makes its own jarring and dissonant inscriptions against these discursive frameworks, displaying an acute awareness of how the Pakistani woman both appears and is erased in their political spaces. Her work is therefore a credible starting point when considering what is at stake in questions of gendered agency in the context of Pakistani romance literature. The dissonant questions raised by her material also emerge as traces in the work of the diasporic authors Shamsie and Abdullah. In refashioning the romance through a transnational lens, the margin appears to be under erasure rather than the site of agency. A novel like *The Holy Woman* thus cannot just be viewed as pastiche. The representational work of the romance in the Pakistani context is, therefore, transformed, especially where the female body is concerned. For so many years the site of literal and epistemic violence, the body in Shahraz's romance is ironically able to inscribe, and to enunciate after it is inscribed upon. The correlation between an activism acutely conscious of a history shaped by violence against the female body and a literary practice that cleverly crafts subversion and agency out of a hegemonic cultural form which seems unsustainable, appears, in my opinion, powerfully coincidental.

Notes

1 For a particularly enlightening study of the way popular culture is consumed and received, see Hanaway and Heston (2006).
2 I have been fortunate enough to be able to consult several works which provide perceptive analysis of the historical period relating to the military ideologue's dictatorship. I am indebted to Ian Talbot (2005) for the bulk of my information, particularly his excellent chapter on Zia's deployment of religious nationalism. Other historical studies include Lawrence Ziring (2003), Mohammad Waseem (1989), and Shahid Burki and Craig Baxter (1991). From a feminist perspective, especially the way the body intersects with religiously based ideas of nationhood, Sadia Toor (2007), Rubina Saigol (1995), and Sadia Toor and Neelam Hussain (1997) are seminal texts.

3 By far the most infamous measure of Zia's nationalist project in this respect was his implementation of the Hudood or Zina ordinances circa 1983, following on from a rigorous campaign to infuse the ideological consciousness of the public with *Chaadar aur Char Diwari*, which literally translates as 'the veil and the four walls', and puts an emphasis on erasure and enclosure. The body, first and foremost, is to be regulated, with the *Chaadar*, derived from an Islamic directive as a head covering, to be mandatory as a form of dress for all women. This message was disseminated and reinforced through a coordinated media campaign.

Bibliography

Abdullah, S. (2005) *Beyond the Cayenne Wall*. Bloomington: iUniverse.
Burki, S. and Baxter, C. (1991) *Pakistan under the Military*. Boulder: Westview Press.
Chaney, D. (1979) *Fictions and Representations: Representations of Popular Experience*. London: Edward Arnold.
Hanaway, W.L. and Heston, W. (eds.) (2006) *Studies in Pakistani Popular Culture*. Karachi: Sang-e-Meel Publications.
Hussein, A. (ed.) (2005) *Kahani: Short Stories by Pakistani Women*. London: Saqi.
Mahmud, A. (1995) *Working with Zia: Pakistan's Power Politics 1977–1988*. Karachi: Oxford University Press.
Radaway, J. (1991) *Reading the Romance*. London: University of North Carolina Press.
Rahman, T. (1991) *A History of Pakistani Literature in English*. London: Vanguard.
Riaz, F. (1990) 'Chaadar aur Char Diwari'. In *Beyond Belief*. Ed. by Ahmad, R. Lahore: ASR Publications, 52–55.
Riaz, F. (2005a) *Four Walls and Black Veils*. Ed. by Hussein, A. London: Oxford University Press.
Riaz, F. (2005b) 'Some Misaddressed Letters'. In *Kahani: Short Stories by Pakistani Women*. Ed. by Hussein, A. London: Saqi, 95–104.
Saigol, R. (1995) *Knowledge and Identity*. Lahore: ASR Publications.
Shahraz, Q. (2001) *The Holy Woman*. London: Arcadia.
Shamsie, K. (2002) *Kartography*. London: Bloomsbury.
Sidhwa, B. (1993) *An American Brat*. Karachi: Sama Publications.
Talbot, I. (2005) *Pakistan: A Modern History*. London: Hurst and Company.
Toor, S. (2007) 'Moral Regulation in a Postcolonial Nation-State: Gender and the Politics of Islamization in Pakistan'. *Interventions* 9(2), 255–275.
Toor, S. (2011) *The State of Islam: Culture and Cold War Politics in Pakistan*. London: Pluto.
Toor, S. and Hussain, N. (eds) (1997) *Engendering the Nation State*. Lahore: Simorgh Publications.
Waseem, M. (1989) *Politics and the State in Pakistan*. Lahore: Progressive Publishers.
Ziring, L. (2003) *At the Crosscurrent of History*. Oxford: Oneworld.

20

CONJUGAL HOMES

Marriage culture in contemporary novels of the Pakistani diaspora

Rahul K. Gairola and Elham Fatma

Contemporary proliferations of Pakistani diasporic fiction in English, mainly post-9/11, have been mapping their way to the global stage of writings about the shared borders and liminal spaces in which people find themselves when moving from their country of ethnic affiliation to that of nationality and vice versa. These narratives of shared borders enfold both the laurels and lapses of diasporic culture, thus serving as empathising counterpoints to the Islamophobic stereotypes that reproduce and expand myths of the closed, static cultural arrangements of Pakistani society. The roll call of Pakistani diasporic writers includes Nadeem Aslam, Mohsin Hamid, Kamila Shamsie, Azhar Abidi, Mohammed Hanif, Hanif Kureishi, Bapsi Sidhwa, and Qaisra Shahraz. According to Claire Chambers, these writers, who are mostly 'living or educated in the West, currently feature prominently on the international literary scene as award winners or nominees, best-selling authors, festival speakers and, increasingly, topics for research students and critics' (2011: 122–123). We agree with Chambers' observation concerning these writers' wide popularity, and would add that they situate their craft around themes of home and family, deploying fiction as a powerful site of contestation of xenophobia. Such narrative strategies include dissent, alternative visions, debunking of myths, resistance of bigotry and Islamophobia, and representing a panorama of identities.

Moreover, many novels from the Pakistani diaspora document various tropes of diasporic life from myriad perspectives that include racialism, alienation, identity crisis, acculturation, gendered Islamophobia, cultural shock, etc. Despite the intellectual finesse with which these writers present issues relating to marriage as an institution that envelops nuanced complexities for partners from disparate cultures, it has arguably not been examined as thoroughly as it might be within the frame of marriage as a recurring leitmotif in contemporary novels of the Pakistani diaspora. Our chapter expands on this theme through an extended comparative analysis of three novels by Pakistani diasporic writers: Sidhwa's *An American Brat* (1993), Abidi's *Twilight* (2008), and, especially, Aslam's *Maps for Lost Lovers* (2004). This contribution, moreover, endeavours to offer insights into the dynamics of sociocultural and religious features that the Pakistani diasporic community assumes to engender through cultural friction between parents and their progeny. It engages, in other words, a dialectic of intergenerational mythos and the resulting conflict of perspectives that debilitate matrimonial relations and exert influence on the matrimonial spaces of domesticity in the Pakistani diaspora.

We also argue that these novels reify their characters' idiosyncrasies, which are instituted by the cultural topographies in which they are situated. They adumbrate the two distinct generations' respective conjugal expectations, beliefs, and views about consent and coercion to sex and marriage against the contradistinction of 'East meets West' tensions. That is, we propose that these three novels narratively represent generational values and the complex ways in which such values are refracted by different characters' geographical positions throughout the Occident and the Orient. In Muneeza Shamsie's appraisal of Pakistani fiction in English, we must be attentive to the 'historical trajectory [...] of the colonial encounter' (Halai 2017: n.p.). We would add to Shamsie's observation that, in these three novels, the various historical links to power relations churned in the crucible of gender dynamics within and between different countries further complicate how home and belonging are refracted by the kaleidoscopic lens of Pakistanis in motion. These diasporic subjects are born and brought up in Western countries and select spouses from those "foreign" countries.

Thus, through the fictive landscapes of *Maps, Twilight*, and *An American Brat*, we critically explore issues including sex, family honour, ritual pollution, purity of lineage, and shame, which foment and complicate the subtleties of intimate relations between spouses and lovers. Different complications arise from both similar and transcultural societies, different religions, and/or transatlantic backgrounds with respect to diasporic, domestic configurations that anchor Pakistani characters while marking them as 'other'. Indeed, the historical trajectory of the colonial encounter as we see it locates precisely in conjugal homes of the Pakistani diaspora a nexus of competing identities and desires that carry and imbibe the loaded traces of skewed power relations based on class, sex, and religion. Despite these variations in narrative and manifestations of themes of 'home' and 'homeland', we propose that the figure of the Pakistani mother is central to understanding the ways in which competing constrictions and avenues of identity liberation are made possible by these three authors. We read the figure of the mother as caught in the crosshairs of a xenophobic nation state even as she is the nexus of kinship that links current and former homelands, various family members, and the past with the present.

In recognising the matriarch as caught in the juxtaposed position of both protagonist and antagonist in these narratives, we also note that these figures embody a number of issues that unfold the dichotomy between their own religious views and their children's secular outlooks. As might be expected, the diasporic offspring of these maternal figures are born and raised under the influence of Western ethos and cultural assimilation. As such, their attitudes and positions do, at times, come into conflict with their mothers' righteous observances of Islamic dogma and how life should be lived. While it would be a sweeping generalisation to claim that religion dictates all such developments in diasporic narratives, we note that it often serves as a guiding beacon for mothers as they negotiate connections to their offspring, on the one hand, and their situatedness in the homeland on the other. For example, Sidhwa underscores the predicament and despondency of a Pakistani Parsee mother in *An American Brat*. Zareen, along with her husband, Cyril Ginwalla, fear that Feroza's Muslim peers influence her conservative attitude and internalised diffidence in Pakistan. The couple resolve to send their sole offspring to the USA to live with her uncle in the hope that a change of culture will mediate against her shyness and shape her into a confident woman with liberal views.

However, her stay lengthens with her admission to university, which exposes her to a new lifestyle in modern America where she drinks, dances, drives, and imbibes her transformation without inhibitions. Feroza's love affair with David offers her an excellent opportunity:

> She gradually exposes herself to varied experiences of life in the new world. Thus, Feroza evolves from an innocent, conservative, and protected life in Lahore to one

that is marked by the experiences of independent spirit and self-confidence of [the] modern American world.

(Sheela and Muthuraman 2013: 19)

The metamorphosis of Feroza's personality, shown in her attitude and attire, confounds her parents' expectations, and her views on sexuality, especially David as her chosen partner, further infuriate her mother. Zareen believes that her objectives and rationale for sending Feroza to the US have led to the loss of her only child to a world that is insensitive to the religious rigidity and *force majeure* of a minority community like the Parsees.[1] Fearing ostracism from the Parsee community, Zareen repeatedly warns Feroza not to go against the family's wishes by marrying a non-Parsee.

But as G. Kain opines, 'Feroza's resistance involves denying dominant ideological constructs from both her Parsee heritage and contemporary American culture. She perceives herself as "other" from either/both of these vantage points, and thus must contend with the turbulence of an unsettled cultural jurisdiction' (2002: 241). Kain's reading of Feroza's self-assessment is parallel to the way in which xenophobic nation states scrutinise the alien other. In Sara Ahmed's evaluation,

> Through strange encounters, the figure of the 'stranger' is produced, not as that which we fail to recognise, but as that which we have already recognised as 'a stranger' [...] The alien stranger is hence, not beyond human, but a mechanism *for allowing us to face that which we have already designated as the beyond.*
>
> (2000: 3; emphasis original)

The exclusionary dis-identification which the logic of xenophobia invests in the diasporic Pakistani outcast seems to be reflected, at the micro level, in Feroza's domestic milieu. Indeed, it is her self-abnegation through the eyes of the new, promised as other, that acts as a psychological fulcrum engendering her own gendered and racialised oppression.

Through Feroza's inclination towards intercommunity marriage, Sidhwa illustrates contrasting views of mothers and their children. She also elucidates the set of repercussions that children invite *vis-à-vis* the unforgiving and unrelenting ways of the Parsee community, irrespective of their modern thinking and advanced ways of living. Sidhwa fashions her fictional diasporic family into a microcosm of the nation, wherein personal battles, competitions, and incentives drive the plot as the maternal figure is both pivot and pathogen as the harbinger of racialised reproduction. The Ginwalla family in *An American Brat* exemplifies the stereotypical disposition of the Pakistani upper class with its liberal education, high status, and wealth, which they have in common with their Muslim counterparts of the same social class who share the same political orientations. Thus, the reader encounters another prototypical family of the Pakistani elite in Abidi's *Twilight*. The Khan family is spearheaded by a matriarch, Bilqis Begum, who faces a difficult time when her only son, Samad, brings a *gori mem* from Australia (*gori* refers to a 'fair skinned' lady: where *gori* means 'white' and *mem* signifies 'madam').

While she accepts Kate as her son's bride, Bilqis struggles hard to face the reality that she is gradually losing her son, whose ideas, thoughts, and choices seem totally Westernised now. For Bilqis, Samad's white wife symbolises his total embrace, both literally and figuratively, of Western culture with little hope of his return to Pakistan. Samad's ostensible rejection of the 'motherland' through a white wife, who has ideologically displaced his mother precipitates a crisis for the characters in both novels, which, moreover, has ramifications for the delicate class structure of contemporary Pakistani society. Rehana Ahmed examines the ways in which class and social space intersect with religion and ethnicity at multicultural sites in *Writing British Muslims: Religion, Class, and Multiculturalism*. Ahmed opines, in that context, that British Muslims 'have been the target of verbal and physical attacks, as a group who tend to want to maintain and assert elements of their culture and religion which are not easily assimilable to a majoritarian British way of life' (2017: 6). Rather, for Ahmed, 'the British Muslim has become a cipher for the excesses of multiculturalism […] the supposed cultural excesses of Muslims provide a useful vehicle for criticising multiculturalism' (2017: 8).

Ahmed's concerted observation of the Pakistani diaspora in the UK resonates with those of Sara Ahmed in her examination of 'the alien stranger' (2000: 3). Like a mirrored echo chamber, the accent of pathological difference fractures the very social discourse that might, even reluctantly, permit assimilation. For Bilqis, then, Samad's white wife is testament to the extent to which the nation state's exclusionary tactics become internalised in the hallowed domestic realm of home and hearth. We witness some of these diasporic tensions between competing sites and sights materialise in the class relations in Abidi's novel. While the dazzling decor of the Khans' mansion – their 'social home', if you will – validates the superior status of its occupants and its visitors, the Ginwallas' evening parties at their residence, peppered by their friends' heated debates on dicey politics in Pakistan, exude their social standing and intellectually nuanced, liberal thinking.

The Khans and the Ginwallas seem to conform to these stereotypes of the Pakistani diaspora, and wish their children to have the best educational qualifications which will allow them to secure excellent careers in Pakistan. Yet, ironically, the same parents are aghast or devastated when their children find their spouses from the Western culture of their education. For example, Bilqis is depicted as dejected; her son Samad is oblivious to her explanations and arguments against marrying a partner from a totally different culture, religion, and racial taxonomy. Samad compels her to accept his choice and attend his low-key marriage ceremony with Kate in Australia because he is struck by her beauty and grace, and it is only in Kate that he can envisage his life partner. Abidi illustrates, through the characters of Bilqis and Kate, how people harbour stereotyped views and doubts about each other's inner essences based on their country of origin (and the more muted 'race projects' – to borrow the useful term coined by Omi and Winant (1994) – that attend them). In another example, Bilqis deems Kate an outsider, one of those who 'don't understand us or our values, and, to be quite honest they are people of whom we know nothing' (2017: 25). Here, Ahmed's notion of the recognisable stranger again rears its xenophobic head, but this time we see the ways in which Bilqis' ability to dis-identify with Kate have already invoked an intimate familiarity with her.

In contrast, Kate has always thought of Pakistan as a failed nation – a barbaric place with strange customs where young girls are forced into marriage, and where poverty, ignorance, and a lack of education are the rule of thumb. However, after coming to Pakistan, she is surprised to discover an unexpected underbelly that defies orientalist stereotypes: this Pakistan is vibrant, colourful, and developed, even ostentatious. The Pakistanis of this realm are wealthy, educated, and eccentric Muslims whose religious convictions do not ultimately stifle their liberal lifestyles. But despite their magnificent mansions, luxurious cars, and hosts of servants, Pakistan does not meet Kate's expectations; Samad finds that Australia meets his, however, and thus attempts to assimilate himself into Australian culture. However, he encounters various difficulties there. Samad experiences, on a regular basis, that Australians do not regard him as part of their society, no matter how hard he strives to assimilate. Here, Samad's social exclusion is an epidermal testament; neither his newly adopted homeland nor his new wife can earn him the impossible pedigree required to belong in Australian society.

We might pause here to meditate on assimilationist discourse as it relates to capitalism. Assimilation, although racially impossible, occurs through a familiar logic of postcolonial commodification since xenophobic foreclosure pre-empts any efforts to truly belong in the new country. Even assimilation into the romantic ideals of marriage, heteronormative ideals of reproduction, the circuits of neoliberal capitalism that buttress them, and all of the pathways in between, cannot bleach away the difference that always marks Samad as a knowable outsider. Such coals on the path to the immigrant's promised land underscore Iain Chambers' observation that:

> Migration, together with the enunciation of cultural borders and crossings, is also deeply inscribed in the itineraries of much contemporary reasoning [...] If exile presumes an initial home and the eventual promise of a return, the questions met with *en route* consistently breach the boundaries of such an itinerary.
>
> (2008: 2; emphasis original)

In the context of conjugal homes of the Pakistani diaspora, Chambers' contention enables us to think of not only migratory and cultural border-crossings, but also of spaces in-between. Heteronormative marriage, and the juridical privileges it affords via citizenship and the rights of offspring born in the host country, becomes the most contestable variable on the borders of the nation and its domestic homes. This is also coloured by labour relations which characterise domestic spaces in South Asia. Back home in Pakistan, Samad's mother is not happy with his choice of Kate, while the latter is a curious novelty for both Samad's relatives and friends in Pakistan. Bilqis' servants gaze upon Kate with surprise and awe as her whiteness, and even accent, is alien to them; the tension produced by this fascination with difference also marks the threshold of class which they cannot breach. Here, the diasporic Pakistani home and hearth is characterised by domesticity, or domestic labour to be more precise, that *must* remain alien, estranged, other, like race, within the comforts of home.

We see this unfold through the novel's plot. The dominant notion upheld by the upper echelon of Pakistanis regarding white women compels Samad to realise, through his friend Asim's belief, that white women surely possess something apart from Asian women, yet they cannot fit into the conventional role of daughters-in-law. Although Asim admires their white skin, blue eyes, and blonde hair, he is too traditional to enter into the sacred institution of marriage with any of them. In these narratives, Abidi and Sidhwa chronicle that even the bourgeoisie of Pakistan are controlling and hypersensitive concerning their children's marriages, and generally fuss over the ramifications of their bringing spouses from alien cultures back to them. However, in *Maps for Lost Lovers*, Aslam engages an array of cultural, emotional, and physical traumas that Pakistani-British women experience in their conjugal homes, when they are forced into marriages arranged by their families in the Islamic state of Pakistan, having been raised in a non-Islamic multi-ethnic space like England.

In *Maps*, Aslam charts out a fictional enclave called Dasht-e-Tanhaii (a metaphorical expression meaning 'a steppe of loneliness'), situated in the north of England, which echoes 'the story of the British Pakistani community and families at the crossroads of liberalism and orthodoxy' (Kanwal 2012: 57). This ethnic enclave is an immigratory counterpoint, and an 'other' home space, that we encounter in contrast to the neoliberal wonderland of Thatcherite 'meritocrats' in Hanif Kureishi's *My Beautiful Launderette* (Gairola 2016: 79) – in which arranged marriage to consolidate capital and kinship is expected and commanded over and above feminist and queer identificatory affiliations and self-affirmations. Rather, the life trajectories of Pakistani immigrants ghettoised in Dasht-e-Tanhaii delineate their superstitions, conservatism, ancestral feuds, and cultural practices brought across seven seas to England, where they impose on their children the social and cultural paraphernalia from Pakistan which complicate their familial relationships.

Ironically, this tendency resembles the British race project, under Margaret Thatcher, which looked to inspire a nostalgia for Victorian ideals enshrined throughout the British Empire while assimilating Pakistani immigrants and their families into the machinery of neoliberal capitalism throughout the 1980s (Gairola 2009: 41). These Pakistani immigrants strive to retain a connection to their lost homeland by adhering to their Islamic faith, abiding by the diktats of Muslim clerics, and subscribing to the endogamous xenophobia that haunts the logic of arranged marriage. Yet, here we encounter a sad contradiction – in yearning to be part of their lost homeland, its languages, beliefs, and cultures, they have rejected the constantly dangled carrot of British integration. Aslam's characters are just as much victims of themselves as they are victims of the cold and calculating homelands between which they exist. For example, the double murder of Jugnu and Chanda unravels the timely issue of honour killings, which point to a more extreme modality of social oppression in close-knit communities that wish to punish women for choosing their own partners. After two failed marriages with cousins, Chanda ends up living with Jugnu in the same neighbourhood in which their families reside.

The residents of Dasht-e-Tanhaii consequently label her as wanton, a source of shame to her family, and so her brothers kill her, along with Jugnu. Kaukab, Jugnu's sister-in-law, believes in the part of Islamic jurisprudence which considers their murder the outcome of their sinful living together, outside marriage. She also finds fault with the ethical and moral values of the cultural system of the West, of which her brother Jugnu, and her own three children, Charag, Mah-Jabin, and Ujala, are by-products. She feels offended by her husband Shamas' condescending views regarding Islam, Jugnu's audacity in living with Chanda, and her children's unabashed assimilation into the decadent and dirty West. As a devout Muslim, while residing in Dasht-e-Tanhaii, Kaukab experiences acute estrangement due to acculturation. Her children do not comprehend her inability to assimilate into the culture of the host country in which they have been raised since birth. This aspect reflects Esra Mirze Santesso's observation that Muslim women characters must 'cope with a more severe divide between the private and public spheres, and their bodies frequently become contested spaces through which to negotiate religious identity – as we see not only in terms of sexual politics but also symbolic politics' (2013: 4).

Kaukab belongs to those *desi*s (people of Indian, Pakistani, and Bangladeshi birth or descent who live in the West) whose fear of moral transgressions is so overwhelming that it prevents them from understanding the culture of the West, which they deem to be morally bereft and corrupt. Moreover, they are antagonistic to their host country and make no attempt to assimilate into it, which creates further mental and emotional distance from their own British-born children. Yet, in the eyes of Britain and its policies, these foreigners are the adopted children of its glorious erstwhile Empire who cannot and will never share the white skin, and thus the same blood, as 'true' Britons. Avtar Brah comments on this stark reality, noting that between the 1950s and 1980s, 'the figure of "the Asian" was constructed in different discourses, policies, and practices [...] South Asian groups appropriated or resisted the meaning of these representations; and the everyday life of Asian people articulated with these discourses' (2006: 35). For example, born and brought up in England, Chanda, Mah-Jabin, and Suraya are expected to establish their marital homes in Pakistan.

The critical account of their forced marriages acquaints readers with the religio-cultural and social issues endured by women like them trapped in arranged (forced) marriages. Indeed, here we see unambiguous links between love and lifestyle, law and libidinal desire, nation and nature. At the age of twenty-five, Chanda has already experienced two failed marriages. Her first, contracted in Pakistan to a cousin, ended in disaster. Her second husband, another cousin brought from Pakistan, leaves her as soon as he procures a British passport. Despite being in the UK, Chanda is subject to traditional Islamic laws which consider her married until she has completed a stipulated period of separation from her husband which may last years. Nadia Butt avers that, regarding marriage in *Maps*, 'the family structure and society at large is brutal and callous with respect to rebellious sons and daughters who dare moving an inch from prescribed boundaries of the supposed Islamic "do's" and "don'ts"' (2008: 159).

Suraya's case parallels Chanda's. Suraya is like a culturally conditioned automaton at the beck and call of her husband, who divorces here by pronouncing *talaq* in a drunken state. Her husband's wish for reconciliation, or *halala*,[2] after *talaq* compels her to face the harrowing experience of marrying another man, who should give her a divorce after spending some time with her. Now, she desperately needs a man who can marry and release her, so that she can reconcile with her husband and son. The predicament of both Chanda and Suraya is grave, since the institution of marriage in Pakistan lays special emphasis on women's *izzat* or honour. Also, male family members' pride and ego are conjoined with their women's *izzat*. Chanda's brothers primarily accuse her for living with Jugnu and sabotaging their family's honour rather than not abiding by the Islamic rules of divorce and marriage. Suraya's husband mentally tortures her, anticipating that she will taint his *izzat* by contracting physical relations with her second husband.

These women's religio-cultural quandaries and socially denigrated states give their close-knit society an opportunity to label them 'loose women' who lack feminine virtues of forbearance, acquiescence, and clemency required to establish conjugal homes.[3] With scrupulous attention to historical record, Aslam efficaciously records religio-cultural realms and beliefs through which several cultural practices are nourished in Pakistan, as well as those engaged in by the Pakistani diaspora in the UK. In *Maps*, Aslam offers readers domestic scenarios that are historical antecedents of, in the words of Ahmed and Sumita Mukherjee, 'the very different contexts informing the struggles of the past 150 years' (2012: xviii). We can extend this notion to recognise that the womanly figure who is at once wife and mother in the Pakistani diaspora in Britain acts as a repository of these struggles. For example, the reason for Mah-Jabin's suffering with her Pakistani husband lies in his male chauvinism; his mindset is rooted in the social dynamics of Islamic patriarchy, which assumes that beating wives is not violent; rather, blood on the hearth is to be expected. The violent way in which he behaves towards Mah-Jabin suggests that his beliefs are based in the religious dictums, social hierarchy, rites of passage, and status of women found in patriarchal culture.

In fact, a number of passages in *Maps* depict various ways in which Pakistani-British women are tortured in their marriages. The daughter of one Muslim family in Dasht-e-Tanhaii does not comply with her husband's wishes, stays aloof, and fails to come to terms with her forced marriage as she cannot detach herself from her Hindu boyfriend. The holy man diagnoses her problem as a spiritual one, that a *djinn* has possessed her, and thus prescribes exorcism. Another girl in love with a Hindu boy is coerced to marry her cousin, brought from Pakistan; when she does not respond to her husband's sexual demands, her mother advises him to rape her. Here, in the crucible of the conjugal home of the Pakistani diaspora in Britain, inter-religious love marks the corrosion of family, nation, home, and homeland; the difference it threatens to bring to the system is an assault on the future as well as the past. In Sara Ahmed's theorisation, 'Differences, as markers of power, are not determined in the "space" of the particular *or* the general, but in the very determination of their historical relation (a determination that is never final or complete, as it involves strange encounters)' (2000: 8–9; emphasis original). Aslam mocks the culture of violence immanent in the homes of diasporic subjects, especially the hypocritical idealism of male perpetrators and the paradoxical attitudes of female family members.

Wives who do not accede to their husbands' (excessive) sexual desires and defy them are often appraised as abnormal and uncustomary. Kaukab also accuses Mah-Jabin of being impatient with her husband. The matrix of her beliefs prevents Kaukab from realising that her daughter's trauma is due to her husband's tortuous means of obtaining sexual gratification. She also shows Mah-Jabin her disappointment at the neighbourhood's two married girls, who unabashedly share dark secrets of their sex lives with their mothers. One seems distressed because her husband wants it from behind, and the other is tormented by her husband's demands to ejaculate in her mouth. Kaukab seems to be a patriarchal character who firmly believes in the idealistic notion that a woman is the embodiment of the family's shame. For women like Kaukab, raising one's voice against men's expectations of marital sex is symptomatic of women's lower levels of endurance. It also implies that one is neglecting one's wifely duties and indulging in gross shamelessness.

Through his vivid characters, Aslam throws into sharp relief oppressive cultural practices based on essentialising notions of kinship and home, which ultimately impoverish the social system while damaging the social links that bind partners in conjugal relationships. Forced marriages, (dis)honour killings, fetishising lavish marriages, honour- and status-certifying ceremonies, and dowry demands primarily victimise women and lead to regression in society, impeding its progress. Moreover, Tishani Doshi writes that

> [Aslam's] narrative is a palimpsest of some vital Islamic issues of (re)marriage, sex, divorce and conflicts of ideas, as well as what he proclaims in his interview, i.e. that he writes about East, and West, tradition and modernity, the global and the local, and about religion and secularism.
>
> (2017: 2)

Through his narrative, Aslam also suggests that the process of assimilating into a new culture is undertaken at the expense of overlooking several characteristics of the culture of origin, but disengaging from the ossified ideology is problematic.

The diasporic subjects' attempts to translocate the culture of the home country into a new demographic space often end in conflict, which they find difficult to resolve. Because of their inability to accommodate or cope with changing subjectivities of morality, paradigmatic shifts in thinking and the volatility of situations traumatise those who largely stay cocooned in ethno-religious shells, avoid moving beyond their stereotypical identities, and follow the trajectory delineated by their religion, society, and culture. Where 'some migrants identify more with one society than the other', the majority seem to maintain several identities that link them simultaneously to more than one nation (Schiller 1998: 231). But the rationale that motivates some migrants to identify and build links with other nations does not diminish the paranoia of miscegenation conspicuous amongst Pakistani families. Miscegenation is a *misdemeanour* against the *nation* as it is both imagined and juridically enshrined. It is perceived as a threat that disrupts the sanctity of 'pure-blooded' families by introducing spouses from other nationalities, languages, religions and cultures. Aslam, Abidi, and Sidhwa show the same fear expressed by the mothers of the elite class of Pakistan, despite their education and purportedly liberal outlooks.

Thus, through the maternal anguish of mothers like Kaukab, Bilqis, and Zareen, who object to their progeny's spouses, a common narrative thread emerges. These plots share the collective experiences of the larger communities of which they form a part as they problematise the whitewashed trust that communities have in 'consanguineous marriages'. However, consanguineous marriage also involves issues, which Nejat Tongur finds are often based on selfish motives. For Tongur, Pakistanis are 'involved in organized crime called arranged marriages', and stubbornly keep their formalities, codes, rituals, customs, and ceremonies intact while the community tries to cover up the crimes and inappropriate behaviour of fellow countrymen to save the face of the community as a whole (2016: 131). We would, moreover, draw the reader's attention to the success of the institution of consanguineous arranged marriage which Bilqis and Zareen probably explain through the notion that 'the closer the relative, [the] more secure the knowledge about the potential spouse, and so the safer marriage is considered to be' (Charsley 2007: 1122). Thus, the fear of marital rupture is eased by unions between relatives from the same social class, culture, religion, caste, language, etc., although Mah-Jabin's marriage to her first cousin in Pakistan fails.

The consciousness of class/status also features as one of the driving forces of (consanguineous) arranged marriage. Abidi takes Bilqis' wish for Samad to marry his cousin as the vested interest of parents seeking to maintain their social status in the society. This reflects a core argument in Gayle Rubin's 'The Traffic in Women', in which she argues that 'kinship and marriage are always part of total social systems, and are always tied into economic and political arrangements' (1975: 207). In the context of conjugal homes in Pakistani diasporic literature, Aslam presents Kaukab's insistence on an arranged marriage for Charag as a remedy which women deploy to cure sons whom they consider to have gone astray. For she believes it is not unusual for

> Muslim men to marry white girls and then divorce them quickly upon learning how difficult and shameless they were, and then having an arranged marriage to a decorous and compliant Muslim girl, preferably a first cousin brought over from back home.
>
> (2005: 57)

Desis' stereotyping of white women as promiscuous and unprincipled in sexual matters criminalises them, whereas they regard their own women as obedience personified in personal, social, and sexual matters, and hence preferred by them for marriage. However, this prejudice disguises and deflects from their subjection to 'the hazards' of 'close kin transnational marriage' (Charsley, 2007: 1127). Robina Mohammad has appropriately identified the predicament of overseas partners, when brought from Pakistan:

> These imported partners simultaneously embody strangeness as well as familiarity, often experienced as a shock. As life-long kin, they *are* seemingly a 'known quantity', as co-ethnics they are ostensibly part of a shared culture and religion. But the newness of the spousal bond combines with their hegemonic gender, social conservatism and sheltered upbringing in Pakistani *dehat* (rural regions) where Islamic practices remain localised, to make them disorientingly different, a difference narrated as incommensurable and drawn on as an explanation for emotional distance and difficulties of communication within the marriage.
>
> (2015: 610–611)

Here, we would argue that the primordial consternation over going against dogmatic religions informing self, society, sexuality, and marriage is traumatic. Kaukab, Bilqis, and Zareen anticipate that their children's drifting away from their religion fused with cultural mores will instigate a new order in their society. These women comprehend that this direction is an affront to their religion and coreligionists, because marriage with people of other religions involves compromises on the religious ideals of either or both partners' religions. Bilqis always winces at the question 'has Kate converted?', about which she conjectures that 'conversions are only partial redemption. It confers the religion but never makes one equal' (Abidi 2008: 25). Zareen surmises that marrying into another's religion weakens one's social standing in one's own religious community, and thus offers Parsee prayers while supplicating for her daughter's disassociation from David.

Although Zareen finds David admirable and appealing, she reasons that 'he would deprive her daughter of her faith, her heritage, her family, and her community. She would be branded an adulteress and her children pronounced illegitimate' (Sidhwa 1994: 289). Beguiled by the American way of life, Zareen thwarts Feroza's courtship with David by insinuating the issues that such unions precipitate. Her harangue over the expenditure incurred by the bridegroom's family while performing the Parsee wedding rituals unnerves David, 'despite his tolerant and accepting liberality' (Sidhwa 1994: 309). He finds the Parsee community unaccommodating and very different from his informal and liberal approach to marriage. His enthusiasm for Feroza and marriage thus cools, and their relationship culminates in separation. The defiance and undermining of traditional practices at home are not expected of women, because conjugal homes are believed to be founded on the premise that women are the transmitters of familial traditions, passing the legacy of cultural practices to subsequent generations. Zareen reprimands Feroza regarding the significance of Parsee cultural heritage, and repeatedly reminds her that 'it's not your culture! You can't just toss your heritage away like that. It's in your bones!' (Sidhwa 1994: 279).

Bilqis opines that 'a family's lineage survived through the continuity of its tradition' (Abidi, 2008: 24); in the same vein, Kaukab firmly believes that children inherit values from their parents, especially the mother; and she foresees a bleak future for her grandson, as he will inherit libertine impulses from his parents, or more precisely from his mother, who is a product of a place where 'the display of wantonness and sex before marriage was the norm and not grave sins' (Aslam, 2005: 309). Society's expectations of women are greater when it comes to preserving the culture, ethics, religious practices, and traditions; even mothers also expect more from their daughters and daughters-in-law than from sons. These diasporic writers' narratives are mired in the quotidian beliefs of South Asian communities concerning the sanctum of the conjugal home, which primarily theorise women's duties as mothers, daughters, and wives, as more stringent and onerous than those of men. They are expected to uphold the honour of the family. Amongst the many virtues expected from them, a restrained sexuality is of primary importance, and bound up with familial regulations. Adherence to this cultural edict enables the residents of Dashte-e-Tanhaii to accept that 'Chanda's murder is labelled as honour killing for bringing shame upon the family, subverting the male dominance, disrupting their life and social values and violating the sanctuary of home' (Karim and Nasir 2014: 132).

In this chapter, we have drawn attention, through Feroza's and Chanda's cases, to the fact that daughters' obstinacy to marry someone they love torments their parents more than sons', while they are more likely to yield to their parents' will than sons. Against popular cultural beliefs regarding marriage, Feroza's, Mah-Jabin's, and Chanda's antagonistic voices are meeker in resisting their parents' moral stance than Charag's, Ujala's, and Samad's and their assertions. Moreover, their obstinate display of their spouses is deemed transgressive by some who cannot stomach the idea of a woman being wedded and bedded by a *gora* (a Hindi/Urdu word meaning a European or light-skinned person), because it is a disgrace for the family and community. Ironically, the same mothers grant space to their *gori bahus* (meaning a fair-skinned/European daughter-in-law) in their homes. Thus, *Maps*, *Twilight*, and *American Brat* explore the complex ways in which some men navigate their way and exercise their right to select and reject prospective brides. Society is arguably more inclined to tolerate their marital choices, and overlook their pre-/extra-marital affairs, than those of women, who in contrast must face more intense gender chauvinism and social conservatism.

Aslam, Abidi, and Sidhwa write against the backdrop of a globalised world shaped by the cross-cultural communication of people through migration, tourism, educational enterprises, etc., in which they perceive the clinging on to notions of purity of lineage, blood, and strict adherence to a caste system to be a sham. Their narratives are a means of appealing for the redress and recalibration of various orthodox, popular religious and cultural tenets in line with universal values that curb the violation of human rights and stimulate peace, harmony, justice, and equal rights. Therefore, through their narratives that also appeal for transformations of cultures that oppress women, we envisage that the growing interspace between religions, especially Islam with its stereotypical readings as a religion of gender inequality, prejudice, and discrimination, will ease and the horizon of tolerance will broaden globally. Especially for brown women, because their conditions worldwide demand and warrant urgent amelioration – especially in their roles as wives, mothers, sisters, and daughters in conjugal homes in and beyond South Asia.

Notes

1 Though we do not have the space here to expound upon them, we would like to recognise from the outset that additional theories from Talal Asad, Tahir Abbas, Mehmood Mamdani, and Akeel Bilgrami give us more sophisticated heuristic tools with which to further analyse Pakistani diasporic texts.
2 *Halala* occurs when a man who has earlier divorced a woman wants to remarry her. Islamic tradition dictates that such a woman must marry another man, consummate her marriage with him and then, after divorcing him, can return to her previous husband.
3 David Lelyveld's discussion of 'Sharif Culture' and the loaded secrecy of the female body in Eastern cultures could be an important reference (1978: 35–92). Suleri too discusses the metaphor of shame with reference to Rushdie's novel in *The Rhetoric of English India* (1992: 186).

Bibliography

Abidi, A. (2008) *Twilight*. 1st edn. New Delhi: Penguin Books.
Ahmed, R. (2017) *Writing British Muslims: Religion, Class and Multiculturalism*. Manchester: Manchester University Press.
Ahmed, R. and Mukherjee, S. (2012) 'Introduction'. In *South Asian resistances in Britain, 1858–1947*. Ed. by Ahmed, R. and Mukherjee, S. London: Continuum, xi–xxxi.
Ahmed, S. (2000) *Strange Encounters: Embodied Others in Post-Coloniality*. London: Routledge.
Aslam, N. (2005) *Maps for Lost Lovers*. London: Faber and Faber.
Brah, A. (2006) 'The "Asian" in Britain'. In *A Postcolonial People: South Asians in Britain*. Ed. by Ali, N., Kalra, V.S., and Sayyid, S. London: C. Hurst and Co., 35–61.
Butt, N. (2008) 'Between Orthodoxy and Modernity: Mapping the Transcultural Predicaments of Pakistani Immigrants in Multi-ethnic Britain'. In *Multi-ethnic Britain 2000+: New Perspectives in Literature, Film and the Arts*. Ed. by Eckstein, L. New York: Rodopi, 153–170.
Chambers, C. (2011) 'A Comparative Approach to Pakistani Fiction in English'. *Journal of Postcolonial Writing* 47(2), 122–134.
Chambers, I. (2008) *Migrancy, Culture, Identity*. London: Routledge.
Charsley, K. (2007) 'Risk, Trust, Gender and Transnational Cousin Marriage among British Pakistanis'. *Ethnic and Racial Studies* 30(6), 1117–1131. Available from <www.tandfonline.com/doi/abs/10.1080/01419870701599549> [14 April 2017].
Doshi, T. (2017) 'Nadeem Aslam: "I Know Him Vaguely"'. *The Hindu Literary Review* [online]. Available from <www.thehindu.com/books/books-authors/nadeem-aslam-i-know-him-vaguely/article18057414.ece> [10 October 2017].
Gairola, R.K. (2009) 'Capitalist Houses, Queer Homes: National Belonging and Transgressive Erotics in *My Beautiful Launderette*'. *South Asian Popular Culture* 7(1), 37–54.

Gairola, R.K. (2011) 'A Critique of Thatcherism and the Queering of Home in *Sammy and Rosie Get Laid*'. *South Asian Review* 32(3), 123–137.

Gairola, R.K. (2016) *Homelandings: Postcolonial Diasporas and Transatlantic Belonging*. London: Rowman & Littlefield International.

Halai, S. (2017) 'Hybrid Tapestries: Why Pakistani Writing in English Is Thriving'. *The Herald* [online]. Available from <http://herald.dawn.com/news/1153783> [10 October 2017].

Kain, G. (2002) 'Rupture as Continuity: Migrant Identity and "Unsettled" Perspective in Bapsi Sidhwa's *An American Brat*'. In *Asian American Literature in the International Context: Readings on Fiction, Poetry, and Performance*. Ed. by Davis, R.G. and Ludwig, S. Berlin: LitVerlag, 237–246.

Kanwal, A. (2012) 'After 9/11: Trauma, Memory, Melancholia and National Consciousness'. In *Consciousness, Theatre, Literature and the Arts 2011*. Ed. by Dinkgrafe, D.M. Newcastle: Cambridge Scholars Publishing, 57–66.

Karim, A. and Nasir, Z. (2014) 'Multiculturalism and Feminist Concerns in South Asian Diaspora Novels'. *3L: The Southeast Asian Journal of English Language Studies* 20(3), 125–134 [online]. Available from <http://ejournals.ukm.my/3l/article/view/6830> [6 May 2017].

Lelyveld, D. (1978) *Aligarh's First Generation: Muslim Solidarity in British India*. Princeton: Princeton University Press.

Mohammad, R. (2015) 'Transnational Shift: Marriage, Home and Belonging for British-Pakistani Muslim Women'. *Social and Cultural Geography* 16(6), 593–614 [online]. Available from <http://dx.doi.org/10.1080/14649365.2014.998268> [14 May 2017].

Omi, M. and Winant, H. (1994) *Racial Formation in the United States: From the 1960s to the 1990s*. New York: Routledge.

Rubin, G. (1975) 'The Traffic in Women: Notes on the Political Economy of Sex'. In *Toward an Anthropology of Women*. Ed. by Reiter, R.R. New York: Monthly Review Press, 157–210.

Santesso, E. (2013) *Disorientation: Muslim Identity in Contemporary Anglophone Literature*. Basingstoke: Palgrave Macmillan.

Schiller, N. (1998) *Towards a Transnational Perspective on Migration: Race, Class, Ethnicity, and Nationalism Reconsidered*. New York: New York Academy of Sciences.

Sheela, G. and Muthuraman, K. (2013) 'Conservative East versus Modernized West: A Study of Bapsi Sidhwa's *An American Brat*'. *Asia Pacific Journal of Research* I(XII), 17–21.

Sidhwa, B. (1994) *An American Brat*. Gurgaon: Penguin Books India.

Suleri, S. (1992) *The Rhetoric of English India*. Chicago: University of Chicago Press.

Tongur, N. (2016) 'City within a City: The Pakistani Ghetto in *Maps for Lost Lovers* by Nadeem Aslam'. In *Interdisciplinarity, Multidisciplinarity and Transdisciplinarity in Humanities*. Ed by Steele, E. Newcastle: Cambridge Scholars Publishing, 122–135.

21

BRITISH-PAKISTANI FEMALE PLAYWRIGHTS

Feminist perspectives on sexuality, marriage, and domestic violence

Aqeel Abdulla

According to the UK's last official census in 2011, British citizens with a Pakistani background are the second largest non-white British ethnic group, only slightly behind British Indians (Office for National Statistics 2012). We also learn from the British Council of Muslims' analysis of the census that 38 per cent of British Asians have a Pakistani background (Muslim Council of Britain 2015). This percentage is particularly significant when we know that British Muslims come from over 150 ethnic and national backgrounds, and that the second largest ethnic-national group amongst British Muslims is from Bangladesh, making up 14.9 per cent of British Muslims, which is less than a third of those with a Pakistani background. Most British Pakistanis either came to the UK at the same time as the large-scale immigration of South Indians in the 1960s, or are descendants of those who came in that wave of immigration; and this makes British Pakistanis not only the largest group within British Muslims, but also one of the longest-existing groups – that is, of course, if we consider waves of immigration to the UK rather than individual cases. Alongside the numbers and facts that establish the strong presence of the British-Pakistani community as a whole, there are many individual stories of high-profile success for British people with a Pakistani background, the latest and most prominent being that of the Mayor of London, Sadiq Khan. The media representation of the British-Pakistani community, however, is usually negative, and links are constantly made, directly or indirectly, between this community and issues including radicalism, forced marriage, and gangs that groom and sexually abuse teenage girls. Whether positive or negative, generalisations are dangerous; at worst, they lead to discrimination and the persecution of people who belong to a certain group due to no fault of their own; at best, treating a group as large as British Pakistanis as a monolith brings with it the danger of taking away agency and establishing assumptions about people's experiences and preferences.

Assumptions about what people from specific minority groups need or prefer are usually not in the best interests of women; Susan Muller-Okin expresses concern that giving special rights and treatment to certain minority groups may lead to patriarchal and misogynistic practices being tolerated, or even encouraged. Okin claims that 'Some proponents of group rights argue that even cultures that "flout the rights of [their individual members] in a liberal society" should be accorded group rights or privileges if their minority status endangers the culture's continued existence' (1999: 11). To further clarify this point, instead of sharing some facts and statistics, I will share an incident that happened to me personally, and very recently, which I think exemplifies the problem perfectly. At acta community theatre company where I work, in Bristol, UK, we decided to do outreach and target members of the refugee community to try to engage them in the drama sessions that we offer. As part of this outreach initiative we paid a number of visits to an organisation that supports refugee women. My co-worker and I made three visits, spoke with many women, and managed to tempt some of them to join our drama group. On the third visit, the manager of the organisation, who had invited us to come and speak to the women, came up to me and asked me very apologetically to wait outside but let my co-worker, a woman, carry on speaking to the women. I immediately complied because I assumed that one of the women present was not comfortable with having a man in the room, and I did not wish to impinge on her comfort during a weekly session that is very useful for women in her situation. I later discovered, however, that the person who asked the manager to request that I step aside is a white Englishwoman who occasionally volunteers at the centre. The same woman approached my co-worker as soon as I left and said to her, quite patronisingly, 'I don't know what kind of cultural training you as an organisation [meaning the theatre company] have. How did you think that it is okay to bring a man into a women's group?' My friend tried to explain to her that we were actually invited by the manager, that this was the third week we had been there, and that every time we came we felt welcomed by the women, that they were keen to listen to what we had to say, and that there were no signs on the door indicating that men were not allowed. The woman replied that 'These women are vulnerable and we need to be sensitive around them. You see, I have been helping refugee women for so long that I now feel I think like a Somali woman, not an Englishwoman!' As for the Somali women in the group, like whom this woman claimed to be thinking, they actually joined our drama group and had been sharing stories and playing drama games and exercises facilitated by me, a man, and my female co-facilitator for months. The group also includes Muslim women from Iran, Iraq, and Ivory Coast. In fact, Muslim women have been heavily involved with acta community theatre for years, and we have created five plays with groups of predominantly Muslim women. The group of women whom the white English volunteer was trying to protect from me are now working with me on a new play, whose topic, which they chose, is women's strength and their ability to overcome challenges and control their future. It is very clear that the volunteer was not thinking like a Somali woman at all, but rather like someone with 'white saviour' tendencies, someone who makes assumptions about Muslim women and patronises them and others in accordance with her views.

It is a sign of maturity in any community to engage in a constant process of internal observation and self-criticism that challenges the status quo, especially when it relates to social and gender issues. This becomes a necessity even, and not just a duty, when one is surrounded in wider society by a colonial mindset that still maintains the right to patronise minority groups, and still gives itself a mandate to 'protect' them. This chapter is an attempt to show how three feminist British-Pakistani playwrights, Alia Bano, Nadia Manzoor, and Emteaz Hussain, are taking on this responsibility to comment on the issue of gender in their society, with all the different layers and definitions of the word 'society' in mind.

Dimple Godiwala writes that 'British Asian theatre is constructed through differences in acculturation, as it is modified through intercultural exchange and socialisation, avoiding the false representation produced by rigidly antithetical and binary categories which lead to a need for "authenticity" and "elitism"' (2006: 103). This is clearly the case with the current wave of new feminist British-Pakistani playwrights to which Bano, Manzoor, and Hussain belong. These playwrights are not trying to speak on behalf of a group or to offer an 'authentic' representation' of them or of the issues that concern them, rather they are trying to offer perspectives and provocations to drive discussion of issues they are passionate about. The current British-Asian theatre companies have all been founded on the principle that British Asians need to be represented and their culture needs to be present within wider British culture. Tara Arts was founded in 1977 as a response to the murder of a Sikh boy by white English fascists (Hingorani 2010: 14), and the founding members were mostly university students who had no experience of drama but wanted to counter political and social racism artistically (Dadswell and Ley 2011: 13). Seeking to represent one's culture and heritage is not, therefore, a problem in itself, but authors, artists, and dramatists need to be careful not to be controlled by a perceived need to represent culture and tradition 'authentically' because, as Godiwala puts it, 'the pursuit of the preservation of these [traditions], fossilizes them' (2006: 12). In short, when the British-Asian community needed a way to remind wider British society that they exist, and that they are neither a marginal nor a temporary presence in the UK, this is exactly what British-Asian theatre companies did, by bringing their culture and art forms to British stages. However, since 9/11 and the 7/7 bombings, a certain section of the British-Asian community (i.e. Muslims, and particularly Muslim women) has faced a different challenge, which is to counter the patronisation and manipulation to which they are subjected by two opposing camps in Britain: one with a colonial mindset that wants to 'liberate' Muslim women, and one with a traditionalist/radical mindset within the Muslim-Pakistani community that wants to 'protect' Muslim women from being Westernised.

After Tara Arts was established in 1977, and Tamasha Theatre in 1989, South Asian women playwrights have seen added support since 1991, when Kali Theatre, who prides itself on being 'the UK's only theatre company dedicated to championing women writers from a South Asian background', was founded. Over the last decade in particular, a new wave of young female playwrights have provided us with plays with strong feminist messages, and I will look at how Bano, Manzoor, and Hussain have engaged with the issues of marriage, sexuality, and domestic violence in ways that defy taboos and expectations.

Sexuality and Marriage

Controlling the sexuality of women is probably the most important, or at least most visible, aspect of patriarchal control over women. I will state the obvious here and say that I find the drive to have dominion over women's sexuality to be a cross-cultural patriarchal practice, and not in any way exclusive to Muslim societies. However, different patriarchal practices have different manifestations and intensities in different societies due to many circumstances, and sexuality is an issue that is undeniably intensely sensitive in Muslim societies. In her attempt to analyse Muslim men's particular fixation with controlling women's sexuality, renowned Moroccan feminist theorist Fatima Mernissi argues that there is an explicit and an implicit theory regarding attitudes towards women's sexuality in Islam:

> The explicit theory is the prevailing contemporary belief that men are aggressive in their interaction with women, and women are passive. The implicit theory, driven far further into the Muslim unconscious, is epitomized in Imam Ghazali's classical work. He sees civilization as struggling to contain women's destructive, all-absorbing power. Women must be controlled to prevent men from being distracted from their social and religious duties. Society can survive only by creating institutions that can foster male dominance through sexual segregation and polygamy for believers.
>
> (2000a: 22)

This explicit theory about women's sexuality in Islam, Mernissi argues, leads to two different rhetorics: the first is the misogynistic belief that women enjoy playing the role of victim, a prey awaiting the hunter, a subordinate awaiting the leader. The other rhetoric accepts the premise that women's sexuality is *fitna* (an Arabic word that means 'seduction', 'disorder', or both in some contexts), but rejects the belief that it is entirely women's responsibility to protect society from this *fitna* by covering up. Proponents of this rhetoric argue that men too have a responsibility to fight this *fitna* by practising self-control, and that focusing only on women covering up is unjust, and also suggests that men, not women, are the weaker sex because they are unable to control their sexual desires.

The sensitivities around women's sexuality in Muslim families in the UK are present in most of the contemporary plays written by British-Pakistani writers, and I will focus on Bano's *Shades* (2009), with a brief reference to *Hens* (2010), to see how her writing deals with issues and tensions related to Mernissi's implicit and explicit theories about women's sexuality in Islam. I will also look at how Nadia Manzoor exposes and satirises these sex-related tensions in a strict British-Pakistani family.

Bano is a London-based British playwright, born and raised in Birmingham by her parents who came to the UK from Pakistan in the 1960s. *Shades*, Bano's first full-length play, was commissioned by the Royal Court Theatre and premiered in January 2009. In an interview I did with Bano in London on 9 March 2012, she said:

> In a way, [the play] was a microcosm of the world I inhabit [...] I tend to write about things that annoy me, or that I have questions about. If I don't know the answer I write a play to see if somebody can give me the answer.

Just like Bano at the time of writing *Shades*, Sabrina, the protagonist, is a Muslim woman in her twenties who lives and works in London, away from her family. She is single and eager to get married, so she tries her luck with Muslim speed-dating! The play actually starts at a Muslim speed-dating event; Sabrina is sitting at a table waiting for the next person to join her, feeling out of place and eager to leave. Her next 'date', Ali, is nice looking, but he is 'the *haram* police', as Sabrina puts it. He wastes no time in addressing how she dresses, and her unconventional job (an events organiser). Proving Sabrina's worries were justified, Ali's questions become a long interrogation:

ALI An events organizer- [...] So, you're a party girl [...] Perhaps another occupation might be more suitable [...] You must work late at nights [...] Aren't you scared as a woman [...] Are you seriously looking? [...] How do you think your partner would feel about you working late? [...] How religious are you? [...] Do you pray? [...] Do you drink? [...] Have you ever been in a relationship? [...] Have you ever been out with someone? [...] I just can't believe someone with your looks and dress hasn't –
SAB Hasn't what?
PAUSE. Ali tries to choose his words carefully.
ALI – attracted the attention of the opposite sex.
SAB Right. (*Beat.*) What about you?
ALI What about me?
SAB Have you ever 'attracted the attention of the opposite sex'?
ALI I don't think I'm going to answer that question.
SAB Then neither am I.

(Bano 2009: 5–7)

This conversation in scene one establishes the main issue of the play; a young, liberal Muslim woman tries to balance the two worlds to which she belongs: her Muslim British-Pakistani family, and her liberal independent life. She does not wish to break away from her Pakistani and Muslim identities, but she is also not prepared to play the role of traditional housewife. Sabrina expresses this inner conflict again in scene two, in a conversation with Zain, her flatmate. Zain asks her what kind of guy she is looking for:

SAB Just a normal guy.
ZAIN There's plenty out there.
SAB Just wish they were Muslim.
ZAIN Stick to wanting diamonds.
SAB I just want someone with a pulse and a brain. And that's hard to find round here. [...]
ZAIN So log onto shaadi.com
SAB [...] I only did it for about five minutes. I was attracting the wrong types. I was attracting the really religious types. God knows why.
ZAIN Just face it: you want to marry a white guy.
SAB Marry a white guy when there's millions of Pakis about? My mother would just love that.

(Bano 2009: 9–10)

In the first few scenes Bano introduces Sabrina as someone who hates being Muslim and Pakistani, someone only looking for a Muslim Pakistani husband because she does not want to upset her family. So far, one can see one-dimensional characters that represent opposite ends of the divide between liberal and traditional British Pakistanis, or British Muslims in general. When Ali asks Sabrina how religious she is, she answers, 'I never know how to answer this question. I mean, how do you measure religiousness?' (Bano 2009: 6). And in scene two, when Sabrina and Zain are contemplating whether she is getting too old to be a suitable Asian wife, Zain says: 'Look, when you hit thirty, just stick on a scarf. Your marriage rating would go up' (Bano 2009: 10). One can sense there is no mutual respect between the two sides of the divide; in fact, when Zain, who also works with Sabrina as an 'events organiser', wants to punish her for being late in scene three, he could not think of a worse punishment than to partner her with Reza, a volunteer who is a devout Muslim, and the son of a scholar. However, building Sabrina's character in this way at the beginning only adds to the intensity and complexity of the plot that ensues. Instead of another judgemental member of the '*haram* police', as she expected, Sabrina finds Reza to be an open-minded, loving, and compassionate person. From their first encounter, Reza acknowledges his differences with Sabrina and talks about them openly and light-heartedly, which immediately puts Sabrina at ease. To complicate things, Ali – from the speed-dating event – is ominously revealed to be Reza's friend. In the following scenes, Sabrina and Reza start falling for each other, much to the disappointment of Ali who, since their first encounter, interpreted Sabrina's attitude, job, and dress as indicators that she is someone with whom he can have casual sex. Ali tries to sabotage the emerging relationship between Reza and Sabrina by telling Nazia, Reza's elder sister, that Sabrina hit on him and he had to push her away. Initially, Ali's plan works, and with the help of Nazia, Reza decides to remove himself from Sabrina's project in order not to get further attached to her. However, the play ends with hope as Reza discovers Ali's lies, so he comes with his parents to the charity event that he was helping Sabrina to organise and asks her to meet them.

Sexuality and all the tensions and stereotypes associated with it in Muslim society are at the heart of the plot of *Shades*. Ali, Nazia, and Reza are clearly threatened and alarmed by elements of Sabrina's lifestyle which they interpret as sexual liberty: her dress code, the fact that she shares a flat with men, and that her job entails working at night. Ali is so sure of his analysis of Sabrina's character that he even asks her, suspiciously, at the speed-dating event whether she was seriously looking for a husband. The hypocrisies and contradictions that Mernissi points out in her explicit and implicit theories are reflected in Ali's simultaneous disrespect for Sabrina because of her sexuality, and his lust after her for the same reason. Moreover, Bano avoids a clichéd ending in which Reza and Sabrina reconcile and get together after he apologises for making negative assumptions about her. Instead, she reluctantly agrees to see Reza's parents after her friends encourage and reassure her that they will be there for her no matter what comes out of meeting them. This ending seems like a commitment from Bano to show the extent of the gap between people with liberal and traditional attitudes towards sexuality in a Muslim community. The ending suggests that reconciliation between the two worlds is a work in progress.

Following the success of *Shades*, Bano won the Charles Wintour Award in 2009 for Most Promising Playwright at the Evening Standard Awards. In 2010, she wrote her second play, *Hens*, which is about a group of young women – three from a Pakistani background, and one white English – on a hen do weekend in Paris. The main theme of the play is the expectation in traditional, conservative Asian families that a woman is supposed to dedicate herself to her husband and his family after marriage, which will naturally affect friendships and individual aspirations, perhaps even destroy them. Another theme is how these women negotiate the boundaries of what is considered acceptable or unacceptable by Muslim standards when it comes to behaviour and dress codes. As in *Shades*, Bano offers a non-stereotypical portrayal of British Muslim women in *Hens*, and addresses the issue in a way that focuses on personal stories rather than a generic representation. The three girls from Pakistani families are portrayed as liberal and outgoing, whereas the white woman, who is married to one of their brothers, is the one wearing a *hijab* and constantly criticising how the others are dressed.

Manzoor's *Burq Off!* takes an in-your-face and uncompromising approach to the subject of female sexuality. It is a one-woman autobiographical play, written and performed by Manzoor, who is also the founder of the company that produced the play, Paprika Productions. The play was first performed in December 2013 in New York, and I saw it at the Cockpit Theatre in London in September 2014. Manzoor tells her life story from when she was a little girl until she left her family home at the age of twenty-one. She offers a comedic narration of her story, exploring themes of identity (British, Pakistani, and Muslim), gender roles, and sexuality. One childhood story early in the play establishes the topic of the paranoia surrounding sex within traditionalist Muslim families. Young Nadia innocently shows her father a letter that she wrote to a boy at school in which she tells him that she wants to lie under silky sheets and 'do sex' with him, just like in the TV show *Dallas*. Nadia mentions earlier in the play that she was always taught not to say the word 'vagina', and every time she says it her mother would say 'shame, shame', so when she shows the letter to her father and he angrily shouts 'where's your shame?', she innocently points to her vagina and says 'Abbu? Shame, Shame?', and she receives a slap in the face.

Sex, according to Nadia the narrator, is not a subject that exists in the Pakistani family, or even in Pakistani movies. She mockingly dances to a song from a famous Pakistani movie, and at the end of the dance mimes how she suddenly has a baby in her hands. The narrator says that this is how babies are born in Pakistani movies: through dance and a spiritual love, but no sex! Later in the play we come to the story of how Nadia loses her virginity at university, and in complete contrast to the way the song and dance portray the physical relationship that produces a baby, Manzoor makes sure her portrayal of Nadia's first sexual experience is as raw as possible (within the limitations of a one-woman show!). Manzoor replicates the positions, the awkwardness, the pain, the intense facial expressions, the noises and moans, and the ridiculousness of a man's face when he climaxes!

There are two very symbolic scenes in the play that depict two different experiences in her life, and represent very well the inner conflict and identity crisis that Nadia has had to deal with throughout the play. In the first, teenage Nadia goes on the *hajj* (pilgrimage to Mecca) with her family, and there she wears a *burqa* for the first time in her life. Nadia says, 'I stepped out, into the dusty streets of Mecca. I was a Muslim in a *burqa*'. She then comes from one corner of the stage, eerie music playing, a spotlight on her, and dimmed light on the stage, walking very awkwardly and obviously self-conscious, and starts moving her hands, which are covered by the *burqa*, as if she is discovering now that she is actually completely covered. Suddenly, she becomes comfortable, the music changes to happy dance music, and Nadia dances around excitedly, including on a table that is a central prop throughout the play. At a later point, adult Nadia lies to her parents about spending a week at her white English friend's home, when actually they were going to Majorca together. There, Katy convinces her to get rid of the burqini that her mother brought her from Pakistan and wear a bikini instead. The moment in the *burqa* in Mecca is repeated again: 'I tied the three pieces of string around my boobs and stepped out, onto the sandy beaches of Majorca. I was a Muslim in a bikini'. Nadia then comes from the other corner of the stage, walking as awkwardly as she had in Mecca, looking very embarrassed, trying to hide her breasts with her hands, and mimes pulling down her bikini bottom to cover more of her bum, while the spotlight is on her and the same eerie music from the Mecca scene plays. Then, again mirroring the scene from Mecca, she suddenly becomes comfortable and repeats the same excited dance as before, around the stage and on the table. Manzoor is clearly trying to depict here the two extremes between which a young British Muslim female is torn, and the contradiction is very visually apparent when it comes to the body of a woman and her dress code. The two scenes also show that Nadia is not completely comfortable in either of the two situations; and indeed, the play ends with her making the decision to leave home after her mother's death. She says that she had to leave,

> Not through imagination and out of the window, not by covering myself up in layers of cloth, nor by taking it all off. But through the front door, of my home, one foot in front of the other, with only one possible destination.

Domestic Violence

In *Feminist Thought: A Comprehensive Introduction*, Rosemarie Tong quotes fellow feminists Alison Jaggar and Paula Rothenberg's five reasons why they and other feminists believe that 'women's oppression is the most fundamental form of oppression' (1989: 71). One of these reasons is that 'women's oppression is the most widespread, existing in virtually every known society' (1989: 71). This concept of the universality of women's causes is never truer than in the very domestic sphere of the family. Patriarchal societies insist on placing the woman in second place, behind the man, and they propagate the idea that it is a necessity for family and society, if they are to function, that men should always lead and protect their women.

In Islam, the position and role of the woman in the family, and the degree of power and control that a man has over a woman, is certainly a thorny and controversial issue where theory and practice can be, and usually are, at odds. The Qur'an and a plethora of stories from the life of the Prophet Muhammad prove that in the historic, social, and geographic context within which Islam emerged, Islamic laws related to women (marriage, family, inheritance, etc.) were actually progressive and a step forward for women. As Ziba Mir-Hosseini points out, the tradition of patriarchy in Islamic jurisprudence comes mainly from classical jurists between the twelfth and sixteenth century, not from the Qur'an. She quotes these jurists who describe marriage as 'a contract whose object is that of dominion over the vagina, without the right of its possession' (2009: 29). Similarly, marriage is described as 'a kind of slavery, for a wife is a slave to her husband. She owes her husband absolute obedience in whatever he demands of her, where she herself is concerned, as long as no sin is involved' (Mir-Hosseini 2009: 30). Mir-Hosseini shows that many misogynistic *fatwa*s and rulings are social, traditional, regional, and archaic, but because of the revered status of the jurists who issued them, they 'were sanctified, and then turned into fixed entities of *fiqh* [jurisprudence]. That is, rather than considering them as social, thus temporal institutions and phenomena, the classical jurists treated them as "divinely ordained", thus immutable' (2009: 33). *Bahishti Zewar* ('Heavenly Ornaments') is a perfect example of what Mir-Hosseini's work describes. It is a book written about a hundred years ago by a famous Indian religious scholar called Ashraf Ali Thanwi, and it teaches women how to be good wives and mothers. Anyone with even a basic knowledge of the Qur'an and *hadith* can easily see as they read through this book that its most misogynistic rulings and *fatwa*s have no basis in these two main sources of Islamic law, in fact it sometimes contradicts key concepts in the Qur'an and *hadith*. Nevertheless, this book is a popular gift for future brides in the South Asian Muslim community.

The line between leadership and protection, on the one hand, and control on the other, can be blurred, and usually is. Similarly, the line between patriarchal control and domestic violence is also blurred. This is particularly evident in communities/cultures that create a direct link between a woman's sexuality and her honour, and then between her honour and the family's/community's honour. Such belief is not in any way exclusive to a certain religion or society, but it has a strong resonance with the more traditionalist components of Muslim Pakistani communities due to the factors mentioned above, and also due to the sensitivities around sexuality that I discussed in the previous section of this chapter.

Arranged, or even forced, marriages and insistence on the woman's pre-marriage virginity are the two main reasons behind the violence and crimes committed against Muslim women. One common reason behind the crimes against Muslim and Asian women in the UK is the rejection of an arranged marriage (Siddiqui 2005). Another common reason for so-called 'honour killings' is the discovery that a bride was not virgin on her wedding night. In fact, Nawal El-Saadawi (1998) recounts a practice in rural areas in Egypt where the wedding party does not end before the mother of the bride proudly displays to the guests a piece of blood-stained white cloth that proves that her daughter was a virgin and has just been deflowered. A forced marriage is often used to hide a family's shame when they discover that their daughter has had a relationship (Carroll 2000: 245). In Syria, it was not rare for me as I grew up to hear stories about families who tried to hide the shame of a daughter losing her virginity before marriage (or sometimes even the shame of her being seen publicly with her lover) by meeting with the lover's family and arranging a quick marriage. As a teenager at school, I personally knew people who were hurriedly and forcibly married this way; in fact, most people married in this way, especially girls, are usually teenagers. In some cases the police will mediate the proceedings and give a young man who has deflowered a teenager the choice of either marrying her or going to jail.

British playwright and performance poet Hussain has personal experience of domestic violence because she escaped the family home to go to a women's refuge at the age of sixteen. Her first play, *Sweet Cider*, produced in 2008 by Tamasha, is about Tazeen, Nosheen, and Jasvinder, three Asian teenagers who run away from their families to a refuge. Jasvinder is Sikh, and she escapes her family because she is in love with a Muslim boy, Aki. She eventually comes to the realisation that Aki is never going to marry her, so she leaves the refuge without telling anyone, which leaves them worried about her fate. Nosheen and Tazeem, the main characters of the play, are both Muslims from Pakistani families. Nosheen escapes because when she tells her family that her uncle tried to molest her, they warned her to keep quiet and not to repeat her claims to anyone. She is saddened by the fact that her family did not make any effort to find her, as if they are relieved that she left. She is a sceptical and angry character who does not trust people easily, and self-harms. We do not know why Tazeem escaped, but we see her father meeting a bounty hunter whom he pays to find her and bring her back. The mood of the play is generally ominous and eerie, and this is particularly apparent in three scenes. First, when Tazeem's father, Fiaz, meets Mahmood the bounty hunter:

FIAZ Hey, they call you the bounty-hunter ey na?
MAHMOOD No, no, no, not the bounty-hunter, not me. Me, me, I'm a community mediator. I keep families together.
FIAZ Don't know who she thinks she is kutee [bitch] breaking up the family, our family, my family [...] these young ones they don't understand, they have no idea how hard we've worked, what we've had to deal with, what we've had to do. Do you understand bhai? They have no idea, they've got it easy, so easy in this country [...] They don't understand bhai, they don't understand what we've been through, our ways, our culture, ey zoroori gal hai [important] so important it's family, it's who we are, izzat you understand is everything, understand, it's who you are. It's who we are, identity, izzat. Got to protect it. Stop it from dying away.

(Hussain in Robson and Gillieron 2013: 208–209)

Mahmood's confidence, tone, and body language are ominous and convey a sense of inevitability, especially as he says, 'Most of the time I don't need to use my stick', and repeats the phrase 'once they're in my car, they're alright' twice in his conversation with Fiaz. Moreover, his conversation with Fiaz, the way he describes himself as a community mediator, and the way he talks about protecting *izzat* ('honour') and family portray him as a representative of the type of oppressive patriarchal system that Tazeem is escaping. When Mahmood eventually finds Tazeem, this sense of inevitability about him and what he represents is present again; he comes face to face with her in the park where she hangs out with Nosheen, she looks behind her and sees another man approaching, then Mahmood signals to her with his finger to come and, as if surrendering to her fate, she goes to him without even attempting to escape.

Hussain's second play, *Blood*, produced in 2015, also by Tamasha, is about a young couple, Caneeze and Sully, who fall in love, but are not supposed to. Caneez's brother, Saif, is a notorious local gangster who has plans for his sister's future that do not include a broke student like Sully. We only see Caneez and Sully in the play, but we are introduced to other characters through their speech, which most of the time is directed straight to the audience as narration.

On his way to the airport, where he is supposed to meet Caneez to travel together to Egypt for a week, Sully is attacked by Saif's thugs. They warn him not to get in touch with Caneez again, or next time they will break her knee caps instead of his. He ends up in hospital and stays away from Caneez, who is ignorant of what has happened, and so thinks that Sully has abandoned her. We are then introduced to another character, Yousuf, Saif's friend and a suitor for Caneez who has the blessing of the family. After initially appearing to be friendly and compassionate, Yousuf ends up taking advantage of a time when Caneez is at home alone, and he rapes her. Caneez escapes with Sully because she realises that her brother and mother are aware of the truth about Yousuf, and yet take his side. In hiding, we see Caneez writing a message to her mother on her laptop, she faces the audience and the message becomes a moving soliloquy:

> Dear Amma,
> I hate you for taking Saif's blood money […]
> I hate that you don't question it
> I hate you for not listening to me
> Thinking about me
> I hate that you put what other people think above what I think or feel […]
> [Yousuf] hurt me bad
> really bad […]
> under our roof […]
> and I hate him for what he did to me
> and what he's doing to you
> and I hate you because you're too fuckin' stupid
> but I know you're not stupid, Amma
> you just don't see […]
> 'n' I hate you for choosing not to see.
>
> (Hussain 2015, 67–68)

Although the topic and plot of *Blood* are as dark as in *Sweet Cider*, one can feel that Hussain made a decision to make this play more optimistic and light-hearted. The first half of the play was pleasant to watch, a feel-good teenage love story between two characters who are funny and adventurous. Obviously, the play takes a bad turn when Sully is attacked and the drama starts to unfold, but the very last action of the play makes the audience smile again: while the couple are in hiding and quite paranoid about Saif and his thugs finding them, they hear something outside their door. Sully goes to check, and when he comes back he acts as if he has been shot or stabbed, Caneez is terrified, then he laughs and we realise he is just teasing her to lighten the mood, and the play ends with the two laughing and kissing.

Reflection

As I said at the beginning of this chapter, Bano, Manzoor, and Hussain emerged among a new wave of feminist British-Pakistani playwrights and, more generally, a wave of British-Muslim feminist playwrights. It is a new genre of Muslim feminist writing that is trying to balance the narratives and debates about Muslim women that have been hijacked by politics, self-appointed community leaders, radical religious speakers, and the manipulative and sensationalist British media.

The general atmosphere within which British-Pakistani feminist playwrights work and produce new writing is one in which Muslim women are being pulled in different directions in what looks like a game of cultural and political tug-of-war. One side is trying to pull them towards a traditional and uncompromising understanding of what it means to be a Muslim woman, an understanding that is patriarchal and misogynistic. The other side is pulling them towards a hegemonic, and also uncompromising, understanding of what it means to be British. Bano, Manzoor, and Hussain are clearly rejecting both camps.

Bibliography

Bano, A. (2009) *Shades*. London: Methuen Drama.

Bhabha, H.K. (2004) *The Location of Culture*. London: Routledge.

Carroll, L. (2000) 'Arranged Marriages: Law, Custom and the Muslim Girl in the UK'. In *Women and Sexuality in Muslim Societies*. Ed. by Ilkkaracan, P. Istanbul: Women for Women's Rights, 245–251.

Daboo, J. (2012) 'Mixing with the Mainstream: Transgressing the Identity of Place'. In *British South Asian Theatre: Critical Essays*. Ed. by Ley, P.G. and Dadswell, D.S. Exeter: University of Exeter Press, 154–169.

Dadswell, S. and Ley, G. (2011) *British South-Asian Theatres: A Documented History*. Exeter: University of Exeter Press.

Gilliat-Ray, S. (2010) *Muslims in Britain: An Introduction*. Cambridge: Cambridge University Press.

Godiwala, D. (2006) *Alternatives within the Mainstream: British Black and Asian Theatres*. Newcastle: Cambridge Scholars Press.

Hingorani, D. (2010) *British Asian Theatre: Dramaturgy, Process, and Performance*. Basingstoke: Palgrave.

Hussain, E. (2013). 'Sweet Cider'. In *Plays for Today by Women*. Ed. by Gillieron, R. and Robson, C. Twickenham: Aurora Metro Publications.

Hussain, E. (2015). *Blood*. London: Bloomsbury.

Mernissi, F. (2000a) 'The Muslim Concept of Active Women's Sexuality'. In *Women and Sexuality in Muslim Societies*. Ed. by Ilkkaracan, P. Istanbul: Women for Women's Rights, 19–35.

Mernissi, F. (2000b) 'Virginity and Patriarchy'. In *Women and Sexuality in Muslim Societies*. Ed. by Ilkkaracan, P. Istanbul: Women for Women's Rights, 203–214.

Mir-Hosseini, Z. (2009) 'Towards Gender Equality: Muslim Family Laws and the Sharia'. In *Wanted: Equality and Justice in the Muslim Family*. Ed. by Anwar, Z. Petaling Jaya: Musawah, 23–64.

Muslim Council of Britain. (2015) *British Muslims in Numbers* [online]. Available from <www.mcb.org.uk/wp-content/uploads/2015/02/MCBCensusReport_2015.pdf > [1 September 2015].

Okin, S. (1999) 'Is Multiculturalism Bad for Women?' In *Is Multiculturalism Bad for Women?* Ed. by Cohen, J.H. Princeton: Princeton University Press, 9–24.

Office for National Statistics. (2012) *Ethnicity and National Identity in England and Wales: 2011*. [online]. Available from <www.ons.gov.uk/peoplepopulationandcommunity/culturalidentity/ethnicity/articles/ethnicityandnationalidentityinenglandandwales/2012-12-11> [1 September 2015].

Saadawi, N. (1998) *The Nawal El Saadawi Reader*. New York: St. Martin's Press.

Siddiqui, H. (2005). 'There is no "Honour" in Domestic Violence, Only Shame! Women's Struggles against "Honour" Crimes in the UK'. In *Honour: Crimes, Paradigms, and Violence Against Women*. Ed. by Welchman, L.A. London: Zed Books, 263–281.

Thanwi, A. (n.d.). Bahishti Zewar. *Islamic Bulletin* [online]. Available from <www.islamicbulletin.org/free_downloads/women/bahishti_1_2_3.pdf> [1 September 2015].

Tong, R. (1992) *Feminist Thought: A Comprehensive Introduction*. London: Routledge.

PART VI

Shifting contexts
New perspectives on identity, space, and mobility

22
IDENTIFYING ISLAMIC SPACES OF WORSHIP IN CONTEMPORARY BRITISH-PAKISTANI MUSLIM LIFE WRITING

Georgia Stabler

Contemporary British-Pakistani Muslim life writing is a literary subgenre that has received considerable interest from major UK literature festivals, the publishing industry, and the media in recent years. These texts are often positioned as a response to major political events concerning British Muslim communities, or as narratives solely concerned with depicting aspects of British-Pakistani life that feature heavily in national debates, such as assimilation, arranged marriage, or the reconciliation of simultaneous 'Muslim', 'British', and 'Pakistani' identities. In addition, the life writing market in the West increasingly propagates narratives about Muslim women that Claire Chambers has categorised as 'misery memoirs' (2013: 81), and male autobiographies about Islamic militancy or fundamentalism. By focusing only on these narratives, the UK publishing industry fails to recognise the genre's diversity and instead presents a simplistic and partial view of British-Pakistani writers and the communities they discuss. This chapter moves away from a negative, homogenising discourse to explore a facet of British-Pakistani Muslim life writing that is often overlooked: the presence and function of private, public, and global Islamic spaces of worship. By drawing attention to the role of particular sites as contexts of negotiation where a range of Muslim identities are negotiated, celebrated, or resisted (including the home, the mosque, and the Ka'ba in Mecca), I analyse how different aspects of British-Pakistani Muslim identity are articulated and present an alternative avenue of investigation into the genre. Further, the foregrounding of 'space' avoids the tendency to overdetermine the homogeneity of Muslim subjectivities or interpret contemporary British-Pakistani Muslim life writing chiefly as a response to Islamic terrorism. The texts explored in this chapter offer insight into how Muslim spaces are connected, the ways in which they shape the British landscape, and also the role they play in the writers' construction of self, and their relationship with Islam. Finally, a discussion about intergenerational outlooks on Islamic spaces of worship, the impact of religious traditions in the home, and the significance of undertaking the time-honoured *hajj* pilgrimage to Mecca will reveal how identities are construed in a constant interplay of one's orientation to the past and the future in these life writing texts.

Although this chapter is primarily concerned with writers of Pakistani heritage, a British Muslim writer of East African descent, Shelina Zahra Janmohamed, will be examined alongside them in order to comment upon the homogenous presentation of Muslim life writing in the UK literary marketplace. Close textual analysis reveals significant parallels between the writers' treatment of formal, public religious sites (i.e. mosques) and informal, private spaces, such as the domestic kitchen. I compare moments of intersection in the texts between public and domestic religious spaces, for example, during the Islamic forty-day period of mourning and the Night of Power.[1] These episodes often inspire revelatory or profound reflections. Mecca emerges as the physical centre of Islam, and as a space that inspires transnational connections, reiterating the idea of the global *ummah*. These readings also support Sidonie Smith and Julia Watson's theoretical approach to autobiographical writing, which highlights the interconnectedness of space and subjectivity. They suggest that we, 'as subjects are bodies inhabiting space; but more important, we are positioned subjects, in and [out] of place' (2010: 42). The focus on both the 'location' and the 'position' of a narrator has importantly reshaped thinking about life writing. These concepts, which are both inescapably spatial, are increasingly understood as the juncture from which self-articulation is formed in life writing texts. Thus, it is timely to observe this juncture in specific life writing texts by British-Pakistani Muslims and investigate the impact of different personal, social, and public places of Islamic worship on British Muslim subjectivity.

The more marketable memoirs by British-Pakistani writers are often texts about Muslims that have been categorised as 'misery memoirs' (Chambers 2013: 81). These popular narratives often describe the abuse, forced marriage, or kidnapping of passive, oppressed Muslim females. Running parallel to the so-called misery memoirs are the male autobiographies about Islamism wherein the individual documents a journey of indoctrination into radical Islam, and subsequent alienation from these movements. Notable examples include Ed Husain's *The Islamist: Why I Joined Radical Islam in Britain, What I Saw Inside and Why I Left* (2007) and Maajid Nawaz's *Radical: My Journey from Islamist Extremism to a Democratic Awakening* (2013). The dominance of these strands of British-Pakistani life writing serve to prop up a discourse in the West about Pakistani Muslim communities that is inherently negative (see Hirsi Ali 2006; Manji 2004). However, numerous contemporary life writing texts by British-Pakistani Muslim writers challenge this presentation. Notable memoirs published in the mid- to late 2000s include Sarfraz Manzoor's *Greetings from Bury Park* (2007), Zaiba Malik's *We are a Muslim, Please* (2011), and Yasmin Hai's *The Making of Mr Hai's Daughter: Becoming British* (2008). These writers, who are also linked by their shared background in journalism, received considerable exposure during a time when postcolonial memoirs were gaining prestige and becoming well-known worldwide (Jelodar et al. 2013: 216). They were also born and experienced childhood in 1970s/1980s Britain, were young adults in the 1990s, and came of age when the so-called 'Salman Rushdie Affair', 7/7, and 9/11 made them increasingly conscious of their cultural and religious backgrounds. Although approached from different angles, these texts are generally perceived as being shaped by a shared thematic preoccupation with family, Britishness, culture, and attempts by the writer to reconcile their composite identities in a way which allows them to be both British and Asian.

Pakistani communities emerged in Britain in the period following the 1948 Nationalism Act, predominantly in industrial towns and inner-city areas with viable employment opportunities, and it was in these areas where settlers created new religious institutions as well as 'transnational cultural and social spaces for themselves' (Hopkins 2007: 3) Investment in these spaces (which include businesses and facilities that serve the needs of the dominant Muslim community) quickly led to certain British inner-city areas being re-envisioned primarily as places of Muslim settlement. One such area is Bradford in northern England, Malik's hometown. In the first chapter of her memoir, entitled 'The Found City', Malik maps out Bradford as a city connected by distinctly Pakistani Muslim places. She describes how cultural and religious infrastructure was establishing itself in 1970s Britain and the ways in which the area, once principally defined through its industrial production and output of worsted wool (Malik labels it 'Worstedopolis' 2011: 37), was being rewritten by its newly settled Pakistani communities as 'Bradistan. A home from home for the Pakistanis' (2011: 37):

> For the thirty thousand or so of us in the city, there was a process of 'settlement by tiptoe' – we took on some aspects of British life by working in its factories and sending our kids to its schools, but preserved Pakistani life through language, religion and culture. [...] We established our own mosques and madrasas; we ran our own businesses – goldsmiths, curry houses, fabric shops; we even set up our own entertainment in the form of Asian record shops and cinemas.
>
> (Malik 2011: 36)

Malik's description corroborates Hanif Kureishi's articulation of Bradford[2] as a place with a significant Pakistani influence: 'If I ignored the dark Victorian buildings around me, I could imagine that everyone was back in their village in Pakistan' (1986: n.p.). Both Malik and Kureishi describe a perceived friction that exists in Bradford between spaces defined by England's industrial past and those being shaped dramatically by and for a growing Pakistani presence. Kureishi notes the businesses from a bygone era, such as 'drapers, ironmongers, fish and chip shops that still used newspaper wrappers', that evoke memories of his 'English grandfather and the Britain of my childhood: pigeon keeping, greyhound racing, roast beef eating and pianos in pubs' (1986: n.p.). This nostalgic image is juxtaposed with the burgeoning infrastructure that caters to Bradford's large Asian Muslim populations:

> the Islamic Library and the Ambala Sweet Centre where you could buy spices: dhaniya, haldi, garam masala, and dhal and ladies' fingers. There were Asian video shops where you could buy tapes of the songs of Master Sajjad, Nayyara, Alamgir, Nazeen and M. Ali Shahaiky.
>
> (Kureishi 1986: n.p.)

These texts acknowledge and reinforce the religious and ethnic identifications that have come to be associated with Bradford as it continues to be shaped by its Pakistani/South Asian communities. Both Malik and Kureishi recognise Bradford as a location of diaspora and settlement, they read the area as a shifting cultural space which has been heavily affected by a process of deindustrialisation and an increasingly significant Pakistani presence. The 'settlement by tiptoe' effect in Bradford in the 1970s and '80s allowed the area to be understood geopolitically as a space of negotiation and of erasure, whereby the remaining post-war 'English' businesses existed alongside, and were boosted by, an economy generated by large-scale immigration and settlement in the area.

Businesses founded by Muslim migrants were often driven by economic motives, rather than religious ones, with religious structures providing an important personal and collective resource 'once settled in Britain' (Gilliat-Ray 2010: 45). As Anshuman Mondal highlights, 'For many Muslims of the older generation, the observance of Islam was less about piety and more to do with participation in communal life' (2008: 4–5). The performance of rituals, attending the mosque, and fasting during Ramadan, whether sincerely undertaken or not, are aspects of Muslim existence which form a social life and a semblance of community for the older generation of Pakistani immigrants. This attitude is certainly true for Sarfraz Manzoor's father, Mohammed Manzoor, who arrived in Britain in 1963 from Karachi as an economic migrant 'consumed with a passion for self-improvement' (2007: 26). Finding Britain to be a hostile environment for a newly settled Pakistani immigrant, Mohammed 'drew his strength from his community' (2007: 7). However, as industry declined, many Muslim communities suffered from mass redundancies, deprivation, and discrimination. In an early episode of his memoir, Manzoor describes how the loss of his father's job impacted the whole family both emotionally and economically. Throughout his unemployment Mohammed made himself useful, assisting other Pakistani immigrants secure mortgages by negotiating with bank managers on their behalf, or by assisting with passport and visa problems (2007: 37–38). Alongside its primary religious function, the mosque provided a space where members of the community could share advice and information and provide administrative assistance. For Mohammed, the mosque became a place of empowerment for marginalised working-class communities where he could meet with a network of Pakistani Muslims who became an indispensable resource in times of economic hardship.

The mosque is an increasingly significant feature in Mohammed Manzoor's later years. Never having previously shown much interest in exploring religion, being preoccupied with his 'relentless quest to achieve and know and gain and become' (2007: 47) in his adoptive country, he explores his faith in later life. Manzoor notes that while he had been going to see Oasis at the Hacienda in Manchester during his years as a student there, his father had developed a more profound understanding of his faith:

> When I rang home from my Manchester home to speak to the family my mother would tell me that he was at the mosque. When I asked why, she would explain that he had said that he found it soothing and inspiring to discuss religion with the imams.
> (2007: 43)

Manzoor suggests that perhaps 'his faith was encouraging him to try fresh ways of reaching out to me' (2007: 43). That Manzoor's memoir only makes reference to Islamic spaces of worship to describe how they impacted on his father's life and his relationship with him suggests that these spaces played only a peripheral part in his own life. By associating these spaces with his father, Manzoor also contextualises how early examples of British mosques served first-generation migrants by providing them with a space in their new locality where they could meet, socialise, and develop a sense of community.

Unlike Mohammed Manzoor, Malik's devout father had always insisted that 'God came first' (2011: 37). As such, he 'spent more time at the mosque than he did at home'. His regular place of worship was 'an old Victorian building that had once been a church' (2011: 37–38). As the mosque is largely an unrestricted archetype, in theory it can take any architectural form and express almost any visual language. The mosque is made significant by the socio-spatial constructions and practices that define it as an Islamic space of worship, not by its physical form. It is hardly significant, then, that Malik recalls her father's preferred mosque as being a repurposed Christian site with a decidedly traditional British architectural style. The adaptability of the mosque structure allows for the '(re)inscription of "old" space with "new" cultural (Islamic) meanings' (McLoughlin 2006: 1045). In her memoir *Love in a Headscarf* (2009), Janmohamed similarly describes mosques in her local area as being a mixture of purpose-built facilities, small converted houses, and old buildings of worship 'that had been closed down or in disrepair and then rescued and revived as a place of worship, but this time as a mosque' (42). The fusion of traditions, histories, and religions in repurposed spaces of worship represents the changeability of place and the emphasis of religious observance over physical surrounding. This is further underscored in Malik's text when she notes if the call to prayer came when her father was elsewhere in the city, 'he would often nip into one of the other 'God's Homes', as he called them' (2011: 38–39). 'God's homes' around Bradford in the late 1970s were mostly converted terrace structures, 'stripped, so that the furniture you would expect to see in a normal residential abode – sofa, bed, table, etc. – had all been removed, but other than that there were few other changes' (2011: 39). Malik's and Janmohamed's descriptions of early converted mosques in Britain suggest that recently settled, concentrated Muslim populations were reconstructing localities to suit a new social function in keeping with a new community identity. This hints at a more sophisticated conceptualisation of the notion of locality or place itself, whereby place as a bounded piece of territory is challenged. As Linda McDowell suggests, geographers 'now argue that places are contested, fluid and uncertain' (1994: 4). This is certainly applied to public spaces of worship in Malik's and Janmohamed's texts, where mosques are encountered in a range of structures, demonstrating that it is socio-spatial practices which define places and result in overlapping and intersecting places with multiple and changing boundaries, constituted and maintained by social relations of power and exclusion.

However, a mosque can also be perceived as a 'very concrete and material sign of domination and power' (Allievi 2003: 344), even more so when it is purpose-built. The bricks and mortar make a 'visual claim on public space' (Eade 1996: 220) and where mosques are permitted to broadcast the call to prayer, often only for the midday and afternoon prayer, there is a further 'acoustic' claim on the non-material spaces of a locality (Gilliat-Ray 2010: 197). The perceived sensory intrusion of purpose-built mosques did little to quell the rising hostility towards immigration and the Muslim community in the 1970s. It was during this time, Malik notes, that the National Front held regular rallies in Bradford, and the Yorkshire campaign against Immigration (2011: 37) (which won around 20 per cent of the vote in some wards in the 1970 general election). Mosque-related conflicts can therefore be read as symptomatic of a national identity crisis that purportedly revealed a tendency within the ethnic majority to interpret the (re)creation of Muslim sociocultural space and a Muslim presence in Britain as an ever-expanding (Islamic) threat. For Kevin Dunn (2001), mosque conflicts are interwoven with dichotomising socio-spatial constructions of identity, belonging, and 'community', resting upon narrow articulations of self-Other binaries. However, the interpretation of repurposed religious sites found in British Muslim memoirs presents a different view of these spaces. That Muslim communities have 'rescued' and 'revived' disused and abandoned existing British buildings, as writers like Janmohamed imply, suggests that they are not only providing for Muslim communities, but helping to improve locations in Britain as a whole.

A second obstruction to mosque development during this time came from within Muslim communities. Malik describes the divisions that were forming during the 1970s between groups with different national, denominational, and geographical affiliations following a period of relative cooperation:

> As 'the community' became more settled in Ingerland, it also became more fragmented, with divisions based on nationality – Pakistani, Bangladeshi, Indian; geography – Mirpuri, Gujarati, Pathan, Punjabi; and denomination – Sunnis, Shias, Deobandis, Barelwis. So deep-rooted were the differences between these factions that they couldn't even agree on the most fundamental things, such as should we class ourselves as Muslims or as Moslems or Mohammedans or Mosalmans, never mind reaching consensus on where to build the next place of worship.
>
> (2011: 40)

This is read as a point of contention for Malik, as she highlights that, according to Islam, the global Muslim population forms a collective community united in faith: 'So much for the

Ummah. So much for "the community". So much for "God's home". Left to the Muslims in Bradford, God would be permanently homeless' (2011: 40). Malik sets up her narrative by detailing the evolution of Bradford from an industrial northern English town to a Muslim-majority area and contextualises the development and disputes involved in that transition before and during her childhood. Later on in the narrative, Malik turns her attention to describing personal encounters and responses to the religious sites that have featured in her life, and how these spaces have affected her relationship with her faith.

Although the mosque is recognised as a significant Islamic space of worship in Malik's text, it is also depicted as a distinctly public place, associated with communal prayer, formality, and for Malik it is a space more befitting male use. Malik's father's enthusiasm for visiting the mosque comes not only from his religiosity, but also because 'the mosque was a place where the Uncles could relax and talk openly without the Aunties snooping. It was hallowed ground for more than the obvious reason' (2011: 41). However, Malik notes that there was a lack of provision at her local mosque for women in terms of prayer and pastoral care (2011: 43). The writer's foremost recollection of the women's section of the mosque is of strong, unpleasant smells and cold conditions:

> The mosque stank of sweaty women and their sandals; the madrasa stank of sweaty teenagers and their pumps. Nobody could afford heating in those places, so the odour froze in the air. Imagine the stench in a Bedouin tent in the middle of the night after twenty nomads have trekked thirty miles across the Sahara in the glaring heat and then devoured a feast of lamb mansaf and gone to sleep. It smelt like that.
>
> (2011: 42)

Malik makes repeated reference to the unpleasant 'odour' of footwear throughout the text, consistently associating it with communal Islamic spaces such as the mosque or the *madrasa*. The writer also places considerable distance between herself and formal Islamic spaces by comparing the smells in her local mosque in Britain to a Bedouin tent in the Sahara, a context completely alien to her own lived experience. This passage is juxtaposed with a description of her preferred space of worship, her childhood home. More specifically, the kitchen, which is the focal setting for several significant religious experiences in the text:

> our kitchen was warmer and it smelt nicer.[...] Umejee spent hours cooking, making masala from scratch [...] patting out chapattis on the smoking *thava*. The spicy aroma of Mum's cooking comforted me. The smell of holy buildings made me retch.
>
> (2011: 42)

The synonymous use of 'odour' and 'aroma' to describe the mosque and the kitchen respectively subtly indicates a sensorial connection between these settings and underscores them both as significant Islamic spaces of worship for Malik. However, Malik compares the mosque to a foreign land, while she personally identifies with the kitchen, which evokes a sense of closeness with a combination of pleasant smells, her mother's presence, home cooking, warmth, familiarity, and comfort. Accordingly, Malik chose to 'learn the rules I needed to know about being a good Muslim at home. From Dad and Umejee and the Koran' (2011: 54). The link between aspects of embodiment and 'place' is well established in Malik's memoir, evidenced by the recurrent association between her mother's presence and the kitchen, and the unpleasant smell that doubly evokes in her mind the local mosque and the Sahara. In this sense, Malik's narrative may be understood in relation to a growing body of materialist-feminist scholarship in the field of 'critical geography' – Notable examples include Gillian Rose's *Feminism and Geography* (1993), Doreen Massey's *Space, Place and Gender* (1994), and Linda McDowell's *Gender, Identity and Place* (1999) – which exemplifies the ways in which women's subjectivities are partly determined by their insertion within a variety of socio-spatial locations.

These interconnected contexts range from global diasporas, through national spaces, cities and neighbourhoods, domestic dwellings, and the body. The body in particular is a site of autobiographical utterance in many life writing texts, it is the focal point through which places are experienced and connected, and where key concepts which construct subjectivity come together. For Malik, this idea is most realised in relation to the domestic context. Throughout *We are a Muslim, Please*, the kitchen table is central to the scene of narration, emphasised through repetition as the nucleus of Malik's positive religious experiences throughout her childhood. She receives her informal schooling in Islam sat 'at the kitchen table with Dad […] listen[ing] to him as he told us about the amazing miracles the Prophet Mohammed had performed' (2011: 52). It is at the kitchen table that Islam first becomes intelligible, accessible, and inspiring to Malik.

Significant events in the Islamic calendar also take place against the backdrop of the kitchen, including the Night of Power, which Malik describes as 'the holiest time in the Islamic calendar' (2011: 102). During this annual event, Malik's father placed copies of the Qur'an in the centre of the kitchen table and he and his children sat around 'in the same positions as at mealtimes' to read and pray from dusk until dawn (2011: 103). It is also during one such episode when Malik experiences a closeness to her faith that reaches transcendent levels. As an adult, this episode is reflected upon in a way which links concepts of memory and embodiment to Malik's Muslim identity, which is primarily how the narrator constructs her broader subjectivity in this life writing text. Malik notes that she often lies awake 'between three and four a.m.', a 'neither-here-nor-there time':

> I wonder if that tingly ethereal feeling I now get in the hour between three and four a.m. when I'm wide awake, of some other presence in the room, some supernatural being, has something to do with the sensation I used to get as a child when I stayed up during The Night of Power and when, for one miraculous night only, I could hear and feel the flutter of Angels' wings […] hovering above us in our kitchen.
>
> (2011: 103)

Malik's insomnia and deep, physical connection to her formative experiences, which are rooted to the specific micro-space of the domestic kitchen, can be understood as part of an important marker of the autobiography genre that Kathleen A. Boardman and Gioia Woods also identify. They assert that autobiographical texts often express a 'preoccupation with place, along with a focus on identity issues directly related to place: rootedness, anxiety, nostalgia, restlessness' (2004: 4). In Malik's text, this becomes even more pertinent in the wake of the domestic acts of terror which attempt to threaten and contradict the narrator's understanding of her religious identity. The influence of the kitchen as a space of worship is reaffirmed in the final passage when she returns to this space like a refuge in uncertain times:

> [T]here were no suicide bombers, no inflammatory clerics, no jihadis, no *kuffirs*, no war on terror, no extremists or fundamentalists, no radicalism or fanaticism, no Islamism, no Islamophobia. Then there was just my father and his four children sat at the kitchen table quietly reading the Koran.
>
> (2011: 276)

Although Malik's text highlights an individual connection to her faith, she contextualises this as being part of a cohesive British-Pakistani Muslim community, strengthened by regular visits to the local mosque for communal worship. It is a sense of collective religious duty that compels the *apney lokhi* (Malik 2011: 41) or *apney log* (Hai 2008: 35), both of which translate to describe 'the community', to offer their support and presence in the event of a bereavement in the Muslim community. This idea is explored in both Malik's and Hai's narratives following a death in the family when members of the community gather at the deceased's home for the observance of a forty-day mourning period. Although approached from different religious perspectives, in both texts the private home is repurposed to function as a markedly public space designed primarily for Islamic worship. In Hai's narrative, the forty days of mourning alter the context of the home as a space once associated with her atheist upbringing and imbues it with new, religious meaning, whereas Malik describes the event as an uncomfortable intersection between two prominent, yet hitherto separate, spaces that are integral to her identity as a practising Muslim.

In Hai's memoir, *The Making of Mr Hai's Daughter: Becoming British*, the family home becomes the centre of an unfamiliar and disorientating Muslim ritual during the forty days of mourning following the death of Hai's father. The late Mr Hai's individuality as a communist freethinker and an atheist is disregarded: 'as far as anyone in the *mahalla* was concerned, my father had been born a Muslim and he would also die a Muslim' (2008: 190). Despite their different backgrounds, in both Hai's and Malik's memoirs the home undergoes a similar cosmetic transformation during the mourning period to suit its new primary function as a temporary religious space. All domestic furniture is pushed aside and covered in 'clean but dull' (Malik 2011: 157) white or beige sheets, and the floor cleared for the guests to sit and read from the Qur'an. In Malik's religious household, the only objects left uncovered following her uncle's death were ones 'that bore God's name – the plaques inscribed with verses from the Koran, the calendar photographs of Mecca and Medina and the huge wall hanging of Kaba' (2011: 157). In both narratives, the home is visually altered and stripped back in a way that more closely resembles a typical and more permanent Islamic space of worship. Accordingly, the guests *respond* to the home in its altered state as a formal religious space. As is expected at a mosque, guests remove their shoes before entering the home, are separated by sex for prayer, and mourners are adorned with religious headwear.

These customs during the forty days of mourning are significant in both Malik's and Hai's text as they qualify the home as a formal space of worship during a religiously significant time. Hai notices that 'without prompting', the guests 'immediately took their shoes off' (2008: 187) in the hallway. At first, this automatic and unspoken conduct is unsettling for Hai, who begins to 'feel like a stranger in my home' (2008: 190). However, over the course of the ritual, the 'Islamic spirit of the occasion' (2008: 190) is embraced and the guests' treatment of her home as a place for worship is welcomed as Hai begins to comprehend the profound meanings behind the customs, noting that 'being around the *mahalla* was opening up a whole new world' (2008: 194). Once the forty-day period of mourning comes to an end, the religious function is removed from the space and the home reverts back to being foremost a domestic environment:

> I came downstairs one morning and saw that the white sheets on the floor had gone and our furniture was back in place. It was as if nothing happened. I stood in the middle of the room, allowing the silence to envelope me.
>
> (2008: 195)

Although cosmetically the space is the same as it was before Mr Hai's death, the religious function of the room during the forty days of mourning is not completely erased. Hai is surprised to see her mother praying in the corner of the room even though 'the room was back to normal' (2008: 195). In Hai's narrative, the event of her father's death is a turning point whereby religion is invited into the home during the ritual period of mourning and the space is permanently altered by this contact. Although Hai never becomes a practising Muslim, she ultimately finds that Islam can play a role in her life without compromising her Britishness. Following the mourning period, Hai self-defines as a cultural Muslim which ultimately connects her to a family past, the present, and provides the 'missing piece in [her] jigsaw identity' (2008: 199).

For Malik, the home during forty days of mourning for her late uncle provides the context where the two significant Islamic spaces in her life meet. The 'dozens of pairs of shoes' (2011: 187) in the entrance of her home create a 'discernible spectrum of smells' that conjure up a physical response that is interchangeable with the one observed in her earlier memories of visiting the mosque: 'Standing near the front door [...] the stench of sweaty footwear made you want to retch' (2011: 159). The smell, made up of many 'sandals, trainers, lace-ups and slip-ons', although unpleasant, recapitulates Malik's presentation of the mosque as being a public place, characterised by communal worship and formality. As the separate smells of discarded footwear and Malik's mother's cooking meet in her hallway, the two scents, and the contexts they have come to represent, are brought into conflict with one another:

> Down the hall, the aroma of curry battled with the stink of footwear. Neither smell won, but they formed an even more sickening union. You had to get to the far end of the corridor near the kitchen before there was any nasal salvation – just the fragrance of tender lamb masala.
>
> (2011: 159)

Although the blend of these smells is repellent, that neither smell 'won' or was able to overpower the other can be read as an affirmation of the equality between these contexts.

The focus of this chapter so far has been on how mosques and domestic spaces in Britain have been presented as significant sites of Islamic worship and as spaces in which subjectivities become decoded in several British-Pakistani Muslim memoirs. In the texts, these spaces make up part of the writers' local context where they are able to comprehend what being a British Muslim means to them personally. The next section turns its attention to the presentation of the Ka'ba in Mecca. Mecca is the birthplace of Islam, the destination of the *hajj*, and the focal point towards which all Muslims orient themselves in prayer. As Muslims from all over the world perform the *hajj* annually, religious affiliations coexist and overlay national ones, and the Muslim *ummah* offers an alternative affiliative space and means of communal identification and transnational connection. The memoirs discussed so far all make reference to the *hajj* but it is not personally experienced, or articulated as a globalised religious space. Janmohamed details her pilgrimage to Mecca in her memoir *Love in a Headscarf*, describing it as a 'physical as well as a spiritual journey' on which all participating Muslims 'found themselves also having to be physically part of the world's most global and diverse community' (2009: 245).

Janmohamed's pilgrimage to Mecca may usefully be discussed in relation to a geopolitical theorisation of identity construction, which is in essence a 'spatial practice', to reiterate Michel de Certeau's central point in *The Practice of Everyday Life* (1984). This involves mapping, routes and routing, borders and border crossings. Susan Stanford Friedman has elaborated on this idea by analysing what she calls 'relational spatialization' (1998: 151) which incorporates the opposing dimensions of the homonym routes/roots.[3] Friedman's position can be summarised as follows:

> Routes are pathways between here and there, two points of rootedness. Identity often requires some form of displacement – literal or figurative – to come to consciousness. Leaving home brings into being the idea of 'home,' the perception of its identity as distinct from elsewhere. Rootlessness [...] acquires its meaning only in relation to its opposite, rootedness.
>
> (1998: 151)

Moreover, routes imply travel, physical and psychical displacements in space, which in turn incorporate the crossing of borders and contact with difference. Janmohamed's articulation of the pilgrimage to Mecca as a devout Muslim demonstrates Friedman's argument that geopolitical identity can be understood through 'recognising the symbiosis between roots and routes and the multicultural encounters they engender' (1998: 152). Being at the 'location for the birth of Islam' (Janmohamed 2009: 244) in order to perform the *hajj* signals a return to an ancestral, spiritual home for Janmohamed. Mecca represents an imagined collective rootedness for the global Muslim population whose members are themselves positioned all across the world but aspire to physically make the journey at least once in their life. Janmohamed's pilgrimage addresses the meanings of location and itinerary in the production of cultural and geopolitical identities. Her position as 'a British East-African Asian Muslim girl in the bubbling ethnic mix of North London in the context of 1980s Anglo-Saxon monoculture' (2009: 34) complicates and disrupts the fixity and implied singularity of 'roots' as an identifier. Janmohamed's physical roots are in North London, her ancestral roots are in East Africa, and, like all Muslims, her spiritual roots are in Mecca; her route is between these equally important coordinates.

The vast mosque that houses the Ka'ba is internationally known as the 'House of God', which in itself indicates its status as the ultimate transnational Muslim space. However, Janmohamed deliberately notes that 'since God has no physical location, it is more a concept for Muslims to focus on than an actual abode for the Divine' (2009: 244). Mecca itself is not sanctified in the text, but performing *hajj* is regarded as an act of Islamic worship. The Ka'ba, then, is encountered simultaneously as a sacred and an unconsecrated space in the narrative. The focus is drawn once more towards the social practices that define place, the ritual itself whereby 'wave upon wave of thousands of thousands of men and women dressed in white [are] slowly walking around the black cube' seven times (2009: 244). The synchronised movement of the crowd is further likened to a body of water in order to signify unity, Janmohamed describes how 'the circulating movement of the ocean of humanity evoked emotions from the very depth of my being' (2009: 244), and how she watched the crowds 'swirling past' and 'flowing into each other' (2009: 245–246). This unification is further emphasised by the dress code: those performing the *hajj* are required to dress in simple white clothing which is intended to erase any 'inequalities of the physical and material world' so that 'Everyone was just a soul' (2009: 246). The scene depicts the *hajj* as an embodiment of the universality of Islam against a background of cultural diversity. This space functions primarily to bring Muslims together at the site of their faith's genesis and facilitates the 'immediate and proximate' interconnections (2009: 245) between believers and their counterparts from all over the world.

The *hajj* ritually and symbolically connects Muslims to a powerful 'chain of (placed) memory' (Hervieu-Léger 2000: 4). Janmohamed considers how the underlying meanings of the long-established rituals may be connected to a collective memory that also applies to a contemporary context:

> Circulating round the Kaba established that the Divine was the focus of being a Muslim [...]. The universe was a repetition of cycles, each one following its set orbit

and finding its place in the Divine order. The two parts balanced each other perfectly and I realised that both the sublime and the mundane fitted together.

(2009: 247)

Janmohamed's own interpretation of the *hajj* is in keeping with her understanding of Islam and how she identifies as a British Muslim. Through the *hajj* ritual she reaches an understanding that 'looking for food and shelter were just as much part of worship as prayer' (2009: 247), and so the mundane and the spiritual aspects of her life as a London career woman and a practising Muslim exist symbiotically and uncomplicatedly as pinnacles of spiritual devotion. Further, the visit to the physical centre of Islam from Britain ultimately functions to underpin Janmohamed's notion that faith is omnipresent and therefore unbound to any physical space:

> For many Muslims from less affluent backgrounds it would be a dream come true to be here. For those of us who had grown up in comfort in the West but outside our Muslim heartland, it created a new view of Islam, one that was holistic, ever present and in the majority.
>
> (2009: 247)

In the texts, performing the *hajj* and experiencing Mecca is presented as an aspiration (Mohammed Manzoor), a realised dream (Janmohamed), an annual event (Malik's father), and, for some, it doesn't feature at all (Manzoor, Hai). The sacred space of Mecca has an omnipresence in the texts, whether it is represented physically through a visit, visually displayed in the home (photographs in Malik's parents' house), or gesturally, in instances when worshippers orient themselves towards Mecca in prayer. In each of the texts, the writer's relationship with their faith and how they identify as a Muslim is unpicked and made clearer.

This chapter has sought to understand the role that spaces of Islamic worship play in writers' lives, how they are connected, and how this impacts on writers' construction of self in their life writing texts. Through its signposting of personal and intergenerational encounters with Islamic spaces in four texts, this chapter has also uncovered how identities are construed in a constant interplay between past and present. For example, the development of Pakistani-run businesses and mosques in the 1970s and '80s helped to establish communal identity and social cohesion amongst newly settled immigrant populations and also created an infrastructure in deindustrialised British towns. As established in Manzoor's and Malik's narratives, the mosques especially functioned as a sanctuary for their parents' generation, a space for socialising, business, and prayer. This generation carried with them the religious rituals and tradition of community gatherings at both the mosque and in the domestic home in times of bereavement. Altering the domestic space to befit religious ritual and adopting certain behaviours in line with Islamic tradition helped Malik and Hai to cope with their grief and understand what place these long-established religious traditions had in their own lives as a practising British Muslim and as a cultural Muslim respectively. Hai in particular describes the forty days of mourning as a transformative episode which ultimately connects her to a past, a present, and provides the 'missing piece in [her] jigsaw identity' (2008: 199). Janmohamed confirms her Muslim identity during her pilgrimage to Mecca, which ritually and symbolically connects all Muslims and takes them to the perennial heart of Islam. Encounters with these spaces are significant in the texts for a number of reasons, but the most significant element is how these spaces are used and understood. The different ways in which the writers respond to these spaces, and the social practices, rituals, prayer, and religious observance that take place within them, and how these responses evolve during the narratives is telling of how the construction of identity is never complete, fluid rather than static.

The marketing material and exposure of Muslim life writing largely excludes the influence of religious spaces and their role in the construction of autobiographical subjectivity in their discussions of the texts in favour of foregrounding the main narrative thrust or responses to acts of terrorism. There is a prevalence of oversimplification and polarisation in popular discourse which highlights the importance of interrogating homogenous representations of British Muslim texts. The presentation of and interaction with the home, the mosque, and Mecca as private, public, and global Islamic spaces encountered in the texts reveal an aspect of each writer's idiosyncratic relationship with Islam, and complicates the idea of a homogenous British-Pakistani Muslim experience. Through a discussion of places of Islamic worship in specific life writing texts, this chapter supports Janmohamed's assertion that 'each of us [Muslims] occupied so many spaces and identities and that made us multiversal not identical' (2009: 246).

Notes

1 In several key texts discussed, a death in a Muslim family or community is followed by forty days of mourning. During this time the community gathers at the home of the deceased, recites the Qur'an, and prays together. The Night of Power commemorates the night when the Qur'an was first revealed to the Prophet Muhammad, it is often considered the holiest night of the year for Muslims.
2 The magazine *Granta* published Hanif Kureishi's article 'Bradford' (1986) as part of a special edition that showcased life writing by authors of Pakistani descent.
3 Friedman is not the only academic to engage with the idea of roots/routes in critical theory. For example, Paul Gilroy's *The Black Atlantic* challenged black nationalism's fixation with roots and exclusive ownership of cultural production, suggesting instead that black diasporic identity is the result of 'a process of movement and mediation […] more appropriately approached via the homonym routes' (1993: 19). Stuart Hall (1996) and Clifford James (1997) have also discussed the homonyms in relation to diasporic identity and travel respectively.

Bibliography

Allievi, S. (2003) 'Relations and Negotiations: Issues and Debates on Islam'. In *Muslims in the Enlarged Europe: Religion and Society*. Ed. by Marechal, B, Allievi, S., Dassetto, F., and Nielsen, J. Leiden: Brill, 331–368.
Boardman, K. and Woods, G. (2004) *Western Subjects: Autobiographical Writing in the North American West*. Salt Lake City: University of Utah Press.
Chambers, C. (2013) 'Countering the "Oppressed, Kidnapped Genre" of Muslim Life Writing: Yasmin Hai's *The Making of Mr Hai's Daughter* and Shelina Zahra Janmohamed's *Love in a Headscarf*'. *Life Writing* 10(1), 77–96.
Delaney, C. (1990) 'The *Hajj*: Sacred and Secular'. *American Ethnologist* 17(3), 515–530.
Dunn, K. (2001) 'Representations of Islam in the Politics of Mosque Development in Sydney'. *Tijdschrift voor Economische en Sociale Geografie* 92(3), 291–308.
Eade, J. (1993) 'The Political Articulation of Community and the Islamisation of Space in London'. In *Religion and Ethnicity: Minorities and Social Change in the Metropolis*. Ed. by Barot, R. Kampen: Kok Pharos, 29–42.
Eade, J. (1996) 'Nationalism, Community, and the Islamisation of Space in London'. In *Making Muslim Space in North America and Europe*. Ed. by Metcalf, D. Berkeley: University of California Press, 217–233.
Ferris, I. (1999) 'Mobile Words: Romantic Travel Writing and Print Anxiety'. *Modern Language Quarterly* 60(4), 451–468.
Friedman, S.S. (1998) *Mappings: Feminism and the Cultural Geographies of Encounter*. Princeton: Princeton University Press.
Gale, R. (2004) 'The Multicultural City and the Politics of Religious Architecture: Urban Planning, Mosques and Meaning-making in Birmingham, UK'. *Built Environment* 30(1), 18–32.

Gilliat-Ray, S. (2010) *Muslims in Britain: An Introduction*. Cambridge: Cambridge University Press.
Gilroy, P. (1993) *The Black Atlantic: Modernity and Double Consciousness*. London: Verso.
Hai, Y. (2008) *The Making of Mr Hai's Daughter: Becoming British*. London: Virago Press.
Hall, S. (1996) 'Who Needs Identity?' In *Questions of Cultural Identity*. Ed. by Hall, S. and Gay, P. London: SAGE, 1–17.
Hervieu-Léger, D. (2000) *Religion as a Chain of Memory*. Trans. by Lee, S. Cambridge: Polity Press.
Hirsi Ali, A. (2006) *The Caged Virgin: A Muslim Woman's Cry for Reason*. London: Free Press.
Hopkins, P. (2007) *Geographies of Muslim Identities: Diaspora, Gender and Belonging*. Abingdon: Routledge.
Ilott, S. (2015) *New Postcolonial British Genres*. Hampshire: Palgrave Macmillan.
James, C. (1997) *Routes: Travel and Translation in the Late Twentieth Century*. Cambridge, MA: Harvard University Press.
Janmohamed, S.Z. (2009) *Love in a Headscarf*. London: Aurum Press Ltd.
Jelodar, E.Z., Yusof, N.M., Hashim, R.S., and Raihanah, M.M. (2013) 'Critical Pedagogy of a Post-9/11 Muslim Memoir'. *International Journal of Applied Linguistics and English Literature* 2(2), 216–222.
Kureishi, H. (1986) 'Bradford'. *Granta* [online]. Available from <https://granta.com/bradford/> [18 May 2017].
Malik, Z. (2011) *We are a Muslim, Please*. London: Windmill Books.
Manji, I. (2004) *The Trouble with Islam: A Muslim's Call for Reform in her Faith*. London: St. Martin's.
Manzoor, S. (2007) *Greetings from Bury Park*. London: Bloomsbury.
Marshall, J. (1994) 'The Mosque on Erb Street: A Study in Sacred and Profane Space'. *Environments* 22(2), 55–66.
McDowell, L. (1999) *Gender, Identity and Place: Understanding Feminist Geographies*. Minneapolis: University of Minnesota.
McLoughlin, S. (2006) 'Mosques and the Public Space: Conflict and Cooperation in Bradford'. *Journal of Ethnic and Migration Studies* 31(6), 1045–1066.
Mondal, A.A. (2008) *Young British Muslim Voices*. Oxford: Greenwood World Publishing Ltd.
Nasser, N. (2005) 'Expressions of Muslim Identity in Architecture and Urbanism in Birmingham, UK'. *Islam and Christian-Muslim Relations* 16(1), 61–78.
Shahed, S. (2012) 'A History of Mosques in Britain'. *An Architects' Journal* [online]. Available from <www.architectsjournal.co.uk/a-history-of-mosques-in-britain/8629263.article> [13 December 2016].
Smith, S. and Watson, J. (2010) *Reading Autobiography: A Guide for Interpreting Life Narratives*. 2nd edn. Minneapolis: University of Minnesota Press.

23
HOMES AND BELONGING(S)
The interconnectedness of space, movement, and identity in British-Pakistani novels

Éva Pataki

Belongingness as a sense of belonging to a particular group, person, or place, or of being a fundamental and vital part of something, is a natural and universal desire. But how does one achieve belongingness? What does it mean to share a sense of belonging and belongings with a fellow community member, immigrant, diasporian, citizen, or human being? Where and how is such a sense created and what factors determine its creation? How do spaces, places, homes, and homelands relate to belongingness and how can movement – in a simplified meaning of not being at home but on the road – generate a sense of belonging? In an attempt to answer these questions, the present chapter investigates notions of home and belonging as common recurring tropes in British-Pakistani diasporic fiction, and as highly relevant issues in our modern world characterised by various experiences of and attitudes to migration and diasporisation. Through the close reading and comparative analysis of three British-Pakistani novels, I examine Pakistani diasporians' experience of belongingness, with a special focus on various ways in which the (trans)formation and construction of identity and space, as well as different forms of movement, interconnect with alternative ways of belonging.

Nadeem Aslam's *Maps for Lost Lovers* (2004) provides us with an insight into the condition of working-class British Muslims alienated and segregated in their exclusively immigrant neighbourhood. Through the story of the honour killing of Jugnu and Chanda, and the focal points of Shamas, Kaukab, and their children, Aslam portrays how British-Asian immigrants create their diaspora space[1] in England and how, despite the shared immigrant experience, a community may be pulled apart by religious, cultural, and generational differences, thus depriving its members of a sense of belonging. Having proposed a new definition of national identity, a 'new way of being British' (1986: 18), Hanif Kureishi gave life to the British hybrid *par excellence*, the protagonist of *The Buddha of Suburbia* (1990). Karim Amir is running away from the rootedness, boredom, and stasis of the white lower middle-class suburb of Bromley; yet, paradoxically, it is the restlessness of the suburbs that makes him fidgety and eventually drives him to engage in perpetual motion between urban and suburban spaces, greatly determining his sense of belonging and identity construction. Suhayl Saadi's *Psychoraag* (2004) has received critical acclaim for its redefinition of Scottish identity and been recognised as the first Scots Asian novel, and may also be marked out for being a contemporary Glasgow novel with an ethnic twist: presenting the city as 'Migra Polis' (Saadi 2004: 310), a postcolonial space reterritorialised and hybridised by the Pakistani diaspora. With its insightful representation, *Psychoraag* provides a new aspect of regional diasporic identity in British-Asian fiction and highlights both traditional and alternative ways of belonging for the diasporian.

The close reading of the maps, spatial positions, and routes of the British-Pakistani protagonists of my chosen corpus – varying from hybridised diasporians on the move to nomads and transcendent selves – reveals how diaspora space is created in an attempt to have a home to belong to, as well as ways in which different spaces and places contribute to or hinder the experience of belongingness. I shall contend that urban and suburban spaces may serve both as confining factors and as motors for movement and transgression, thereby becoming significant loci of belonging and what Simone Weil calls 'rootlessness' (1952),[2] as well as points of departure for so-called 'mobile subjectivities', for whom Britain itself becomes a multicultural, lived diaspora space appropriated, practised, and travelled.

Aslam's multifocal narration exposes the underlying patterns of a universal(ised) diaspora experience – the loss of the homeland and the unavoidable feeling of unbelonging and loneliness in an alien land – as he describes the Pakistani diasporians' (im)migration: 'Roaming the planet looking for solace, they've settled in small towns that make them feel smaller still, and in cities that have tall buildings and even taller loneliness' (2004: 9). The immigrants' consciousness is characterised by repeated moments of awakening to the fact that, although one is part of a global network of worldwide diasporas, part of a community and culture, one will forever feel the loneliness and uprootedness of a scattered people – isolated, unbelonging, displaced. The general description of diaspora experience as displacement entails a sense of placelessness[3] or '"unhomeliness" which can be defined as the obscure feelings that simultaneously draw and repel a person in her relations to a place' (Leon 2009: 15). To resolve this ambiguous feeling, the diasporic community in Aslam's *Maps for Lost Lovers* tries to create a sense of belonging by re-christening places 'to give the map of this English town a semblance of belonging' (2004: 156): with each new immigrant arriving in the town, place names are changed to resemble well-known streets, squares, and hills back in the homeland (India, Pakistan, Bangladesh, etc.). The only name equally accepted by each immigrant group in the neighbourhood is the name of the town: 'Dasht-e-Tanhaii. The Wilderness of Solitude. The Desert of Loneliness' (2004: 9).

The renaming and reappropriation of space suggests the possibility of interpreting both immigration and the creation of diaspora as a result of 'deterritorialisation' and, as a compensation for the lost homeland, the 'reterritorialisation' of the place. The two terms were originally coined by Gilles Deleuze and Félix Guattari as part of their theory of nomadology: deterritorialisation denotes 'the movement by which "one" leaves the territory', it is 'the operation of the line of flight' and 'may be overlaid by a compensatory reterritorialisation obstructing the line of flight' (1987: 508). In diaspora studies (not entirely in the spirit of Deleuze and Guattari), deterritorialisation and reterritorialisation denote the loss of an old territory (in the homeland) and taking possession of a new one (in the host country) (cf. Kalra, Kaur, and Hutnyk 2005: 32). Since the immigrants in Aslam's novel yearn for roots, stability, and a certain symbolic identity, their rootlessness in England is not the symptom of deterritorialisation in a Deleuzian sense, but an indicator of an attempt 'to unsettle and unpack the problems associated with having multiple belongings or no sense of belonging at all' (Kalra, Kaur, and Hutnyk 2005: 4), and of their failed attempts to achieve reterritorialisation and a fixed place/identity associated with it. Therefore, in their case, deterritorialisation becomes a spatial metaphor of identity formation, while reterritorialisation may indicate the diasporian's wish for a fixed identity, manifested in their inability to secede from the homeland, but also in attempts to create a certain sense of belonging in the host country by renaming and various cultural practices. The latter, according to Anne-Marie Fortier, are 'collective performances of identity and belonging' (2000: 6) (such as going to the mosque or the Hindu temple, celebrating religious festivals like Eid and Ramadan, and visiting cultural events such as a performance by the renowned Sufi singer Nusrat Fateh Ali Khan in the local bookshop), which 'mark out spatial and cultural boundaries for the immigrant population' (Fortier 1999: 42) – boundaries which simultaneously protect and confine.

Boundaries and belonging (or the lack thereof), as well as de- and reterritorialisation are also emphatic tropes in Saadi's *Psychoraag*, which depicts postcolonial Scotland as a place still perceived by the English as a 'dusty frontier post' (2004: 178) and Glasgow as 'Migra Polis' (2004: 310). Saadi's description of the Pakistani diaspora in Glasgow is confined to racialised inner-city spaces and the 'petit bourgeois Punjabi folk of Glasgae' (2004: 334). Saadi's immigrant community, like the diaspora subjects in Aslam's novel, attempts to fight the feeling of transience and placelessness by reterritorialising the cultural space of the city through various cultural practices and renaming its neighbourhoods: Kinning Park, for instance, is known as 'Wee Faisalabad' (2004: 102), named after a village some immigrants came from but simultaneously indicating the influence of the host country.

Another thought-provoking aspect of renaming is that besides suggesting a yearning for the lost homeland and for belonging, it may in fact intensify a self-induced sense of being isolated, excluded from, and not belonging to the cultural space surrounding them. The Pakistani immigrants in *Psychoraag* live 'hermeneutic lives' (Saadi 2004: 205) in their neighbourhood, while the Pakistani Muslim characters of Aslam's novel form a closely-knit community which marks its own territory and creates its diasporic space within urban space by trying to isolate itself from both 'white' England and other diasporic communities. In doing so, *Maps for Lost Lovers* metaphorises otherness and cultural isolation by the somewhat paradoxical tropes of 'the country within the city', and the alleged (or hoped) cultural purity of diaspora subjects and diaspora space.

A slightly different approach to and appropriation of diaspora space is depicted in Saadi's description of Kinning Park, a place where 'the Changezi Family ruled [...] Big shoes, bhangra boots, markin out territory. The pavements hereabouts were all Punjabi' (2004: 373). While the immigrant neighbourhood in *Psychoraag* seems to be just as exclusive as the one in Aslam's novel, Kinning Park is reterritorialised and terrorised primarily by the second-generation 'Kinnin Park Boys [...] a gang of about thirty or so lads' from the '*baratherie*',[4] a 'mini Cosa Nostra' (2004: 102–4) who, 'not knowing what mask tae wear, had acquired those of East Coast Gangstas' (2004: 253) and taken over the crime scene in the immigrant neighbourhoods. Not for a sense of belonging but for the sake of belongings, the Kinnin Park Boys treat Glasgow as their personal territory, defined by invisible yet clearly marked boundaries and a certain power over space, which is also apparent in their exercise of a form of ownership and control by crime, having a hold on various enterprises and the media (including Radio Chaandni). As Ali Madanipour points out, such a sense of territoriality is 'derived from emotional attachment and familiarity' (2003: 44); conversely, by renaming and reterritorializing, the immigrants may achieve emotional attachment, which enables them to appropriate and control the place as their own primary territory and may offer a sense of belonging. Territorial behaviour, then, may be a third aspect of diasporic belonging, besides cultural practices and renaming.

The protagonist DJ Zaf's primal territory, the home where he belongs, is his childhood neighbourhood, Pollokshields: an immigrant ghetto; a confined, peripheral space where all the houses 'faced inwards [...] built to be blocked off' (Saadi 2004: 376) from which young diaspora subjects yearn to run away, since 'growin up in the Shiels in those days wis purgatorial and, for years, Zaf had existed in a state of unrequited life' (2004: 377). Zaf's experience of home indicates not only isolation and confinement but also a concomitant identity crisis, which strongly affects the diasporian's sense of belonging: it is manifested in the first generation's inability to belong to their current location or to return to their country of origin, and the second generation's unwillingness to accept their parents' birthplace as their home. In *Maps for Lost Lovers*, one of the neighbourhood women wonders 'why her children refer to Bangladesh as "abroad" because Bangladesh isn't abroad, *England is abroad; Bangladesh is home*' (Aslam 2004: 46; emphasis original). For the first generation, Dasht-e-Tanhaii may be a reterritorialised space but it will never be home; it may seem to be a replica of the homeland but merely an imperfect, fractured one. For the second generation, however, it is indeed home but a home they are bound to leave: in *Maps for Lost Lovers*, Kaukab and Shamas' older son Charag moves out and marries a white woman, their daughter Mah-Jabin has the looks and the life of an independent young woman in London, while in *Psychoraag* Zaf claims to have 'grown up and away' (Saadi 2004: 272) from his diasporic community and neighbourhood, only to find himself in an equally ambivalent space and position at Radio Chaandni.

DJ Zaf's cubicle is a small confined and divided space where he feels safe from the ghosts of his past but also imprisoned; it is a cultural space which both manifests his identity crisis and serves as a place of and a motor for movement, as the following quote suggests:

> By the end of every six-hour session, Zaf would have become the room. And, as the weeks had gone on, he had found it more and more difficult to define an existence outside of Radio Chaandni and his life on the air [...] He felt suffocated. Trapped [...] He had the sudden urge to get up and walk out.
> (Saadi 2004: 13)

Instead of engaging in perpetual movement like Karim in *The Buddha of Suburbia*, Zaf opts for mental movement (in the form of recollections, visions, and hallucination) and his perception of becoming the cubicle – spinning silently and standing poised – results in a ritual pacing:

> Zaf moved round and round the cubicle, slowly [...] and as he walked, he trailed the end of his fingers along the grey cones so that, by the end of the whirls, his skin would be electric and [...] a hazy brown line had formed, at waist level, [...] like a border, dividin the room into two separate halves.
> (Saadi 2004: 62)

Pacing in the cubicle may be a movement to mark out his territory, a personal space which, according to Madanipour, 'may start from the person's mind and extend to the personal space of the body' (2003: 46), which then 'locates an individual in the physical world' and 'marks out a personal territory, enabling the individual to develop a sense of identity' (2003: 30) and belonging. Furthermore, the division produced by pacing in the cubicle may be interpreted as the spatial manifestation of his identity performance[5] as a diasporian (i.e. emphasising his Asianness to match the image of the radio) and his cultural positioning as a hybrid.

Such identity performances are also highly emphatic and significant in Kureishi's novel, which starts off with Karim's trenchant self-identification and – positioning as a cultural hybrid:

> My name is Karim Amir, and I am an Englishman, born and bred, almost. I am often considered to be a funny kind of Englishman, a new breed as it were, having emerged from two old histories. But I don't care – Englishman I am (though not proud of it), from the South London suburbs and going somewhere. Perhaps it is the odd mixture

of continents and blood, of here and there, of belonging and not, that makes me restless and easily bored. Or perhaps it was being brought up in the suburbs that did it.
(Kureishi 1990: 3)

In claiming to be 'going somewhere', Karim both foreshadows the undetermined routes he shall take and displays a sense of inbetweenness generated both by his mixed-race origins and the suburbs. Furthermore, Karim's words suggest several aspects of hybridity: first, he is a hybrid in a biological sense, as a man of mixed-race (Anglo-Indian) origin; then, as a second-generation immigrant born and brought up in Britain, he is hybridised by the dominant culture; thirdly, he is also a hybrid in the sense of being a representative of Kureishi's vision of a new kind of Britishness; and, fourthly, as a suburbanite – the child of a hybrid, liminal space.

Without any palpable cultural roots inherited from and imposed on him by his father, Karim does not long for the lost homeland and the belongingness it may entail; nor does he admit belonging to suburbia, despite having lived there all his life. What makes his sense of unbelonging to the space he is most rooted in so contradictory is that, in a way, the suburbs can be interpreted as the spatial manifestation of Karim's hybridity. In the introduction to his collection *Visions of Suburbia*, urban theorist Roger Silverstone claims that the modern suburb and its culture are both socially and culturally hybrid and that suburbia is 'revealed, as well as masked, in all its overblown hybridity' (1997: 4). For Julien Wolfreys, the hybridity of the suburb is manifested in 'a certain ambiguity of identity, the result of its hybrid borrowing from more than one source or location' (2010: 97), hence it may only be described by means of a set of dichotomies: 'Instantly recognizable though never entirely familiar. Ubiquitous but invisible. Secure but fragile. Desired but reviled' (2010: 4). Suburbia is, then, forever intertwined with the concepts of inbetweenness, liminality, and hybridity, and it is the quintessential metonymy of these notions.

Although Karim does not seem to be able to escape the feeling of inbetweenness in suburbia, nor his 'destiny, which is to be a half-caste in England' (Kureishi 1990: 141), every so often he manages to turn his hybridity into an advantage as he continues to engage in 'direct mimicry', a concept Roger Caillois (2003: 91) defines as a conscious decision to use a disguise. In Karim's case, this intention and behaviour manifest in a constant role-play, performing his identity as suits the situation; for instance, he tries to fade into his environment by applying the 'hip' look and language of Western youth or emphasises his exotic appearance by wearing a 'scarlet Indian waistcoat with gold stitching around the edges' (1990: 5) which, according to James Procter, is nevertheless a hybrid look, because it is borrowed from 1960–1970s London fashion and its 'fetishization of the orient' (2003: 129). Karim's Indianness, similarly to his father's orientalism (Haroon Amir is the Buddha of the title), has little to do with connecting to the roots or yearning for belongingness – it is a theatrical performance given for an expected benefit, while the identity it suggests is a staged identity, a 'staged exoticism' (Procter 2003: 129). With all its narrow-mindedness, pretentiousness, and emphasis on the facade, suburbia appears in the novel as a theatre or a stage for acting out various roles and performances, which Karim consciously plays upon, yet simultaneously despises and wants to escape. Interestingly, it is exactly these performances and masks that make him a suburbanite and indicate his inevitable belonging to the suburban space from which, with the help of these very performances, he hopes to be able to break out, just as he wants to do away with his monolithic image as a hybrid and inbetweener.

As opposed to the inbetweenness and liminality of the suburbs, the city represents for Karim 'a house with five thousand rooms, all different; the kick was to work out how they connected and eventually to walk through all of them' (Kureishi 1990: 126). Since Karim has always considered the suburbs as merely temporary accommodation, 'a leaving place, the start of life' (Kureishi 1990: 117), Bromley becomes a point of departure in contrast to the city, the place of arrival, the place where he can finally 'be himself'. Karim's move to the city is, seen from this aspect, an instance of 'local migration' (Nasta 2002: 181) or what Clement Ball calls 'a small-scale migration' (2004: 233) to a new long-term residence. However, Karim's new residence in the city centre proves to be anything but a permanent location and his efforts to leave the suburbs behind are doomed to failure: whether in West Kensington or in Bromley, he is in-between what he has and what he wants to have, who he is and who he appears to be, and at times he is *in-between* in-between spaces: on the way.

Similarly to Aslam's protagonist Shamas, who frequently walks from the immigrant neighbourhood to the city centre and back, making journeys between the two cultural worlds and within the neighbourhood, Karim does not settle permanently either in the suburbs or in the city, but makes ceaseless journeys between the two. However, where journeying serves the purpose of mapping space for Shamas who as a hybrid embodies the border zone of the cultural spaces, Karim's perpetual motion is, in Procter's view, 'symptomatic of his desire to uproot himself' (2003: 150) and he is the quintessential hybrid of suburban space. Although I agree with Procter and also read Karim's perpetual movement as a wish to uproot himself and as a metonymy of his unstable identity, I interpret his journey as an indicator that he is a 'mobile subjectivity' – a term coined by Kathy E. Ferguson to denote subjects that are 'temporal', 'relational', 'ambiguous', 'messy and multiple', refusing 'to stick consistently to one stable identity claim' (1993: 154). While my understanding of the term draws on Ferguson's definition, it also involves the subject's ability and desire to be constantly on the move. Apparently, even when Karim leaves the suburbs for the city, he keeps returning to the suburbs, and especially to Bromley, the magnetic field of his roots, only to leave it again, fed up with the stasis it denotes. This undecidedness and the movement it generates may in fact indicate the lack of a home or the possibility of multiple 'temporal' abodes, as well as the contradictory yet simultaneous sense of longing for belongingness and not being able to truly belong anywhere at all.

The only instance when Karim settles in one location for a relatively long period of time is when he goes to New York as part of a theatrical production and decides to stay there for a while. In Karim's experience, New York is an even more enabling space than London, and he is perceived not as an exotic other or a half-caste but just 'an English boy'; that is, he is identified based on his permanent physical location and the concomitant nationality it entails. What I find most ironic about this perception is that both the suburbanite identity he has fled and the Englishness he is identified with here are place-bound identities (and for Kureishi they are practically synonyms), which may indicate that Karim has returned to the start line here in terms of his perceived belonging.

In contrast, in *Psychoraag* there appear to be three basic levels where belonging is experienced and manifested: the locale (the city of Glasgow), language (polyglottism), and music. Zaf the DJ claims that he 'Wanted to share himself with the whole of Glasgow' (Saadi 2004: 330), that he needs his voice 'goin out to millions (well, hundreds) of people, all over Glasgow and beyond' (2004: 328) and hopes that 'his breath, his being, would go out to the silent ones' (2004: 128). His words imply that he wishes not only to be heard and to be able to share himself but also to achieve a renewed sense of belonging to the diaspora and, even more importantly, to create his own community of listeners as well, which points to the understanding of belonging as both self-identification and 'a sense of shared imaginary possessions or "belongings"' (Ferreday 2009: 29). Zaf's emphasis on the shared attribute of being Glaswegian suggests the possibility of building a community not on the basis of kinship, diasporic experience, religion, or nationality but on a regional identity. His aim to share himself reveals a desire to overcome his inbetweenness and identity crisis by connecting with Glaswegians and creating a community through music and language, thus manifesting Saadi's conception of music as 'a unifying force, both in the individual and society at large' (2006b: n.p.), which Zaf translates as a relationship of love: 'They were his. An he wis theirs forever. Lovers on the ayre' (Saadi 2004: 333–334).

When Zaf calls out to his '*Junnunies*' (Saadi 2006a: 97), the final night of *The Junnune Show* becomes a manifesto of his 'striving for unity' (Saadi 2006a: 131), for the shaping of a community on a basis other than ethnicity and cultural identity – a community that can influence the social and spatial composition of space, and, as Zaf claims, 'redraw aw the maps' (Saadi 2004: 208) and build a bridge between East and West, white Scottish and Scots Asian, based on the premise that 'in our hearts, we are all Glaswegian' (Saadi 2006a: 360). In my view, the most thought-provoking aspect of this identification is that it signals a considerable shift from the first generation's clinging to what Salman Rushdie calls 'imaginary homelands' (1992) (as portrayed in, for example, *Maps*) and a second-generation individual's sense of belonging to a particular location (Karim of *The Buddha* as a Londoner) to the possibility of belongingness for a whole community – including diasporians *and* white British – in the host country that has become home.

The concept of home is decidedly different in *The Buddha*, since Karim appears to be unable to settle permanently in any location or to experience belongingness *per se*. In fact, even before his 'official' departure from the suburbs for London, he refers to himself as an 'itinerant' (Kureishi 1990: 94), a free spirit leading a bohemian lifestyle, setting up makeshift homes at his relatives' and friends' houses:

> [T]here were five places for me to stay: with Mum at Auntie Jane's; at our now empty house; with Dad and Eva; with Anwar and Jeeta; or with Changez and Jamila […] I now wandered among different houses and flats carrying my life-equipment in a big canvas bag and never washing my hair.
>
> (Kureishi 1990: 93–94)

Being on the road between various locations – Chislehurst, Bromley, Beckenham, Penge, Peckham, and West Kensington – Karim marks out his own nomadic territory in Greater London: 'I was not too unhappy, criss-crossing South London and the suburbs by bus, no one knowing where I was. Whenever someone – Mum, Dad, Ted – tried to locate me, I was always somewhere else' (Kureishi 1990: 94). These locations serve as stages in his process of identity formation, as points of endless departures and as temporary resting places on a perpetual and ultimately non-teleological journey.

Karim's interim homes and routine paths may be understood more clearly in the light of Deleuze and Guattari's nomadology. In *A Thousand Plateaus: Capitalism and Schizophrenia*, Deleuze and Guattari differentiate their concept of the nomad from both the conventional anthropological definition and the migrant as the diasporic subject. They argue that while the migrant 'reterritorializes on its interior milieus', the nomad is 'the Deterritorialized par excellence' (1987: 381), he 'has a territory; he follows customary paths; he goes from one point to another' (1987: 283) and, in a way, he exists inbetween these two points, two places or locations. It follows that as a nomad and an inbetweener, Karim's life, like 'The life of the nomad[,] is the intermezzo' (Deleuze and Guattari 1987: 284). Karim's inbetweenness is thus both a cultural and – perhaps even more emphatically – a physical, geographical, and spatial condition which consequently determines, if not redefines, his individual sense of belonging.

Karim may also be perceived as a nomad in a Braidottian sense, transgressing the borders of sexuality, race, and social roles, repeatedly deconstructing and reconstructing his own identity. Drawing on Rosi Braidotti's theory, I argue that Karim exists in 'transitory attachment' (1994: 25), in permanent fluidity, mental, and spatial movement: he is on the move from adolescence to young adulthood, from one home to another, in transit between identities, performances, and locations. As opposed to the stereotypes of ethnic minorities in Britain, Karim's subjectivity is one that has little to do with migrants' displacement or with their desperate attempts to hold on to their roots; rather, he is a subject with no desire for fixity; his desire is for an identity of transitions and changes (Braidotti 1994: 22–23). Karim's *being*, then, is a case of perpetual *becoming*, that is, what Elspeth Probyn (drawing on Deleuze's nomadic approach to movement and becoming) refers to as 'the inbetweenness of belonging' and 'belonging in constant movement' (1996: 19).

When, at the end of the novel, Karim leaves New York for London, he does not return home *per se*, nor does he finally settle in a fixed mode of existence – his free-spirited, transgressive, dynamic nomadism persists. Although Kureishi portrays his protagonist as resisting any commitment or attachment throughout the novel, and Karim never admits to himself that his ceaseless wandering and identity performance are symptoms of his desire to belong, eventually he realises that he is very much rooted – not in suburbia as such, but in his nomadic territory of Greater London; he is not a mere suburbanite but first and foremost a Londoner. London, his contentious and ambiguous home, is, in Karim's words, 'where you start from' (Kureishi 1990: 249), and also the place to return to over and over again. By acknowledging London as his marked-out nomadic territory, he can finally locate himself in the world, 'reterritorializing and renaming' (Nasta 2002: 197) the spaces of the city and the suburbs and can achieve his own personal sense of belonging.

Another alternative way of belonging is suggested by Saadi, introduced in the musical narrative style and special language of *Psychoraag*, through which the novel positions itself as a hybrid cultural production. Music occupies a central position in the novel, as a means of getting in touch with the audience (and the readership), of evoking memories, conveying thoughts and various mental states, and indicating a carnivalistic, almost chaotic hybridity and cultural diversity, as the following quote implies: 'In places, the notes would merge and, from somewhere, there would arise a third tune, one that nobody had ever written but which sounded better than either of its component parts' (Saadi 2004: 239). This 'third tune' sounds like a vocal counterpart of Homi Bhabha's (2005) concept of third space and hybridity as a third entity,[6] and indicates Saadi's alternative take on identity construction: although Zaf initially claims to be a sample, that is, a fragmented, faulty representation both in Scotland and in Pakistan, he later realises that his identity 'lay not in a flag or in a particular concretization of a transcendent Supreme Being but in a chord, a bar, a vocal reaching beyond itself' (Saadi 2004: 210). While Zaf previously identified himself according to his region (as a Glaswegian), his words here suggest an identity position beyond spatial concerns since it is music that describes and defines him; when he claims, 'music an soang [...] That's whit Ah'm aboot' (Saadi 2004: 208–209), he lays claim to an identity constructed and positioned in and through music.

On the radio, in the open space of the ether, Zaf finds his own voice which 'belonged to the whole world' and a self which 'wis immortal. Invisible, formless, perfect' (Saadi 2004: 85). This formless and invisible existence points to Aristotle's theory of the ether as the sphere of 'the divinely changeless' and of the soul consisting of ether, which may explain its perpetual movement (Merlan 1967: 40), and also evokes the Platonic concept of the immortal soul, 'an entity whose kinship to eternal, changeless beings occurs alongside its capacity to undergo radical and ceaseless transformation' (Brill 2013: 2–3). Through music and the rebirth it generates, Zaf in a sense divorces himself from the physical world and becomes the metonymy of an immaterial, spiritual substance in a state of perpetual movement, transformation, and transfusion, belonging nowhere and everywhere at the same time – he becomes perfect and immortal, a 'new and improved' diasporian *without* a diasporic consciousness and belonging.

Eventually, however, Zaf's voice may be 'conjoinin wi the magical, geometric dance ae the spheres' (Saadi 2004: 402) for the duration of the show, but it cannot maintain a transcendence of the self for good. Zaf's transcendent self is a complex but by no means divine self, since through the novel he remains decidedly human, with all the attendant bodily sensations, faults, desires, and attachments. Therefore, it is perhaps more expedient to view Zaf's transcendent self as one strand of his multiple identities, one stage in his process of identity formation and construction, as well as one possible alternative way of belonging.

My analysis of *Maps for Lost Lovers*, *The Buddha of Suburbia*, and *Psychoraag* revealed the diasporians' deep need for a sense of belonging which, especially for first-generation immigrants, appears to be a primary factor in the creation of diaspora spaces: a place may be produced as a diaspora space by a diasporic community's acts of renaming and reterritorialisation, cultural practices, and various other attempts to achieve belongingness. Similarly to immigrant experience, diaspora experience – encompassing the creation of hybrid diaspora space and subjects – necessarily brings about a sense of dislocation, placelessness, and inbetweenness, generated by the discrepancies between the dominant culture and the roots. These spatial aspects of the diaspora experience may necessarily involve diverse ways in which diasporians search for a sense of belonging to a place, a community, a human relationship, or even to an ideology or abstract idea.

In *Maps for Lost Lovers* the diasporic community displays a strong attachment to the lost homeland and a certain Weilian rootlessness, that is, unbelonging in their own diasporic community, while for the young diasporians of *Psychoraag*, belonging is first and foremost understood as control of space, as a means of self-identification, and as imaginary shared belongings. While *Maps* and *Psychoraag* portray the diasporian's search for a sense of belonging to a certain ethnic, religious, or local community through mapping, exclusion, and territorial behaviour, Karim of *The Buddha* chooses belonging in movement in his own nomadic territory of London, whereas DJ Zaf of *Psychoraag* calls out for a shared Glaswegian identity as a means of achieving belongingness and also experiences belonging in music and, for a brief period, transcendence. A shared characteristic of these divergent forms of belonging is their interrelatedness with a certain kind of movement – whether mapping, following nomadic paths, pacing, or mental movement – in order to resolve or erase the problematics of belonging.

In the novels discussed in this chapter, diaspora space, suburbia, and the metropolis, with their safeguarded, transgressable or fluid and permeable borders, and the multitude of routes to take within and across these borders both literally and metaphorically, invite various forms of movement and various strategies of identity (re)construction, the creation of mobile subjectivities: the figures of the nomad and the transcendental self. These mobile subjectivities may thus be interpreted as the metonymy of an identity in the process of perpetual (trans)formation and re-construction, encompassing and reformulating their cultural roots, diasporic experience, and identity crisis, as well as their own perception and sense of home and belonging(s).

Notes

1 In cultural studies, diaspora space is defined as 'the intersectionality of diaspora, border, and dis/location' (Brah 1996: 208) and as such a liminal zone, while in human geography it is a space of 'ambiguity and discontinuity', 'a source of anxiety', and 'a zone of abjection' (Sibley 1995: 33). I use the term in both senses, to designate the contested concept of home and physical location of a diaspora in the host country.
2 Weil's concept of rootlessness refers to the loss of a collective communal spirit, that is, the loss of a common past and common ancestors (see Dietz 1988: 154).

3 I use the term 'placelessness' in relation to the diasporic condition to denote what Carol E. Leon refers to as 'a loss of place or context' (2009: 3) or Steve Pile as being 'out of place' (1996: 6), that is, being displaced or misplaced.
4 According to the novel's glossary, *baratherie* is an Urdu word denoting a person's extended family or a clan. Hereafter the translations of the Urdu in the text are drawn from the glossary.
5 I use the term 'identity performance' as a concept at the intersection of social performance as role-play and Butlerian performativity (2011), a construction and a display of a gendered cultural identity, with diasporians as both the subject and the agent of their own performative actions.
6 Hybridity for Homi Bhabha becomes a 'third space' of the 'in-between' – a liminal third term, the metaphor not of sameness, but of cultural difference (2005: 38, 115). The concept of third space enables Bhabha to make direct links between colonial and postcolonial hybridity, and between the hybrid nature of colonial and contemporary culture.

Bibliography

Aslam, N. (2004) *Maps for Lost Lovers*. London: Faber.
Bhabha, H.K. (2005) *The Location of Culture*. New York: Routledge.
Brah, A. (1996) *Cartographies of Diaspora: Contesting Identities*. New York: Routledge.
Braidotti, R. (1994) *Nomadic Subjects: Embodiment and Sexual Difference in Contemporary Feminist Theory*. New York: Columbia University Press.
Brill, S. (2013) *Plato on the Limits of Human Life*. Bloomington: Indiana University Press.
Butler, J. (2011) *Bodies that Matter*. New York: Routledge.
Caillois, R. (2003) 'Mimicry and Legendary Psychasthenia'. Trans. by Shepley, J. In *The Edge of Surrealism: A Roger Caillois Reader*. Ed. by Frank, C. Durham: Duke University Press.
Clement Ball, J. (2004) *Imagining London: Postcolonial Fiction and the Transnational Metropolis*. Toronto: University of Toronto Press.
Deleuze, G. and Guattari, F. (1987) *A Thousand Plateaus: Capitalism and Schizophrenia*. Trans. by Massumi, B. London; New York: Continuum.
Dietz, M.G. (1988) *Between the Human and the Divine: The Political Thought of Simone Weil*. Totowa: Rowman.
Ferguson, K.E. (1993) *The Man Question: Visions of Subjectivity in Feminist Theory*. Berkeley: University of California Press.
Ferreday, D. (2009) *Online Belongings*. New York: Peter Lang.
Fortier, A.M.F. (1999) 'Re-membering Places and the Performance of Belonging(s)'. In *Performativity and Belonging*. Ed. by Bell, V. London: Sage, 41–64.
Fortier, A.M.F. (2000) *Migrant Belongings: Memory, Space, Identity*. Oxford: Berg.
Innes, K. (2007) 'Mark Renton's *Bairns*: Identity and Language in the Post-*Trainspotting* Novel'. In *The Edinburgh Companion to Contemporary Scottish Literature*. Ed. by Schoene, B. Edinburgh: Edinburgh University Press, 301–309.
Kalra, V., Kaur, R., and Hutnyk, J. (2005) *Diaspora and Hybridity*. London: Sage.
Kureishi, H. (1986) *My Beautiful Laundrette and The Rainbow Sign*. London: Faber.
Kureishi, H. (1990) *The Buddha of Suburbia*. New York: Viking.
Leon, C.E. (2009) *Movement and Belonging: Lines, Places and Spaces of Travel*. Oxford: Lang.
Madanipour, A. (2003) *Public and Private Spaces of the City*. New York: Routledge.
Merlan, P. (1967) 'Greek Philosophy from Plato to Plotinus'. In *The Cambridge History of Later Greek and Early Medieval Philosophy*. Ed. by Armstrong, A. H. London: Cambridge University Press, 114–132.
Mir, S. (2007) '"The Other within the Same": Some Aspects of Scottish-Pakistani Identity in Suburban Glasgow'. In *Geographies of Muslim Identities: Diaspora, Gender and Belonging*. Ed. by Aitchison, C. et al. Aldershot; Burlington: Ashgate, 37–77.
Nasta, S. (2002) *Home Truths: Fictions of the South Asian Diaspora in Britain*. London: Palgrave.
Pile, S. (1996) *The Body and the City: Psychoanalysis, Space, and Subjectivity*. New York: Routledge.
Probyn, E. (1996) *Outside Belongings*. New York: Routledge.
Procter, J. (2003) *Dwelling Places: Postwar Black British Writing*. Manchester: Manchester University Press.
Rushdie, S. (1992) *Imaginary Homelands: Essays and Criticism, 1981–1991*. London: Penguin.
Saadi, S. (2004) *Psychoraag*. Edinburgh: Black & White.
Saadi, S. (2006a) 'Songs of the Village Idiot: Ethnicity, Writing and Identity'. In *Ethically Speaking: Voice and Values in Modern Scottish Writing*. Ed. by McGonigal, J. and Stirling, K. Amsterdam: Rodopi, 117–137.

Saadi, S. (2006b) 'Suhayl Saadi: *Psychoraag*: The Gods of the Door'. *Spike Magazine* [online]. Available from <www.spikemagazine.com/0206-suhayl-saadi-censorship-in-the-uk.php> [13 February 2013].
Sibley, D. (1995) *Geographies of Exclusion: Society and Difference in the West*. London: Routledge.
Silverstone, R. (ed.) (1997) *Visions of Suburbia*. London: Routledge.
Weil, S. (1952) *The Need for Roots. Prelude to a Declaration of Duties towards Mankind*. Trans. by Wills, A.F. London: Routledge.
Wolfreys, J. (2010) 'Literature'. In *Theory: Tropes, Subjectivities, Responses and Responsibilities*. London: Continuum.

24
COMMITTED AND COMMUNIST
Negotiating political allegiances in the diaspora

Miquel Pomar-Amer

Pakistani migrants in Britain are often associated with low levels of cultural and economic capital and this narrative of economic and intellectual precariousness is also extensively applied to their offspring, diasporic subjects who may not have experienced any migratory process but whose physical appearance or family name still mark a history of migration. In response to this stagnating situation, typical experiences of diasporic subjects have been reinterpreted in cultural products which aim 'to encourage solidarity among those with a group affinity, and a sense of political agency in making justice claims to the wider society' (Young 2000: 103).

This chapter will focus on the development of two characters, namely Shamas in Nadeem Aslam's novel *Maps for Lost Lovers* (2004) and Syed Samsamul Hai (hereafter Mr Hai) in Yasmin Hai's memoir *The Making of Mr Hai's Daughter* (2008). The aim is to see how their characterisation engages with this 'identity politics' to reveal and subvert the narrative of precariousness which is indiscriminately assigned to diasporic subjects. The evolution of these characters will be used to show how the initial adversities associated with migration are overcome and a higher social position is eventually consolidated. This raises the paradox of an author taking a counter-hegemonic stance through characters who exert themselves in order to occupy positions closer to hegemony. Despite this exercise of mimicry, these characters become the object of a 'repetition that will not return as the same' (Bhabha 1994: 162) because their possession of a similar economic or cultural capital does not guarantee their inclusion in the hegemonic group.

Even though the decision to migrate is often ingrained in the pursuit of social mobility (Appadurai 2006: 589), the political instability of Pakistan throughout the 1950s, 1960s, and 1970s was another good reason for which many decided to migrate. Aslam had to leave Pakistan with his family and move to Huddersfield in 1980 because President Zia's regime persecuted his father, a communist film-maker and poet writing under the pen-name of Wamaq Saleem. This personal experience certainly inspired Shamas in *Maps for Lost Lovers* – he migrates after Ayub Khan's coup. Mr Hai in *The Making of Mr Hai's Daughter* also leaves Pakistan after General Zia's coup and his escape is portrayed like a James Bond film as he fools the Pakistani secret services that try to arrest him.

Regardless of the reason behind migration, Tariq Modood notes that, in the case of Asian migrants, 'their occupational levels were depressed by migration effects and discrimination in the labour market' and, as a consequence, they 'often suffered a downward social mobility on entry into Britain' (2004: 93). This association is not arbitrary because it serves the interests of the hegemonic group. As Michel Foucault states, 'Every relationship of power puts into operation differentiations which are at the same time its conditions and its results' (1982: 792). Hegemonic discourses operate precisely on this principle of differentiation which is materialised in 'subtle everyday discriminatory practices sustained by socially shared representations' (van Dijk 2000: 48). Hence, the initial economic fallout experienced by migrants is used to construct and sustain a narrative of precariousness that is applied indiscriminately across generations so that the existing social structure remains unaffected.

Even though hegemonic discourse has the capacity to overcome hermetic conceptions of social class because it operates on what Antonio Gramsci calls a 'historical bloc' (1971: 263), this does not imply that hegemonic discourses dissolve social stratification in any way as their aim is precisely to preserve the social order and ensure that it is unaffected. For instance, the leading classes may appeal to aspects such as ethnicity or religion with a double aim. On the one hand, a common ethnic/religious background is often used to establish bonds with sections of the subaltern classes; on the other, the association of diasporic subjects with precariousness has effects on conviviality because they may be perceived as direct competitors by other members of the subaltern class, not just in the labour and housing markets but also in the allocation of social services such as health or benefits. Worryingly, in Britain these attitudes are not just engaged by overtly anti-migration parties such as the National Front, British National Party, or UK Independence Party, they also appear in statements by mainstream politicians and media.

Hence, the development of a subaltern class consciousness beyond ethnic and religious affiliations is prevented by representing diasporic subjects as a competing and homogeneous social body suffering from different forms of deprivation. This situation has been contested by diasporic authors like Aslam or Hai, who have attempted to dismantle the tenets of this pervasive logic in their texts. They have endorsed their cultural difference to write 'from the perspective of the signifying position of the minority that resists totalization' (Bhabha 1994: 162) and to propose alternatives to the dominant narrative of precariousness.

Migrants often have menial jobs because of the negative effects of migration. By extension, diasporic subjects are often imagined as unskilled workers with little chance of prospering. This disadvantaged situation is justified by claims of allegedly low levels of education and an absence of qualifications that, at the same time, slip all too easily into assertions of ignorance and/or laziness without considering that these qualifications are often not 'recognised' in the immigration country (Modood et al. 1997: 141–2; Collett and Zuleeg 2008: 5). The assumption of this cultural capital deficit, amplified by the media portrayal of migrants as 'underachievers' and a 'burden' on the educational system (Lipsett 2008: n.p.; BBC 2011b: n.p.), explains the reluctance of local parents to school their children in institutions with high numbers of diasporic students. Sometimes, this discourse transcends political correctness and is replicated by public personalities such as the former Chichester councillor John Cherry (Conservative), who suggested that Pakistanis would not 'rise to the top' as 'There are certain nationalities where they are uncertain what this hard work is all about' (Hughes 2013: n.p.). Thus, the hegemonic discourse operates as a 'reciprocally confirming' practice (Williams 1977: 110) when it appeals to academic results to argue that the alleged economically precarious situation of the diasporic subject is a direct consequence of his/her ignorance and/or laziness.

Certainly, economic and cultural capitals are interrelated and the possession of the former usually implies a greater amount of free time that can be invested in the acquisition of cultural capital. For this reason, we should not submit to the illusion that meritocracy blurs all inequalities because those with a more advantageous economic situation have usually had more opportunities to increase their cultural capital as well. Considering this, I will use Pierre Bourdieu's distinction between the embodied and institutionalised states to discuss the characters analysed in this chapter. Bourdieu describes the embodied state as that existing 'in the form of long-lasting dispositions of the mind and body' (1997: 47), which refers to the skills and knowledge acquired by a person. When these skills and knowledge are objectified and turned into an academic qualification, Bourdieu argues that we are dealing with an institutionalised state so that 'a certificate of cultural competence […] confers on its holder a conventional, constant, legally guaranteed value with respect to culture' (1997: 50). Hence, the main difference between these two states of cultural capital lies in the fact that those who do not possess a valid academic qualification are not backed by the state and are more vulnerable to the fluctuations of the labour market.

According to Mike O'Donnell and Sue Sharpe, many young ethnic minority men in Britain must cling to their 'own cultural resources against the grain of a still significantly prejudiced and discriminatory society' to survive (2000: 131). These cultural resources are an example of what Bourdieu would call the embodied state of cultural capital and it is precisely this experience as a diasporic subject that the characters discussed in this chapter exploit. Shamas and Mr Hai use their cultural and social capital to cope with the social downgrading that migration often entails. Their aim is not to become rich but to act as mediating agents between their respective diasporic communities and society as a whole. For this purpose, they appeal to their cultural background and their position as diasporic subjects to improve their social position and become a kind of organic intellectual. My analysis will look at their trajectories in terms of social position taking into account two important features shared by both. First, their cultural capital turns them into referents within the diasporic space as their assistance is requested when someone needs to deal with bureaucratic issues, a position as facilitators of knowledge which appears in other texts by British-Pakistani authors such as Mr Manzoor in Sarfraz Manzoor's memoir *Greetings from Bury Park* (2007: 37) or Mr Shah in Almas Khan's novel *Poppadom Preach* (2010: 31).

Second, their political commitment signals their advantageous position in terms of cultural capital because 'it is not sufficient to consider the capacity to understand, reproduce, and even produce political discourse, which is guaranteed by educational qualifications' since 'the (socially authorized and encouraged) sense of being entitled to be concerned with politics, authorized to talk politics' must also be considered (Bourdieu 1984: 409). In addition, the characterisation of these politically committed diasporic subjects also aims to question the two predominant images of migrants in relation to politics: either they are not supposed to show an interest in 'local' politics or, if they do, their interest is perceived with suspicion and accusations of corruption are too easily made (Laville and Muir 2006: n.p.; Quinn 2013: n.p.; Liddle 2013: n.p; Malnick 2013: n.p). Lower levels of electoral participation among British ethnic minorities have been reported but 'The key barrier to participations is […] registration not turnout' (Heath and Khan 2012: n.p.). As Parveen Akhtar highlights, the reasons for not registering include 'doubts over eligibility criteria, language difficulties, general alienation from politics, fear of racial harassment and racial attacks from extreme right-wing groups who identified Asian names on the register, concerns over anonymity, […] and doubts about residence status' (2014: 18).

Moreover, the left-wing inclinations of the two characters discussed here comply with the dominant voting pattern among minorities. In Britain, more than two-thirds of ethnic minority voters (68 per cent) voted Labour in 2010 and Anthony Heath and Omar Khan's data show that migrants 'have high levels of political involvement in terms of identification with a political party (primarily Labour), high levels of turnout and participation in conventional politics, and they feel that Labour represents their interests reasonably well' (2012). In a more recent study on the 2015 elections, Khan states that even though around 60 per cent of black and minority ethnic voters still support Labour, Conservatives have increased their ethnic minority vote to 25–30 per cent (Khan 2015). The political allegiances exhibited by Shamas and Mr Hai also suggest a challenge to an economic structure based on inequality. Therefore, their involvement with politics proposes an alternative discourse based on equality, emphasising the importance of the public over the private and, ultimately, blurring the differences among individuals within and beyond the diasporic space.

According to John Hutnyk, this left-wing political involvement among some British-Asian subjects is concealed in the dominant ethnographical approach and that is why he aims to 'reconstruct this absent history' by resorting to published biographies, living memory accounts, and selected historiographical works (2005: 348). The portrayal of the selected characters is intended to overcome these limitations by stressing their political allegiances and representing alternative models of politics of difference. Indeed, it is their politically motivated decision to migrate that poses a challenge to the hegemonic discourse, by not fitting in with the picture of the migrant whose migratory project is motivated by economic precariousness and whose main aim is to overcome it. Instead, emphasis is placed on the negotiation of their left-wing allegiance with a particular position regarding the politics of difference and which always places cultural capital in a predominant position.

First, Mr Hai's involvement with communism is a result of a class consciousness awakening after his experience of poverty in early life. His increasing notoriety in the first years after Pakistani independence forced him to go underground when the Party was banned, and he eventually migrated to England in 1964 (Hai 2008: 10–11). Second, Shamas was a promising poet involved in political discussion groups before migrating and his decision to leave is presented as a way of escaping political persecution after Ayub Khan's coup in 1958 (Aslam 2004: 80). In this regard, Amina Yaqin's discussion stresses the parallelisms between Shamas' characterisation as an organic intellectual, a poet, and an activist and Faiz Ahmed Faiz's biography (2013: 69).

The case of Mr Hai is probably the most paradigmatic example because his cultural capital resisted the financial constraints he faced even though his life trajectory shows a series of ups and downs in terms of social position. Mr Hai was born into one of the richest families in colonial India, but they wasted their fortune and Syed needed to study hard to win a scholarship that allowed him to attend university (Hai 2008: 9). Even though 'to delay entry into the labor market through prolonged schooling [is] a credit which pays off, if at all, only in the very long term' (Bourdieu 1997: 54), this investment in cultural capital is only possible when supported by economic capital. Mr Hai thus had to apply for alternative funding to pursue his university education. However, his elders might have converted a part of their former fortune 'into an integral part of the person' (Bourdieu 1997: 48), thus bestowing certain cultural capital that can be transmitted in the domestic sphere, such as manners or a determinate way of thinking, for example. Consequently, one could infer that family status is still an important aspect that raises expectations to follow predictable occupational routes (Savage 2002: 63)

In the absence of economic capital, Mr Hai's brother developed his religious capital and became a 'prominent religious figure in Pakistan', while Mr Hai became 'Professor of English at the prestigious S. M. Law College in Karachi' (Hai 2008: 98, 10). Nevertheless, it is his political activism that granted him recognition. Appointed as Chairman of the Pakistan Peace Committee and summoned to China for talks with the communist leaders, Mr Hai seemed to excel in this political role. However, political changes in Pakistan eventually forced him to go into hiding because communism was persecuted, and then to England afterwards when he was almost caught by the Pakistani Secret Service. Mr Hai's process of adaptation and the description of his first years in England provide an unusual representation of the migratory experience. He was already in his late forties and shared a house with men of a similar profile to his own: they were all South Asian diasporic subjects belonging to the elites of their respective countries and faced impoverished conditions in England as a side effect of defending their left-wing ideas (Hai 2008: 12).

Their crusade against 'the shackles of the British Empire and the dark forces of religion, poverty and feudalism' seems to be impaired by the romantic idea of England that they still hold (Hai 2008: 10, 9, 15, 31). This image is doubtless linked to the introduction of English literature in the curricula of the former colonies, which 'marks the effacement of a sordid history of colonialist expropriation, material exploitation, and class and race oppression behind European world dominance' (Viswanathan 1989: 20). Nevertheless, Mr Hai does not seem to be aware of the imperial connotations of the hegemonic values he endorses and supports through a politics of assimilation. In this case, 'the rôle of literature in the production of cultural representation should not be ignored' (Spivak 1999: 113) because, as an operation of colonial discourse, 'it interpellates colonial subjects by incorporating them in a system of representation' (Tiffin and Lawson 1994: 3). Despite his political ideas, Mr Hai was brought up in a rather conservative family and it should not come as a surprise that he feels more comfortable with the values of 'modesty and reserve' (Hai 2008: 129) which he presumably associates with Victorian literature. In fact, he disapproves of many aspects of the contemporary British lifestyle as the result of 'westernization' (Hai 2008: 77), a broad term used by Mr Hai that is often tied to notions of sexual permissiveness and rebelliousness.

Yasmin Hai depicts her father as a man who mimics the white English by focusing on the assimilatory efforts he enacts in an old picture of himself: 'He looks the picture of a model English gentleman. Or is it more like the picture of a foreigner playing at being English – dressing more English than the English?' (Hai 2008: 11). It is this excess that places him in a space of difference he did not intend to inhabit but cannot avoid because, 'as one who has just arrived from the outside, he is, by definition, not admissible at all' (Guha 1998: 157). His liminal position in relation to Englishness is visible in the reaction of the 'blurred faces [that] peer curiously out of an Austin Minor in the direction of the brown-faced man leaning against the railing' (Hai 2008: 11). Mr Hai plays with what Bhabha refers to as 'a difference or recalcitrance which coheres the dominant strategic function of colonial power, intensifies surveillance, and poses an immanent threat to both "normalized" knowledges and disciplinary powers' (1994: 86). It is in order to efface this difference that the embodied state of cultural capital intervenes as a source of respectability and a tool for upward social mobility. Devoid of the volatility of economic capital, Yasmin Hai's description of the picture also refers to her father's cultural capital when she notes the pen that 'casually juts out of my father's left breast pocket, a signal to the world that he is also a man of books' (2008: 11).

However, Mr Hai's approach to cultural capital is particularly biased and he privileges whatever he considers to epitomise Britain. Consequently, he negotiates his communism and his praise of British values by endorsing what Young calls the socialist critique of the politics of difference (2000: 85–86): Mr Hai discourages any position alluding to multiculturalism or ethnic pride because they undermine class solidarity and 'only perpetuate the ghetto mentality and hold minorities back' (Hai 2008: 175). Instead, he promotes the acquisition and domestic transmission of cultural capital by demanding a good command of English and an interest in politics from his future wife (Hai 2008: 20). Extending the James Bond-like anecdote which opens *The Making*, Hai entitles the chapters describing Mr Hai's settling down 'Operation X', and 'Operation Wife' is just one of many others he undertakes to come closer to the hegemonic position that he covets in Britain.

For this purpose, Mr Hai highlights any feat of his family as a cultural capital generator and leaves the economic capital or status that such action could produce in a secondary position. Geographic mobility is presented as a chance 'to become something better' (Hai 2008: 37) but this desire is frustrated by the lack of appropriate English role models in the area (Hai 2008: 43). For this reason, Aunt Hilda, an Englishwoman married to Mr Hai's best friend, is a crucial influence in the fulfilment of this narrative of becoming because she is 'a guide to life in England' (Hai 2008: 135). She embodies the 'authentic' English, the 'connoisseur' who has 'an unconscious mastery of the instruments of appropriation which derives from slow familiarization and [...] a practical mastery which [...] cannot be transmitted solely by precept or prescription' (Bourdieu 1984: 66). At the same time, she is free of Mr Hai and his former housemates' idealised view of Britain and her opinions are highly considered whenever it comes to the improvement of cultural capital and the routes that must be taken to achieve it. Indeed, the investment in cultural capital as a way to disavow, or at least elude, the negative typifications associated with Pakistani diasporic subjects is clearly portrayed during a meal, when Yasmin is scolded by Aunt Hilda for taking some food with her hands, because 'only Pakis eat with their hands' (Hai 2008: 51). The use of the abusive term 'Paki' unleashes a series of synonyms involving a lack of cultural capital that young Yasmin identifies with 'being uncivilised, primitive, savage, ignorant, backwards, uneducated, illiterate and uncultured' (Hai 2008: 51). Therefore, table manners is a basic principle in the acquisition of the 'legitimate culture' – the English, in this case – 'to dispense with the labour of deculturation, correction and retraining that is needed to undo the effects of inappropriate learning' (Bourdieu 1984: 71) and to come closer to the aim of the becoming narrative: '"this" thing you had to become [...] was called "English"' (Hai 2008: 37).

This aspiration makes Mr Hai put aside his political commitment for the sake of his daughter's education and approve of Yasmin's new school because of its 'middle classness', which he perceives as the epitome of Britishness and, consequently, cultivated – '[middle class girls] spent all their spare time reading Shakespeare or playing the flute' (Hai 2008: 128). In fact, Mr Hai's decision responds to his own experience: the stability of embodied cultural capital and its eventual convertibility into economic capital makes it useful to go through difficult situations. Mr Hai thus encourages this choice because he conceives cultural capital as the best path towards a hegemonic position, whose legitimacy is independent from ethnicity and religion (Hai 2008: 333). In fact, this stability is traceable in his professional career in England. After working in a factory for a while, he progressed thanks to his knowledge and taught basic literacy to immigrant children (Hai 2008: 47). Mr Hai's job as a teacher was relatively better than the manual jobs of his neighbours. However, the social position of an individual is relational and Mr Hai's position is not so highly valued when his neighbours start 'running their own small business ventures, supported by the expanding Asian network' (Hai 2008: 161). The other diasporic families show their economic capital by refurbishing their houses but Mr Hai rejects such things: 'It's all about showing off' (Hai 2008: 163). As with the pen in the photograph discussed above, the characterisation of Mr Hai challenges the image of the migrant as ignorant and only interested in either economic or symbolic capital because the only innovation he allows in his house is the purchase of more bookshelves (Hai 2008: 163).

Unlike Mr Hai, Shamas is reluctant to move to better-off areas despite his financial capacity to do so, because moving away from a neighbourhood described as a 'sink area' (Aslam 2004: 210) would imply a betrayal of his political ideas. Even though Kaukab blames her husband for the limitations that such geographical immobility might have imposed on their children's social mobility (Aslam 2004: 328–329), Shamas perceives his decision as an unavoidable effect of his integrity. In this sense, Ujala accuses both his parents of neglecting their responsibilities to their children, because Kaukab was 'too busy longing for the world and the time [her] grandparents came from' and Shamas 'was too busy daydreaming about the world and the time his grandchildren were to inherit' (Aslam 2004: 324). Ujala's accusation appeals to the 'temporal dilemma' that a migrant may face in his/her attempt to participate in the host society: 'whatever is anticipatory and futural about it is liable to make him appear as an alien, and whatever is past will perhaps be mistaken for nostalgia' (Guha 1998: 159). For this reason, although Shamas looks to a utopian future, this future becomes 'a space of intervention in the here and now' (Bhabha 1994: 7) and this requirement of immediacy cannot leave notions of difference and alienation aside. In fact, Shamas' communist ideas are imbricated in the anti-colonial struggle, as is shown by his unwillingness to be granted an OBE (Aslam 2004: 328). This perspective may encourage an interlocked view of ethnicity and class since some of the racial prejudices of colonial discourse are still recurrent in the hegemonic discourse. For this reason, whenever interethnic conflicts arise, Shamas brings forward a shared history of exploitation for all diasporic subjects, be it under a colonial regime in the past or under a neoliberal mode of production in the present.

The urban space of Dasht-e-Tanhaii, translated as 'The Wilderness of Solitude' or 'The Desert of Loneliness' (Aslam 2004: 29), is represented as a place where 'strangers are thrown together' (Young 2004: 198) so that distress, alienation, and isolation become chronic features of the city because the complex divisions of labour determine that:

> social life is structured by vast networks of temporal and spatial mediation among persons, so that nearly everyone depends on the activities of seen and unseen strangers who mediate between oneself and one's associates, between oneself and one's objects of desire.
>
> (Young 1990: 237)

In his positions as the director of the Community Relations Council and a member of the Commission for Racial Equality, Shamas is a mediator who is 'the person the neighbourhood turns to when unable to negotiate the white world on its own' (Aslam 2004: 15). However, he rejects any privilege that may come from such a position because his communist ideals prevent him from pursuing the convertibility of cultural capital into economic capital (Bourdieu 1997: 47) and he is not interested in enhancing his status. This disinterested attitude is not understood by many of his neighbours because migration is only considered worthwhile when it is in the pursuit of better economic prospects. Yet Shamas does not conceive of his migratory project as such but as a temporary exile, since his desire to return is still alive (Aslam 2004: 60) because, ultimately, 'His aim is to change conditions in Pakistan, for which he was expelled, and not to settle in Britain simply for financial reasons' (Lemke 2008: 181). Thus, the political is more important than the economic in Shamas' scale of priorities although his political ideas are based on the idea of a new economic order.

Unlike Mr Hai's assimilatory approach, Shamas advocates a multiculturalism that he understands as a competition between the hegemonic and the subaltern groups so that bonds of solidarity are established with other diasporic subjects who may face racist and class confrontation on an everyday basis. Consequently, an oppositional view of society is eventually suggested by conceiving the white English and the Asian as configuring two different social spaces (Lemke 2008: 181), especially when interethnic conflict arises. Thus, Shamas is involved in what Pnina Werbner calls ethnic politics, 'a field in which the primacy of the social, cultural, symbolic, or political is asserted over the purely economic; in which the economic is culturally and politically constituted' (1991: 34). This does not necessarily imply underestimating the importance of the economic as the requirement for the establishment and reproduction of a group's hegemony (Gramsci 1971: 269).

Indeed, as Gramsci anticipates, the intellectual's relationship with 'the world of production is not as direct as it is with the fundamental social groups, but is, in varying degrees, "mediated" by the whole fabric of society and by the complex of superstructures, of which the intellectuals are, precisely, the "functionaries"' (1971: 12). In other words, Shamas' attempt to subvert the existing hegemony is engaged with the actual state apparatus in which he is employed and which has been promoted by the cosmopolitanist turn that, paradoxically, Timothy Brennan attributes to the fall of communism (2006: 213). The problematic that this situation may involve for Shamas' long-term political project is not acknowledged, however, as he regrets the break-up of the Soviet Union (Aslam 2004: 156), while he frames his empathetic relationship with other diasporic subjects within the institutionalised delegation formations that he recognises. For instance, he encourages a bus driver who is racially harassed to report it to his superiors and to start a record of racial abuse of bus drivers (Aslam 2004: 179), and he also thinks of ways to bring Suraya's son to England by resorting either to the legal (Aslam 2004: 244–245) or religious fields (Aslam 2004: 234). In other words, Shamas relies on the state's superstructure and frames his mediating position in the field of bureaucratic consultancy but he often neglects interpersonal relations when these imply a compromise of his political ideas.

Consequently, Shamas is depicted as a dreamer who embodies 'a position of hope' but 'also suggests immaturity and a failure to engage with the reality of the world' (Gunning 2010: 89). However, Shamas' sense of reality should be considered excessively optimistic rather than defective. Although his political ideas function as a lens through which he makes sense of the world, he fails to reconcile them with some of the functions that his family expects from him. For instance, Kaukab accuses him of being irresponsible because he said that saving money for his first child's future was not necessary as 'by the time this child grows up the whole world would have become Communist, and things like education, healthcare and housing would be free' (Aslam 2004: 324). This quote shows that there is a mismatch between what each of the spouses sees as the appropriate depository of social capital and provider of economic capital: Kaukab considers that her husband must perform his role as head of the family, but Shamas delegates this duty to the communist state, which he perceives as having ultimate responsibility for the welfare of its citizens. Positioning the state thus reveals Shamas' universalist demand for the eradication of any form of social stratification and his rejection of those measures that contribute to it. In other words, a common well-being is preferable over an exclusive well-being, even when this minority is his own family as he 'neither seek[s] honour among men nor kingship over them' (Aslam 2004: 328). Shamas thus insists on denying that his cultural capital works as a source of distinction (Aslam 2004: 225; Bourdieu 1984: 63) but in vain because, despite his wishes, he is considered 'someone quite prominent and respected' (Aslam 2004: 368), even posthumously.

The two characters analysed in this chapter excel and are able to turn their knowledge of the bureaucratic maze into economic and/or symbolic capital. In fact, their position as intellectuals is certainly affected by, and cannot exist without, acknowledging their mediating position between their diasporic status and certain hegemonic demands: 'Without that turn [to the West,] we would not in fact have been able to make out a life ourselves as intellectuals' (Spivak 1990: 8). The representations of these characters place cultural capital in the foreground but also highlight how problematic their positions are despite their attempts to balance them with different social models and politics of difference (i.e. assimilation, multiculturalism, interculturality), hence emphasising the complexity of the notion of precariousness. The dominant narrative of precariousness does not simply encompass a limited economic status but also refers to alleged social, legal, and even intellectual deficits that are uncritically assigned to diasporic subjects. Rather than categorically denying the statements that characterise these diasporic subjects as ignorant and backwards (Aslam 2004: 312; Hai 2008: 51), the representations analysed here construct the figure of the Pakistani migrant in Britain as an intellectual, with a much more productive and engaging outlook that supplements the hegemonic discourse and exposes its reductiveness.

Bibliography

Akhtar, P. (2014) *British Muslim Politics*. Basingstoke: Palgrave Macmillan.

Appadurai, A. (2006) 'Disjuncture and Difference in the Global Cultural Economy'. In *Media and Cultural Studies: KeyWorks*. Ed. by Durham, M.G. and Kellner, D.M. Oxford: Blackwell, 584–603.

Aslam, N. (2004) *Maps for Lost Lovers*. London: Faber and Faber.

BBC (2011a) 'Immigrants Have Children for Benefits, Says Asian Peer'. *BBC News* [online]. Available from <www.bbc.co.uk/news/uk-politics-14909062> [22 May 2013].

BBC (2011b) 'Pakistanis and Bangladeshis Underachieving?'. *BBC Asian Network* [online]. Available from <www.bbc.co.uk/programmes/b01179w9> [28 May 2013].

Bhabha, H.K. (1994) *The Location of Culture*. London: Routledge.

Bourdieu, P. (1984) *Distinction: A Social Critique of the Judgement of Taste*. Trans. by Nice, R. Cambridge, MA: Harvard University Press.

Bourdieu, P. (1997) 'The Forms of Social Capital'. In *Education, Culture, Economy, Society*. Ed. by Halsey, A.H., Brown, P., and Wells, A.S. Oxford: Oxford University Press, 46–58.

Brennan, T. (2006) *Wars of Position: The Cultural Politics of Left and Right*. New York: Columbia University Press.

Collett, E. and Zuleeg, F. (2008) *Soft, Scarce, and Super Skills: Sourcing the Next Generation of Migrant Workers in Europe*. Washington, DC: Migration Policy Institute.

Foucault, M. (1982) 'The Subject and Power'. *Critical Inquiry* 8(4), 777–795.

Gramsci, A. (1971) *Selections from the Prison Notebooks*. Ed. and trans. by Quintin, H. and Smith, G.N. New York: International Publishers.

Guha, R (1998) 'The Migrant's Time'. *Postcolonial Studies* 1(2), 155–160.

Gunning, D. (2010) *Race and Antiracism in Black British and British Asian Literature*. Liverpool: Liverpool University Press.

Hai, Y. (2008) *The Making of Mr Hai's Daughter: Memoirs of his Daughter*. London: Virago.

Heath, A. and Khan, O. (2012) *Ethnic Minority British Election Study – Key Findings*. London: Runnymede Trust [online]. Available from <www.runnymedetrust.org/uploads/EMBESbriefingFINALx.pdf> [6 October 2013].

Hughes, D. (2013) 'Tory Councillor John Cherry Resigns over "Openly Racist Language" after Saying "there are Certain Nationalities where they are Uncertain what this Hard Work is all About'. *Independent* [online]. Available from <www.independent.co.uk/news/uk/home-news/tory-councillor-john-cherry-resigns-over-openly-racist-language-after-saying-there-are-certain-8581755.html> [12 February 2018].

Hutnyk, J. (2005) 'The Dialectic of Here and There: Anthropology "at Home" and British Asian Communism'. *Social Identities: Journal for the Study of Race, Nation and Culture* 11(4), 345–361.

Khan, A. (2010) *Poppadom Preach*. London: Simon & Schuster.

Khan, O. (2015) 'Diversity and Democracy: Race and the 2015 General Election'. London: Runnymede Trust [online]. Available from <www.runnymedetrust.org/uploads/GE2015.pdf> [8 July 2015].

Laville, S. and Muir, H. (2006) 'Secret Report Brands Muslim Police Corrupt' [online]. Available from <www.theguardian.com/uk/2006/jun/10/race.topstories3> [12 February 2018].

Lemke, C. (2008) 'Racism in the Diaspora: Nadeem Aslam's *Maps for Lost Lovers* (2004)'. In *Multi-Ethnic Britain 2000+. New Perspectives in Literature, Films and the Arts*. Ed. by Lars, E., Korte, B., Pirker, U., and Reinfandt, C. Amsterdam: Rodopi, 171–183.

Liddle, R. (2013) 'Rod Liddle: The Truths You Can't Tell in Today's Britain'. *Spectator* [online]. Available from <www.spectator.co.uk/2013/11/you-cant-say-that/> [12 February 2018].

Lipsett, A. (2008) 'Ethnic Minority Students "Still Underachieving"'. *Guardian* [online]. Available from <www.theguardian.com/education/2008/jan/22/highereducation.uk3> [28 May 2013].

Malnick, E. (2013) 'Minister Apologises for Pakistani 'Corruption' Remarks'. *Telegraph* [online]. Available from <www.telegraph.co.uk/news/politics/10470450/Minister-apologises-for-Pakistani-corruption-remarks.html> [21 February 2014].

Manzoor, S. (2007) *Greetings from Bury Park: Race, Religion and Rock 'n' Roll*. London: Bloomsbury.

Modood, T. (2004) 'Capitals, Ethnic Identity and Educational Qualifications'. *Cultural Trends* 13(2), 50, 87–105.

Modood, T., Berthoud, R., Lakey, J., Nazroo, J., Smith, P., Virdee, S., and Beishon, S. (1997) *Ethnic Minorities in Britain: Diversity and Disadvantage*. London: Policy Studies Institute.

O'Donnell, M. and Sharpe, S. (2000) *Uncertain Masculinities: Youth, Ethnicity and Class in Contemporary Britain*. London and New York: Routledge.

Quinn, B. (2013) 'Politicians Need to "Wake Up" to Corruption in Minority Communities'. *Guardian* [online]. Available from <www.theguardian.com/politics/2013/nov/23/dominic-grieve-electoral-corruption-pakistani-community> [21 February 2014].

Savage, M. (2002) 'Class and Labour History'. In *Class and Other Identities: Gender, Religion and Ethnicity in the Writing of European Labour History*. Ed. by Voss, V., Heerma, L., and Linden, M.M. New York: Berghahn Books, 55–72.

Spivak, G.C. (1990) *The Post-colonial Critic. Interviews, Strategies, Dialogues*. ed. by Harasym, S. New York: Routledge.

Spivak, G.C. (1999) *A Critique of Postcolonial Reason: Toward a History of the Vanishing Present*. Cambridge, MA: Harvard University Press.

Tiffin, C. and Lawson, A. (1994) 'The Textuality of Empire'. In *De-Scribing Empire. Post-colonialism and Textuality*. Ed. by Tiffin, C. and Lawson, A. London: Routledge, 1–11.

Van Dijk, T.A. (2000) 'New(s) Racism: A Discourse Analytical Approach'. In *Ethnic Minorities and the Media*. Ed. by Simon, C. Milton Keynes: Open University Press, 33–49.

Viswanathan, G. (1989) *Masks of Conquest: Literary Study and British Rule in India*. Oxford: Oxford University Press.

Webster, C. (2003) 'Race, Space and Fear: Imagined Geographies of Racism, Crime, Violence and Disorder in Northern England'. *Capital & Class* 27, 95–122.

Werbner, P. (1991): 'Black and Ethnic Leaderships in Britain. A Theoretical Overview'. In *Black and Ethnic Leaderships: The Cultural Dimensions of Political Action*. Ed. by Werbner, P. and Anwar, M. London: Routledge, 15–37.

Williams, R. (1977) *Marxism and Literature*. Oxford: Oxford University Press.

Yaqin, A. (2013) 'Cosmopolitan Ventures during Times of Crisis: A Postcolonial Reading of Faiz Ahmed Faiz's "Dasht-e-tanhai" and Nadeem Aslam's *Maps for Lost Lovers*'. *Pakistaniaat: A Journal of Pakistan Studies* 5(1), 62–78.

Young, I.M. (1990) *Justice and the Politics of Difference*. Princeton: Princeton University Press.

Young, I.M. (2000) *Inclusion and Democracy*. Oxford: Oxford University Press.

Young, I.M. (2004) 'The Ideal of Community and the Politics of Difference'. In *Contemporary Political Theory: A Reader*. Ed. by Farrelly, C. London: SAGE, 195–204.

PART VII

Unsettling narratives
Imagining post-postcolonial perspectives

25
NON-HUMAN NARRATIVE AGENCY

Textual sedimentation in Pakistani anglophone literature

Asma Mansoor

This chapter focuses on depictions of non-human narrative agency that blend with human narratives to create alternative conceptions of human subjectivities in Pakistani anglophone literature. My contention is that a post-postcolonial selfhood[1] can initiate a reconstruction of social and individual practices that see humans enmeshed within their immediate material contexts that temporally predate and outlast anthropocentric epistemologies. It is for this reason that I read Pakistani anglophone poetry and fiction to theorise a concept of Pakistani subjectivities which are constructed in terms of their engagement with their agentic material environment. I argue that Pakistani anglophone literature reflects the country's material environment in terms of a semiotic environment wherein diverse material phenomena engage in meaning-making processes which intervene in human, historical, and geopolitical narratives, and vice versa. Thus, Pakistani anglophone literature invites a rereading of representations of Pakistan's material environment within which Pakistani selfhood, in all its diverse forms, may be rethought. Interweaving the theoretical arguments of Karen Barad, Peter Sloterdijk, Felix Guattari, Michel Serres, Wendy Wheeler, Jeffrey Jerome Cohen, and Timothy Morton, this chapter explores how fossils, rocks, and mountains function in the selected texts as narrative-generating 'nobjects' (Sloterdijk 2011: 467) whose intra-actions with humans permit the sedimentation (i.e. layered superimposition) of multiple stories and histories. The texts selected for this discussion reflect how human and non-human layers are enfolded and sedimented in each other. Thus, both human and non-human phenomena function intra-actively as historical archives, narrating stories together, framing an alternative sense of the self that exceeds anthropocentric history. The texts that I consider here are Uzma Aslam Khan's *The Geometry of God* (2014) and Kamila Shamsie's *A God in Every Stone* (2014), as well as selected poems written by Ilona Yusuf, Harris Khalique, and Rizwan Akhtar that are pertinent to this discussion. My argument begins by delineating the notion of post-postcolonial subjectivities in terms of the material environment. It then uses relevant theoretical tenets to define Pakistani post-postcolonial subjectivities, as evinced in Pakistani anglophone literature, by presenting the material environment as a reference point for theorising a post-postcolonial selfhood.

Therefore, in this discussion, the focus remains on Pakistani subjectivities that are heterogeneous due to various ideological, ethnic, and class factors. These subjectivities have generally been defined in terms of glocal power structures, which range from Pakistan's economic, regional, and social engagements with countries like India, China, the United States of America, and Saudi Arabia, to its complex multi-ethnic spectrum, its unstable democracy,[2] and the complexities engendered by its participation in the ongoing war on terror.[3] Contrary to this, my theorisation posits the non-human material environment as a new referent for rethinking Pakistani identities. Therefore, this chapter focuses on the material-discursive resonances of non-human phenomena represented in the selected texts. It highlights the audibility of these resonances as they constitute Pakistani subjectivities outside the binaristic framework provided by postcolonial theories which, in turn, operate within the paradigm of colonisation and its aftermath in former colonies. My argument centralises the Baradian notion of material-discursive resonances as it foregrounds the entanglement of biological, social, and cultural discourses with processual materialisations of matter and their 'agential contributions' (Barad 2007: 66) spanning the human and non-human spectra. I play with the idea that not only are entanglements of materiality and knowledge co-constitutive of each other, they are also co-responsible in accounting for a historicity of the land and a fluid human subjectivity. The main contention is that Pakistani subjectivities are constituted in terms of their material environment whose open-ended enunciations exceed hierarchal anthropocentric enclosures, as well as the exclusionary binaries that have outlined postcolonial discussions in South Asian contexts.

In the context of a postcolonial subject, which is haunted by the spectre of colonialism and its binaristic hierarchy, the realisation of belonging to such an open-ended world is extremely important. This is because this world functions as a reference point for thinking about one's subjectivity outside the referential plane of colonialism. This realisation also enables one to think of 'alternative futures' (Harari 2016: 59), particularly in the context of Pakistan's medial environment that functions as a 'semantic plasma' (Sloterdijk 2011: 316) which surrounds us Pakistanis and our narratives like an 'intra-uterine butler' that remains close and at the periphery, nourishing us, 'privy to all our secrets' (Sloterdijk 2011: 357). It generates an awareness that being-in-the-world does not merely mean recognising the materiality of the world, but also realising its semantic agency. Pakistan's specific topography, smells, sights, and embedded memories continue to frame the postcolonial subject's subjectivity, just as the womb functions as a sphere wherein sounds and nutrients catalyse the development of an inchoate subjective being. The realisation that the world is the non-human companion of our subjectivity, therefore, functions as a starting point for rethinking the subjectivity of postcolonial subjects. Post-postcolonialism could completely discard the idea of subalternity and rethink human subjectivities in terms of material *logoi* articulated by the material environment. In doing so, it would allow the juxtaposition of numerous temporal frameworks in one moment in time, thus displacing the primacy of any particular politico-historical phase, such as the age of colonialism, as the dominant referent of human identity. Post-postcolonialism would not see human subjectivity as a singular, positive ideological outcome of a particular epistemic phase in history alone, but rather as a processual product of multiple material histories.

This idea has not been investigated by either Pakistani or international theorists in the context of Pakistani anglophone literature, despite the fact that it could prove to be a means of opening up debates regarding Pakistani subjectivities in an era when we are aiming to move beyond the Empire and its aftermath. It is precisely this reason that makes my work timely, as it explores the 'intimate-spheric enclosedness' (Sloterdijk 2011: 542) between the human and the non-human, as evinced in Pakistani anglophone literature. This intimacy is evident in Shamsie's *A God in Every Stone* whose main character, Viv Spencer, sees a stone statue of Buddha in a Peshawar museum as articulating a 'humanity beyond all other humanities' (2014: 226), a humanity that enunciates itself through the non-human, and vice versa. The non-human statue is a concrete articulation of a human belief system which, in turn, functions as a symbolic buttress for humans reinforcing their belief in eternal wisdom, rebirth, and peace, as well as a reminder of the region's 5,000-year history. The statue, in its interface with humans, gains unique semantic agency as it coalesces with their belief systems. *The Geometry of God* also depicts this intimacy through a blind girl, Mehwish, who is immersed in an audible semantic plasma, a fact covered at length later in this discussion. In these texts, being-in-the-world implies recognition of the environment as a relationship in itself, where the perpetual interwovenness of all phenomena outlines the state of 'being-in' (Sloterdijk 2011: 579) the world and its multiple narratives. Within these works, all bodies are 'storied bodies' (Phillips and Sullivan 2012: 5). As storied bodies, the non-human phenomena in the selected texts counter anthropocentrism, which proclaims human uniqueness on the grounds of humans' ability to speak. I argue, therefore, that if anthropocentrism claims exclusivity on the basis of speech, then the textual enactments of nobjects in Pakistani anglophone literature negate anthropocentric exclusivity on account of their being articulate storied bodies enfolded in each other. Here, Peter Sloterdijk's idea of 'nobjects', which functions as a concept generator within this theorisation, merits some elaboration. Nobjects are things, persons, or media that function as 'intimate augmenters' (Sloterdijk 2011: 467) and allow the transformation of a subject within their frame, such as the placenta or the womb. Being neither subjects nor objects, nobjects, such as rocks, mountains, ores, winds, seas, etc., are medial mechanisms with which the human race is intimately enmeshed through a reciprocal process of reading and interpreting each other. The texts discussed in this chapter indicate this reciprocal narrative agency. If this agency is evinced in narrative enunciations, then phenomena like the Circlet of Skylax, which galvanises the plot in *A God in Every Stone*, the fossil in *The Geometry of God*, and other non-human phenomena in the selected poems are storied agents that continue to move across time and space, blending into malleable individual and collective human histories.

The literary texts discussed in this chapter reflect this malleability of non-human phenomena and histories. Embedded within them, human subjectivity also functions as an irreducible singularity, allowing one to question the fixity of epistemological enclosures and their exclusionary politics. This realisation of being enmeshed within the material world opens up a space to recast one's sense of the self outside racial and cultural binaries, since the world and human bodies function as emergent phenomena, constantly opening themselves up to new futures.

Therefore, venturing in the direction of a post-postcolonial discourse, my discussion sees the present as a multi-'medial' (Sloterdijk 2011: 397) narrative in which phenomena generate asemiotic narratives intra-actively. Both Karen Barad and Sloterdijk characterise the world as a combination of multiple 'intra-actions' across diverse enmeshed media, or agentic phenomena (Barad 2007: 33). Barad argues, on the basis of quantum theory, that all bodies are radically interconnected, and thus challenge all restrictive categorisations. Her neological term 'intra-actions' accounts for *'the mutual constitution of entangled agencies'* (Barad 2007: 33; emphasis original) which emerge from phenomena interfacing with each other. Her idea of intra-actions differs from the idea of interaction, in the sense that intra-action posits the 'ontological inseparability' of phenomena across the spectrum of existence while interactions stem from a preconceived idea of their existence as separate entities (2007: 128). In short, her major idea is that agency does not precede interactions; rather, malleable phenomena are produced as a result of their intra-actions and account for the world's 'differential becoming' (Barad 2007: 149). Through these modes of differential becomings, material and discursive phenomena function as 'actants' (Latour 2004: 75), configuring the world's syntax which exceeds any linguistic, ontological, or epistemological enclosure. The term 'actants' refers to non-human agentic interventions within the ecological web, as well as to human actions that affect all modalities of knowing and mattering in the world. These fluid, intra-active narratives require a blending of 'new micropolitical', 'microsocial', 'aesthetic', and 'analytic practices' (Guattari 2000: 51) that see the human and the non-human immanently enmeshed.

Pakistani anglophone literature and material textuality

As established above, humans and non-humans exist in a state of intimacy as they mutually engage in both material and semiotic meaning-making practices. Customs, ideologies, experiences, landscapes, histories, expressions, etc. are all congealed as assemblages across an extended geological time span (Ahmed 2010: 246). Pakistan's topographical changes across various historical epochs bear witness to this congealment. As Buddhist, Hindu, Muslim, and British rules succeeded each other, the material landscape changed and medially articulated the fluctuant ideological patterns of changing times. The rise of stupas, temples, mosques, churches, and changing cityscapes at the behest of succeeding dynasties have all functioned as indicators of such changes that repeatedly framed the political, social, and economic infrastructure of the country over the centuries. Such changes are evident even today, as Pakistan enters a vital trade link, the China-Pak Economic Corridor (CPEC), with a neighbouring country. Under the umbrella of the CPEC, it is the material infrastructure of the country that is altered as it operates as a vital participant catering to the needs of this corridor which, in turn, impacts on the lifestyles of people in the region. As wealth comes in and new business opportunities arise, the materiality of the land and the people become participants in the country's changing geo-strategic partnerships as Pakistan moves away from the USA and inclines more towards the economic patronage of China.

In this process of material meaning-making and exchange, language, and by extension textuality, becomes an extended concept suffused with an 'ecological consciousness' (Cohen 2015: 6) in a confined sense, as well as imbued with a material force that allows a constant de- and reterritorialisation of signs, both material and conceptual, so that new narratives are generated. This de- and reterritorialisation is evident in *A God in Every Stone*, which focuses on a British archaeologist, Viv Spencer, and her search for a historical artefact that moves across time and space. From the Persian invasion of India under Darius, which pushed as far as Caspatyrus, modern-day Peshawar, the artefact finally falls into the hands of a revolutionary Pashtun woman, Zarina, who is fighting the British colonisers. In each era, the artefact has been a site of struggle for the natives of the land against foreign invaders. The circlet thus undergoes a constant de- and reterritorialisation as it moves from one spatial and historical context to the next. During this movement, it becomes a part of the lives of the humans who discover it, and an integral component of their ongoing narratives. This is evident in the character of Viv's assistant, Najeeb, another participant in a long line of historians and storytellers who have chronicled the events shaping the land since the accounts of the Indus Valley Civilisation given by Herodotus in the fifth century BCE. Historical narratives undergo constant de- and reterritorialisation through both human and non-human phenomena (i.e. through the artefact, Herodotus, Zareena, Viv, and Najeeb) across millennia. Pakistanis, therefore, are not defined by narratives constituted by those in power alone. Their subjectivities are constituted through their material heritage too. What *The God in Every Stone* indicates is that the material world is intra-actively alive, composed of 'Stone made flesh; no, stone made bone and skin', and seemingly a 'heart beating within' (Shamsie 2014: 139), thus interfacing with the people intra-actively embedded within this material frame. What this movement affirms is that humans and non-humans have a shared 'placenta' of existence (Sloterdijk 2011: 44), owing to the medial power of non-human actants in the constitution of their world views as they reconceptualise their relationship with their material environment. In doing so, they rethink themselves as actors situated within a matrix of transtemporal material, cultural, historical, and economic institutions, in dialogue with actors that are not human. The medial power of non-human actants reminds us of a heritage that precedes our cultural and socioeconomic beginnings. The material-semiotic agency of our landscape thus becomes the predominant factor framing our living mechanisms and our perceptions of whom we are as subjects within a history that is mobile.

Khan's *The Geometry of God* also focuses on this agency of non-human actants as it depicts the suppression of independent thought during Zia's Islamisation. Revolving around two sisters, Mehwish and Amal, their palaeontologist grandfather, and a whale fossil, their stories coalesce with the epochal narrative of evolution and its conflict with obscurantist religious interpretations. As the fossil travels through time, it gets wrapped up within multiple histories, ranging from the pre-human era to the present time, when it interweaves with the debates regarding human evolution in modern-day Pakistan and becomes the fulcrum of political conflicts. While the fossil vindicates the belief of palaeontologists like Amal and her grandfather that the human race evolved out of the animal kingdom, they come into direct conflict with government-backed religious zealots who believe in the divine origin of the human race. Thus, the fossil is a sedimented archive of historical narratives, both individual and collective, geological and political, as Amal establishes 'co relation(s)' among bones extending across time different times (Khan 2014: 171). These texts show these natural formations and cultural artefacts telling their own stories, rhizomatically weaving across the grid of history[4] and thus exceeding the official historical narratives imposed by those who have been in power in the country in different eras, both before and after its independence in 1947.

The material world, in its reciprocal relationship with evolving human narratives, thus functions as the site where changes in human subjectivities manifest themselves. Khan and Shamsie use the fossil and the Circlet of Skylax, respectively, as points where multiple histories converge and new senses of the self emerge. As Amal reads the fossil, and Zareena re-buries the circlet, the novels raise important questions pertaining to who we are as citizens with specific material histories that rhizomatically interweave with various historical narratives of the world at large, and who we are as humans in relation to non-human actants. What they suggest is that, as Pakistanis, we are more than what our official histories say we are. We are at one with our land and vice versa; and as our 'entangled state of agencies' (Barad 2007: 23) with the non-human world shifts, our awareness of the self also undergoes a diffraction. In presenting the artefact that originated in Darius' court around 515 BCE and the whale fossil emerging out of an age preceding human beings, these texts open up avenues into rethinking what it means to be Pakistani, while Amal's grandfather declares, 'Pray five times a day and be a *real* Pakistani! Speak Urdu and be a *real* Pakistani!, or English and half as Pakistani! Well, here's my answer. Study whales and be Pakistani!' (Khan 2014: 5; emphasis original). Being Pakistani is not about complying with a particular ideology; Pakistani subjectivities rise out of the land in which the fossil was embedded. They predate politics and history, and thus are inherently malleable. In studying the whale, we study ourselves across millennia, not centuries or decades. Pakistan is a geopolitical enclosure of land that predates geopolitics and its assigned nomenclature. As inhabitants of this land, we too are like the whale fossil; we are also sedimented beings moving through time. The whale fossil is in motion, and so are Pakistani subjectivities.

In highlighting this mobile materiality of the environment, Pakistani anglophone literature presents history as an ongoing narrative, defying completion and resisting confinement within any political, human discourse, and thus granting mobility to human subjectivities. As the whale fossil and the Circlet of Skylax move through time, they participate in different historical events, suggesting an ongoing continuity of history, even when human actors are no longer there to call the shots. In *A God in Every Stone*, Zarina's act of burying the Circlet does not signify an end to history; rather, it reaffirms the fact that the Circlet will continue on its travels through time. During their historical itineraries, these actants illustrate the malleability of political identities by disrupting and extending the concept of time. Since human subjectivities emerge out of specific historical narratives, they do not remain embedded within political history alone, they become embedded within a cosmological history that provides a wider space to think of ourselves not only as citizens of a political and religion domain, but as citizens of a much more extensive geological domain. Since geological time is mobile, it cannot be reduced to a stagnant value. Pakistani subjectivities are thus defined in terms of this geological time.

As civilisations died out in the region, such as the Indus Valley Civilisation, the Buddhist dynasty in Northern Pakistan, followed by numerous invasions by the Huns that were succeeded by the arrival of Persians and Turks, the subject identities of inhabitants of the land varied as belief and political systems underwent alterations as new masters replaced each other. The only factor that remained constant was the land in all its ongoing material configurations. These configurations created 'thingly' narratives (Cohen 2015: 4) that could neither be shut down nor confined within rigid ideological enclosures. It is these 'thingly' memories embedded within these artefacts that allow the excavation of deleted historical narratives, producing different asemiotic narratives that blend with the numerous historical narratives of the land. Thus, the material phenomena defy their supposed subalternity and no longer remain silent participants in the ongoing history of Pakistan and the region. As the materiality of the landscape changes, so do meanings and their enunciations, which demands a discarding of history seen only in human terms. It is for this reason that the non-human material environment and textual practices function as reference points to redefine a Pakistani selfhood.

Entangled agencies and transversal subjectivities

I have already established that the world is a compendium of 'enunciative assemblages' that articulate themselves in multiple 'registers'. As a consequence, all these assemblages remain in a state of 'transversality', intra-acting across expressive substances which are both linguistic and non-semiotic (Guattari 1995: 24), such as DNA helices, computer algorithms, information-laden photons and quanta, fossils, and tree rings. This transversality, or transindividual intra-actions, is evident in many Pakistani anglophone poems. Elements of Yusuf's poems, such as 'images from the Karakoram', 'slum', 'cloudscape', 'history', and 'modern times', present different modes of transversality as the human and the non-human come together in the ecologically diverse Pakistani landscape. In her poems, memory is a narrative whose syntax is constituted through Yusuf's intra-action with the material environment and its internalisation. Yusuf's history resides in her alloyed genes, transversally transferred from a Western mother and an Eastern father:

> So folded am i in my own complexity
> Folded as a foetus upon itself.
> (2001: 34)

Pakistan and its landscape are internalised, prompting Yusuf to learn another language, as she decodes the language of the material world in the context of her own situation. The language that she registers is encoded in different physical stimuli with which she intra-acts by way of 'cognitive transference' (Guattari 1995:101). Subjectivities are medially transformed as different bodies engage in an intersubjective transference in her work. The human and the non-human enunciate each other differentially as the forbidding layered mountains of the Karakoram move in a fluid syntax along fault lines where the subcontinent collides with the Eurasian plate. All the while, the human has 'sketched his fingers his path his mark / along the map of centuries' (Yusuf 2001: 76). What becomes evident is that, as time moves on, the 'medial' (Sloterdijk 2011: 295) environment of Pakistan continues to shape human subjectivities. This is also evident in Khalique's poetry. His poem 'Lahore Airport' defines life as a multilayered 'running text' (2012: 34), and all that people leave behind is articulate imprints of their departure on a tarmac runway. In Khalique's poetry, trees and rivers remain active reminders of the country's paradoxical problems, such as class stratification, political uncertainties, and ideological conflicts. With the country's 'liquid history flowing everywhere' (Khalique 2012: 84), the material world appears to be spreading 'rumours of happiness / in a nation brooding on despair' (Khalique 2012: 56), while the radioactive mountains of Chaghi and Pokhran symbolically inscribe the volatile relations between India and Pakistan at the time of their nuclear tests in 1999. History is thus a malleable narrative composed of flowing material-semiotic encoding and decoding practices.

In similar manner, the Circlet of Skylax in Shamsie's *God in Every Stone* enacts this material-semiotic coding and recoding through time. Material and discursive stories connect histories embedded in the material and sociopolitical worlds. As the Circlet moves across geo-temporal scales from Caria to India, passing through the hands of Alexander, Asoka, Maya the Buddhist Nun, Najeeb, and finally Zarina, multiple narratives are sedimented within the artefact. It is more than a thing; it is a conveyance device that, in Jeffery Jerome Cohen's terms, can be described as a 'storied materiality that lasts' (2015: 57). This lasting materiality is also evident in Akhtar's depiction of the landscape in his poem 'Lahore 2009'. Lahore presents a melting of human and non-human phenomena into each other, displaying a conscious energy that creates meanings. This is also evident in his poem 'Noise', where a whining crow, screeching cars, and screaming vendors all become a comment on the beggar who is flanked on all sides by a world of material wealth and indifference (2017: 199). In 'Lahore 2009', Akhtar reminisces about Lahore, a city embedded in his family's history and in his blood, and he writes how 'Words drop into another's words' while the '*azan* / throbbed at our door'; sounds and words, bound in a 'lingual embrace' (2017: 138; emphasis original), collectively create a symphony specific to a city. Cities like Lahore are quilted in poems; therefore, the city speaks and is spoken to. The acoustics produce a material-semiotic symphony that wafts into the human consciousness, as he writes in his poem 'Behind Rain': 'Cicadas' tymbals deny evening of its privacy suddenly I woke to sounds behind windows … a euphoric rain over-weeps broadcasting a bawling melee of consonants each tree effuses its pitter-patter' (Akhtar 2017: 95). In a country where freedom of speech has been rigidly curtailed by successive military and democratic governments, human language becomes 'a mutilated wick' (Akhtar 2017: 127), an aspect that Akhtar depicts in 'The Porcelain: In Memory of Faiz Ahmed Faiz'. In such a scenario, it is the world of matter that becomes a spokesperson for the human condition, as depicted by Akhtar's poem 'Ways of Reading':

Deep in winter's trees
a slow story of leaves
finds your hands
poking words on pages …
These are ways of reading
lost treasures of silence
same as bodies do not yell
and become interpretations.
        (2017: 23)

In this game of mutual interpretations, Akhtar's work reflects how sights, sounds, and smells all synchronise to establish a vibrant material syntax of the world, which the human mind processes to create new combinations of meanings that allow one to reread oneself in terms of one's individual self as embeddedness within an articulate material world.

In this material environment, meanings continue to be deposited within various embodied material forms, so that all phenomena function as open-ended hypertextual environments imbricated together, a factor evinced in Akhtar's 'The Maids of the City of Dust'. Here too, all phenomena are speaking in different codes. As Lahore's 'layers and layers of litter' (Akhtar 2017: 40) are swept away by its 'women of dust', it reflects an interwoven changing materiality that also speaks of class hierarchies, as the people travelling on those roads treat these women's labour with a snobbish nonchalance. The cityscape of Lahore thus presents a history in which economic, political, and material alterations remain intricately entangled, articulating its multiple problems and complexities that define how people live their lives.

Matterphor: rereading meanings and materiality in Pakistani anglophone literature

In order to further read the eloquent agency of matter as depicted in Pakistani anglophone literature comprehensively, I coalesce two concepts, 'matterphor' and 'biosemiosis', expounded by Cohen and Wendy Wheeler, respectively. Cohen argues that material structures like stones and mountains function as archives of mobile narratives or material metaphors. While biosemiosis foregrounds 'biological meaning' and the 'embodied nature' of intra-acting agencies and meanings (Wheeler and Westling 2015: 216), a matterphor is a conversation between the biological and the non-biological. Therefore, in the world at large, matter and metaphor enunciatively come together as 'matterphor' (Cohen 2015: 4), that is, a semiosis across ontological and epistemological differences, thus producing material stories. An author does not, strictly speaking, give voice to non-human phenomena; rather, an author adds to the symphonic play of semiotic differences which constitute the world. In this play of differences, semiotics gains an ecological texture as both biological and non-biological material phenomena disseminate their own narratives in a language that exceeds logocentrism through biosemiotics and matterphoric exchanges.

This matterphoric exchange is evident in Akhtar's poem 'Houbara Bustards', named after endangered migratory birds that arrive in Pakistan from Central Asia in winter. Hunted by Arab princes for its supposed aphrodisiac qualities, the Houbara Bustard's narrative ends in Pakistan as its life's story is cruelly interwoven with the story of the country's geopolitical dependence on Arab oil (2017: 36). The poem is a scathing criticism of the special dispensations that the Pakistani government grants to Middle Eastern royals to hunt this endangered bird in exchange for political and economic perks. The Houbara Bustard moves across a vast terrain of material and ideological differences, both materially and symbolically, to be metabolised within the vast maw of the vested political interests of the human race. Folded within this complicated web of materiality, ideologies, and political gimmickries, it is not only non-human phenomena, like the Houbara Bustard, that are impacted upon – the vectors of human subjectivity also undergo a shift. As Pakistan's political elite pander to the whims of Middle Eastern oil magnates, such as Qatari princes and the Saudi royal family, permitting them to hunt down these rare birds, the Houbara Bustard becomes more than a bird; it functions as a comment on the condition of a nation that is exploited by many masters, despite the fact that it has cast off the yolk of colonialism.

As medial metaphors, non-human actants in Pakistani anglophone literature depict a sliding of material-discursive enunciations across the medial world in a manner that constantly modifies the praxis and 'theory of knowledge' (Serres 1982: 65), so that new histories are created which connect diverse bodies in a joint trans-temporal narrative. For instance, both the human and the non-human function as equal participants in Pakistan's determination to consolidate its economic connections with China and the Central Asian countries that lie to the north, linked via the Karakoram mountain range. Yusuf's poem 'Images from the Karakoram' depicts 'wide sweeps of sand and boulder / fanned down years of mountainside' in the Karakoram mountain range. This rocky syntax of mountains then merges into a 'new road that winds and twists' through the 'blasted-out overhangs' (2001: 75–76), which are the result of human engineering. In addition, this road, the Karakoram Highway, re-etches the ancient Silk Road that connected the subcontinent to China in ancient times. The road and the mountains are thus trans-temporal bodies functioning as sites of new historical inscriptions that remain fluid as new socioeconomic necessities compel alterations to the country's topography. With the CPEC, as mentioned above, the ever-developing road links between China and Pakistan make physical alterations to the layout of the land inevitable. In the present time, these material alterations hint at the further consolidation of Pak-China economic links in the future. The Karakoram Mountains, as well as the slum areas in Yusuf's poetry, are connected in a joint, trans-temporal narrative. Each of these material phenomena functions as an 'exchanger of time' (Serres 1982: 72–73) bound in matterphoric intimacies. The enunciations of the material world thus remain open-ended and, by extension, so do their historical interpretations. Human and non-human bodies, like those of Mehwish, the fossil, the Karakoram Highway, and the Circlet, act, therefore, not only as exchangers of time, but also as exchangers of meanings and narratives.

To conclude, one of the major insights that one draws from Pakistani anglophone literature is that as the material world changes, narratives and history continue to change, too. Shifts in human subjectivities also emanate within the medial space of nobjects. For instance, the nobjects constituting Mehwish's material environment functions as meaning-making intimate augmenters of her ability to comprehend herself through her physical experience. Similarly, in the works of Shamsie, Yusuf, Akhtar, and Khalique, the fossil, the circlet, the buildings of Lahore, etc. all signify an open-ended, transtemporal, and multi-medial exchange of meanings. As a result of this material-semiotic fluidity, history is recast in terms of a malleable symbiotic intra-action with the material world. This intra-action prevents placing phenomena within exclusive categories, which liberates the definition of one's identity from the narrow confines of race and gender alone, allowing it to be rethought in terms of an agentic materiality that functions as an audibly resonant archive of narratives. It is through depictions of such agentic materiality that Pakistani anglophone literature provides a viable site for a post-postcolonial reframing of Pakistani subjectivities, thus liberating this selfhood from the spectre of its colonial past.

Notes

1 While colonial and postcolonial discourses focus primarily on dealing with the coloniser-colonised binary, my idea of a post-postcolonial discourse initiates a mode of thinking that goes beyond this binary in terms of a mutual osmosis of ideas that pre-empts the reinstallation of rigid, hierarchised categorisations. From my perspective, the idea of post-postcoloniality is different from decoloniality, which focuses on an epistemological disconnect from colonial mental models. Conversely, post-postcoloniality is a means of amalgamating Western and non-Western epistemological models without alienating either of these thinking patterns, in order to conceptualise ourselves as glocal citizens with a diversely mobile selfhood.

2 In the seven decades since its independence, Pakistan's democracy has been overturned by three military coups. Martial law was first imposed in 1958 by Major General Iskander Mirza, who was exiled by General Ayub Khan. Ayub Khan's rule ended in 1971. The second military coup was led by General Zia-ul-Haq in 1977 against Prime Minister Zulfiqar Ali Bhutto, who was subsequently hanged. General Zia's reign ended in a plane crash in 1988, allowing the country's shaky democracy to establish itself again under Benazir Bhutto's premiership. However, the next eleven years saw Benazir Bhutto and Nawaz Sharif taking the helm twice, since both their governments saw repeated dissolutions due to conflicts between the army and the presidency. In 1999, Nawaz Sharif forcibly removed the then Army Chief, General Pervez Musharraf, which led to a military coup and the expulsion of Nawaz Sharif from the country. Musharraf's rule lasted until 2008, when he resigned under public pressure.
3 With the collapse of the World Trade Center in New York, Pakistan's ties with the Taliban came under global scrutiny. As Pakistan's links to various *jihadi* groups in the region attracted US ire, it joined the Global War on Terror, and since then has been a key ally of the United States.
4 We find a similar traverse across millennia effected by material objects in the poetry of Akhtar, Yusuf, and Khalique. Their works reflect how life is all about intra-active textual becomings; however, due to space constraints, they cannot be encapsulated in detail here. The reader can nevertheless refer to their collections (i.e. Akhtar's *Lahore, I Am Coming*, Yusuf's *Picture This ... Poems*, and Khalique's *Between You and Your Love*) for further analysis.

Bibliography

Ahmed, S. (2010) 'Orientations Matter'. In *New Materialisms: Ontology, Agency and Politics*. Ed. by Coole, D. and Frost, S. Durham: Duke University Press, 234–257.
Akhtar, R. (2017) *Lahore, I Am Coming*. Lahore: Punjab University Press.
Barad, K. (2007) *Meeting the Universe Halfway: Quantum Physics and the Entanglement of Matter and Meaning*. Durham: Duke University Press.
Cohen, J.J. (2015) *Stone: An Ecology of the Inhuman*. Minneapolis: University of Minnesota Press.
Guattari, F. (1995) *Chaosmosis*. Trans. by Bains, P. and Pefanis, J. Indianapolis: Indiana University Press.
Guattari, F. (2000) *The Three Ecologies*. Trans. by Pindar, I. and Sutton, P. London: Athlone Press.
Harari, Y.N. (2016) *Homo Deus: A Brief History of Tomorrow*. London: Harvill Secker.
Khalique, H. (2012) *Between You and Your Love* [online]. Available from <http://harriskhalique.com/book.php?title=between> [30 December 2016].
Khan, U.A. (2014) *The Geometry of God*. Lahore: ILQA Publications.
Latour, B. (2004) *Politics of Nature: How to Bring the Sciences into Democracy*. Trans. by Porter, C. Cambridge, MA: Harvard University Press.
Morton, T. (2015) 'Spectres of the Non-human'. In *For They That Sow the Wind*. Ed. by Charrière, J. London: Parasol Unit, 64–67.
Phillips, D. and Sullivan, H.I. (2012) 'Material Ecocriticism: Dirt, Waste, Bodies, Food, and Other Matter'. *Interdisciplinary Studies in Literature and the Environment* 19(3), 445–447.
Serres, M. (1982) *The Parasite*. Trans. by Schehr, L.R. Baltimore: Johns Hopkins University Press.
Shamsie, K. (2014) *A God in Every Stone*. London: Bloomsbury.
Sloterdijk, P. (2011) *Bubbles*. Trans. by Hoban, W. Los Angeles: Semiotext(e).
Wheeler, W. (2011) 'The Biosemiotic Turn: Abduction, or, the Nature of Creative Reason in Nature and Culture'. *Ecocritical Theory: New European Approaches*. Ed. by Goodbody, A. and Rigby, K. Charlottesville: University of Virginia Press, 270–282.
Wheeler, W. and Westling, L. (2015) 'Biosemiotics and Culture: Editors' Introduction'. *Green Letters: Studies in Ecocriticism* 19(3), 215–226 [online]. Available from <http://dx.doi.org/10.1080/14688417.2015.1078973> [30 December 2016].
Yusuf, I. (2001) *Picture This ... Poems*. Islamabad: Alhamra Publishing Pakistan.

26
POST-POSTCOLONIAL EXPERIMENTS WITH PERSPECTIVES

Hanji Lee

This chapter looks at a few narratological curiosities among recently published Pakistani anglophone novels. Mohsin Hamid's *The Reluctant Fundamentalist* (2007) and *How to Get Filthy Rich in Rising Asia* (2013) and Bilal Tanweer's *The Scatter Here is too Great* (2013) are all intriguing novels about Pakistan and its social, economic, and political realities as they are affected and complicated by the global politics. They are noteworthy for their experiments with narrative perspectives. *The Reluctant Fundamentalist* presents its main narrative in the form of a dialogue between an American-educated Pakistani resident in Pakistan and his silent American listener. *How to Get Filthy Rich* and a chapter in *The Scatter Here* are told from the unusual second-person perspective and feature authorial characters involved in the act of writing self-help literature. In the course of reading Hamid's and Tanweer's novels, the reader is constantly faced with baffling questions with regard to the narrative points of view: From whose perspective is the narrative being told? To whom is the narrative voice addressing? Are the narratee(s) in the novel and its actual readers the same people? How reliable is the narrative perspective – its assumptions, beliefs, agendas, and judgements – being presented in the novel? How reliable are readers' own assumptions and assessments about the narrative perspectives? The overall effect of radical narrative instability on readers is one of disorientation.

So why disorient readers with narrative instability? To answer this question, I start with the authors' delicate position as Pakistani anglophone novelists who write local stories for a global readership. Paul Jay, in his book *Global Matters*, heralds the emergence of 'post-postcolonial' generation of writers 'whose experiences grow out of the postcolonial condition but are informed even more by the forces of globalization' (2010: 96). There is no doubt that these authors belong to this post-postcolonial generation of writers who deal with the pressing issues of globalisation in the local context in their fiction. But their own relationship to globalisation is a conflicted one. In an immediate practical sense, globalisation has opened doors for them, making their work available to a wide readership in the English-speaking world and perhaps beyond. As they narrate local stories to the global audience, however, they confront the age-old problem of representation. After all, these authors represent only a tiny portion of the whole Pakistani population who have received an elite education and enjoy a marked position of privilege and prestige. No matter how comprehensive their understanding of Pakistan's local issues may be, the narrative point of view they adopt for their fiction is bound to be partial and incomplete. Hamid and Tanweer are acutely conscious of such limitations on their choice of perspective.

Through the fragmentation of perspectives in their fiction, they have chosen to radically dismiss the possibility of privileging one particular perspective over others. Their experiments with narrative perspectives fictionalise multiple points of view in flux and formation. This narrative unsteadiness, in turn, represents the authors' own Pakistani subjectivity caught in a tension between the local and the global. Readers, too, are implicated in the process of this unfolding of new points of view: they are invited to re-examine their own assumptions, beliefs, agendas, and judgements even as they question those of the narrative perspectives.

Narrative perspective as a system of relations

According to Susan Lanser, 'Unlike such textual elements as character, plot, or imagery, point of view is essentially a relationship rather than a concrete entity' (1981: 13). The dictionary entry for 'point of view' includes two main potentially contradicting definitions. The first is 'angle of vision' and denotes an objective position from which one makes observations; the second is 'attitude of a person' and indicates one's subjective mindset. Lanser understands this rather ambiguous dual nature of narrative perspective – both objective and subjective at the same time – in terms of a relationship. She writes, '[the] first designates an "objective" position, the subject's relation to some external reality; the second denotes some "subjective" response or evaluation of that reality' (1981: 16). In short, point of view is the narrating subject's relationship to the external world. Through narration, readers gain access to the external world of the narrator and the changes in the internal world of the narrator as the external world influences it. This is not to say that the narrating subject is the only one being affected by the relationship. A relationship is an interactive process which transforms all parties involved. In the act of perceiving and being perceived, and narrating and being narrated, the narrating subject and the object of narration influence and shape each other. Wrapped up in the concept of narrative perspective is an intimate intermingling of subjectivity and objectivity.

Narrative perspective is a difficult concept to theorise because of its two-way, interactive aspect. Since neither the narrating subject nor the external world is a singular static object, it is furthermore difficult to define the narrator's subjective identity and outline the parameters of her external world. In the real world, numerous factors make up one's subjectivity and external surroundings. This is no less true of fictional subjectivity and objectivity. Just as an individual is subject to the rules and regulations of the society in which she lives, a narrating subject is bound to the larger literary system by which the text operates. Therefore, point of view in narrative opens up a whole web of complex relations. Lanser notes how this relationship between the subject and her objective world in fiction could explode into multiplicities of relations:

> If we understand point of view to concern the relations between narrating subjects and the literary system which is the text-in-context, then we confront a complex network of interactions between author, narrator(s), characters, and audiences, both real and implied [...] Even a single narrating subject can be expected to engage in simultaneous multi-leveled relationships with various textual characters, events, and addressees. Moreover, because narrative has the capacity to be multi-discursive – that is, to integrate the discourse of any number of personae within a single text – works of narrative often involve numerous subject/system relationships. In such cases, the textual perspective may become a superstructural synthesis of the various voices and perspectives – points of view – encoded in the discourse.
>
> (1981: 13–14)

Narrative is 'multi-discursive' and simultaneously deals with 'numerous subject/system relationships'. Perspective in narrative represents the development of the interactions between multiple discourses and 'numerous subject/system relationships'. There is no way of stabilising such a complex network of relations, and the unfolding of a perspective will always be an ongoing process. Narrative perspective can, then, be considered as a testing ground for multi-layered interactions between subject and system, or subjectivity and objectivity. Any attempt at constructing a particular narrative perspective would automatically involve an experimentation of some degree.

Who is speaking to whom in *The Reluctant Fundamentalist*?

Pakistani anglophone writers actively experiment with narrative perspectives to make sense of their own complex relationships to the nation and the world, and the nation's relationships to the local and the global. In his essay, 'My Reluctant Fundamentalist', Hamid says that he wrote his second novel to 'help [him] understand [his] split self and [his] split world' (2014: 67). Hamid characterises the perspectives with which he wrote his first two novels as follows:

> *Moth Smoke* had for me been a look at Pakistan with a gaze altered by the many years I had spent in America. *The Reluctant Fundamentalist*, I thought, would be a look at America with a gaze reflecting the part of myself that remained stubbornly Pakistani.
> (2014: 67)

The novel finds a fitting subject in a secular Pakistani Muslim who undergoes an identity crisis over his failed American dream. From the very beginning, *The Reluctant Fundamentalist* was to be an experiment on perspective.

It is interesting to note that Hamid had completed his first draft of the novel before the historic attack on the World Trade Center even took place, although his work is now conveniently referred to as a 'post-9/11 novel' in literary studies. Hamid remembers the response of puzzlement that his first draft incited in his agent, who 'upon reading' the draft asked, 'why would so secular and westernized a Muslim man feel such tension with America?' – to which the author answered, 'there [is] deep resentment in much of the rest of the world towards the sole remaining superpower' (2014: 68). The rest of the world may indeed have resented the unrestrained economic and military power that America exercised on a global scale as a modern-day empire. Such resentment, however, could have been easily dismissed by people like Hamid's agent as a harmless eccentric attitude adopted by some non-Americans.

Things changed when September 11 hit. The traumatic events of the day completely transformed the external and internal worlds of Hamid and his readers. When revising his draft, Hamid concluded that his original idea of setting the events of *The Reluctant Fundamentalist* the year before September 11 was no longer possible:

> I had initially chosen to keep it set in the year before September 11, so that my characters would not be overwhelmed by an event that spoke so much more loudly than any individual's story could. I grew personally more divided, saddened and dismayed by the heavy-handedness of the Bush administration's conduct abroad [...] Eventually, I realized that, just as in my exterior world, there was no escaping the effects of September 11 in the interior world that was my novel. The story of a Pakistani man in New York who leaves just before that cataclysmic event would inevitably be bathed in the glare of the reader's knowledge of what would happen immediately after.
> (2014: 68–69)

The 9/11 attacks and America's war on terror which followed exacerbated sentiments of racial division among the general public. The sociopolitical changes which took place during this period deepened the author's inherent sense of alienation living as a Muslim Easterner in the West. His readers' perspectives on Muslim Americans, Islam, Afghanistan, and Pakistan were fundamentally altered too. The forceful intermingling between the internal and external worlds of the author led him to rethink the novel's narrative perspective. He had written his first draft in the style 'of a fable, of a parable, the kind of folk or religious story one looks to for guidance' (2014: 68). A few years after the 9/11 attacks, Hamid returned to his draft and went through several rounds of trial and error to find the most incisive narrative voice for the novel. He tried 'variations of minimalism in the third person, with voices ranging from fable to noir'. He also experimented with 'the comforting oral cadences of an American-accented first person'. The problem with the American voice was that 'there was not enough of Pakistan' in it, and 'it felt wrong somehow both to [his] ear, in its sound, and to [his] eye, in its architecture' (2014: 69–70). The novel's perspective had to be perfect in both its subjective *voice* and objective *structure*.

The Reluctant Fundamentalist eventually took on 'the frame of a dramatic monologue in which the Pakistani protagonist speaks to an American listener, and a voice born of the British colonial inflections taught in elite Pakistani schools and coloured by an anachronistic, courtly menace that resonates well with popular Western preconceptions of Islam' (2014: 70). Hamid's arrangement consciously invokes the multiple dimensions of communication involved in his narrative act: the interactions between the narrator, the narratee, and the reader with their respective cultural backgrounds, political attitudes, and national loyalties. The novel's Pakistani narrator is perfectly bilingual and has a unique perspective developed through his Pakistani upbringing and years of living in the West. He is also a savvy communicator who adjusts his approach to narration and representation according to his understanding of the narratee's American sensibilities. The motivations behind the two parties' engagement in the conversation are deliberately made unclear, which leaves enough room for readers to project their own assessments and expectations of the narrative situation in the course of their reading. This intricate dramatic setup of the narration seeks to maximise the narrative's potential to be multi-discursive by embodying the complex context of the production and consumption of the novel within the novel's own narrative structure.

Hamid opens *The Reluctant Fundamentalist* by having the Pakistani protagonist locate and address an American visitor in Lahore. The narrator immediately recognises the narratee as an American disoriented in a foreign city and offers his assistance:

> Excuse me, Sir, but may I be of assistance? Ah, I see I have alarmed you. Do not be frightened by my beard: I am a lover of America. I noticed that you were looking for something; more than looking, in fact you seemed to be on a *mission*, and since I am both a native of this city and a speaker of your language, I thought I might offer you my services.
>
> (2007: 1)

The narrator's injunction to not be 'frightened by [his] beard' invokes the common Western stereotype of what an Islamic fundamentalist looks like. Unlike the stereotype, however, he is a fluent speaker of the English language and a lover of America. Interestingly, the narrator's injunction is not just directed to the fictional narratee but also to the readers as they find themselves implicated in the narrator's address to the silent 'you' – albeit a very specified 'you'. Having invoked the cultural prejudices of the narratee (and readers) against bearded Muslims, the narrator starts playing a complex stereotyping game with his American companion. How does the narrator know that the narratee is an American? It is not his 'skin colour' although he is white. It is not his suit although the 'single vent' on his jacket is characteristic of American suits. It is not his broad chest although such a chest is 'typical of a certain *type* of American' who 'maxes out well above two-twenty-five' (2007: 1). 'Instead', it is his '*bearing*' that gives his nationality away, which means that there is something distinctively American in the narratee that people like the narrator can pick up on right away. The narrator sees that the narratee's face 'harden[s]' at the word 'bearing' to express his displeasure at being a target of stereotyping. He does not mean it as an 'insult' though; it is a mere 'observation'. Whereas both readers and the narratee are encouraged to hold off their prejudices and biases before properly getting to know the narrator, the latter himself objectifies and characterises his American listener based on his initial observations of him. In this narrative setup, an interesting reversal of cultural othering occurs. A strange Pakistani native, who looks like a religious fanatic, claims to know intimately and love America. America, more than Pakistan, is going to be the object of his scrutinising gaze.

The narrator of *The Reluctant Fundamentalist* tells his American interlocutor that 'a certain familiarity with the recent history of our surroundings [...] allows us to put the present into much better perspective' (2007: 45). As a Pakistani Muslim with an intimate knowledge of America, the narrator, Changez, appoints himself as a mediator between the two conflicting world views and perspectives, and presents an alternative 9/11 narrative from an outsider's point of view. He reflects on the American reaction to the 9/11 attacks:

> As a society, you were unwilling to reflect upon the shared pain that united you with those who attacked you. You retreated into myths of your own difference, assumptions of your own superiority. And you acted out these beliefs on the stage of the world, so that the entire planet was rocked by the repercussions of your tantrums, not least my family, now facing war thousands of miles away.
>
> (2007: 168)

America's parochial retreat 'into myths of [her] own difference' and assumptions of her 'own superiority' are allegorised by the character of Erica, who has an unhealthy relationship to her past. Erica represents the emotional dimension of Changez's tension with America. Martin Randall notes the close proximity of her name to 'America' in his book *9/11 and the Literature of Terror* (2011: 142). Despite Changez's ardent courtship, Erica continues to pine after her dead lover, Chris, whom she describes as 'a good-looking boy' with an '*Old World* appeal' (2007: 27; emphasis original). Anna Hartnell suggests that Chris' name not only represents 'Europe's Christian roots' but also 'Christopher Columbus' encounter with the Americas, and the continent's status in the European imagination as an object of its own discovery'. Subsequently the memory of Chris, which Erica dearly holds onto, represents a form of 'American nationalism that looks back to a European past, a past that [in reality] only partially captures the nation's roots and the make-up of contemporary America' (Hartnell 2010: 343). In the end, Erica disappears and is suspected to have committed suicide. After her disappearance, Changez obtains the manuscript of Erica's novel and is puzzled to find it to be 'no tortured [...] autobiographical affair' (Hamid 2007: 166). Instead he finds 'a tale of adventure of a girl on an island who learns to make do' (2007: 188) – a kind of female Robinson Crusoe! Her manuscript makes it clear that there is no part for Changez to play in her narrative. With no hopes of uniting with Erica or returning to his former work in finance with the same passion as before, Changez's personal American dream reaches its inevitable ending.

The frame narrative, however, does not conclude with the ending of Changez's American narrative. Readers are yet to decide what to make of the narrator's and the narratee's identities and their relationship. The narrator tells his American listener that he has become a sort of rallying point for political activists on his university campus where he works as a finance professor. The demonstrations his students organise to advocate 'greater independence in Pakistan's domestic and international affairs' have descended into violent scuffles and been labelled 'anti-American' by the foreign press (2007: 179). One of his activist students has recently been 'arrested for planning to assassinate a coordinator of [America's] effort to deliver development assistance to [Pakistan's] rural poor' (2007: 181). The narrator denies any connection to the supposed plot, and disapproves of such a violent plan. He is also 'certain that the boy in question had been implicated by mistake' (2007: 181). 'But how "could he be so certain?"' his American interlocutor asks'. The narrator senses 'a decidedly unfriendly and accusatory tone' in his voice and reassures him that 'you should not imagine that we Pakistanis are all potential terrorists, just as we should not imagine that you Americans are all undercover assassins' (2007: 183).

But what do *readers* make of it? Do they think that the narrator is an anti-American terrorist? Is his American interlocutor an undercover agent on a mission to assassinate the narrator? On their way to the hotel where the American is staying, a group of men ominously closes in on them. Are they just coming to 'say goodbye' or about to jump on the narratee? Is the 'glint of metal' the narrator detects in the narratee's jacket a gun or 'from the holder of [his] business cards'? Hamid writes in a later essay that he wanted to 'push the boundaries of what [he knew] how to do with "you" with his second novel'. He wanted to experiment with 'how feelings already present inside a reader – fear, anger, suspicion, loyalty – could colour a narrative so that the reader, as much as or even more than the writer, is deciding what is really going on'. He wanted the novel to act as a 'mirror, to let readers see they are reading, and, therefore, how they are living and how they are deciding their politics' (2014: 78). Would it even be possible that readers might change their views on post-9/11 politics and Pakistani Muslims after reading the novel? Would the experience of reading bind readers to the perspective of the novel 'by a certain shared intimacy' (Hamid 2007: 184)?

'Who are you?' in *How to Get Filthy Rich in Rising Asia* and *The Scatter Here Is too Great*

As evident in Hamid's detailed profiling of the American listener in his novel, Pakistani anglophone novelists are all too aware of the unique positioning of their global audience attempting to relate to the local context. They work with Pakistani raw materials for their fiction, but a substantial number of their readers live in the English-speaking world outside Pakistan. Hamid's *How to Get Filthy Rich in Rising Asia* and Tanweer's *The Scatter Here is too Great* seek to bridge readers' distance from the local Pakistani context by adopting the second-person point of view as their narrative voice. The direct address to readers in the second-person voice involves readers as active participants in the creation of the story and thus challenges the cultural differences between readers and the writer 'as a barrier of [their] communication'[1] (Paul 2003: 364).

Hamid's *How to Get Filthy Rich* is written in the form of a self-help book and directly addresses the reader as 'you'. An interesting conflation of identities occurs in the novel as the second-person voice blurs the distinctions between the subject positions of author, narrator, protagonist, and reader. Is the narrator the same person as the protagonist? Is the person addressing the 'you' in the novel, in fact, the 'I' of the 'you'? The key to understanding this conflation lies in what the narrator calls the 'slippery' nature of the self, associated with the self-help genre. Taken literally, the name of the genre 'self-help' conveys an oxymoronic message that problematises the divide between the self (reader) and the other (author). How can a book be called a 'self-help' book when the person who is actually helping you is the author, not you yourself? According to the narrator, this means that 'the idea of self in the land of self-help is a slippery one. And slippery can be good. Slippery can be pleasurable. Slippery can provide access to what would chafe if entered dry' (Hamid 2013: 3–4). The sexual undertone used in the passage is a direct nod towards Roland Barthes' idea of *Jouissance* – the sexual-like pleasure that arises from reading a text that defies literary conventions and thus challenges the stable subject position occupied by readers (Abrams 2005: 311). There is also a nod to Hamid's deliberate engagement with formal play. The text's genre-bending playfulness invites the self of the reader to temporarily mingle with the self of the 'you' in the narrative as in a romantic affair.

Thus begins Hamid's tale of the nameless 'you' who rises to obscene wealth through entrepreneurship from a humble rural beginning in a nameless country that looks much like Pakistan. On the one hand, the power of the second-person pronoun draws the readers into the narrative and fills the void of the protagonist's subjecthood left by his namelessness. On the other hand, the highly specified and narrativitised position of the nameless protagonist alienates readers from their efforts to identify with the protagonist. As the plot advances, readers begin to read the story more like a third-person narration which focalises on one character. In fact, throughout the novel, the narrator actively reminds readers of their material alienation from the protagonist and his world. At the beginning of the narrative, the narrator finds 'you huddled, shivering, on the packed earth under your mother's cot one cold, dewy morning' (Hamid 2013: 4). He compares 'Your anguish' to that of 'a boy whose chocolate has been thrown away, whose remote controls are out of batteries, whose scooter is busted, whose new sneakers have been stolen'. All these comparisons are vaguely helpful but completely misplaced as 'you've never in your life seen any of these things' (Hamid 2013: 4) and highlight the disparity between the economic situations of the impoverished protagonist and the readers. The narrator would also make reference to the physical process of writing and reading that is involved in the production and consumption of the text. In the beginning of Chapter 10, the narrator says, 'As my writer's fingers key and your reader's eyes flick, you stand at the cusp of the eighth decade of your life' (2013: 179). Even as he tells readers to fast forward their clock and picture themselves as the protagonist who is approaching his seventies, he reminds them of their physical position as readers and jerks them out of their immersion in the assumed role. These reminders about the extra-textual world disturb readers' stable positioning from the fictional role of the protagonist. Readers' position remains unsettled either in identification with or in distancing from the 'you' of the protagonist.

Readers' unsettling relationship to the narrative's second-person voice opens up interesting ways of thinking about connections between people who are utterly unrelated, dissimilar, and foreign to each other. In thinking about such connections, the narrator makes an appeal to our common humanity and does so by using the discourse of science and technology:

> We are all information, all of us, whether readers or writers, you or I. The DNA in our cells, the bioelectric currents in our nerves, the chemical emotions in our brains, the configurations of atoms within us and of subatomic particles within them, the galaxies and whirling constellations we perceive not only when looking outward but also when looking in, it's all, every last bit and byte of it, information.
>
> (Hamid 2013: 159)

The narrator veers away from his usual second-person voice and uses 'we' in this passage. He first recognises the distinctive identities of the subjects involved in the narrative act – readers, writers, or you or I. Despite 'our' distinctiveness, 'we' are made up of the same building blocks that constitute each other in our world and 'the galaxies and whirling constellations' in the universe. From the smallest unit of the matter that makes up your person to the entire expanse of the universe, it is 'information' and every 'bit and byte' of it governs the arrangements and behaviours of life and matters. What is outside is in you, and what is inside of you is outside. There is internality in externality, and externality in internality.

This language of information technology resonates closely with the narrator's discussion of globalisation. In the age of global finance, the protagonist's business becomes 'quantified, digitized, and jacked into a global network of finance, your activities subsumed with barely a ripple in a collective mathematical pool of ever-changing current and future cash flows' (Hamid 2013: 183). When the protagonist is hospitalised in his old age over shock and stress, his body, not just his business, is jacked into a global network of industries and people: 'To be a man whose life requires being plugged into machines, multiple machines, in your case interfaces electrical, gaseous, and liquid, is to experience the shock of an unseen network suddenly made physical, as a fly experiences a cobweb' (Hamid 2013: 185). The protagonist finds his consciousness connected to his body and life, which are connected to a cobweb of electrical strands connected to the hospital's power system, 'informational technology infrastructure', and 'the unit that produces oxygen', which are connected to the people who labour to make the systems work and supply them with necessary materials and medications, which are connected to the factories where they are made, which are connected to the mines where raw materials are dug up (185–186). According to Angelia Poon, who analyses the same passage, the realisation of one's dependency on the interconnectedness between people and machineries is 'part of the moral transformation of the protagonist and the reader'; what they learn from this interconnectedness is 'sympathy, the ability to feel for someone else' (2017: 146–147). The interior system of the body, both mental and physical, is connected to a complex external system of interconnected people, industries, and machines. It is a picture of how subjectivity relates to objectivity, and the local to the global, and readers to the nameless protagonist in a nameless country. Brian Richardson posits that the 'hypothetical you', the kind used in *How to Get Filthy Rich*, is a 'protean one' and prone to 'ontological slippage'. And 'This "you"' can embrace almost all of us' (2006: 30).

Interconnectedness is also an important theme for Tanweer's *The Scatter Here is too Great*. The novel is a web of interconnected stories of characters whose lives are collectively affected by bombings at a train station in Karachi, Pakistan. The fourth story, 'Lying Low', is written in the second-person voice and tells a story of a successful entrepreneur in the game industry, a self-made man who is much like the nameless protagonist in *How to Get Filthy Rich*. Unlike Hamid's novel, however, the story is not written in the form of a self-help book although the protagonist is in the process of writing one and frequently makes references to lines from his work in progress. The story opens right after the bombing. The protagonist is at his mother's apartment with his mother and another elderly woman. The force of the explosion has shaken the house, shattered the windows, and banged open the door of the fifth-floor apartment. In a state of shock, the protagonist panics over what he should do to protect himself and the women in the house in case of further terrorist attacks. The external and internal shock of experiencing the bombing puts the protagonist in a rather self-reflective mood in which he thinks about his estranged son and his own father, a communist poet, who has abandoned him for political activism.

Unlike Hamid's novel, which is downright playful and transgressive in its use of the second-person voice, Tanweer's narrative perspective faithfully sticks to the protagonist's viewpoint without any direct address to the reader or intrusion by a narrator. In other words, the 'you' in 'Lying Low' could be replaced by a third-person pronoun. So what effects does Tanweer's use of the second-person voice achieve in this narrative? I find a clue in Richardson's discussion on the 'rich ideological possibilities' of second-person narration when it is used to make sense of the coexistence of multiple conflicting discourses in one's consciousness. The second-person voice 'helps dramatize the mental battles of an individual struggling against the internalized discourse of an oppressive authority'. It also opens up a philosophical discussion on the idea of selfhood and '[expresses] the unstable nature and intersubjective constitution of the self' (Richardson 2006: 36). Richardson's discussion is highly relevant to the second-person narration of 'Lying Low', which portrays the main protagonist's conversation between his split selves.

The protagonist admits to having started working on his autobiography 'out of a desperation' to 'make sense of [his] life'. This book was going to be a kind of self-help book about his 'successful career' and his 'humble beginnings' and the ways in which he 'faced those challenges and rose to where [he was] now' (Tanweer 2014: 47). The protagonist has been successful with his game business since he has lived his life like he played the game of Pac-Man: 'get the dots, avoid the ghosts, move up one level at a time. no shortcuts, no exits, and absolutely no pauses whatsoever' (2014: 49). He has believed in 'a relentless cutting down of the unnecessary – thoughts, imagination, ideas – which had been the reason of your success' (2014: 49), the kind of American financial fundamentalism with which Changez in *The Reluctant Fundamentalist* is disillusioned. In writing, however, the protagonist starts to notice the presence of different voices within himself. Before writing, he 'had clear ideas', but 'what made it onto paper was circular and loopy and joined at the wrong ends with everything else. It messed up the whole picture' (2014: 51–52). The second-person voice effectively expresses the process through which he is distancing himself from the two-dimensional economic discourse that used to dominate his consciousness.

The external shock of the explosion further breaks the firm grasp which the restrictive economic discourse previously had on the protagonist's consciousness. The shattered windows in his mother's apartment are a great metaphor for the changes taking place in his perspective. In the aftermath of the explosion, his usual self-absorbed inward-looking glance shifts its focus to the outward reality and other people's pains. Towards the end of the story, the protagonist 'peep[s] through the side of the [broken] windows and see[s] a lot of fire and dispersing men' (2014: 58). Observing the mayhem caused by the explosion, the protagonist becomes conscious of his own internal wounds and experiences an epiphany regarding the true reason of his estrangement from his father:

> [Y]ou have suddenly become conscious of wounds you carried but could not see. Now looking out this broken window at people rushing toward sources of smoke, throwing water over burning cars and buses, you realize that what you had felt for your father was much worse than hate: it was a kind of love where it's impossible to know what you want, and where every act of reaching out lacerates you more deeply, and expression is impossible because no matter how hard you try you'll inevitably fall at odd angles to each other's needs.
> (Tanweer 2014: 59)

He used to hate his father's poetry since it epitomised for him his father's selfish idealism. He realises now that 'your father wrote poetry to find a language for his wounds. Yes: you in your own way have become your father' (2014: 59). In a moment of great communal ordeal, he becomes aware of others' pains, which allows him to put his own internal suffering into perspective. At the end of the story, he hears another crash. This completely smashes the remaining glass of the windows, and they make 'a huge mess on the floor'. In the meanwhile, he notices that 'the door is still open'. The complete destruction of the windows signals to the protagonist that it is time for his book to be 'rewritten' (2014: 61). As the windows go missing and the door remains open, the boundary between the self and his objective world becomes porous and permeable. Something of him is now outside, and something of the outside is now inside of him. The newly found interconnectedness between him and others forces him to open up, expand, and transform his perspective. In the narrative, all of this is happening not to the third-person 'him' but to the second-person 'you'. The second-person voice draws the readers both internally into the subjective side of the broken window and externally to others' sufferings in the real world. Readers are invited to feel the pain of the protagonist and to empathise with those who suffer the violence which breaks out all too often in the author's beloved city of Karachi, which he describes as 'broken, beautiful, and born of tremendous violence' (2014: 1).

Conclusion: an open invitation to an ongoing conversation

No scientist goes into an experiment knowing exactly what the outcome will be. Writers start from a similar position of uncertainty when they engage in a creative project. Hamid and Tanweer experiment with narrative perspectives in their fiction to make better sense of the connection and tension between the local and the global, and their subjectivity and the world outside. Through experimenting with perspectives, they start a conversation between their own split selves and a world marred by corruption and violence. Writing in itself is not an end to the experiment though. Readers play an important part in the complex system of relations that is narrative perspective. The novels examined in this chapter seek to meaningfully implicate readers in the construction of their perspectives. As such, the conversation remains open and ongoing, and the novels' points of view still in flux.

Note

1 This quotation is taken from Premila Paul's essay 'The Master's Language and its Indian Uses', where she discusses the mature reception of Arundhati Roy's novel among the English-speaking readership: 'Readers both in India and abroad also have come a long way in their relationship with English. There is growth towards maturity in this relationship. A practitioner of English is no longer dubbed a traitor to the Indian cause. Roy's novel has shown that the basic difference between the culture of the writer and the culture of the reader is no barrier to communication' (2003: 364).

Bibliography

Abrams, M.H. (2005) 'Structuralist Criticism'. In *A Glossary of Literary Terms*. 8th edn. Boston: Thomson, 381–384.
Hamid, M. (2007) *The Reluctant Fundamentalist*. Toronto: Bond Street Books.
Hamid, M. (2013) *How to Get Filthy Rich in Rising Asia*. New York: Riverhead Books.
Hamid, M. (2014) *Discontent and its Civilizations: Dispatches from Lahore, New York, and London*. London: Hamish Hamilton.
Hartnell, A. (2010) 'Moving through America: Race, Place and Resistance in Mohsin Hamid's *The Reluctant Fundamentalist*'. *Journal of Postcolonial Writing* 46(3–4), 336–348.
Jay, P. (2010) *Global Matters: The Transnational Turn in Literary Studies*. Ithaca: Cornell University Press.
Lanser, S. (1981) *The Narrative Act: Point of View in Prose Fiction*. Princeton: Princeton University Press.
Paul, P. (2003) 'The Master's Language and its Indian Uses'. In *The Politics of English as a World Language: New Horizons in Postcolonial Cultural Studies*. Ed. by Mair, C. New York: Rodopi, 359–365.

Poon, A. (2017) 'Helping the Novel: Neoliberalism, Self-help, and the Narrating of the Self in Mohsin Hamid's *How to Get Filthy Rich in Rising Asia*'. *The Journal of Commonwealth Literature* 52, 139–150.
Randall, M. (2011) *9/11 and the Literature of Terror*. Edinburgh: Edinburgh University Press.
Richardson, B. (2006) *Unnatural Voices: Extreme Narration in Modern and Contemporary Fiction*. Columbus: The Ohio State University Press.
Tanweer, B. (2014) *The Scatter Here is Too Great*. New York: Harper Collins.

27
PERIPHERAL MODERNISM AND REALISM IN BRITISH-PAKISTANI FICTION

Asher Ghaffar

In *Beginnings: Intention and Method*, Edward Said emphasised the importance of style as:

> a necessary part of the status and volume of a text […] which for the author producing his text is the language of his career. Syntactically, style is the extended signature of a writer, his characteristic way of connecting signs […] style is not the origin of a text, but that which the beginning of a text intends.
>
> (1985: 254)

Since the Indo-Pakistani novelist and poet Zulfikar Ghose has spent his entire career experimenting with style, this feature can be viewed a part of his identity, which is also non-identical with it. Style connects to the labour of his art, obscured by the weave of the novel's mimetic spell. This chapter will first focus on unpacking the logic of the conceptual arrangement of Ghose's novels that resist identification with a national form, but where nation is still uncannily present. Ghose's work is then compared with Hanif Kureishi's novels, where identity predominates in the *Bildungsroman* form. Kureishi's novels can be rethought if the *Bildungsroman* is not understood to be reflective of the author's ideology, or the subjective position of the novelist in a psychological theory of writing, which is what Bart Moore-Gilbert's (2001) genre analysis amounts to. Instead, the *Bildungsroman* should be grasped as part of this broader social and historical process that internalises a series of generic problems shaped in the compositional process. These antimonies persist and are internalised by a specific genre which is their aesthetic 'repository'.

Ghose's challenging aesthetics is, of course, modernist. However, literary scholars have not understood his work through *peripheral* modernism. His non-canonical status in postcolonial studies is in part due to his experimental style, which pushes against identity and modernism. Kureishi is canonical because his style, or 'extended signature' (Said 1985: 254), is recognisable within postcolonial studies where identity, difference, and irony predominate in autobiographical forms.

Indo-Pakistani

In Ghose's autobiography, *Confessions of a Native-Alien* (1965), names not only summon political violence but also evoke the nameless and placeless. At one point in *Confessions*, Ghose recounts that his family's decision to change their Muslim surname to a Hindu one may have prevented them from being killed in the communal violence of 1946: 'I feel certain that if four hundred million other people had a name as queer as mine, there would have been no bloodshed' (1965: 6). History leaves traces in the body, preserved as fossils that return to language with the memory of their origin as condensed, liquid fire.

In *Confessions*, Ghose refers to himself as 'Indo-Pakistani' – clearly problematic when viewed beside the geopolitical tension between India and Pakistan following the violence of Partition and the nuclear testing that has come to define the relationship since the late 1990s. Indo-Pakistani is something of a historical contradiction – a persistent, jarring memory that shapes Ghose's work. In his autobiography, the novelist metonymically links his strange circumstance to his stammering in early childhood – existing in a historical reality, language, and form that have yet to arrive. In an interview with Bruce Meyer, Ghose remarks that literature is a search for a lost place: 'Ever since having been uprooted from India, I seem to have been looking for the landscape which would relieve me from the sense of that traumatic loss' (Meyer 1991: 99).

Literature is a landscape; and Ghose's stylistic experiments represent a search for the new in given historical forms such as realism and magical realism. His work also depicts an Indo-Pakistani and Muslim subject that resists national and religious commodification through an interweaving of styles that disavows the autobiographical form. *The Triple Mirror of the Self* (1992) echoes Paul Valéry's notion that 'My worth comes from what I lack' (2000: 117). Ghose's 'real' autobiography is clearly a representation of distinct styles in *The Triple Mirror* that is simultaneously irreconcilable with autobiographical forms and the *Bildungsroman*, which predominates in postcolonial studies.

Ghose's marginality within postcolonial studies is partially due to his own vehement resistance to the categories that shape the field, particularly narrative modes and styles associated with autobiography and realism, which are often associated with national representation. According to him, minority literature is judged through a nativist lens; in opposition to this, Ghose attempts to evade the nation and its subject matter, particularly in his criticism. This modernist critique extends to the formal features of Ghose's novels.

In this respect, Ghose's late interpreter, Chelva Kanaganayakam, highlights the contradiction between realism and magical realism (or 'counterrealism') in Ghose's work, which has resulted in 'a critical dilemma' for literary theorists. In *Structures of Negation: The Writings of Zulfikar Ghose*, Kanaganayakam states:

> Even in the more ambivalent Brazilian Trilogy, the fabulosity does not eclipse the colonial experience of Brazil. The critical dilemma for the reader of *Torments* and *Don Bueno* is the degree to which these novels adopt a realistic mode, a difficulty that has led to both misunderstanding and adverse criticism.
>
> (1993: 136)

Zulfikar Ghose's peripheral modernism

For the most part, postcolonialists have abandoned modernity as a colonial relic (Lazarus 2011), or as a quaint and anachronistic return to Eurocentrism (Huggan 2001). Contrary to popular belief, Neil Lazarus suggests an affinity between literary modernism and anticolonialism:

> while colonialism is commonly taken as intrinsic to the socio-historical project of modernity, modernism is not typically viewed – for all its 'dissidence' – as featuring an anticolonial dimension. On the contrary, modernism is typically viewed, for all that

it says 'no' to modernity, as a Eurocentric projection, as itself latently if not explicitly colonialist in character.

(2011: 28)

The modernist dimension in Ghose's work lends itself to Theodor Adorno's philosophical aesthetics, particularly *Aesthetic Theory* and *Notes to Literature*, where the politics of form is emphasised – challenging representational politics. Timothy Brennan (2014) has recently reinterpreted peripheral aesthetics through the Neapolitan humanist Giambattista Vico and emphasised orature, the sheer physicality of language, and the philologist's critique of irony. These peripheral aspects both draw on and push literary modernism's configuration to something unfathomed.

The Triple Mirror is a world novel narrated through magical realism, realism, and modernism, which correspond to the geopolitics of the world during the Cold War. The Suxavat section draws on magical realism. The section set in the UK shifts to a kind of stream of consciousness that evokes Ghose's *Crump's Terms* and is reminiscent of Woolf. The final, Indo-Pakistani, section is written in a realism that resembles the novelist's *The Murder of Aziz Khan*, which is set in Pakistan, and other Urdu and anglophone Pakistani (and Indian English) post-Partition novels. That is, different styles relate to distinct narrative modes that are also *national* forms that clash with one another.

The overall effect between these different styles is a dissonance within the 'unity' of the world novel. These styles are also constitutive of Ghose's 'autobiography' and his own working through formal problems. As such, *The Triple Mirror* is a mimesis of Ghose's other works, and arguably a culmination of sorts – not a grand synthesis, but a representation of aesthetic antimonies in their uncompromised form, which is distinct from the *Bildungsroman* and other autobiographical forms, where compromise is a defining feature (Moretti 2000).

In Ghose's novel, names summon political violence, while also invoking cross-religious identities that serve as a response to the religious violence of Partition. While Ghose is stridently secular, he approaches art with a religious intensity. Religious and oral elements are realism's after-effects reverberating in the novel's lyrical cauldron. The negation of the self does not affirm orature, but develops into a critical position in the formal cells of the work that is ambiguous, future-oriented, and historical.

Ghose represents familiar Buddhist, Muslim, and Hindu concepts to depict the composite character of pre-Partition India. In some ways, the cross-religious style of his work echoes the short stories of the great Urdu writer Intizar Husain, who bridges Islam with Hinduism in *A Chronicle of the Peacocks: Stories of Partition, Exile and Lost Memories* (2006). While Husain's work is an important nostalgic representation of pre-Partition India, Ghose's work focuses on what is not yet (Bloch 1988). Despite not belonging to the same literary tradition, the Partition shaped both writers. They are both haunted by the same moment; and the juncture serves as a primal scene in *The Triple Mirror* whose tremors can be felt throughout Ghose's corpus.

In *The Triple Mirror*, oral culture is not a mystical antithesis of political subjects emerging out Partition's trauma, but an absent presence that circulates in this work. Oral culture is powerful in the novel because it is unnamed. By evoking oral culture without commodifying it, Ghose preserves an important feature of peripheral aesthetics. Oral culture does not become a facile affirmation of a false universality that resolves religious tension. This absence animates as the after-effect of the realist representation of historical trauma that resists objectification.

Ghose's identification with the 'Indo-Pakistani' concept is ambiguous and does not slip into a facile cosmopolitanism that sutures memory from its visceral physicality, which is registered in densely figurative prose. 'Indo-Pakistani' always exists as a historical possibility – the intimacy of the self and the other, rather than their objectification. In his fiction, Ghose does not seem to reconcile with a place – whether it be a specific nation or the world abstractly conceived. This differentiates him from Salman Rushdie's notion of immigration as an affirmative process of 'translation' (1991). In his study on Rushdie, Brennan highlights that exile and nationalism are two oppositions that relate to 'more traditional aesthetic conflicts: artistic iconoclasm and communal assent, the unique vision and the collective truth' (1989: 23).

In *The Triple Mirror*, this aesthetic conflict manifests in the clash between modernism and realism, which results in a uniquely peripheral modernist style. On the one hand, the writer of the contemporary world novel focuses on specific national experience, predominantly through a realism that self-consciously represents national experience. On the other hand, this conspicuous form strives to reach the global market through firmly entrenched and urbane magical realism. This aesthetic often evades the novelistic setting and tends to challenge the nation as a narrative construct.

In his attempt to evade subject matter, Ghose vehemently affirms the modernist ideology of art for art's sake. In *Aesthetic Theory*, Adorno argues that modernism is an attempt to transcend the historical; and he also saw realism as a recurrence of the nineteenth-century rationalism that did not break its spell, particularly after the rationalisation of the Holocaust. He suggested that form underlies political content, while political content or subject matter is an effect of form, or 'epiphenomenal' to it. Subject matter is important insofar as it is also developed at a formal level too.

Ghose echoes Adorno when he remarks that 'form is all there is' (personal communication, 24 August 2009). His attempt to reject subject matter in his criticism and interviews is likely a response to critics whose sole focus is reconciling subject matter and placing it within an appropriate critical paradigm. Since the novelist is unable to locate a language to link his formalist and political concerns, he often simplistically opposes them. Adorno provides the critical link to bridge form and politics and to grasp the 'truth-content' of Ghose's work – its social and political meaning – while Ghose's development of modernism requires one to rethink realism. That is, if peripheral modernism entails a disavowal of realism, must not the latter re-enter the sphere of literary and cultural criticism in a renewed form to understand its object?

For Ghose and Adorno, literary form is a central means of resisting the course of the world. As literary critics, they both analyse the universalising tendencies of theories that attempt to extrinsically grasp artwork which affirms the world as it is, rather than showing how artwork negates social reality in its form. Ghose reinforces this point in *The Art of Creating Fiction*:

> What is being praised is not literature but the fact that the East European or West African is deemed worthy of warm sympathy because his body or his mind has been tortured by the rulers of his native land or because there is some other socio-political consideration that is generating universal debate or because the work briefly enchants us with some exotic myth.
>
> (1991b: 37)

Ghose's own insistence on 'things' – the sheer necessity of style to put vigorous pressure on subject matter – rather than a false imposition of subject matter on the movement of style – draws on William Carlos Williams' modernist poetics.

Despite Ghose's somewhat predictable recoil from representational aesthetics in his vehement affirmation of art for art's sake, realism returns in his work. Ghose's work thus also develops Adorno's ideas further because in *The Triple Mirror* the narrative does not do away with realism in Part Three ('Origins of the Self') of the novel. One of the recurring images in the novel's opening section, 'The Burial of the Self', is the jaguar which, as Wilson Harris notes, has symbolic importance in a broadly conceived Latin American and Caribbean culture (2005). This image appears in a synchronous dream of each member of the Suxavat 'tribe', suggesting a kind of muted and mythic collectivity; yet the jaguar eventually disappears in more predicable sentences: 'We lost our way. There was no jaguar' (Ghose 1992: 67). A myth that does not necessarily possess a seamless relationship with 'the people' is a retrospective gaze at the fragmentary past. Like a sinuous snake circling its tail, the magical realist form searches for its antithesis in the realism of the novel's final section.

In Ghose's work, peripheral aesthetics registers in the return of realism, which is a yearning for the lost totality of the Indian nation that is metonymically linked to his childhood and oral culture – the latter emphasises the conjunction between myth, history, and a kind of progress. Ghose's longing for the impossible crystallises into novel categories such as 'native-alien', 'Indo-Pakistani', and 'the scattered one', which reflect both disunity and unity, what is and what has not yet arrived.

The return of realism

The Triple Mirror of the Self mediates representational and modernist aesthetics, which as Fredric Jameson remarks, have returned as a central conflict in aesthetics. He remarks:

> Nowhere has this 'return of the repressed' been more dramatic than in the aesthetic conflict between 'Realism' and 'Modernism,' whose navigation and renegotiation is still unavoidable for us today, even though we may feel that each position is in some sense right and yet that neither is any longer wholly acceptable.
>
> (2002: 196)

The Triple Mirror extends modernism through an immanent critique, using the strength of its own concept, to move it forward.

The distinctive modes in Ghose's work also correspond to overlapping styles that critique one another – questioning the global commodification of magical realism and, more recently, the 'national' realist mode into 'the unfortunate feel of ready-mades' (Brennan 1997: 203). Some critics have been quick to denounce the composite character and lack of unity in Ghose's work. Brouillette more accurately understands it as a 'pastiche' of his prior works (2007). Then again, if pastiche is viewed as evidence of a loss of historicity (Jameson 1991: 25), Ghose's work cannot be seen simply as a mere mixing of modes and forms to produce a distinctive formalist experiment. Pastiche overlooks the historical dimension of style, which is one of the novel's most compelling features and not random in the logic of its conceptual arrangement.

When describing his own experience of geographical space, Ghose uses the modernist term 'montage':

> There are a good many images, especially of landscapes, where there is a sort of montage effect in my mind: I've only got to look hard at the superimposed Brazilian landscape and I can see an Indian landscape showing through it.
>
> (Ghose qtd. in Brouillette 2007: 151)

His work is a montage of styles – each of which reflects a place that correlates to a specific literary history and mode. Ghose's work straddles national forms to provide a critical phenomenology of the world. Emphasising postcolonial categories, such as pastiche, irony, and artifice, undermines the historical dimension of *The Triple Mirror* and its affective sense of loss, which is physically registered at the level of style, particularly in the realist section. Although irony is clearly at play in the novel, particularly in the Suxavat section, it is 'epiphenomenal' to the novel's form, in Adorno's sense.

Unlike the *Bildungsroman*, which is concerned with the self's formation, Ghose's *The Triple Mirror* is also a fractured autobiography that in its stylistic movement generates a modernist twilight. Literary style is the aesthete's identity – but also presents the minority, secular Muslim self, under threat of annihilation. No style emerges uncompromised. There is no pure, disinterested narration that is held together in a single stylistic medium. Identity is disavowed and remains only as a residue of the work's movement – which can be understood in relation to the real threat of the annihilation of the stateless individual and the refugee condemned to a placeless place.

Autobiography and style come together, but Ghose represents the self as an aesthetic effect that clashes and converges with other stylistic divisions that are national in character. The movement against identity is not only a function of content, but also of Ghose's engagement with form, which is non-representational, moving away from identity like Islamic mosaic art. This creates a stylistic texture that remains unnamed, but is present as the 'embodiment' of a stylistic 'vigour' in Erich Auerbach's historical sense.

The uncanny return of realism haunts Ghose's engagement with literary modernism. This return of the repressed points to modernism's insularity which becomes open to the world and non-synchronous temporalities that interrupt it, while also dispelling Jameson's (1986) notion that the peripheral novel does not provide aesthetic enjoyment of the modernist classics. In juxtaposing the dominant modes that have come to shape the post-Cold War novel, the novelist provides a more deeply critical form for the world novel that emphasises the problem of form.

Realist dissonance

The aforementioned critical dilemma to which Kanaganayakam alludes has led to accusations that Ghose has 'always been avowedly elitist in his artistic aims' (Sanga 2003: 75). It is important to understand *The Triple Mirror*'s fragmentary form as interrelated to the novel as a whole. Adorno understood the form of the fragment as opposing the idea's totality and not as the manifestation of a particular idea (1997). After all, *The Triple Mirror* is, in part, about a scholar attempting to locate the meaning of a magical realist fragment written by the world's greatest realist.

The failure to produce unity is intentional and somewhat predictable on Ghose's part; what is less expected is that the dissonance between different narrative modes and styles occurs within the 'unity' of the world novel – questioning it as a mode, style, and a chronotope. Ghose's work is a disavowal of the world novel that challenges its concepts through stylistic heterogeneity, which is the novel's historical 'braille' that requires further exploration.

Adorno understood the dissonance of form as constitutive of the work's truth-content, which is social; and thus his philosophical aesthetics mediates the false opposition between form and content in the reception of Ghose's work. Thus, for Adorno, artwork does not 'resolve objective contradictions in a spurious harmony, but […] expresses the idea of harmony negatively by embodying the contradictions, pure and uncompromised, in its innermost structure' (1997: 31).

The Triple Mirror represents a dissonant unity of unresolved styles – two of which have come to define the post-Cold War world novel: magical realism and realism. *The Triple Mirror* juxtaposes magical realist, modernist (stream of consciousness), and realist styles to dispel their individual auras, while regrouping old aesthetic categories within the forms of the time (Buck-Morss 1977) to intimate another world novel. This is precisely what makes this a far-reaching work – more so because the work is not merely a fleeting experiment, but a mimesis of Ghose's aesthetic labour throughout his life.

In *The Historical Novel* (1962), Georg Lukács suggests that realism arose out of the experience of the French Revolution. Likewise, magical realism emerged out of a specifically Latin American colonial experience, which ended with the boom novels. Literary scholars do not often consider the worlding of styles; and yet what is most striking about Ghose's *The Triple Mirror* is the stylistic interplay in sharp juxtaposition. Putting both together speaks to two discontinuous temporalities and uneven literary processes in the world that continue to shape the contemporary world novel, while also articulating identity as an after-effect of stylistic experimentation, capturing the linguistic braille of dislocated experience: identity becomes non-identity, and it is clear that the novel is obsessed with annihilation of the self in a myriad of ways.

Said identifies the harrowing underside of global experience in the bewildering style of Palestinians dispossessed of their land and stripped of their rights. In this narrative style, Said suggests that Palestinian writers experience: 'an urgent need to reconstitute their roots, usually by choosing to see themselves as part of a triumphant ideology, or restored people' (2002: 177). Echoing Lukács, Said reiterates that the novel represents the 'transcendental homelessness' of modernity, as compared to the 'rounded totality' of the epic that reflects the Homeric world where the self is not yet differentiated from the world (1962: 29). In Said's iteration, however, the exile's 'jealousy' results from their lack of recognition as a collectivity. Ghose's distinct styles juxtapose serial and non-serial time in the shattered image of the 'whole'. Through the juxtaposition of serial and non-serial time, the novelist captures the felt sense of the tension of the Cold War and the decolonising world's appeal to represent itself.

Similarly, Jameson suggests that in developing countries representational aesthetics predominates because of 'the possibility of forgetting, or repressing, the political altogether, at least for a time; of stepping out of the "nightmare of history": into the sealed spaces of a private life' (1989: vii). In peripheral countries, this nightmare seeps into everyday life, perhaps not in the diffuse sense that Jameson suggested, but there is a clear distinction between the US and Pakistan with regard to the separation of private and public space – certainly as it manifests in the secular and religious divide.

The dizzying narrative styles and modes correspond to Ghose's forced migration to Pakistan. He captures this displacement in a counterpoint of style, which is the texture of his native-alien experience. This is reflected stylistically in the rapid movement of sentences such as when the narrator moves from Baltimore, to London, to Karachi in a single paragraph to reflect Proustian convolutions of memory:

> No, this was not the last fortnight before the rainy season ended but much earlier, a decade perhaps before I arrived in the rain forest, a memory prior to experience, its images constituted by the force of a conceit while I stood in the museum in Baltimore in front of the painting of a girl in Tahiti [...] Or much earlier still [...] that moment of hallucination that possessed me as I lay in a cousin's house in Karachi after the flight from London.
>
> (1992: 11)

Ghose's experiment is not gimmicky, as dislocated experience sediments in the novel's form and represents his *labour* with style throughout his career. Experimentation does not signal the new for Ghose, but the recurrence of prior forms that he has reorganised. In his work, magical realism and realism are presented in fragmentary form through sharp contrasts resisting the commodification (and totality) of each form – providing an after-image of the world and the self between the Cold War and 'the end of the age of three worlds' (Denning 2004: 3). Even if realist plot appears to abandon itself to modernist formal concerns, the plot's social function is still present, as it often is in Ghose's compulsively readable novels. Hence, his major novels are both experimental and realist, preserving both a political function of plot in a Lukácian sense of representing the socio-historical movement, in the midst of decolonisation – along with a modernist aesthetic. However, due to their juxtaposition, modernism becomes something other to itself, and the peripheries appear strange in the latter's twilight.

Despite Ghose's vehement rejection of realism in an essay published in *The Art of Creating Fiction* (1991b) a year prior to the publication of the novel, the mode uncannily returns in the final section of *The Triple Mirror of the Self*, published the following year after a trip to Pakistan. Realism signals the return of the repressed – the nation – which haunts Ghose's work, particularly in its depiction of the Partition riots. Even if Ghose rejects realism in his criticism, his rejection is epiphenomenal to the formal concerns of *The Triple Mirror*. The disavowal of realism estranges modernism, realism, and magical realism and places them under critical scrutiny. In his disavowal of the world novel, Ghose provides another conceptual form for writing the nation and the world. The experimental nature of the work is one reason why Ghose could not initially find a publisher for *The Triple Mirror*, and why his work is not considered canonical in the way that Kureishi's novels are.

Nietzsche and the postcolonial *Bildungsroman*

Kureishi's novels are modern in their content and their critique of identity, but demotic in mode; Nietzschean in their de-individualising notion of subjectivity, but anchored to realism in the *Bildungsroman* form – the only novelistic form that Kureishi has really grappled with to date. Friedrich Nietzsche is not so much internalised in postcolonial fiction, but 'impersonated' (Noys 2018). In *The Buddha of Suburbia* (1991), Nietzsche functions through the hardness of Kureishi's powerful characters' determination to overcome all odds to reach artistic success. Kureishi's work seems most liberating in his ironic and almost Dadaesque attack of identity politics. However, the de-individualising creativity of his characters conflicts with the *Bildungsroman*, which documents the growth and formation of an individual. In this form, Kureishi represents the self's revolt against Thatcherism.

At the end of the Cold War, the British lost their imperial status as a nation; Thatcher offered Britain a simplistic national identity, poised between its colonial past and its diminishing role in the world. This period 'found compensation in a cynical hedonism that found lavish outlet in the overconsumption boom of the eighties' (Anderson 1998: 81). Many scholars saw the corresponding cultural turn as entailing a loss of even the possibility of social democracy. The ensuing vacuum caused by the demise of socialism resulted in a transition from 'communities of political belief' to 'communities of being' (Brennan 2007: 11–13).

While contemporary British multiculturalism celebrated the nation as a diverse community, it simultaneously undermined the very communities that represented the ideal of 'diversity' (Sivanandan 1990). Kureishi opposes both the turn to identity and Thatcherism with hedonistic individualism, bereft of a community in the process of becoming. As one of Kureishi's characters states in *Intimacy*, 'If Marx had been our begetter, the ideologue of the century's first half, Freud was our new father, as we turned inwards' (2002: 59).

Kureishi draws on hedonism to critique Thatcherism and the liberal moral order, particularly the politics of identity, but he continually returns to a literary form that is about affirming identity. This contradiction between form and content is a defining feature in Kureishi's work. Herbert Marcuse understood hedonism as the possibility to challenge the morality of reason and thus important to consider for any critical theory of society. However, its limitation was that 'its happiness can be derived only by abstracting from all universality and community' (2009: 125). In Kureishi's novels, racial individualism is extolled at the expense of a collective social body under attack by Thatcher, who upheld thrift as virtue and famously declared that society had ended.

If the *Bildungsroman* describes how one can live fully, the *Künstlerroman* ('Artist's Novel') asks how one could live a life and remain true to one's art. Emerging out of the Romantic era, the *Künstlerroman* depicts the maturation of an artist through childhood into an autonomous subject. In his dissertation on the German *Künstlerroman*, Marcuse remarks that in the Artist's Novel, the protagonist must overcome twoness:

> The artist must overcome this twoness: he must be able to configure a type of life that can bind together what has been torn asunder, that pulls together the contradictions between spirit and sensuality, art and life, artists' values and those of the surrounding world. This is the fundamental problem and theme of the artist novel: it generally presents us with the attempt of an artist to reconcile this dichotomy in some manner.
> (2007: 85)

In the opening of *The Buddha*, the protagonist declares:

> My name is Karim Amir, and I am an Englishman born and bred, almost [...] perhaps it is the odd mixture of continents and blood, of here and there, of belonging and not, that makes me restless and easily bored.
> (Kureishi 1991: 53)

In the racial Artist's Novel, the contradiction between identity and change is complicated because of the tension between belonging and not belonging in a social world dominated by race. In *The Buddha*, Karim remarks:

> Yeah, sometimes we were French, Jammie and I, and other times we went black American. The thing was, we were supposed to be English, but to the English we were always wogs and nigs and Pakis and the rest of it.
> (1991: 53)

For the mixed-race character Karim Amir, this 'twoness' already presupposes the objective negation of the subject, a kind of double negation that must be worked through. The double character of his mixed identity complicates the form, but does not generate a dissonant formal pressure that pushes the form in radically new directions. The excitement that begins the promising novel harkens back to the adventure novels, precursors to 'the baroque novel of ordeal' (Bakhtin 1986: 13–14). The adventure in 'the odd mixture of continents and blood' (Kureishi 1991: 3) is developed in relation to tedium that connects to religion, the past, as well as Changez's disability, failed sexuality, and many of the female characters who are not integral to the plot movement, except as foils for the protagonist's ascent. The facile closures of Kureishi's novels clash with the characters' initial doubleness.

After the Cold War, the decolonising world, the West, and the Soviet Union, became one, mass culture transformed into anticolonial resistance on the one hand, and also the remarkable weightlessness of popular culture on the other (Denning 2004). *The Buddha* links celebrity culture to resistance, and works against a long-standing concept of community where 'black' was non-racial and socialist (Sivanandan 1990). The performative self becomes equated with resistance and cunning is the key to upward mobility. In *The Black Album* (2009), the narrator's encyclopaedic knowledge of pop culture becomes a literary style. Allusions to popular culture give sentences apparent weight, even if they are hollow. For example, Shahid's brother Chili 'drank only black coffee and Jack Daniel's; his suits were Boss; his underwear Calvin Klein, his actor Pacino' (Kureishi 2009: 43). Kureishi's attempt to critique identity is often sacrificed to script-like writing. This unfinished quality of *The Black Album* renders characters chess pieces in an ideological game, as though the novel is surrendering to filmic realist representation.

Discussing Haroon's gift in *The Buddha of Suburbia*, Bruce Robbins alludes to the way in which irony functions in an ambivalent manner:

> On the one hand, the cures are real, and [the novel] treat[s] the guru's prescribing of a curative dose of irresponsibility with at least some irony, the effect is far from ironic. There is a real if reluctant approval for the euphoric escape from over individualized responsibility.
>
> (2009: 95)

The ambivalent function of irony affirms what it attempts to negate. Irony functions as a kind of assent to racial reification. While Robbins' reading of *The Buddha of Suburbia* situates it in the upward mobility genre of the Artist's Novel, he does not address how upward mobility is enabled through racial charisma.

Herbert Marcuse developed the Weberian concept of charisma, derived from the Christian *charism*:

> This image expanded to the vision of the charismatic leader whose leadership does not need to be justified on the basis of his aims, but whose mere appearance is already his 'proof', to be accepted as an undeserved gift of grace.
>
> (2009: 30)

While race and gender identity are expressions of exclusion in *The Buddha of Suburbia*, they are linked to charisma and the commodity form – possessing a mystical and fetishistic quality. In Kureishi's work, characters attempt to overcome the reification imposed by prevailing British ideologies attributed to Thatcherism, such as entrepreneurial individualism and the demise of the welfare state; and yet the plot's movement relies on hedonistic individualism at the expense of community.

Charisma is explored in all of Kureishi's novels through celebrity culture. In the nihilistic and masochistic figure of Charlie Hero, subculture is merged with celebrity culture: 'He had a smart head, Charlie; he learned that his success, like that of other bands, was guaranteed by his ability to insult the media' (Kureishi 1991: 153). The punk celebrity, who sports a swastika, is not unlike a populist leader such as Thatcher. When Karim wins the role of Mowgli in *The Jungle Book*, he yearns for the same mythical status as Charlie.

Race and affirmative culture

In the *Bildungsroman*, the spontaneous and youthful self encounters a cold, calculating, and rational world. The protagonist develops in relation to the world, rebelling against it, but also making compromises towards a greater integration of the particular with the universal. Lukács traces the form to the historical compromise between the bourgeoisie and aristocracy after the French Revolution which left its imprint on modern novelistic structure.

The classical *Bildungsroman*, or novel of education, with Goethe as its romantic prototype, often instructs a young person how to live life through a humanistic education. Goethe's *Wilhelm Meister's Apprenticeship* (1796) was unprecedented precisely because the 'hero emerges along with the world and reflects on the historical emergence of the world itself' (Bakhtin 1986: 23). Bakhtin suggests that the post-Goethean *Bildungsroman* concentrates the idealism of a period within the consciousness of the hero against the calculating and utilitarian world. By contrast, the modern *Bildungsroman* is more often ironic and anti-humanist.

In *The Buddha*, cunning is implicit in the protagonist's ascent of the social ladder towards Nietzschean artistic freedom. Even if such charisma is parodied, Karim ultimately succumbs to it:

> After seeing it work for so long, I began to perceive Charlie's charm as a method of robbing houses by persuading the owners to invite you in and take their possessions [...] it was false and manipulative and I admired it tremendously. I made notes on his techniques, for they worked.
>
> (1991: 119)

Despite this, the protagonist progresses towards a reintegration with the social order. As Marcuse suggests in his understudied dissertation on the *Künstlerroman*, negation is implicit in the protagonist's initial decision to leave the family and community and form their identity, but resolution is frequently its outcome. The character is also irrevocably changed through his experience and reconciles with the world and its contradictions and learns the ultimate bourgeoisie lesson, compromise (Moretti 2000: 69).

Prior to the French Revolution, the protagonist was conceived in a static sense moved along by plot and history, as though by fate, but not yet a force that could transform the world (Bakhtin 1986: 22–23). According to Lukács, the central character of the historical novel is the 'maintaining individual' who is contrasted with drama's revolutionary 'world-historical individuals'. This liminal protagonist mediates between the bourgeoisie and the aristocracy. While historical change concentrates in the being of the 'world-historical figure' (Lukács 1962: 89–170), the social totality is reproduced in the world-maintaining individuals, and is more reflective of the class-based society that emerged following the French Revolution.

In sharp contrast to Homi Bhabha's celebration of the liminal as resistance, Said draws on Lukács' idea of 'maintaining individuals' in Kipling's *Kim*. As Said explains: 'The liminal figure helps to maintain societies, and it is this procedure that Kipling enacts in the climactic moment of the plot and the transformations of Kim's character' (1994: 141). Said's historical reading of liminality draws on Victor Turner's anthropological theories, which suggest that the liminal figure serves a mediatory function knitting together society to reproduce the totality of social relations in his being. Fransco Moretti suggests that the *Bildungsroman* is the 'symbolic form of modernity' that internalises objective contradictions such as identity and change, freedom and happiness, security and metamorphosis, and so on:

> When we remember that the *Bildungsroman* – the symbolic form that more than any other has portrayed and promoted modern socialization – is also the most contradictory of modern symbolic forms, we realize that in our world socialization itself consists first of all in the interiorization of contradiction. The next step being not to solve the contradiction, but rather to learn to live with it, and even transform it into a tool for survival.
>
> (2000: 9–10)

In his new prologue to his work, Moretti reiterates the centrality of compromise in shaping this important form:

> And so, in the same decades as Faust, the enormous and unconscious collective enterprise of the *Bildungsroman* bears witness to a different solution to modern culture's contradictory nature. Far less ambitious than synthesis, this other solution is compromise: which is also, not surprisingly, the novel's most celebrated theme.
>
> (2000: 9)

In Kureishi's *The Buddha of Suburbia*, Karim becomes marketable as an artist and attains upward mobility in part due to racial charisma. When Eva sees him, she exclaims: 'Karim Amir, you are so exotic, so original!' (1991: 9). Even though this is parodied, there is a silent assent as Karim is also cast in Shadwell's play 'for authenticity and not for experience' (1991: 147). Eva becomes a mentor who teaches him that 'compliments [are] useful tools in the friendship trade' (1991: 92). In *The Black Album*, Deedee's erotic desires are shaped by Shahid's skin colour: 'I love that café-au-lait skin' (1991: 217). Racial charisma is sexualised and ultimately celebrated – even if it is parodied. In the racial *Bildungsroman*, compromise is ultimately about racial integration – a structural feature of the racial *Bildungsroman* that constitutes a contribution to the European form.

Kureishi's writing prefigures multicultural Britain, culture administered from above, rather than developed out of plebeian material from below. The novelist's treatment of the *Bildungsroman* prefigures the contemporary post-race discourse that resolves race, disguising its psychic trauma with the triumph of liberalism. Karim moves up the social ladder by his own merit, but also because of his skin colour. In the process, he becomes integrated into post-war Britain against traditional and relatively changeless and more important figures such as Jamila.

Through humour, parody, and Nietzschean masking, Kureishi's characters develop a romantic concept of art premised on sensuality to resist Thatcher's Protestant views. In Karim, race converges with charisma, despite Jamila's reminders of the racial attacks in her less affluent neighbourhood. Karim is ultimately profoundly calculating as a character, prefiguring the modern racialised artist whose skin colour and national affiliation are their wares – the means by which they enter into the marketplace. Irony serves the dual purpose in simultaneously critiquing colonialism and racism, while also reinforcing the affirmative culture it sets out to critique – particularly through individualism that converges with race and celebrity authorship in the formal cells of the *Bildungsroman*.

Bibliography

Adorno, T. (1997) *Aesthetic Theory*. Trans. by Hullot-Kentor, R. Minneapolis: University of Minnesota Press.
Adorno, T. and Horkheimer, M. (2002) *Dialectic of Enlightenment: Philosophical Fragments*. Trans. by Adorno, T.W. and Noerr, G.S. Stanford: Stanford University Press.
Adorno, T. and Jameson, F. (2007) *Aesthetics and Politics*. London: Verso.
Adorno, T.W., Tiedemann, R., and Nicholsen, S.W. (1991) *Notes to Literature*. New York: Columbia University Press.
Adorno, T.W., Weber, S., and Nicholsen, S. (1981) *Prisms*. Cambridge, MA: MIT Press.
Ahmad, E. (2006) *The Selected Writings of Eqbal Ahmad*. Ed. by Bengelsdorf, C., Cerullo, M., and Chandrani, Y. New York: Columbia University Press.
Anderson, P. (1998) *The Origins of Postmodernity*. London: Verso.
Auerbach, E. (2003) *Mimesis: The Representation of Reality in Western Literature*. Princeton: Princeton University.
Bakhtin, M. (1986) *Speech Genres and Other Late Essays*. Trans. by McGee, V. Austin: University of Texas Press.
Bhabha, H.K. (2012) *The Location of Culture*. London: Routledge.

Bloch, E. (1988) *The Utopian Function of Art and Literature: Selected Essays*. Trans. by Zipes, J. and Mecklenburg, F. Cambridge: MIT Press.
Brennan, T. (1989) *Salman Rushdie and the Third World: Myths of the Nation*. London: Palgrave Macmillan.
Brennan, T. (1997) *At Home in the World: Cosmopolitanism Now*. Cambridge, MA: Harvard University Press.
Brennan, T. (2007) *Wars of Position: The Cultural Politics of Left and Right*. New York: Columbia University Press.
Brennan, T. (2014) *Borrowed Light: Vico, Hegel, and the Colonies*. Stanford: Stanford University Press.
Brouillette, S. (2007). *Postcolonial Writers in the Global Literary Marketplace*. London: Palgrave Macmillan.
Buck-Morss, S. (1977) *The Origin of Negative Dialectics: Theodor W. Adorno, Walter Benjamin and the Frankfurt institute*. Hassocks: Harvester Press.
Denning, M. (2004) *Culture in the Age of Three Worlds*. London: Verso.
Ghose, Z. (1965) *Confessions of a Native-Alien*. London: Routledge & Kegan Paul.
Ghose, Z. (1967) *Jets from Orange*. London: Macmillan.
Ghose, Z. (1969) *The Murder of Aziz Khan*. New York: John Day Company.
Ghose, Z. (1972) *The Violent West: Poems*. London: Macmillan.
Ghose, Z. (1981) *Hulme's Investigations into the Bogart Script*. Austin: Curbstone Press.
Ghose, Z. (1983) *The Incredible Brazilian: The Native*. Woodstock: Overlook Press.
Ghose, Z. (1984) *A Memory of Asia New and Selected Poems*. Connecticut: Curbstone Publishing.
Ghose, Z. (1986) *Figures of Enchantment*. London: Hutchinson.
Ghose, Z. (1991a) *Selected Poems*. New York: Oxford University Press.
Ghose, Z. (1991b) *The Art of Creating Fiction*. Houndmills: Macmillan.
Ghose, Z. (1992) *The Triple Mirror of the Self*. London: Bloomsbury Publishing.
Harris, W. (2005) *Selected Essays of Wilson Harris*. Ed. Bundy, A.J. London: Routledge.
Hitchcock, P. (2010) *The Long Space: Transnationalism and Postcolonial Form*. Stanford: Stanford University Press.
Huggan, G. (2001) *The Postcolonial Exotic: Marketing the Margins*. New York: Routledge.
Husain, I. (2006) *A Chronicle of the Peacocks: Stories of Partition, Exile and Lost Memories*. Trans. by Adil, V. and Bhalla, A. Oxford: Oxford University Press.
Jameson, F. (1986) 'Third-World Literature in the Era of Multinational Capitalism'. *Social Text* 15, 65–88.
Jameson, F. (1989) 'Foreword'. In *Caliban and Other Essays*. By Retamar, R.F. Trans. by Baker, E. Minneapolis: University of Minnesota Press, vii–xii.
Jameson, F. (1991) *Postmodernism, or, the Cultural Logic of Late Capitalism*. Durham, NC: Duke University Press.
Jameson, F. (2002) 'Reflections in Conclusion'. In *Postmodernism, or, the Cultural Logic of Late Capitalism*. Ed. by Bloch, E. and Jameson, F. London: Verso, 196–209.
Kanaganayakam, C. (1993) *Structures of Negation: The Writings of Zulfikar Ghose*. Toronto: University of Toronto Press.
Kureishi, H. (1991) *The Buddha of Suburbia*. New York: Penguin Books.
Kureishi, H. (2002) *Intimacy and Midnight All Day: A Novel and Stories*. New York: Simon and Schuster.
Kureishi, H. (2009) *The Black Album*. London: Faber and Faber.
Lazarus, N. (2011) *The Postcolonial Unconscious*. Cambridge: Cambridge University Press.
Lukács, G. (1962) *The Historical Novel*. London: Merlin Press.
Lukács, G. (1971) *The Theory of the Novel: A Historico-philosophical Essay on the Forms of Great Epic Literature*. Trans. by Bostock, A. Cambridge, MA: MIT Press.
Marcuse, H. (2007) 'The German Artist Novel: Introduction'. In *Art and Liberation: Collected Papers of Herbert Marcuse, Vol. 4*. Trans. by Reitz, C., ed. by Kellner, D. New York: Routledge, 71–81.
Marcuse, H. (2009) *Negations: Essays in Critical Theory*. London: MayFly Books.
Meyer, B. (1991) 'From an Interview with Zulfikar Ghose'. In *Selected Poems*. By Ghose, Z. Karachi: Oxford University Press, 99–113.
Moore-Gilbert, B. (2001) *Hanif Kureishi*. Manchester: Manchester University Press.
Moretti, F. (2000) *The Way of the World: The Bildungsroman in European Culture*. London: Verso.
Nietzsche, F. (1977) *The Portable Nietzsche*. London: Penguin.
Noys, B. (2018) 'Übermenschen and Untermenschen: Global Nietzsche and Postcolonial Fiction'. In *History, Imperialism, Critique: New Essays in World Literature*. Ed. by Ghaffar, A. London: Routledge.
Robbins, B. (2009) *Upward Mobility and the Common Good: Toward a Literary History of the Welfare State*. Princeton: Princeton University Press.
Rushdie, S. (1991) *Imaginary Homelands: Essays and Criticism 1981–1991*. New York: Penguin Books.
Said, E. (1983) *The World, the Text, and the Critic*. Cambridge, MA: Harvard University Press.

Said, E. (1985) *Beginnings: Intention and Method*. New York: Columbia University Press.
Said, E. (1994) *Culture and Imperialism*. London: Vintage.
Said, E. (2002) *Reflections on Exile and Other Essays*. Cambridge, MA: Harvard University Press.
Sanga, J.C. (ed.) (2003). *South Asian Novelists in English: An A to Z Guide*. Westport: Greenwood Publishing.
Sivanandan, A. (1990). *Communities of Resistance: Writings on Black Struggles for Socialism*. London: Verso.
Valéry, P. (2000) *Notebooks, Vol. 1*. Bern: Peter Lang.
Vico, G. (1999) *New Science: Principles of the New Science Concerning the Common Nature of Nations*. New York: Penguin.

PART VIII

New horizons
Towards a Pakistani idiom

28
'BRAND PAKISTAN'
Global imaginings and national concerns in Pakistani anglophone literature

Barirah Nazir, Nicholas Holm, and Kim L. Worthington

Who can or should be counted as a Pakistani anglophone author? This seemingly innocent question raises many issues, such as relations of belonging and community under globalisation, the role of literature in nation-building, and even the status of the Pakistani nation itself. Is a Pakistani (anglophone) author a product of location or ethnicity, communal imagination or Western imperialism, the nation state or the global literary market? These enormously complex questions are not limited to the scope of Pakistani literature, of course, but speak directly to claims made about 'national literature' and the way it is promoted and read across the globe. This chapter will explore the complications and contradictions inherent in defining contemporary Pakistani anglophone authorship in a global context. Employing a cultural materialist framework, it will then argue that claims about Pakistani anglophone literature need to be understood as bound up with the marketing strategies adopted by global publishers and that this has ramifications not just for the way this literature is marketed and the authenticity it claims or is claimed for it, but also for the literature and authors that are afforded international acclaim.

Defining a Pakistani author

The anxieties and controversies that animate discussions about Pakistani authorship are particularly evident in the case of anthologies and overviews of Pakistani writing. Clearly, not everyone who writes about Pakistan will be immediately accepted as a 'Pakistani writer', nor can assumptions/attributions of this title be a straightforward question of self-affiliation or critical reception, which are often at odds. Muneeza Shamsie, in her introduction to the anthology *A Dragonfly in the Sun* (1997), raised the problem of defining a 'Pakistani' writer when primordial means, such as blood and genetics, are not the only criteria, while her more recent collection, *Hybrid Tapestries* (2017), has been criticised on social media for the inclusion of Tariq Ali and Salman Rushdie, who are denounced as insufficiently Muslim. Tariq Rahman justifies his inclusion of texts/authors in *A History of English Literature in Pakistan* on the basis of criteria that are 'loose rather than strict, cultural rather than political' (1991: 11). As Rahman's inclusion of authors is premised on their Muslim identity or their tendency to lean towards Islamic ideology, he identifies writers like Khwaja Ahmad Abbas, Ahmed Ali, and Mumtaz Shahnawaz as Pakistani, even though they wrote prior to the creation of the Pakistani state. Elsewhere, in multiple anthologies, Zulfikar Ghose has been identified as a Pakistani writer, despite having never lived in Pakistan (Hashmi 1978; Shamsie 2017). Ghose himself has openly disassociated himself from any nationality, claiming that such identifications are constricting (Brouillette 2011: 9). Regardless, his work has been consistently claimed as that of a Pakistani author (Hashmi 1992, 1993; Brian Shaffer 2006: 26; Shamsie 2012, 2013) and he received the Lahore Literature Festival's Lifetime Award in 2015.

The uncertain nature of Pakistani authorship has also been evident in conversations and assumptions regarding the status of prominent individual authors, despite them not having lived in Pakistan for many of their formative and/or adult years. Mumtaz Shahnawaz is widely claimed to be a Pakistani writer by nearly all local and international critics because of her Muslim identity and her novel, *The Heart Divided* (2004), which favours Partition, despite the fact that she lived in the newly born Pakistan for just two years. Daniyal Mueenuddin, hailed within Pakistan and globally as a 'Pakistani writer', migrated to America as a child and only returned to Pakistan after several decades. Mohsin Hamid, perhaps the writer most decidedly claimed to be 'Pakistani' in recent years, is simultaneously linked to Pakistan, America (where he studied and worked but left after 9/11), and the UK (he holds a British passport and lived in England for many years). Nadeem Aslam, a Pakistani-born (Gujranwala) British writer, emigrated to the UK as a teenager; Kamila Shamsie, a Karachiite by birth, is a British national who studied in New York; Uzma Aslam Khan was born in Pakistan but studied in the USA, and periods of her childhood were spent in the Philippines, Japan, and England; Bapsi Sidhwa lived most of her life in Pakistan, but is now an American citizen. Even more controversial is the status of Rushdie, who was born in British India, two months prior to Partition, to a Muslim family, briefly lived in Pakistan in 1964, and finally emigrated to England. Among the major reasons why Rushdie is not considered a Pakistani writer by most local critics are his atheist leanings, his celebration of hybridity, his self-identification as a 'mongrel', and his claim to disaffiliate from the 'ghetto mentality' of those writers who limit themselves to national borders (1991: 19).[1] Unashamedly, he flaunts his international status noting that 'one of the more pleasant freedoms of the literary migrant is to be able to choose his parents' (Rushdie 1991: 434).

It's clear, then, that the majority of the current generation of 'Pakistani' anglophone writers are best understood as either transnational or cosmopolitan in their outlook. This prompts a question: which 'parents' have they 'chosen'? They cannot be exclusively defined as 'Pakistani' in any localised, geographically-constrained sense as nearly all of them have been educated or have lived outside Pakistan for lengthy periods. Most Pakistani anglophone fiction writers writing today continue to shuttle between Pakistan – their country of (familial) origin – and their adopted homes in North America and the UK. It could be argued that rather than looking out from Pakistan to the wider world, these writers assume the authority to 'look into and on' a nation they have not lived in for long or no longer live in – and to do so from a Western perspective. At best, they live in 'in-between' spaces, occupying a liminal status due to privileged international mobility while staying connected to their country of birth (or of their parents' birth); they are (or claim to be) paradoxically both 'local' and 'cosmopolitan'. Understood in positive terms, it could be claimed, as Pakistani-American writer and critic Anis Shivani does, that 'they are injecting their country into world literature' (2013: n.p.). Others, however, suggest that such writers betray their nation in numerous ways, as we shall discuss below.

Questions of Pakistani authorship are further complicated by their implication in wider conflicts regarding the nature of the Pakistani nation. Ever since its creation, Pakistan has grappled with the issue of defining its identity in ways symptomatic of Benedict Anderson's concept of a nation as 'an imagined political community' (1991: 6): premised not on disputed geographical boundaries (drawn by departing colonisers), but connectedness in a cultural and ideological sense. Traditionally (and this proviso is important) the Western concept of a nation has been associated with the sharing of one language and one religion – a criterion which Pakistan apparently fulfils via the binding forces of Urdu and Islam (despite multiple provincial languages and dialects and the existence of other religious minorities). But French political scientist Christophe Jaffrelot, among many others, highlights the conflicts that lurk beneath Pakistani nationhood. He argues that Islam has been used to produce and nurture nationalistic sentiments among diverse ethnicities (e.g. Punjabis, Sindhis, Balochs and Pakhtuns) who do not share ideological, cultural, or ethnic values (2002: 36). In this sense, Pakistan is a mosaic, like so many postcolonial nations – a synthetic product of various ethnicities with small fractions of minorities conjoined under the banner of Islamic Pakistan. Interethnic tensions have existed as long as the nation has. Yet, despite awareness of the interethnic differences that exist within Pakistan, there is also a strong desire to possess a distinct, and globally understood, national identity, as Mubarak Ali suggests:

> Since the beginning, Pakistan has been confronted with the monumental task of formulating a national identity distinct from India. Born out of a schism of the old civilisation of India, Pakistan has debated over the construction of a culture of its own, a culture which will not only be different from that of India but one that the rest of the world can understand.
>
> (2000: n.p.)

Global imaginings, national concerns

Given Ali's assessment of this 'monumental task', it seems important to ask not only *if* the world 'understands' Pakistan, but *how*? In global media, especially since 9/11, Pakistan is often characterised by images of terrorism and extremism; the patriarchal denial of women's autonomy ostensibly underwritten by religion; sectarian division; and by ignorant, camel-riding people traversing vast deserts. Pakistani anglophone fiction, taken as a whole, both challenges and reinforces such representations. It is also, perhaps inevitably, received and read in terms of its conformity with (internal and international) readers' expectations, that it does one or the other. On the one hand, the nation's anglophone literature is a platform which serves to showcase its diversity and dispel negative representations; on the other, it is vulnerable to the charge that it reinforces and replicates precisely these mediated assumptions. It is no small irony that many authors who are claimed, or claim, to be 'Pakistani' arguably partake in the dissemination of precisely the kinds of stereotypical representations that reconfirm, at least to some degree, Western assumptions about the nation. Claims about authorial national identity are therefore a particularly nuanced and unstable issue in the context of Pakistan, complicated by Western mainstream media (mis) representations of the nation, and by the very form and content of the literature that is claimed to be 'Pakistani'. To be sure, questions about the relationship between authorial identity, (authentic) literary representation, and nationhood are not unique to Pakistan – indeed such concerns are shared by many postcolonial nations – but they take on particular resonance in the context of Pakistan's ongoing attempts to affirm its unique national identity in the face of Western (media) representations, especially since 9/11. Yet, surprisingly, to date, the issue of Pakistani authorial national identity has received very little serious attention from readers, critical or popular.[2]

Cara Cilano uses the term 'transnational' to describe the new generation of Pakistani writers as global citizens (2009: 193). She suggests that the work of these writers merges local and global concerns and marks a break from the (predominantly) nationalistic fiction produced in

Pakistan in the 1990s. Madeline Clements makes similar claims in *Writing Islam from a South Asian Muslim Perspective*:

> Rushdie, Hamid, Aslam and Shamsie orient themselves towards the 'global' in their internationally disseminated novels, both in terms of their geopolitical subject matter and selection of settings which are of symbolic and strategic significance to world powers.
>
> (2016: 9)

A brief consideration of some recent contemporary South Asian (including Pakistani) fiction appears to confirm this claim about 'global orientation'. Aslam's first novel, *Season of the Rainbirds* (1993), is set in rural Pakistan, while his *Maps for Lost Lovers* (2004) is set in a fictional British locale called Dasht-e-Tanhaii, and *The Wasted Vigil* (2008) in Afghanistan. Although he returns to a western Pakistani/eastern Afghani setting in *The Blind Man's Garden* (2013), the novel looks out on the world, exploring the 'War on Terror' from the perspectives of local, Muslim characters. Shamsie's first two novels, *Kartography* (2002) and *Broken Verses* (2005), are set in Pakistan, but *Burnt Shadows* (2009) deals with global issues in a wide variety of international settings in different periods of the twentieth century, culminating in 9/11. The action in Hamid's debut novel, *Moth Smoke* (2000), takes place in Lahore, and while this is also the setting for his second novel, *The Reluctant Fundamentalist* (2007), the majority of the latter details the narrator's experiences of living in the USA and his decision to return to Pakistan following 9/11. Increasingly, then, the works of these 'Pakistani' writers portray locales and concerns that extend beyond the borders of the nation. This is to be expected and lauded: a writer from a certain nation, culture, or ethnicity should not be expected to write only about that nation, culture, or ethnicity. Why can't a New Zealander write about New York or a Canadian novelist situate her work in Multan? A great deal depends, however, on how such writers position themselves in national/cultural terms and, just as importantly, how they are positioned by their publishers, publicists, and reviewers.

'Brand Pakistan'

An alternative way of exploring questions about the nationalistic labelling of writers is to suggest that it has to do as much (or more) with the marketing of the work, rather than with the ostensibly autonomous writer herself. In simplistic terms, the politics of identity has been moved into, and is subsequently shaped by, the marketplace. John and Jean Comaroff, in *Ethnicity, Inc.*, argue that 'Cultural identity […] represents itself ever more as two things at once: the object of choice and self-construction, typically through the acts of consumption, and the manifest product of biology, genetics, human essence' (2009: 1). They maintain that in an era of capitalist globalisation, cultures are essentialised as brands (through patenting customary ways of living and items, for example) and the most sustainable and successful are the ones who brand the best. In the current geopolitical context, a substantial number of writers have thus emerged who are marketed, or market themselves, as representatives of *authentic* cultures (or nations), and benefit from this. This is an idea shared by Aijaz Ahmad, who argues that 'Third World' English literary texts are a product of imaginings of the West (or authors imagining such Western imaginings), so that 'the Third World' and its literature has been successfully fashioned into a global merchandising tool/product (1992: 13). Maximum sales are achieved through marketing tactics such as authors' commercial appearances and managed interviews, mass-market sales of affordable paperback editions, and the development of carefully courted relationships between publishers, reviewers, and the newspapers/magazines in which reviews appear (such as *TLS*, *London Review of Books*, *New York Review of Books*, *New York Times Book Review*, *Boston Globe*, *Village Voice*, *Guardian*, *Salon*). Understood in the terms proposed by the Comaroffs and Ahmad, the term 'Pakistani writer' has become a kind of geographical and political marker for writers whose work is marketed as *representative* of their place of origin, even if they are dealing with a wide variety of topics and places. Pakistan and its literature are far from alone in this regard: J.M. Coetzee, for example, has lived in Australia for many years, and much of his fiction is allegorical or without a clear 'national' setting, dealing instead with transnational issues of racial and gender oppression. However, he is almost always referred to as a 'South African' writer, a reference to the country in which he was born and lived for the first six decades of his life. Coetzee accounts for this situation with references to a 'vast and wholly ideological superstructure constituted by publishing, reviewing and criticism that has forced on me the fate of being a "South African novelist"' (qtd. in Morphett 1987: 460). To highlight the extent to which Pakistani writing is implicated in just such an 'ideological superstructure', we will use the term 'Brand Pakistan' in the remainder of this chapter.

The rise of 'Brand Pakistan' needs to be understood within the geopolitical context of the post-9/11 'War on Terror', and globalisation more broadly. Indeed, one reason for its 'boom' in the past decade or so is a global desire to 'know' about Muslim nations, and Muslim identity, following the 11 September 2001 attacks on the World Trade Center. Pakistani writer Aamer Hussein argues in an interview that Pakistani writers were writing well before 9/11, but this event 'gave them a particular label' and encouraged them to be read in certain ways – ways that sell, globally if not locally (Hussain and Piracha 2013: n.p.). In a similar vein, Shamsie draws attention to the relationship between Pakistan's currently position 'at the centre of geopolitical conflict' and the simultaneous 'flourishing of new [Pakistani] cultural expressions in music, art and literature [in international circles]' (2017: 256). Bina Shah insightfully suggests that:

> the Western world is dying to understand Islam, Muslim people, and the cultures that go with them. And since Pakistan is the only Muslim country in the world with so many English speakers, and a tradition of writing in English, it seems that Pakistani writers are meeting a fortuitous demand by being in the right place at the right time.
> (2010: n.p.)

In an interview in *The New Yorker*, Mueenuddin sardonically notes that 'there must be Lithuanian writers who are not getting the attention they deserve because their country is not in the news' (Habib 2009: n.p.). Others are wary of the 'fortuitous demand' noted by Shah. Pakistani writer Bilal Tanweer criticises the 'anthropological approach' evident in an interview given by Jamil Ahmad to CNN about his book *The Wandering Falcon*, in which Ahmad was asked eight questions about the political situation in Pakistan and only one related to his writing (2011: n.p.). In an interview entitled 'Occupational Hazards', published in the *Guardian*, interviewer Decca Aitkenhead pushes Hamid to comment on Rushdie's *fatwa* and any similarity he might see between Rushdie and himself, hinting at the precarious political situation in Pakistan. When Hamid innocuously replies by equating the risks involved in being a writer to any other job, like that of a pilot, the interviewer declares he is 'wary of commenting' (qtd. in Aitkenhead 2007: n.p.).

It is appreciable that if 'Brand Pakistan' is premised on the promise of insights into Muslim people and cultures, in turn fed by international (media) portrayals of Muslim terrorism, then many Pakistani cosmopolitan writers might choose to offer counter-narratives to global political representations. Ironically, however, in a bid to explain Pakistan as something more than a breeding ground for religious extremism, or a place where men mistreat women under the guise of religious sanctions, such writers may potentially bring more attention to these as key aspects of Pakistani life. Tanweer claims that the Western world is so obsessed with the 'factual information' which Pakistani anglophone fiction might provide that the artistic credibility or aesthetic merit of work is given little attention: 'Fiction from Pakistan is not supposed to have artistic engagements – it's required to provide information, not an experience. In other words, it must be a reliable Dispatch from the Terrorists Lair' (2011: n.p.).

For all this acknowledgement of writers' possible capitalisation on the West's desire to 'know' Pakistan via literary representation, there are some benefits too. Arguably, the desire to 'understand' Pakistan resulted in the publication of *Granta*'s significant issue on Pakistani literature in 2010. International support and interest has been particularly advantageous, given that the local publishing industry is impoverished (*Alhamra Literary Review* had to stop after two issues and the Pakistani branch of Oxford University Press largely focuses on educational titles). It may well be that *The Wandering Falcon* finally found a publisher in 2011, decades after it was written and after numerous attempts by Ahmad to get it into print, precisely because of the new climate of contemporary global interest in Pakistan. Ironically, though, the decades-old tribal focus of his collected stories, which are set in the North Western Frontier Province, which borders Afghanistan, may do a great deal to feed mistaken Western assumptions about Pakistan and pander to notions of 'exoticness' that would be unfamiliar to many living in the larger cities, or the south of the nation.

Authenticity, essentialism, and exoticism

As we have noted, one of the major consequences of the transformation of Pakistan (or its literature) into 'Brand Pakistan' is the potential of a turn towards reductive essentialism and exoticism. Graham Huggan, an early voice in such discussions (albeit not in relation to Pakistani writing), describes the commodification of cultural difference or otherness as a feature of what he terms 'the alterity industry' (2001: x). He cautions against assuming that the fictional representation of cultural 'alterity' offers real-life access to the lived reality of 'exotic' others:

> [T]he exotic is not, as is often supposed, an inherent quality to be found 'in' certain people, distinctive objects, or specific places; exoticism describes, rather, a particular mode of aesthetic perception – one which renders people, objects and places strange even as it domesticates them.
>
> (2001: 13)

Huggan uses the terms 'staged marginality' and 'strategic exoticism' to describe the 'domesticating' work of (postcolonial/decolonised) authors who fetishise difference through cultural/locational mystification in order to benefit via global promotion and sales (2001: 19, 87). Here, it is worth noting Rushdie's much earlier claim that cultural/national 'essentialism is the respectable child of old-fashioned exoticism' (1991: 67). For Rushdie (and many others), national essentialism 'has re-emerged with a vengeance in the packaging of several recent Indo-Anglian [and, we suggest, Pakistani] novels, as well as in the type of uncritical response to them that highlights their provenance, symbolic if not material, from an "exotic culture"' (1991: 75). Thus understood, the alterity industry could be imagined as a gigantic (Western) parasite feeding off cultural difference packaged as 'exotic'. A great deal of critical debate on such issues has taken place since Rushdie made this comment. Indeed, extensive scholarly attention has been devoted to precisely those issues of 'exoticism'/'essentialism' raised by Rushdie and complicated by others in the past few decades. In the South Asian literary context, however, almost all of this work has been focused on Indian anglophone texts and authors. Hence there is an urgent need to attend to contemporary Pakistani literature in similar ways.

One of the charges that have been levelled against writers from formerly colonised nations, or the margins more generally, is that many make use of their ex-centric position to 'sell' an exotic image of their nation (or culture, or religion). This is a claim that is quite routinely made with respect to contemporary Indian anglophone literature, perhaps most vehemently in discussions of Arundhati Roy's *The God of Small Things* (1997). Why this novel in particular has attracted such criticism is open to debate; it may be precisely because of its enormous international success. Critics such as Huggan, Alex Tickell, and Padmini Mongia (who coined the term 'the Roy phenomenon') attribute Roy's success, to a greater or lesser degree, to her cosmopolitanism, which helped her sell 'authentic' India through a book which reeks of exoticness. Tickell squarely chastises Roy for the 'exoticising' exploitation of regional 'difference', and thus of 'staged authenticity' (2007: 161). Lisa Lau offers a more nuanced approach to the question of the 'authentic' (or not) representation of India in Indian writing in English ('IWE'), posing important questions about the very notion of authentic representation itself, questions that are deeply relevant to discussions about contemporary Pakistani anglophone writing: 'a significant flaw in these accusations of inauthenticity and discussions of the "real" [is] the presumption that there exists somewhere an authentic account against which everything else can be measured (and found wanting)' (2011: 28). Similar claims are made by Aamir R. Mufti in the article 'The Aura of Authenticity', where he argues that, paradoxically, if 'authentic' local narratives are intended to 'interrupt the manner in which something called *the West* narrates itself and its others', then we need to be alert to the ways in which the very idea of (postcolonial) localised authenticity is in fact the product of 'Orientalist descriptions' (2000: 100; emphasis original). This is an idea Mufti develops at much greater length in *Forget English!* (2016), where he argues that the naming and lauding of culturally/nationally 'authentic' texts in the 'canon of world literature' in fact depends on 'an Orientalised consciousness' which is the result of a colonial imposition of 'narrowly conceived ethnonational spheres' that have become 'units' of international exchange (2016: 146). Mufti's larger critique is of (naive or exploitative) 'World Literature' studies/consumption; he warns against the 'ascription of authenticity to "local", instead of examining and denaturalizing the historical processes of vernacularization and indigenization, which will reveal their colonial genealogy' (2016: 149). Interestingly, despite being born and raised in Pakistan, Mufti's focus in his discussions of South Asian literature is almost always on texts from India. The relative lack of such a focus on Pakistani literature, to date, may well be due to the relative 'newness' of the emerging 'canon'. For all of this, there is now a considerable body of anglophone literature that is produced and marketed under the banner of Brand Pakistan, and this deserves critical attention of the kind discussed above.

A recent essay by Rohma Saleem begins to address this critical gap by exploring the extent to which two contemporary works of Pakistani anglophone fiction might be guilty of pandering to Western desires for the reconfirmation of stereotypical, essentialist notions about the nation and Islam, particularly with respect to the portrayal of women. This is certainly a welcome intervention. However, Saleem's argument, focused on Aslam Khan's *Trespassing* (2003) and Qaisra Shahraz's *Typhoon* (2007), is arguably informed by precisely the kind of 'Orientalised consciousness' that Mufti explores with such care. The novels are reduced to texts which *simply* 'appease the Western thirst for the mysterious and elusive East' and reiterate 'vilifying tropes of [the] East as necessarily backward, steeped in poverty, corruption, conservatism, a natural antithesis of the liberated West' (Saleem 2017: abstract); in short, they are described as 'deliberately

[...] appealing to the voyeuristic demands of the western reader' (Saleem 2017: 140). Pakistani anglophone writers (via brief analyses of Khan's and Shahraz's novels) are accused of attempting 'to stand in as intermediaries, as translator on one culture for the other', which 'suits them to perfection, since it gives their role heightened significance' (Saleem 2017: 141). Saleem uncritically adopts Lau's suggestion that *some* Indian writers may be 'guilty of skewered, partial, and selective representation, or wilful misrepresentation altogether [...], or outright betrayal' and asserts that 'The scenario is not much different [in the] Pakistani literary scene' (Saleem 2017: 142). She argues that Pakistani writers have just two options: '*either* exotic presentation of [the] Orient *or* an engagement in subversive criticism of one's traditions' (Saleem 2017: 142; emphasis added); they are *either* 'native informers' beguiled by the prospect of international fame and financial reward, *or* 'authentic' (a word that haunts the essay) representatives of their nation. This is an unfortunate reinscription of the kind of either/or logic that dogs and stymies some postcolonial and neocolonial critical discourses; it appears blind to the hybrid or 'mongrel' (self-)positioning of so many contemporary Pakistani writers, including those branded as Pakistani. As Lau and Mufti suggest, the notion of 'authenticity' itself needs to be probed much more carefully, as does the subversive potential of what Homi K. Bhabha terms 'sly mimicry' to unsettle notions of the 'real' (2004: 85).

Saleem thus dismisses Khan's and Shahraz's novels as exemplars of literary 'betrayal' – not only of (authentic) Pakistan but also of Islam (both of which are problematically, monolithically conceived): she reads them as anti-Muslim texts produced for 'anti-Muslim (Western) consumers' (Saleem 2017: 148). The inclusion of local language phrases in novels is dismissed as pandering to 'occidental tastes' (Saleem 2017: 151);[3] cosmopolitan authors are reduced to the role of outsiders 'peeping' in on Pakistani culture (Saleem 2017: 152) and accused of 'rehashing the same worn out themes' of 'marginalised women, the almost unbridgeable gaps between privileged and non-privileged, [...] riots, chaos, [...] lack of security, strikes, lockouts, shutter downs' (Saleem 2017: 153). In sum, then: 'Pakistani English fiction writers are playing a second fiddle to their western counterparts who *deem* Pakistan primitive in every sense of the word' (Saleem 2017: 154; emphasis added) and Pakistanis as 'irredeemably different from, more backward than, and culturally inferior to those who construct and consume the picturesque product' (Saleem 2017: 157); 'This kind of literature is lavishly praised for its miniaturist description but *its intention* is nothing more than to feed the western desire of knowing the east' (Saleem 2017: 155; emphasis added). As these comments suggest, broad and undefended assumptions are made – with respect to how the West 'deems' Pakistan, and about authorial 'intention' – that fly in the face of extensive critical debates that flag up issues of both intentionality and reader response as problematic. Saleem concludes with an assertion that, unfortunately, undermines her critical authority: 'One can only hope that [...] given time', Pakistani anglophone fiction will 'mature and [...] be completely independent of its former mentors' (Saleem 2017: 159). The fact that this fiction is written in English by often self-declared 'mongrels' and marketed internationally (as Mufti discusses so eloquently) renders this vision of autonomous, authentic 'independence' very dubious.[4]

For all her admirable passion, Saleem's essay highlights the perils inherent in uncritical (essentialist) assumptions about Pakistani authorial identity and Pakistani literature. It glosses over important relationships between notions of authenticity, exoticism, and cosmopolitanism that should, we believe, inform analyses of Pakistani anglophone literature – and its relationship with Western publishers, publicists, and readers. Critical debate reverts far too easily to convenient assertions about 'insider' and 'outsider' representational veracity, assertions of 'betrayal' or 'selling out', assumptions about 'real'/'authentic' or 'posturing'/'inauthentic' national or cultural or ethnic identities, complicated by discussions about whether or not the author(s) in question really *are* Pakistani or qualified to write as such, given their physical Western situation or assumed Western audience. When a text crosses the nation's borders, to what extent does its author *intend* to 'feed' Western desires for knowledge about the East? Regardless of intention, to what extent is it *read* by international readers as merely an entertaining information manual about a far-off land, or a means of understanding the relationship between 'us' and 'them'? Is Shamsie naive, misguided, or on the mark when she writes, 'I don't think a good novel works if you are trying to pander to a particular kind of market' (qtd. in Bilal 2016: 149)? This invites some tricky questions for 'Brand Pakistan'. Do anglophone Pakistani cosmopolitan writers anticipate an ideal reader based in the West? To what extent might they deliberately write for such a reader? Can they be accused of 'selling out' their culture and nation for fame and money? Alternatively, to what extent might they deliberately 'censor' their works in the ways Chandra suggests in the quotation provided at the start of this chapter?

Materialist critical approaches: avoiding a regressive return

The problem with accusations of cultural 'selling-out', via capitulation to the 'alterity industry', is that it lays the blame for negative aspects of 'Brand Pakistan' at the feet of Pakistani *authors* (as does Saleem) without fully accounting for the ways in which they are constructed as saleable entities in wider circuits of global cultural and capitalist markets. In a capitalist context, writing is a paid occupation. A writer writes to get published and thus be remunerated, and remuneration depends on meeting publishers' requirements, which in turn involve catering to market demands. No matter how much writers might resent this, these are the facts. Writing in response to Huggan, Bhabha elaborates on the modern phenomenon of 'global cosmopolitanism' in the new preface to *The Location of Culture*, emphasising that its ostensible celebration of a multicultural, diverse world and peoples located at the periphery is utterly conditional on neocolonial expectations of profit from the region (2004: xiv–xv). The 'diversity' of people from ex-peripheries is acceptable only if this diversity is *marketed* to ensure they are contributing economically, politically, and socially to the neocolonial centre (2004: xiv). In such terms, the (saleable) positionality of the author matters more than the quality of their work, let alone any claims (however complex) that may be made about their representational validity or 'authenticity'. In short, this emphasis on the geographic positionality of a literary work (or its author) keeps alive earlier orientalist and now cosmopolitan desires for readily consumed and assimilated 'otherness'. It also invites questions about the culpability of authors who may use their cosmopolitan identity/positioning to prioritise profit at the expense of representational 'authenticity' – if this is indeed possible. The extent to which they might knowingly or deliberately conform to such 'positioning' is one that demands much more attention and research.

In *The Postcolonial Exotic*, Huggan argues that it may be possible to 'truthfully' represent cultural difference in ways that are not exploited by market forces. Simply put, he pitches the idea that postcolonial authors can maintain cultural autonomy if they consciously avoid manipulating and exploiting what is unique and different about their culture (2001: 32). He uses the term 'postcolonial exotic' to describe the deliberate domesticating process through which commodities are taken from the margins and absorbed into mainstream culture (Huggan 2001: 22). In contrast, Sarah Brouillette rejects this distinction between authentic and 'staged' representation, insisting that there is no such thing as 'authentic'. She suggests that writers' 'exoticist' strategies/positionings are always already determined by their reception in the eyes of 'global reader(s)' to whom their work is directed (consciously or not), and by the 'publishing industry' which decides on the viability of content in a metropolitan market (2011: 23–24). Brouillette's account is more nuanced than the above comments suggest. She retains Huggan's touristic analogy (of readers visiting briefly) but goes a step further when she distinguishes, for example, between a number of kinds of 'cosmopolitan' reader (compared with Huggan's singular category, the 'global reader') – say, market reader, ethnographer, cosmopolitan, and tourist – while acknowledging that they all, to some degree, assume that they gain access to foreign cultures by reading texts produced in the margins. Huggan and Brouillette agree that postcolonial authors, in *staging* otherness, become trapped in a circuit of commodification which compromises any (subversive, especially anti-colonial) political function the author of the text might have envisaged.

The 'foreignness' of author's names, their unfamiliar accents, and their often darker skin all contribute to the idea that they are essentially 'other' – and yet their impeccable English, smart Western dress, educational credentials (and so on) mark them out as reliable commentators on the places they have *come from*. Timothy Brennan suggests that these authors are clearly marked as writers of a 'transnational class'. More, he suggests that 'being from "there" in this sense is primarily a kind of literary passport that identifies the artist as being from a region of underdevelopment and pain' (1997: 38). As transnational corporations are strongly grounded in Anglo-American centres, diversity is thus a result of a commodified literary marketplace in which the very location of authors serves an integral role.

Given these concerns, we believe it is important to analyse the (partial) role of Pakistani anglophone writers and of the international publishing market in the formation of the recent canon of Pakistani anglophone fiction. Materialist writers like Huggan, Brouillette, and Brennan clarify that the contemporary periphery is not simply 'writing back' (in the popular term established by Ashcroft, Griffiths, and Tiffin) but rather writing in ways which ensure that their work will be packaged and promoted by the centre, even if this means resorting to exoticist strategies, consciously or not. Globalisation, in this sense, emerges as a sanctioning neo-colonising force which restricts the emancipation of ex-centric narratives from the exotic bandwagon of otherness. Quite ironically, this restriction is itself an enabling process: by making texts palatable and familiar to readers, this strategic exoticism garners global visibility for Pakistani anglophone fiction.

Quite simply, post-9/11 and the War on Terror, 'Brand Pakistan' is likely to sell, due to the Western fascination with Muslim identity and terrorism. If this is true, the extent to which writers who are branded as 'Pakistani' confirm, undermine, or exploit marketing assumptions (and readership appeal) is clearly what is at stake. How do Pakistani writers respond to this allegation of exoticism in contemporary Pakistani anglophone literature? Most of them rebuff this kind of critique. When asked about this, Mohsin Hamid briefly responded: 'I try not to mention the minaret, because when I'm in Lahore, I don't notice it' (Khan 2015: n.p.). Muhammed Hanif, author of *A Case of Exploding Mangoes* (2008), dismisses any such pressure from market forces by downrightly asserting that he freely writes whatever he wants (Bilal 2013: 4). Mueenuddin is apparently happy with the international acclaim he has received and does not even consider local reception important. He disregards Pakistani readership as too small and limited, declaring that he has no interest in 'selling four thousand copies [...] in Pakistan' (Habib 2009: n.p.). In a *Guardian* interview with Natalie Hanman, Shamsie insists that Pakistani writers are telling stories that are no different from other writers across the globe, but nonetheless acknowledges the demands of international readers, stating that 'there will be journalists who come to you and they want to find the Muslim in you, the Pakistani in you' (2014: n.p.) In contrast, Khan speaks of the pressure Pakistani writers face in having to conform to popular Western clichés, but she believes they can choose to resist these practices (Aftab 2012: n.p). In sum, Pakistani anglophone fiction appears to face a complex interplay with market forces, especially given the latter's enchantment with 'Brand Pakistan'. This invites a far more nuanced discussion about (and anticipation of) textual reception in international markets than has currently been undertaken if we are to avoid a regressive return to the binaries that inform colonial orientalism. It also makes clear that writing as a representative of 'Brand Pakistan' entails walking a fine line between cultural/religious essentialism and 'truthful' representation, if the latter is at all possible.

Notes

1 Of the *Satanic Verses*, Rushdie wrote: 'Those who oppose the novel most vociferously today are of the opinion that intermingling with a different culture will inevitably weaken and ruin their own. I am of the opposite opinion. *The Satanic Verses* celebrates hybridity, impurity, intermingling, the transformation that comes of new and unexpected combinations of human beings, cultures, ideas, politics, movies, songs. It rejoices in mongrelisation and fears the absolutism of the Pure. *Mélange*, hotchpotch, a bit of this and a bit of that is *how newness enters the world*. It is the great possibility that mass migration gives the world, and I have tried to embrace it. *The Satanic Verses* is for change-by-fusion, change-by-conjoining. It is a love-song to our mongrel selves' (1991: 394). Mohsin Hamid similarly uses the term 'mongrel' to describe himself in an interview with Harleen Singh published in *ARIEL* (2012: 149).
2 For the most part, Western discussions of 'Pakistani' literature pay scant attention to issues that animate internal Pakistani discussions about nationhood or interpretations of Islam (say), or that engage with concerns such as home-grown terrorism (say). While we acknowledge these important concerns, a full discussion is beyond the scope of this chapter.
3 This flies in the face of so much that has been written about the way in which the inclusion of indigenous, non-English words and phrases might function to challenge (Western) readers' attempts to homogenise and appropriate the culture/ethnicity portrayed in postcolonial texts. The extensive 'African Language Debate', played out between Chinua Achebe and Ngũgĩ wa Thiong'o, and commentators on their respective works, is just one example.
4 In a comment about why Indian Booker Prize winning novels (by Roy, Kiran Desai, and Aravind Adiga) received negative or lukewarm responses in India, Vijay Nair provocatively asks: 'Is it because they hold a mirror to realities we refuse to acknowledge?' (qtd. in Lau 2011: 30). Put another way, is it the role of anglophone writers to represent only the 'good' and incontestable aspects of a culture/nation? Is this authentic? Do they not have a right, and responsibility, to write about what is not so good, or even wrong (in their estimation), about their culture/nation?

Bibliography

Aftab, A. (2012) 'If this were a Civilized Land, Faith Would be Private'. *The Friday Times* [online]. Available from <www.thefridaytimes.com/beta3/tft/article.php?issue=20121026&page=20> [25 November 2017].
Ahmad, A. (1992) *In Theory: Classes, Nations, Literature*. London: Verso.
Ahmad, J. (2011) *The Wandering Falcon*. New York: Riverhead Books.
Aitkenhead, D. (2007) 'Occupational Hazards'. *Guardian* [online]. Available from <www.theguardian.com/books/2007/aug/11/fiction.bookerprize2007> [25 November 2017].
Ali, M. (2000) 'In Search of Identity'. *Dawn Magazine*. 7 May.
Anderson, B. (1991) *Imagined Communities: Reflections on the Origin and Spread of Nationalism*. London: Verso.
Aslam, N. (1993) *Season of the Rainbirds*. London: André Deutsch Ltd.
Aslam, N. (2004) *Maps for Lost Lovers*. New York: Vintage.
Aslam, N. (2008) *The Wasted Vigil*. London: Faber & Faber.
Aslam, N. (2013) *The Blind Man's Garden*. London: Faber & Faber.
Bhabha, H.K. (2004) *The Location of Culture*. London: Routledge.
Bilal, M. (2013) '"I Don't Think I Am Addressing the Empire": An Interview with Mohammed Hanif'. *Postcolonial Text* 8(3–4), 1–11.
Bilal, M. (2016) *Writing Pakistan: Conversations on Identity, Nationhood and Fiction*. Noida: Harper Collins.
Brennan, T. (1997) *At Home in the World: Cosmopolitan Now*. Cambridge, MA: Harvard University Press.
Brouillette, S. (2011) *Postcolonial Writers in the Global Literary Marketplace*. Basingstoke: Palgrave Macmillan.

Choudhury, C. (2009) 'English Spoken Here: How Globalization is Changing the Indian Novel'. *Foreign Policy* [online]. Available from <http://foreignpolicy.com/2009/10/15/english-spoken-here/> [12 December 2017].

Cilano, C. (2009) '"Writing from Extreme Edges": Pakistani English-Language Fiction'. *ARIEL: A Review of International English Literature* 40(2–3), 183–201.

Clements, M. (2016) *Writing Islam from a South Asian Muslim Perspective: Rushdie, Hamid, Aslam, Shamsi*. New York: Palgrave Macmillan.

Comaroff, J.L. and Comaroff, J. (2009) *Ethnicity, Inc.* Chicago: University of Chicago Press.

Dwivedi, O.P. (2013) 'Tabish Khair: Marketing Compulsions and Artistic Integrity'. In *Postliberalization Indian Novels in English: Politics of Global Reception and Awards*. Ed. by Viswamohan, A.I. New York: Anthem Press, 103–112.

Habib, S. (2009) 'The Exchange: Daniyal Mueenuddin'. *The New Yorker* [online]. Available from <www.newyorker.com/books/page-turner/the-exchange-daniyal-mueenuddin> [20 December 2017].

Hamid, M. (2000) *Moth Smoke*. New Delhi: Penguin.

Hamid, M. (2007). *The Reluctant Fundamentalist*. Boston: Houghton Mifflin Harcourt.

Hannan, N. (2014) 'Kamila Shamsie: Where is the American Writer Writing about America in Pakistan? There is a Deep Lack of Reckoning'. *Guardian* [online]. Available from <www.theguardian.com/culture/2014/apr/11/kamila-shamsie-america-pakistan-interview> [10 October 2017].

Hashmi, A. (1978) *Pakistani Literature: The Contemporary English*. Islamabad: Gulmohar.

Hashmi, A. (1989) 'Prolegomena to the Study of Pakistani English and Pakistani literature in English'. Paper Presented at the International Conference on English in South Asia, Islamabad.

Hashmi, A. (1992) 'Pakistan'. *Journal of Commonwealth Literature* 26(2), 93–100.

Hashmi, A. (1993) 'Pakistan'. *Journal of Commonwealth Literature* 28(3), 95–103.

Huggan, G. (2001) *The Postcolonial Exotic: Marketing the Margins*. New York: Routledge.

Hussain, S. and Piracha, M. (2013) 'Spotlight Writer: Aamer Hussein'. *The Missing Slate* [online]. Available from <http://themissingslate.com/2013/08/08/spotlight-writer-aamer-hussein/> [23 December 2017].

Jaffrelot, C. (2002) *Pakistan: Nationalism Without a Nation?* New York: Palgrave.

Kanwal, A. (2014) *Rethinking Identities in Contemporary Pakistani Fiction: Beyond 9/11*. London: Palgrave Macmillan.

Khan, A.R. (2015) 'Mohsin Hamid – The Reluctant Novelist'. *Herald* [online]. Available from <https://herald.dawn.com/news/1153272>[15 October 2017].

Lau, L. (2011) 'Re-Orientalism in Contemporary Indian Writing in English'. In *Re-Orientalism and South Asian Identity Politics: The Oriental Other Within*. Ed. by Lau, L. and Mendes, A.C. London: Routledge, 15–39.

Masterton, J. (2013) 'Aravind Adiga: The White Elephant? Postliberalization, the Politics of Reception and the Globalization of Literary Prizes'. In *Postliberalization Indian Novels in English: Politics of Global Reception and Awards*. Ed. by Viswamohan, I.A. New York: Anthem Press, 51–66.

Mongia, P. (2007) 'The Making and Marketing of Arundhati Roy'. In *Arundhati Roy's The God of Small Things*. Ed. by Tickell, A. New York: Routledge, 103–109.

Morphett, T. (1987) 'Two Interviews with J.M. Coetzee, 1983 and 1987'. *Triquarterly* 69, 454–465.

Mufti, A.R. (2000) 'The Aura of Authenticity'. *Social Text* 18(3), 87–103.

Mufti, A.R. (2016) *Forget English! Orientalisms and World Literatures*. Cambridge, MA: Harvard University Press.

Pal, A. (2013) 'I'm Very Comfortable as a Hybridized Mongrel'. *The Progressive* [online]. Available from <http://progressive.org/dispatches/i-m-comfortable-hybridized-mongrel/> [20 May 2017].

Rahman, T. (1991) *A History of Pakistani Literature in English*. Lahore: Caravan.

Rushdie, S. (1991) *Imaginary Homelands: Essays and Criticism 1981–1991*. London: Granta.

Saleem, R. (2017) 'Marketing Otherness: A Re-Orientalist Gaze into Pakistani Fiction with a Focus on *Trespassing* and *Typhoon*'. *Journal of Research (Humanities)* 53, 139–160.

Shaffer, B.W. (2006) *Reading the Novel in English: 1950–2000*. Oxford: Blackwell.

Shah, B. (2010) 'The Pak Pack Takes Over the Literary World?'. *Hindustan Times* [online]. Available from <www.hindustantimes.com/books/the-pak-pack-takes-over-the-literary-world/story-qElm4U4NLcjasMUv6gZZIK.html> [26 October 2017].

Shah, B. (2012) 'Paperback Writers'. *Critical Muslim* 4, 143–154.

Shahnawaz, M. (2004) *The Heart Divided*. New Delhi: Penguin Books.

Shamsie, K. (2002) *Kartography*. Karachi: Oxford University Press.

Shamsie, K. (2005) *Broken Verses*. Orlando: Harcourt.

Shamsie, K. (2009) *Burnt Shadows*. New York: Picador.
Shamsie, M. (1997) *A Dragonfly in the Sun: An Anthology of Pakistani Writing in English*. Karachi: Oxford University Press.
Shamsie, M. (2007) 'Complexities of Home and Homeland in Pakistani English Poetry and Fiction'. In *Interpreting Homes in South Asian Literature*. Ed. by Lal, M. and Kumar, S.P. New Delhi: Pearson, 127–139.
Shamsie, M. (2012) 'Pakistan'. *Journal of Commonwealth Literature* 47, 561–575.
Shamsie, M. (2013) 'Pakistan'. *Journal of Commonwealth Literature* 48, 555–570.
Shamsie, M. (2016) 'Pakistan'. *Journal of Commonwealth Literature* 51, 644–659.
Shamsie, M. (2017) *Hybrid Tapestries: The Development of Pakistani Literature in English*. Karachi: Oxford University Press.
Shivani, A. (2013) 'What is World Literature?'. *The Missing Slate* [online]. Available from <http://themissingslate.com/2013/08/22/what-is-world-literature/view-all/> [13 August 2017].
Singh, H. (2012) 'Deconstructing Terror: Interview with Mohsin Hamid on *The Reluctant Fundamentalist* (2007)'. *ARIEL* 42(2), 149–156.
Tanweer, B. (2011) 'Cover Story: Wilderness, Wilderness'. *Dawn* [online]. Available from <www.dawn.com/news/635824> [15 June 2017].
Tickell, A. (2007) *Arundhati Roy's The God of Small Things*. London: Routledge.

29
COMPETING HABITUS
National expectations, metropolitan market, and Pakistani writing in English (PWE)

Masood Ashraf Raja

Now that Pakistani fiction writers are better known in the West, it seems, at least to South Asian literature scholars in metropolitan cultures, that Pakistani writing in English (PWE) has finally 'arrived'.

The case of any postcolonial author, and that includes Pakistani writers in English, is peculiar: these authors use native raw materials to write works aimed at metropolitan audiences. Such writing is thus strongly overdetermined even before a book is conceived, written, and published. The expectations and interests of the metropolitan reader are, in a way, preinscribed in an act of writing performed by a postcolonial author. These pre-existing determinisms that decide the kinds of work about and by authors of the global periphery being published in the metropolis are wonderfully explained by Aijaz Ahmad:

> Analogous procedures of privileging certain kinds of authors, texts, genres and questions seem to be under way now with regard to 'Third World Literature' [...] The range of questions that may be asked of the texts which are currently in the process of being canonized within this categorical counter-canon must predominantly refer, then, in one way or another, to representations of colonialism, nationhood, post-coloniality, the typology of rulers, their powers, corruptions, and so forth.
>
> (1992: 124)

In the same work, Ahmad also goes on to suggest that because of this metropolitan practice of privileging certain specific tropes in Third World writing addressed to metropolitan audiences, certain other works 'which do not ask those particular questions in any foregrounded manner would then have to be excluded from or pushed to the margins of this emerging counter-canon' (1992: 124). Ahmad was writing at a time when postcolonial studies had just started to emerge as a viable academic field of study; one could say that we have now reached a stage in Third World cultural production where no demands need to be made of postcolonial authors: those attempting to address metropolitan audiences have already, in most cases, internalised the expectations of metropolitan publishers and readers, and their writings are overdetermined by these internalised concerns. These determinisms play an important role in all acts of cultural representation, and while writers might find it apt and well within their authorial rights to compose such stories, the native reader's expectations of these texts become irrelevant. There is, therefore, a tension between national expectations of PWE and its reception beyond the nation. Most Pakistani authors writing in English must traverse this perilous terrain of two binaristic and often contested domains: national expectations and the demands of the metropolitan publishing market.[1] Some general examples of this contested terrain can be seen in the works of leading contemporary Pakistani authors: Mohammed Hanif's *A Case of Exploding Mangoes* (2008), for instance, comes laden with all the expected tropes – the military dictator, supine politicians, and the like. Similarly, of all the characters to choose from in the city of Lahore, Mohsin Hamid's Changez, in *The Reluctant Fundamentalist* (2007), offers yet another simplistic take on the transcultural aspirations of a Pakistani male subject: if America fails you, your only option is to become a 'reluctant' fundamentalist. In Daniyal Mueenuddin's highly acclaimed short story collection, *In Other Rooms Other Wonders* (2009), we encounter feudal Pakistan with all its ills and possibilities. Though Mueenuddin's stories do complicate the existential choices within the power dynamics of rural Pakistan, the major metropolitan tropes of oppressive patriarchs, feudal men, victimised women, and struggling peasants still seem to be centre stage. Of course, not all PWE relies on these general tropes, but in one way or another these metropolitan-preferred tropes do find their way into most, if not all, works of PWE.

This chapter builds on my previous work on this subject and attempts to articulate a mode of reading and writing about PWE with an understanding of both these poles of representation and reception within the nation and abroad.[2] In other words, one could argue that while Pakistani writers use Pakistani raw materials to compose their fiction, they inhabit a peculiar transnational habitus and their Pakistani readers, on the other hand, read the same works with the predetermined expectations of their own particular habitus. This leads one to account for the most important conundrum of PWE: what constitutes these two competing habitus and what is at stake if we do not account for the authorial and reader expectations governed and constructed by these two overlapping but distinct habitus? To explain my point better, I will use the concept of habitus as theorised by Pierre Bourdieu in reading the works of Pakistani writers published in the special issue of *Granta* on Pakistan edited by John Freeman (2010), with a specific focus on one story. First, my discussion of habitus, which Bourdieu defines as:

> both the generative principle of objectively classifiable judgements and the system of classification (*principium divisionis*) of these practices. It is in the relationship between the two capacities which define the habitus, the capacity to produce classifiable practices and works, and the capacity to differentiate and appreciate these practices and products (taste), that the represented social world, i.e., the space of life-styles, is constituted.
>
> (1984: 170)

To unpack this, a habitus both produces the system of judgements (of taste and art etc.) and provides a classification, or hierarchy, of these judgements. For example, the distinction between high and low art would, in this sense, be constituted by the habitus and then explained and formulated within the same logic of the habitus. And, as Bourdieu suggests, it is within the gap between these two corresponding functions of the habitus that one can learn the governing system of appraisal within a specific lifestyle. This aspect of the habitus is important to bear in mind while dealing with PWE and its reception within and without Pakistan.

Obviously, then, a question arises: where does the habitus itself come from? Bourdieu's explanation of the term suggests that habitus is, in a way, produced by the living conditions of a certain time and space, but acknowledging the existence of a habitus as a productive and evaluative force enables one to understand the given positions and tastes of individuals within a life field. In a schematic diagram provided in his book *Distinction: A Social Critique of the Judgement of Taste*, Bourdieu suggests that 'Objectively classifiable conditions of existence create a habitus, which in turn generates systems of schemes generating classifiable practices and works and taste. These classifiable practices and works then constitute a lifestyle' (1984: 171).[3]

But, in essence, the whole movement is, to me, circular, though ascribing our cultural practices and values to a habitus makes it easier to understand differences in tastes as well as in the reception and evaluation of various works. Bourdieu further argues that the 'habitus is necessity internalized and converted into a disposition that generates meaningful practices and meaning-giving perceptions', and if we agree with this premise then it is easier to agree with Bourdieu when he suggests that 'different conditions of existence produce different habitus' (1984: 170), and these differences in habitus end up affecting our judgements and evaluations of works of art.

With this cursory discussion of habitus, I would like to suggest that PWE and its critique within Pakistan can be better understood by taking a deeper look at the habitus that determines writing and that which structures the expectations and aspirations of Pakistani readers critical of PWE.

Not only are most Pakistani authors writing in English determined by a particular habitus – I call it the 'cosmopolitan habitus' – they also unconsciously forestall and incorporate the expectations of the metropolitan market within their writing. Thus, while they may physically inhabit their social and class habitus within Pakistan, their imaginative habitus, which sometimes overdetermines their writing, is already placed in an elsewhere, an elsewhere that comes across as natural but is determined by the metropolitan publishing industry and its financial and artistic imperatives. These writers, I suggest, are not actively seeking to write in a certain way: instead they write from within the logic of this habitus, and their actions, therefore, must appear to them natural and uncontrived.

Similarly, Pakistani readers who find these representations unfair, anti-Pakistani, or unpatriotic also bring to bear upon these texts the value judgements and critical expectations pertinent to their particular habitus which, for want of a better word, I will call the 'nationalistic habitus'. Note that using 'habitus' instead of 'class' already broadens the two constituencies of readers and writers, as sometimes readers from drastically different classes share the same value judgements about PWE. For example, in my conversations with highly educated Pakistani students, who would normally have aesthetic 'tastes' inspired and shaped by a Westernised canon, often find the works of Pakistani authors deeply troubling as, in their opinion, they tend to represent Pakistan very negatively. Now, class alone cannot explain these views, for the same people who pose this problem are also from the so-called Westernised upper middle class. Only a deeper understanding of habitus can render their views somewhat understandable. My ensuing discussion, however, is not based on any empirical research into the reading habits of Pakistani scholars and students. In fact, the structuring of my entire argument is based on these two large philosophical abstractions: the nationalistic and the cosmopolitan habitus.

Let me first explain the nationalistic habitus. A majority of Pakistanis do not or cannot read anglophone fiction. It would be safe to suggest that only the upwardly mobile bourgeoisie educated in what is termed the 'English medium' system of education can read PWE. Traditionally, as has been asserted by so many postcolonial scholars, when colonised natives acquired the language of their colonial masters, they also acquired and internalised their aesthetics and often their politics. Ngũgĩ wa Thiong'o expresses this impact of colonial education as follows:

> In my view language was the most important vehicle through which the power [of the colonizers] held the soul [of the colonized] prisoner. The bullet was the means of the physical subjugation. Language was the means of the spiritual subjugation.
>
> (1986: 9)

Thiong'o further illustrates this argument by pointing to his own experience as a colonial child in a colonial school, where the children were forced to speak in English and any act of speaking in the local 'vernacular' was derided and often punished (1986: 11–12). Thus, while colonial children learned British or French language and literature, they also internalised certain aspects of this experience as natural: that the colonial languages were superior, and thus the cultures of those languages were also somehow superior to native cultures. These children also internalised a certain distrust and disdain for their own primary cultures. One could say that the colonial educational system was acting as a 'habitus-shifting' mechanism, with which it achieved what Lord Macaulay had hoped for: the creation of human subjects who are 'Indian in blood and colour, but English in taste, in opinions, in morals, and in intellect' (2005: 130). The Pakistani bourgeois elite are, in my opinion, in so many ways still part of this colonial legacy, at least when it comes to their fascination with English literature and language, and their cultural and literary tastes can be attributed to this particular habitus and its attendant tastes and aesthetics. This 'training' of cosmopolitan methods of education and reading habits can be surmised from the English department curricula of most Pakistani universities, which still privilege the traditional English canon.

Thus, one would imagine that this particular class of Pakistanis, being so deeply immersed in the so-called Western way of things, would not be so troubled by PWE. One would usually assign negative views of PWE to more atavistic and Urdu-speaking citizens of Pakistan. But in my discussions about PWE with Pakistani students and scholars, most of the people from this particular social class tended to express deeply critical views of PWE texts and authors. This can only be explained in terms of their nationalistic habitus and not simply in terms of class. Let us dwell a little on the particulars of the nationalistic habitus. What could it possibly mean and what kind of cognitive and meaning-making structuring does it perform?

The nationalistic habitus works as both a structure and a structuring mechanism; it constructs not only the expectations of its inhabitants about the nature of their national identity, but also how that national identity is represented and perceived elsewhere in the world. In this structuring, national anxieties become part of Pakistanis' collective view of themselves as Pakistanis. Thus, those enmeshed in this particular habitus do not experience PWE simply as literary representations, they also see it from the point of view of its reception in the world and in terms of the kinds of national stereotypes which such representations normalise for metropolitan audiences. It is no secret that within metropolitan circles a view of Pakistan as a 'dark place' or as a place riven with despotic patriarchy, terrorism, and interethnic conflicts already exists. In fact, this view of Pakistan had already been normalised by major postcolonial authors. Salman Rushdie, for example, suggests that he couldn't have written *Shame*, his novel about Pakistan, in the same style as *Midnight's Children*, for 'that kind of exuberant, affectionate book about Pakistan [...] would be a false book' (Haffenden 2000: 54). So, it seems that there is no shortage of negative stereotypes of Pakistan, either in Europe or the rest of the North Atlantic world.

Against this pre-existing literary stereotyping of Pakistan, the nationalistic habitus forces the reader not just to dwell on the text, but to ponder more over what the text does. What does it normalise? Any work of fiction produced by PWE thus becomes suspect, as it either represents Pakistan in congruence with its current stereotypes or simply represents Pakistan in overly damaging terms. Needless to say, this way of receiving PWE is deeply connected to issues of recognition, but also to issues of national anxiety as a nation and as a people within the world. This reaction, however, does have a silver lining: readers, even though sceptical of the representation itself, in challenging the representations unconsciously concede the importance and significance of literary representation, for if they did not recognise the importance of PWE, they would not assign it the power of representation that they find troubling.

The question of authenticity is also often posed: I have had to answer questions about these anxieties over 'authentic' representations of Pakistan in many a public talk in Pakistan. For my interlocutors, authors not living permanently in Pakistan somehow lack the capacity or, in some cases, do not have the right to write about Pakistan. This approach confuses the act of 'living' with the act of 'dwelling'. And it presupposes that if one were to live in Pakistan, one would be more attuned to the nuances of Pakistani culture, which is partially true. But even those living in Pakistan cannot always write experientially, for those living in Islamabad probably have absolutely no idea about the lives of people in Gilgit-Baltistan or Kashmir. In all such representations, even when writers residing in Pakistan travel to areas they might want to represent, writing would still involve an act of imagination; and besides the lived experience, they would also have to learn about these Pakistani subcultures through textual research. Authenticity, on the other hand, is also a myth, for if our views of culture are determined by our lived experience, then the particular habitus that we occupy sometimes overdetermines our own views of the real and material world.[4]

Let us now move on to what I have termed the 'cosmopolitan habitus' which, in my view, sometimes overdetermines the kind of literary works that are offered to the world by PWE. I am drawing on the work of Bruce Robbin who, besides a thorough discussion of the concept of cosmopolitanism/cosmopolitics, gives us a succinct understanding of it as a world view, according to which 'we *value* the move away from ethnocentrism' (1998: 260; emphasis original). Pakistanis writing in English are, in so many ways, determined by the structuring imperatives of the cosmopolitan habitus. Thus, while their place of writing and the setting of their works happen to be Pakistan, the stories they tell come across as meant only for a transnational, cosmopolitan audience. This emphasis on the audience also forces them to choose topics that should, in one way or another, interest their metropolitan reading audiences. Hence, it is no surprise that one finds in PWE the very tropes that Ahmad lists in his critique of postcolonial and, in this case, cosmopolitan writing. Writers, of course, have an absolute right to represent what they deem important, and critiques of national cultures and politics are an established genre within postcolonial studies. Thiong'o, for example, provides a convincing reason for representing the national ills to a larger audience in the opening pages of his novel *Devil on the Cross* (1982). The novel uses the figure of a *gīcaandī* player as the narrator and a framing device, which forestalls any critique of exposing national ills to a global audience; he proffers the following reason for telling the story:

> Certain people in Ilmorog, our Ilmorog, told me that this story was too disgraceful, too shameful, that it should be concealed in the depths of everlasting darkness.
> There were others who claimed that it was a matter for tears and sorrow, that it should be suppressed so that we should not shed tears a second time.
> I asked them: How can we cover up pits in our courtyard with leaves or grass, saying to ourselves that because our eyes cannot now see the holes, our children can prance around the yard as they like?
> Happy is the man who is able to discern the pitfalls in his path, for he can avoid them.
> (1982: 1)

In the same vein, one could argue that if Pakistani authors write about the ills of their national or regional cultures, it is part of their job as socially engaged artists and writers. But, sadly, these ills are also stereotypical views of Pakistan upon which depend global perceptions of Pakistan. Furthermore, my Pakistani critics would argue, the Urdu novel and other generic forms are already offering, and have always offered, potent critiques of all forms of oppression and injustice within Pakistan. But when this act of critique is performed in Urdu, only the immediate Urdu-reading audience is aware of it, which is precisely the audience that can read a text within its specific context without generalising it into a whole and uncomplicated view of Pakistani culture. Thus, by writing in English, some authors take the risk, even when they are genuinely challenging national ills and highlighting the complicity of Western nation states in what goes on in the global periphery, of either being misread or blamed for being in service to metropolitan, cosmopolitan audiences. Hence, not all PWE is somehow complicit in the project of empire, and even a cursory look at the huge variety of PWE is enough to disprove any simplistic assumptions. It is, however, quite obvious that when a work does rely heavily on the expected tropes and stereotypes of Pakistan, it is likely to further concretise pre-existing perceptions of Pakistan and Pakistanis stereotypes, as such works come across as more authentic because they are written by so-called 'authentic' cultural informants.

With these two competing habitus at work, it is easier to understand the conflictual nature of PWE: the writer's right to represent and the reader's right to object to such representations. The most striking example of this 'choice' to represent Pakistan as if nothing other than bad things are happening in Pakistan, is evident in the special issue of *Granta* published in 2010.

Let us think about it: an esteemed magazine dedicated to the creative arts offers selected authors from Pakistan a chance to offer some 'representative' Pakistani writing for a global audience. There is no need to unconsciously write overly determined narratives to appease that global audience. The selected authors, it seems, must have had the freedom to write about Pakistan any way they liked: they could have resented Pakistan as a place where so many other things, some life-affirming things, were also happening besides the daily bombings, beheadings, and terrorist attacks. What the authors chose to represent on a global stage, therefore, is not just fiction and art, but art that has the power to concretise or complicate views about Pakistan. In this case, sadly, most of the stories included in the collection ended up supporting the very stereotypes about Pakistan that need to be challenged and disrupted. Here is a rough catalogue.

The collection includes a story of enduring love framed around a ritualistic, transgenerational gang rape (this is the lead story that I discuss below in detail); another about Kashmir and its 'Forever War'; an essay by Intizar Hussain, one of the great Urdu novelists, about the incremental erosion of Pakistani civic society; and yet another story by Hamid, entitled 'A Beheading'. The general picture of Pakistan that emerges through a reading of the collection is that of a nation on the brink, with degrading civic norms and little hope for the future. This gathering of bleak fictional and non-fictional 'representative' texts was obvious to pretty much all the early reviewers of the collection.

In a *New York Times* review entitled 'Midnight's Other Children', Isaac Chotiner finds the collection lacking 'the whimsy that Americans simplistically identify with India', and describes 'Granta's Pakistan' as 'a country of jihadists, anti-Americanism and increasingly misogynistic and brutal forms of Islam'. Chotiner nevertheless acknowledges that 'for all the violence and brutality, the reader does get glimpses of a less visible Pakistan' (2010: n.p.), by which, I guess, he means a Pakistan of natural beauty and some cultural value. In another review in *The Wall Street Journal*, entitled 'Tales of Love and Gore', Mira Sethi opines that 'Violence – physical, emotional, state-inflicted – preoccupies nearly every writer here' (2010: n.p.).

Even the editorial description on the collection's Amazon listing is instructive of the kind of expectations created in its reading audience:

> Brought into nationhood under the auspices of a single religion, but wracked with deep separatist fissures and the destabilizing forces of ongoing conflicts in Iran,

Afghanistan and Kashmir, Pakistan is one of the most dynamic places in the world today. It is also at the forefront of a literary renaissance.[5]

Thus, the metafictional aspects of the collection already suggest that, despite the problems that Pakistan faces, the ability of its writers to produce fiction is somehow, in itself, a redeeming quality, for it proves the exceptionality of the authors themselves. One could also argue that this collection offers itself as a testament to the creative arts and their possibilities, even under adverse conditions. One could also read it as a redeeming narrative of the resilience of Pakistan, which manages to produce world-class authors even under such harsh problems both originary and current. What is not clear, of course, is whether Pakistan can be represented without these attendant modifiers. But if one views the readers' comments in the same Amazon entry, one can guess that most people read the collection as an accomplishment in itself from a country that might be courting disaster but can still produce art. One online reviewer, for example, offers the following view:

> Wonderful writing gives a glimpse into this complex and often misrepresented country. The rawness of many writings reflects the turmoil this country has been in and the suffering its inhabitants go through every single day of their lives. It is a description of a country of contradictions, loaded with nukes, insane religious fanatics, non-existent education or infrastructure and the resilience of its people who continue to produce world-class writers and artists![6]

It seems that the actions of writers become larger than a nation of over one hundred and seventy-five million people: they become the ultimate redeeming quality of an entire nation. Of course, nowhere in such descriptions can one see that, despite these problems, Pakistanis live rich lives, love and care for each other, and maintain normal day-to-day relations.

While I completely understand that Pakistanis writing in English have the absolute right to represent Pakistan as they see fit, I am, as a teacher of these texts within a metropolitan public university, more concerned with what these texts do. How do they come across to our students? Most American students are required to take at least two world literature courses; these courses are often not taught by specialists, but rather by either part-time adjunct professors or graduate students. While I acknowledge that most of these teachers are hardworking, enthusiast teachers, not many of them are trained to teach beyond the text. Thus, what PWE authors write has the potential to become the ultimate window into Pakistani culture for many American students. The chances are that these students will encounter only one or two stories about Pakistan, and what their reading construes from these stories will to some extent inform their views about the country. While no one story or work of art can 'carry the burden of an entire culture',[7] most of the stories included in the *Granta* collection are likely to take on a life larger than mere works of fiction. In this sense, then, I understand the concerns of those Pakistani readers who are sceptical of PWE, for the reason that instead of informing the world about the complex and rich realities of Pakistani lives, some of these writers end up offering rather more plausible stereotypes of Pakistani culture to an already hostile audience of global readers.

The question that Pakistani critics of PWE should be asking is not whether these works are authentic, for authenticity itself is socially constructed, but rather, to misquote Stanley Fish, 'what do these texts do?' (1980).[8] I hope this is also the question that PWE authors ask of themselves whenever they proffer their works to their global audiences. Only this complex way of looking at their own creativity would enable these writers to foresee the kinds of stereotypes that their works mobilise and then crystallise in the minds of their metropolitan readers.

To further elaborate my point, I will discuss the lead story, 'Leila in the Wilderness' by Nadeem Aslam, taking a two-pronged approach. First, I will discuss the conceptual inconsistencies within the story, which indicate that even the author fails to grasp certain subtleties of his own social culture, and in turn allow him to proffer certain unacknowledged stereotypes, stereotypes that metropolitan readers would immediately accept as 'truths' without having either the tools or the knowledge to dwell on the conceptual inconsistencies of the statements or utterances of several characters.[9] My point here is not to prove that the author has somehow not represented the truth, for truth itself is also contextual and socially and ideologically constructed, but that some of the assertions in the story are incongruous with the particular religious ideology assigned to the characters. Such inconsistencies, I suggest, would not have been possible within an Urdu story, as the reader would have immediately grasped them and pointed them out, but in a story written in English, proffered to a Western audience, the same inconsistencies add an additional layer of intrigue to the characters.

Secondly, I will read and discuss the story in terms of its reception within the metropolis and focus primarily on the kind of perceptions of Pakistan that the story instils or reinforces. By far, the setting of the story is the most perplexing aspect and also prone to making the story into an ideal exoticised and orientalised representation of Pakistan: since neither a specific place nor a specific time is indicated, the story places its characters, and by extension Pakistan, into a timeless and unchanging place where modernity has had no impact on day-to-day life. Of course, this view of the orient, and the rest of the Muslim world, is, *à la* Edward Said, an established trope in orientalist writing, but now that a so-called cultural insider is representing his own culture in the same vein, without any irony or playful parody, this view of Pakistan and its 'unchanging' culture comes across as authentic and valid. For the metropolitan reader, then, this story is likely to become unmoored from its spatial and temporal context and thus serve as an allegory of Pakistani culture in its entirety, whether or not such was the intention of the author.

Similarly, the simple plot includes an oppressive feudal lord married to a young woman who cannot produce male children and is thus treated brutally. Instead of offering an incisive critique of a specific locus or class of Pakistani culture, the story comes across as an allegory of the entire patriarchal culture of Pakistan, and that is how it is likely to be read by metropolitan readers. The conceptual inconsistencies also end up distorting or misinforming the reader about the nature of religious practices in Pakistan. For example, at one point, while talking about the 'miraculous mosque', the mother, Razia, suggests that Timur should 'find a way to get the Saudi Arabians involved', for they, according to her, are a 'blessed race' (Freeman 2010: 18) and thus could lend the kind of support that Timur needs to sustain the miraculous mosque. However, in the real-life cultural divide of Brelvi and Wahabi sects, a Brelvi would never suggest seeking the support of the Saudis, as the Brelvi believe in the intercession of saints and their miracles and the Saudis are opposed to any such worship of miracles or shrines. While this incongruent insertion within the text may seem pertinent and display how Pakistani people view the Saudis, it also ends up sanctifying an erroneous belief about the nature of Saudi involvement in Pakistan.

Similarly, at one point, while describing the people flocking to the miraculous mosque, we find the 'gentle mendicants as well as *jihadists* who fantasized about nothing but what they'd do to the American president if ever they got hold of him' (2010: 22). This, of course, is a stylistically convenient but absolutely misleading and ill-informed assertion, for *jihadi* groups are known for their hostility to this form of mystical Islam, and Sufi shrines often become their targets. So, scattering these 'gems' throughout the narrative might serve some aesthetic purpose, and they are flagged up by neither critics nor reviewers because the story is primarily proffered to and written for a Western audience, most of whom will not pick up on these subtle slippages and inconsistencies.

So, what we learn is that Timur had just suddenly 'picked' Leila to marry, just as she was fleeing her would-be rapists. And this brings me to an entirely other dimension of the problematic back story that the author creates about Leila and her mother's past.

In my opinion as a scholar working at a metropolitan university and engaged in teaching literary texts from the global periphery, there are several problems with the back story about Leila's life up to the moment she is randomly picked by Timur, all of them connected to the question of reception and perceptions of Pakistani culture among my metropolitan students and general readers of the story.

What we learn is that Leila's father has died in debt, and as a consequence: 'The [village] council of the wise and the powerful [...] decided that, to make up for the loss, the men of the moneylender's family could possess the debtor's widow one hundred times' (2010: 28). To be clear, what we are being told, in a normative, non-alarming and matter-of-fact way, is that the men from the moneylender's family have been granted the right to rape the widow – Leila's mother – one hundred times as payment of the debt owed by her husband. This rationale is offered nonchalantly in the most benign statement possible within the story. The tone does not offer this as an aberrant or abhorrent act, but rather an everyday occurrence within this generalised picture of rural Pakistan. What are we to make of this?

How would this passage come across to an unwary or ill-informed reader? In other words, what does this text do to the reader's perception of Pakistani culture? It offers, in one simple statement, a generalised Pakistan as the story has no specific location, a place where powerful men can sanction the mass rape of a woman without any legal or moral consequences, and the men so permitted would then openly descend on the woman to exact their 'due' share of her body. Here is how this act of potential gang rape is described:

> The seven boats that converged on her bore a total of thirty men, silhouetted in the fine grained vapour. Some of them leaped over the water like panthers even before the boats connected. She fought them, surrounded, numbed by shock but with her eyes screaming the outrage of her solitude. The only escape was upwards and that was what she had chosen, willing the wings into existence upon her body, the emptiness of mist closing behind her as she rose.
>
> (2010: 28–29)

Let us unpack this carefully. A woman's husband has just died in debt in an unknown, possibly rural, location in Pakistan. The village elders have given their verdict that the moneylenders can claim payment of their 'debt' through an act of collective rape against the widow. The widow, being sexually assaulted by thirty men, has no recourse to any worldly systems of justice or cultural norms and her only escape is to somehow 'magic' herself out of this world. The magic part of the story is quite understandable, as it is an acceptable trope in the specific genre of magical realism, but I find the realistic part of the text quite far-fetched: a whole village council ordering the rape of a widow. Have there been instances of such acts of collective rape in Pakistan recently? Yes, in very remote areas and always as a cultural transgression and an aberration, never necessarily as a norm. The case of Mukhtaran Mai is one example of such a brutal transgressive act (see e.g. Masood 2017). But within the story, this transgressive act of sexual violence is offered as an accepted and normalised practice, and thus to any unaware reader, Pakistan becomes a place where such things happen not as extraordinary acts of violence but as a normative practice of tribal justice. Furthermore, as the story develops, we learn that since the mother could not pay the debt and 'magically' escaped the verdict, the same men are given another option: 'The council of the wise and powerful decided the moneylenders must wait for Leila to grow up to be compensated – with the interest on the original debt accumulating till then' (2010: 29). Thus, we learn that since the mother escaped this raw justice magically, the daughter now must 'legally' become the gang rape victim-in-waiting. And this, to any reader interested in Pakistan, is supposed to be the everyday ultimate reality of the state of women's rights in Pakistan: it certainly becomes so within the logic of the story. Thus, it is while escaping her would-be rapists that Leila is 'seen by Timur' and, we are told, 'they were married within ten days' (2010: 29).

So, Leila's entire life, until we meet her at the beginning of the story, is based on choices that have already been made for her by powerful men in her culture, which is not far from the truth, but the brutality of the elders, as well as that of her husband and mother-in-law, also serves to sanctify one important stereotype of Pakistani patriarchal society generally believed in the West, and even though a Pakistani is writing the story, the story still serves the purpose of normalising Western views of Pakistani culture. Of course, the author has the right to represent what he or she deems appropriate and important, but Pakistani writers in English, if they care about politics of representation and reception, cannot hide behind the absolute right to represent; they must also bear in mind the cultural and political consequences of their acts of representation, especially since their works are proffered to metropolitan reading audiences.

So, within the cosmopolitan habitus, all these authorial choices make perfect sense: on the one hand, a writer has the right to represent all aspects of his or her culture and he or she must guard this freedom at all costs; on the other, though, the nationalistic habitus structures not only national expectations about representation but also anxieties about perceptions of the nation elsewhere in the world. To those who can read them from a nationalistic habitus, the stories come across as a sort of cultural violation, as they present to Western audiences what is already considered the stereotypical view of Pakistan. Thus, to such Pakistani readers, PWE becomes yet another instrument in the hands of the metropolitan culture and publishing industry to bash Pakistan, but now with the added advantage of using native voices to do so.

Similarly, what is done to Leila, under both religious and cultural registers, while giving one a convincing picture of her victimhood, also normalises certain other views of Pakistani culture. I am not suggesting that any critiques of the ills of the patriarchy are sacrosanct, but rather that by offering such brutal treatment of a female protagonist without contextualising it within a specific spatial and temporal setting, the representation takes on the aura of 'authentic' universality. The reader, therefore, will read it not just as an aberrant situation of violent and oppressive males against powerless women, but rather as an allegory of Pakistani culture where the man stands for all men and the woman stands for all women. Thus, there is no room in the story to even imagine a Pakistani life that is not brutal and in which women are not victimised by powerful men. The simple question one must ask is whether there is a possibility of kindness, love, and compassion within Pakistani culture? Such possibilities are never really explored, and since the story has no viable physical or temporal habitus, it becomes an all-encompassing representation of Pakistan; and thus, while the reader might marvel at the mastery of the writing style, the represented space, because of its lack of specificity, is likely to be generalised to the whole of Pakistan.

So, as a concluding thought, I would like to suggest that there is a need in Pakistan to develop the kinds of reading and writing practices where those within the nationalist habitus acknowledge the rights of those within the metropolitan habitus. Only this kind of nuanced understanding of the act of writing and representation would enable the reader to read PWE more sympathetically and further equip writers to write with a better understanding of their own responsibility as writers and of the consequences of their authorial works for general perceptions of Pakistan in the world.

Within the global arena of cultural representation there are no unmotivated texts or transparent representations; all acts of representation come with cultural and political baggage and are read and consumed within the larger context of socially produced knowledge about broader and specific cultures. Writers, of course, have the absolute right to write what they deem important and there is always a need for critique of the ills of the nation, a job that most PWE addresses quite well. But within this realm of cultural exchange, Pakistani writers of English must also bear in mind that the stories they tell are not just stories but also windows into their primary culture, and these windows cannot just be opened onto the very worst vistas of that primary culture, they must also provide a wider and deeper look at what is loveable and salutary about that culture.

Notes

1 This binaristic division of reception of PWE is completely arbitrary and should not be taken as a fixed and immutable position. As far as the national expectation is concerned, my views here are based in the public and private conversations that I have had with several Pakistani scholars and students of literature about the issues of representation of 'their' nation to a global audience.
2 I have argued in a previous article that both Pakistani writers and readers need to be aware of more nuanced modes of writing and reading in order to experience PWE in a fair and balanced way. For more details, please see Raja (2014).
3 Here I am rendering elements of the schematic diagram in simple paragraph form. For details of the entire diagram, please consult Bourdieu (1984).
4 This way of perceiving the real through ideology is quite similar to Althusser's explanation of ideology and 'transposition' of the real through ideology. I think the major difference here is that, for Bourdieu, this transposition is larger than individual acts of agency. Thus, a habitus is a structure but also a structuring structure which can, in my opinion, subsume individual acts of agency and somewhat overdetermine them.
5 *Granta* 112: *Pakistan*. <www.amazon.com/Granta-112-Pakistan-Magazine-Writing/dp/1905881215/ref=sr_1_fkmr0_1?ie=UTF8&qid=1498931061&sr=8-1-fkmr0&keywords=granta%3A+pakistan+issue> [1 July 2017].
6 Shakil's review, 'Pakistani writing (English) at its best'. 7 February 2012. www.amazon.com/gp/customer-reviews/R2LYAL4DT7RWYS/ref=cm_cr_dp_d_rvw_ttl?ie=UTF8&ASIN=1905881215 [4 July 2017].
7 Kobena Mercer discusses the question of the burden of representation with reference to the first ever Black Arts Festival organised in England. In his study, it becomes obvious that the diasporic population somehow expected the organisers to carry the burden of the entire African cultural tradition, and so people faulted them for not thoroughly representing Africa. In Mercer's view, this expectation is peculiar to those groups who have traditionally been on the margins of a dominant culture. For further details on the concept of the burden of representation, see Mercer (2016).
8 This is a slightly rephrased version of the very question that Stanley Fish poses in his most famous work, 'Interpreting the Variorum' (1980), about reader response criticism and the role of readers and interpretive communities in construing the meanings of a work.
9 In a 2013 survey conducted among Americans by the Pew Research Center, only about 10 per cent trusted Pakistan. See Wike (2013).

Bibliography

Ahmad, A. (1992) *In Theory*. London: Verso.
Althusser, L. (2001) *Lenin and Philosophy and Other Essays*. Trans. by Brewster, B. New York: Monthly Review Press.
Bourdieu, P. (1984) *Distinction: A Social Critique of the Judgement of Taste*. Trans. by Nice, R. Cambridge, MA: Harvard University Press.

Chotiner, I. (2010) 'Midnight's Other Children'. *New York Times* [online]. Available from <www.nytimes.com/2010/10/03/books/review/Chotiner-t.html?pagewanted=all> [6 June 2017].

Fish, S. (1980) 'Interpreting the Variorum'. In *Reader Response Criticism*. Ed. by Thompkins, J. Baltimore and London: Johns Hopkins University Press, 164–184.

Freeman, J. (ed.) (2010) *Granta: The Magazine of New Writing* 112. Special Issue: Pakistan.

Haffenden, J. (2000) 'Salman Rushdie'. In *Conversations with Salman Rushdie*. Ed. by Michael, R. Jackson: University Press of Mississippi, 30–56.

Macaulay, T. (2005) 'Minute on Indian Education'. In *Postcolonialisms: An Anthology of Cultural Theory and Criticism*. Ed. by Desai, G. and Nair, S. New Brunswick: Rutgers University Press, 121–131.

Masood, S. (2017) 'Pakistani Village Council Arrested after Ordering Teenage Girl's Rape'. *New York Times* [online]. Available from <www.nytimes.com/2017/07/27/world/asia/pakistan-girl-rape-council-arrest.html?rref=collection%2Ftimestopic%2FMai%2C%20Mukhtar&action=click&contentCollection=timestopics&region=stream&module=stream_unit&version=latest&contentPlacement=1&pgtype=collection> [30 November 2017].

Mercer, K. (1994) *Welcome to the Jungle: New Positions in Black Cultural Studies*. New York: Routledge.

Raja, M. (2014) 'The Pakistani English Novel and the Burden of Representation: Mohsin Hamid's *How to Get Filthy Rich in Rising Asia*'. *The Ravi* 150, 81–89.

Robbins, B. (1998) 'Comparative Cosmopolitanisms'. In *Cosmopolitics*. Ed. by Chea, P. and Robbins, B. Minneapolis: University of Minnesota Press. 246–264.

Sethi, M. (2010) 'Tales of Love and Gore'. *The Wall Street Journal* [online]. Available from <www.wsj.com/articles/SB10001424052748703860104575508901565361546> [30 November 2017].

Thiong'o, N. (1982) *Devil on the Cross*. New York: Penguin Books.

Thiong'o, N. (1986) *Decolonizing the Mind*. Oxford: James Curry.

Wike, R. (2013) 'Few Americans Trust Pakistan'. Pew Research [online]. Available from <www.pewresearch.org/fact-tank/2013/10/23/few-americans-trust-pakistan/> [30 November 2017].

30
DE/RECONSTRUCTING IDENTITIES
Critical approaches to contemporary Pakistani anglophone fiction

Faisal Nazir

Edward Said, in *The World the Text and the Critic*, remarks that 'the critic is responsible to a degree for articulating those voices dominated, displaced, or silenced by the textuality of texts' (1983: 53). Expounding on this in *Culture and Imperialism*, Said enjoins the critic to 'connect these different [artistic and political] realms, to show the involvements of culture with expanding empires, to make observations about art that preserve its unique endowments and at the same time map its affiliations, [...] and set the art in the global, earthly context' (Said 1994: 5). Thus, according to Said, the task of criticism is to deconstruct textual structures which privilege some voices while suppressing others, and to reconstruct the worldly affiliations of artistic works to highlight their political concerns. In opening this chapter with the words of Said, I treat critical approaches to contemporary post-9/11 Pakistani fiction as aligning with his view of literary criticism given in the quotes above. My argument is that critical works on contemporary Pakistani anglophone fiction focus on the theme of identity in fiction and discuss fictional works as engaging in the deconstruction of an exclusivist and hegemonic national identity and the reconstruction of this identity in a more inclusive national and/or global cosmopolitan frame. To conceptualise and discuss the deconstructive and reconstructive strategies used by Pakistani anglophone writers, the critics draw upon various strands of postcolonial theory, historicist, poststructuralist, and nationalist, and particularly the cosmopolitan strand dominant in theory today (see Brydon 2004; Spencer 2010; Mishra 2015). In this way, critical studies of Pakistani anglophone fiction engage with some general theoretical questions and debates in postcolonial theory, particularly those regarding cultural and political representation, the use of poststructuralist approaches in postcolonial theory, the cosmopolitan turn in postcolonial theory, and the Eurocentrism of postcolonial theory.

The chapter is divided into three sections. Section I contextualises criticism of Pakistani anglophone fiction within ongoing debates on questions of identity and representation in postcolonial theory; Section II discusses various extended critical studies of Pakistani anglophone fiction published since 2011 (the year in which *Journal of Postcolonial Writing* published a special edition on Pakistan), and highlights their distinctive approaches to contemporary Pakistani anglophone fiction; Section III reviews these critical approaches in light of general theoretical questions regarding identity and representation, and discusses how the critics engage with these questions in their studies of contemporary Pakistani anglophone fiction.

Pakistani, Muslim, human: Towards a humanistic cosmopolitanism

Critics who have analysed Pakistani anglophone fiction have largely followed Said's advice and example, treating these novels not simply as 'literary' texts which ask for a purely formalist approach, but as interventions in ongoing debates on identity, culture, and politics which, therefore, need to be studied politically as well as aesthetically. The critics have seen it as their task to bring out the political implications of fiction, particularly for contemporary discussions of gender issues, politico-religious questions, and cross-cultural interaction. More specifically, the Muslim identity of Pakistani writers has led many critics to place Pakistani anglophone fiction within the larger category of 'Muslim fiction/writing' (Chambers 2011; Ahmed, Morey, and Yaqin 2012). In this sense, Pakistani anglophone fiction is seen as a rich resource for debating issues of Muslim identity and culture, which have become prominent since the 9/11 terrorist attacks. This approach appears to be highly relevant, as the writers themselves have taken up the themes of religious and cultural identity in their fictional works and have acknowledged in their interviews and non-fiction writing their engagement with the burning political questions of the present times (Chambers 2011; Kanwal 2015; Clements 2016; Bilal 2016).

In the context of recent developments in postcolonial theory in which all monolithic identities, particularly national identities, are deconstructed and migrant, diasporic and cosmopolitan identities are celebrated, critical engagements with Pakistani anglophone fiction appear to follow a general pattern: identity deconstruction through an emphasis on diversity, and identity reconstruction through an inclusive national, religious, and/or cosmopolitan approach. Critical studies of Pakistani anglophone fiction seek to highlight how fiction deconstructs binary oppositions in which Pakistani identity is usually constructed in political and cultural discourses. The binary opposition identified and deconstructed in fiction and its criticism is generally between Pakistan and the West. The conflict of identity in Pakistani anglophone fiction is frequently presented and debated as one between an Eastern, Islamic identity and a Western, liberal/secular one. Literary critics often praise Pakistani writers for staging this conflict of identity in their works and for challenging monolithic constructions of it in historical, cultural, and political discourses emanating both from within Pakistan and abroad (Morey 2011; Cilano 2013; Clements 2016). Pakistani identity, as it is constructed in these historical, political, and journalistic discourses, is identified as overwhelmingly male, Muslim, and national (as opposed to gendered, ethnic, or class-based identities, as represented in literary/critical discourses) (Jalal 1995). In critical accounts, fictional works from Pakistan are often shown to deconstruct this unified and homogenous identity by foregrounding suppressed and neglected groups in Pakistan, such as religious and ethnic minorities, women and secular-minded people largely belonging to the upper or upper-middle classes. According to Mushtaq Bilal,

> Identity politics is another theme which runs across the works as well as the interviews of these [Pakistani] writers. Shah, Hanif, Tanweer, Khan and Sidhwa have often written about the lives of Pakistanis who are marginalized either because of their religious or political identities. In these works, one finds an attempt towards devising an alternative to the jingoistic and fundamentalist mainstream narrative of the Pakistani state and society. By writing about working-class Christians, indigenous peoples and Pakistani leftists, these writers explore a Pakistan that is unfamiliar to many a Pakistani.
>
> (2016: 18)

However, since most fictional works in English from Pakistan engage with the question of identity in a global, transnational context, as invoked or evoked within the texts, critics also identify the presence of a cosmopolitan outlook in them. While the Pakistani identity is shown to be deconstructed by fictional works, from a monolithic identity to a multiple one, recent critical works on Pakistani anglophone fiction describe writers as attempting to redefine the Pakistani identity in cosmopolitan terms by emphasising global allegiances and affinities (Cilano 2013; Kanwal 2015; Clements 2016). Aroosa Kanwal states:

> The novels [...] share a common focus on home and identity while historically contextualising domestic themes and issues in relation to a global setting. In terms of identity discourses, there is a gradual transition from national to transnational identity and from transnational to postnational identity.
>
> (2015: 13)

According to Ahmed Gamal, recent works of 'Anglo-Pakistani writers' like Kamila Shamsie and Mohsin Hamid demonstrate features of 'post-migratory literature', a concept he has borrowed from Elleke Boehmer's book *Colonial and Postcolonial Literature: Migrant Metaphors* (2005), in 'constructing transcultural contact zones grounded in reconcilable compatibilities' (Gamal 2013: 596). For Gamal, 'post-migratory literature can be described as that type of postcolonial literature that fundamentally problematises the condition of migrancy by deconstructing the binarism of home and the world and linking the global to the postcolonial' (2013: 598). While post-migratory literature is open to being characterised as 'fundamentally cosmopolitan', what differentiates post-migratory literature from earlier theorisations of the migrant experience is the 'manifest oppositional stance that might be unavailable in unconditional cosmopolitanism' (2013: 598).

Gamal's preference for the term 'post-migratory' over the more conventional 'cosmopolitan' to describe contemporary postcolonial literature identifies a sceptical attitude among literary and cultural critics towards cosmopolitanism. Described as elitist and superficial, cosmopolitanism has earned a bad name in certain critical circles (see Brennan 1997; Gikandi 2010). The critics discussed in Section II of this chapter reflect these concerns over the exclusiveness of cosmopolitan theory. They not only highlight the brutalities and violence presented by the transnational encounters in the novels they study (Cilano 2013; Clements 2016), they also call for a definition of transnationalism and cosmopolitanism in more inclusive humanist terms. That is why critics like Cilano use alternative terms to describe fictions that seek to transcend narrow approaches to identity, particularly national identity. In the introduction to her book *Contemporary Pakistani Fiction in English: Idea, Nation, State*, Cilano describes the book as 'advocating the end of national identities' (2013: 1). However, she clarifies at once that: 'This argument [...] doesn't lobby for cosmopolitanism or hyphenated identities' but, through a reading of Shamsie's *Burnt Shadows*, emphasises a '"human" identity that takes shape through the recognition of historical experience as an equalising force, suggesting along the way that historical narratives can bear meaning outside of national confines' (Cilano 2013: 1). In contemporary English fiction from Pakistan:

> Migrancy as a concept [...] takes on a different inflection from its more conventionalized usage over the past twenty years in postcolonial discourse. These novels' deployment of migrancy has none of the free-floating or archimedian privileges associated with cosmopolitanism or certain versions of transnationalism. This migrancy isn't about hybridity or translation, either. Instead, these fictions figure and, in some cases, ironize migrancy as a brutal encounter that is, because of its emphasis on a longer historical

perspective, neither a pre-determined, inevitable clash nor a necessarily optimistic exchange.

(Cilano 2013: 194)

As the above discussion shows, while the critics do reflect the 'cosmopolitan turn' in postcolonial theory in their studies of Pakistani anglophone fiction, they also *reflect on* this recent turn in the theory and thus remain alert to the charges of elitism levelled against the cosmopolitan approach, very often by critics working within postcolonial theory. In Section II, I will examine four extended critical studies of contemporary Pakistani anglophone fiction in light of this general cosmopolitan drift in postcolonial theory and its relation to critical readings of Pakistani anglophone fiction. As Section II will show in more detail, critical studies of Pakistani anglophone fiction approach the theme of identity in four distinct though interrelated ways: global/cosmopolitan (Morey 2011), national (Cilano 2013), religious (Chambers 2011; Kanwal 2015), and regional (Clements 2016).

Framing Pakistani Muslims: global, national, religious, and regional approaches

Published in 'Beyond Geography: Literature, Politics and Violence in Pakistan', a special issue of the *Journal of Postcolonial Writing* (May 2011), Peter Morey's article on Hamid's *The Reluctant Fundamentalist* (2007) treats the novel as a parody of the post-9/11 confessional statements made by some 'reformed' terrorists, particularly the one by Ed Hussain. Describing the novel as a 'hoax confession', Morey highlights in his article how Hamid has masterfully deconstructed in his novel such narratives that came out in the wake of the 9/11 attacks and the subsequent 'war on terror'. Morey's article

> argues that, in employing the hoax confessional and dramatic monologue forms, the novel not only effectively parodies the cultural certainties encouraged by those 'true confessions' of former radicals, in destabilizing the reader's identification through hyperbole, strategic exoticization, allegorical layering and unreliable narration, but also defamiliarizes our relation to literary projects of national identification, forcing us to be the kind of deterritorialized reader demanded by the emerging category of world literature.
>
> (2011: 136)

On the one hand, Morey considers Hamid's novel to be a postmodern, parodic narrative, deconstructing and decentring the narratives it parodies, which places the novel 'firmly in the camp of postcolonial literature that "writes back" to both imperial and neo-imperial centres' (2011: 142). On the other hand, Morey also considers the novel to be an example of 'world literature' demanding the readers to forego their national identity, to become 'deterritorialized' (2011: 142). Thus, the deconstructive-reconstructive pattern is visible in this article – nationalist and religious identities are challenged and deconstructed to bring about global, planetary identities defined not by 'conflicting interests and positions' but by an in-between space that makes the text 'a site of struggle for these different versions' (Morey 2011: 138). However, as Morey notes, there is nothing celebratory about the global encounters the novel presents except for the first half, in which the narrator seems pleased to consider himself solely as an employee of Underwood Samson. But, as Morey states, 'the story comes to be about the impossibility of maintaining this globalized, post-political identity position' after 9/11 and the 'resurgent nationalism' coming in its wake, forcing people to define which side they were on (2011: 143).

In contrast to Morey's approach, which sees identity through a postmodernist parodic framework, Claire Chambers brings a comparative approach to the discussion of identity and narrative in the English-language works of Pakistani authors, 'situating them alongside writing by authors of Muslim heritage in other parts of the world' (2011: 123). Justifying her use of religious instead of national identity to classify Pakistani writing, Chambers states that such developments, like the Rushdie Affair, the two Gulf Wars, 9/11, 7/7, and the 'war on terror', have made 'Muslim identity' a 'useful valence for understanding Pakistani texts' (2011: 124). She acknowledges that identity is a fluid thing and that religious/Muslim identity always intersects with other aspects of identity (such as national, regional, gender) and clarifies that, in her article, 'it is the reified figure, and cultural category, of the Muslim that is under analysis' (2011: 124).

The first difficulty to be faced in using this approach, as Chambers acknowledges, is that a significant majority of the writers regarded as having a Muslim identity are 'secular, agnostic, atheists, or [...] were not brought up as Muslims or come from other religious communities' (2011: 124). Chambers' solution to this problem, after Amin Malak (2004), is to claim that these writers, even when they do not appear to be practising Muslims, have access to what she calls 'Muslim civilizational heritage' (2011: 124). Chambers' comparative approach, as the above discussion shows, also focuses on the deconstruction of the narrowly defined Muslim identity in the novels she studies, and a reconstruction of this identity into a more inclusive and diverse framework of 'Muslim civilizational heritage'.

Moving away from this specifically religious construction of identity, Cilano opens *Contemporary Pakistani Fiction in English: Idea, Nation, State* with the 'spoiler' that the book 'concludes with an argument advocating the end of national identities' (2013: 1). However, Cilano's argument against national identities does not necessarily mean an argument for 'cosmopolitanism or hyphenated identities' (2013: 1). Instead, Cilano reads contemporary Pakistani anglophone fiction as offering 'myriads of possibilities [regarding Pakistani identity], creating a spectrum that runs from a reinforcement of dominant modes of belonging to a reinvention of the terms of collective attachments' (2013: 1). She describes her approach in the introductory section of the book:

> *Contemporary Pakistani Fiction in English* explores how literary texts imaginatively probe the past, convey the present, and project a future in terms that facilitate a sense of collective belonging. The three terms listed in my subtitle – idea, nation, and state – motivate these explorations, as they attract or repel the attachments necessary to formulate a collective identity or sense of belonging to Pakistan.
>
> (2013: 1)

Though her design includes approaches to Pakistani identity that 'reinforce the dominant modes of belonging', Cilano's focus is mainly on texts that 'offer an imaginative alternative to dominant forms of identification' (2013: 1). It is in this light that Cilano sees Shamsie's *Burnt Shadows* (2009) as exploring 'the possibility of a nationless belonging' for, in her view, the novel 'effectively dismisses the violence associated with national belonging' (2013: 222). Considering that the novel may be seen by the reader as advocating a conventional form of migrancy and cosmopolitanism, she clarifies that 'although Shamsie's novel posits as an ideal a deeply humanist subjectivity, it is produced through historical relations rather than outside them' (Cilano 2013: 222). Among the various migrant experiences which Cilano analyses in the novel, she considers the experience of Hiroko Tanaka to represent this 'humanist subjectivity' in an exemplary way. According to Cilano, through Hiroko's character and experience, 'the novel presents an alternative type of belonging that seeks to rise above the nation' (2013: 227). Hiroko comes to realise that national belonging has been the cause of some of the worst crimes against humanity, such as the nuclear bombing of Japan during the Second World War and in realising this, she learns that 'to be human is to be recognizable in terms outside of national identities' (2013: 228). Moreover, this human subjectivity is not based on merely personal or individual identity, rather it is constructed out of historical experience and ethical reflection: 'Rather than positing individuals as unproblematized incarnations of national identities […] Hiroko's idea of the "human" demands historical contextualization and accountability' (Cilano 2013: 228).

Kanwal also insists on the importance of historical contextualisation for a better understanding of the complexities of Pakistani Muslim identities in the post-9/11 era. As she states in the Introduction to *Rethinking Identities*, her 'purpose […] is to provide a historical depth to current negotiations of national, Muslim and diasporic identities, and to historicise contemporary encounters between the West and Muslims/Islam' (2015: 2). She is particularly interested in how Pakistani anglophone writers 'problematise identity crises'. For this she 'draw[s] upon numerous interlinking contexts to illuminate a spectrum of locations (local, regional and global; national, transnational and international) that are mutually informative in the construction of post-9/11 (Pakistani) Muslim identities' (2015: 2). In keeping with her aim to historicise the identity crisis depicted in Pakistani anglophone fiction, and thus to challenge the stereotypical ways in which this identity is represented in post-9/11 political and cultural discourses, Kanwal pays particular attention to post-9/11 fictional works by Pakistani writers that use a pre-9/11 setting for, in her view, such works present 'a compelling critique of reductive nationalisms among Pakistanis' (2015: 12). The second-generation Pakistani writers she studies represent 'a more inclusive view of life' than the one found in 'conservative nationalism and monolithic definitions of Islam', as these writers 'arguably seek to define or speak for a community' and 'dismantle negative stereotypes of Muslims and Islam in the West' (2015: 13). Kanwal thus identifies a work of identity deconstruction and reconstruction in the works of such major Pakistani writers as Hamid, Shamsie, Uzma Aslam Khan and Nadeem Aslam. These writers are seen as deconstructing the stereotypical identities of Pakistani Muslims constructed by political and cultural discourses. (Kanwal discusses these discourses in the Introduction with reference to the work of such scholars and critics as Morey and Yaqin, Mahmud Mamdani, Tariq Modood.) Along with carrying out this deconstruction of stereotypical identities, works of Pakistani anglophone fiction 'take 9/11 discourses in new directions whilst recognizing the need to negotiate identities in the wake of contexts beyond 9/11' and respond to this need 'by creating a third space beyond East/West cultural boundaries' (2015: 7). In Kanwal's view, this 'third space' is reflected in the emergence of the idea of a 'non-territorial global *ummah*' in place of nationally or regionally defined identities.

Though Clements' (2016) focus is, like Kanwal's, also on religious identities, she adopts a regional framework to present her thesis on the theme of identity in contemporary 'South Asian' English fiction. Her book 'explores the hypothesis' that the 'international novels' of Salman Rushdie, Hamid, Aslam, and Shamsie 'can be read [as] part of a post-9/11 attempt to revise modern "knowledge" of the Islamic world, using globally disseminated literature to reframe Muslims' potential to connect with others' (2016: 2). Describing their fiction as a contribution to 'world literature', Clements analyses how this fiction 'maps spheres of Islamic affiliation and affinity' and examines the 'inter-cultural and intra-cultural affiliations and affinities the characters pursue in these texts, asking what aesthetic, historical, political and spiritual identifications or commitments could influence such connective attempts' (2016: 2). Clements uses 'affiliations' and 'affinities' as key terms in constructing her argument, and defines them respectively as 'the more active and selective of the modes of Islamic connection' and 'a more natural, unplanned or even involuntary sense of being drawn to a particular community grouping, geographical area or imaginative realm' (2016: 3). While claiming that the writers she studies in her book represent a diversity of 'Muslim experiences of ordinary cosmopolitan contact, co-operation and conflict', Clements argues that the novelists do not attempt a 'simplistic revival' of exoticising 'commercial multicultural fiction' and also resist 'cosmopolitan perspectives' which may homogenise the diversity of experiences represented by the writers (2016: 10). Clements' concluding remarks on the fictional works of Aslam, Hamid, Rushdie, and Shamsie further highlight the deconstructive/reconstructive framework used in her study:

> Considered together, the fictions in English produced by South Asian authors of Muslim background provide a nuanced perspective on contemporary Islam, unsettling crude stereotypes and pessimistic East-West binaries, and writing rather of a world defined by ambiguities and even – occasionally – of hope.
>
> (2016: 158)

Rising into theory: identity, deconstruction, reconstruction

Though Muneeza Shamsie (2017) has discussed the long history of critical engagement with Pakistani anglophone literature in her recent book, it is only since the beginning of the twenty-first century that Pakistani anglophone writing, particularly fiction, has received extensive critical attention. The brief overview in Section II shows that identity deconstruction and reconstruction are the central concern of critics in their analyses of Pakistani anglophone fiction. In this section, I will discuss the significance of this particular reading of fiction in the context of the debates around the question of identity in contemporary literary and cultural theory. I will then pose some critical questions regarding Pakistani anglophone literature and the critical studies I have examined in this chapter and suggest how a more rigorous deconstructive reading of Pakistani anglophone fiction can contribute further to debating questions of identity and representation in critical studies.

Globalisation, transnationalism, and cosmopolitanism are some of the key terms in contemporary literary and cultural theory and various critics have described a 'transnational' and a 'cosmopolitan' turn in theory in recent years (Jay 2010). Postcolonial theory has likewise engaged with these issues and, according to Robert Spencer, 'postcolonialists are currently refining a variety of cosmopolitanism capable of reconciling seemingly contradictory objectives' (2010: 40). Postcolonial critics are constructing a 'distinctively postcolonial cosmopolitanism' which is 'conscious of the need to think and campaign at the local and national levels, whilst at the same time thinking and campaigning at the level of transnational institutions and arrangements' (Spencer 2010: 40). Critical studies of contemporary Pakistani anglophone fiction also demonstrate what Spencer calls a 'dialectical understanding of cosmopolitanism' (2010: 40) in their focus on the deconstruction and reconstruction of Pakistani Muslim identities in fiction. At local and national levels, critics appreciate writers' attempt to deconstruct the dominant discourses of identity which have marginalised some aspects of Pakistani identity while privileging others.

Thus, the deconstruction and reconstruction of Pakistani Muslim identity in contemporary Pakistani anglophone fiction are, according to the critics discussed above, a highly valuable intervention in the context of global political conditions since 9/11 and theoretical and critical developments in the twenty-first century. For their part, the critics' use of various frameworks to theorise this deconstruction and reconstruction of identity is a significant contribution to the ongoing debates around Pakistani Muslim identity in literary and cultural theory. However, in the concluding paragraphs of this chapter, I would like to raise some essential questions regarding critical reflections on identity and representation in Pakistani anglophone fiction with reference to Gayatari Spivak's 'Can the Subaltern Speak?' It is my opinion that engaging with these questions can be helpful in reassessing the representation of identity in contemporary Pakistani anglophone fiction.

In her celebrated and influential essay 'Can the Subaltern Speak?', Spivak identifies a conflation of the two different meanings of the word 'representation' in critical discourse and in critics' self-definition of their role as critics (1993). As Spivak describes, there is a political interpretation of the word 'represent' which, in political discourse, is taken to mean to stand in place of the people, to become their 'representative'. And then there is an aesthetic or literary/artistic interpretation of the word, an interpretation in terms of mimesis, an imitation or re-presentation of reality. This conflation can be observed in much postcolonial literary criticism, particularly that under discussion in this chapter. In the critical works discussed in Section II, Pakistani anglophone writers are supposed to 'represent' Pakistan in both these different senses: in the literary/artistic sense, to describe or portray Pakistani identity and culture, but in the political sense to speak for and to become the voice of that identity and culture. Thus, Pakistani anglophone writers become representatives of Pakistani identity because they re-present that identity. This conflation of the two senses of representation leads to some problematic assumptions about the 'insider' status of Pakistani anglophone writers and their deconstruction of Pakistani Muslim identity in their fiction.

Pakistani anglophone writers are supposed to provide an inside view of Pakistani (Muslim) identity and culture. There are some very strong reservations in postcolonial theory regarding this claim of deriving an 'inside view' of a writer's native culture from his or her works. These reservations are based on sociocultural as well as aesthetic grounds. From a sociocultural perspective, a gap is identified between the identities of the authors and their identification with their native culture. Most of the anglophone writers from the postcolonial world belong to an elite, educated, English-speaking minority and many do not even live in their country of origin. As Bilal notes,

> Importantly, the few contemporary writers who are generally considered 'Pakistani' in the Anglophone publishing world are not just 'Pakistani'. For example, Hamid, Shamsie, Mohammed Hanif, Nadeem Aslam and Aamer Hussein are all British nationals. Writers like Bapsi Sidhwa and Daniyal Mueenuddin are American nationals, and Musharraf Ali Farooqi holds a Canadian passport.
>
> (2016: 2)

Their contact and interaction with the people and the culture they write about, and therefore their experiential knowledge of these people and their culture, is very limited. In this sociocultural sense, then, their 'insider' status is considered highly suspect. As Spivak states, 'Certain varieties of the Indian elite are at best native informants for the first-world intellectuals interested in the voice of the Other' (1993: 79). Pakistani anglophone writers can also be seen to be approached as 'native informants' by theorists and critics located mostly in the West and in this way being burdened with a duty of representation which the writers may not be able, or even willing, to carry.

Moreover, while critics appreciate the deconstruction at work in the novels they study, they do not read the novels deconstructively. Deconstructive reading as practised by the major theorists of deconstruction, Jacques Derrida, J. Hillis Miller, Derek Attridge, and Spivak, attempts to open up fissures and gaps *in* the texts under study and not just those fissures and gaps identified *by* the texts. Such a reading often approaches a text from its margins and digs up elements that lie buried beneath its surface. In the criticism discussed in this chapter, the critics note the various deconstructive strategies used by writers – how writers destabilise and decentre nationalist and religious identity discourses – but, in doing so, restrict themselves to being observers and commentators on writers' deconstructive practices. Thus, critics do not engage in deconstructive reading of texts, they only highlight the deconstruction already at work in them. If the texts they have analysed were read deconstructively, they would no longer be seen as constructed upon a preconstituted essentialised otherness which can be called upon to deconstruct dominant discourses by a simple shift of focus from one kind of identity to another kind – from national to ethnic, cultural to class-based, religious to minority/sectarian, male to female. To read deconstructively would mean to see othering at work in each text specifically, to see how each creates and secures its own margins, without which it cannot constitute itself as a specific, bounded text. In 'Postcolonial Remains', Robert Young expresses his dissatisfaction with how postcolonial criticism has made use of the concept of the other and advises postcolonial critics to 'rethink' it in accordance with the philosophy of Emmanuel Levinas, Jean-Luc Nancy, and Giorgia Agamben (2012: 39). As Young describes, in the works of these philosophers, the other is not someone external to the self but rather a constitutive part of the self. While the critics discussed in this chapter do appreciate writers' efforts to emphasise religious, cultural, ethnic, class, and gender diversity in Pakistan, they do not address the essentialism that this strategy often involves.

When read with the understanding of otherness recommended by Young, it will be seen that in Pakistani anglophone fiction the desire to bring a specific marginal identity (e.g. ethnic, gender, class) to the centre of the narrative from the periphery is also the desire to remove an identity (e.g. national, religious, male) from the centre to the periphery. Deconstructing a narrative, through writing or reading, does not mean replacing one identity by another at the centre of the narrative, but rather displacing the centre itself. For the writer, it means acknowledging that s/he can only 'mix writings [or mix identities], to counter the ones with the others, in such a way as never to rest on any one of them' (Barthes 2003: 149). For the critic, it means never taking the identities represented in a text as unified and absolute, but always intertwined with their 'others', to whom they must hold fast for their own survival and recognition. Thus, the binary oppositions in which identities are constructed in Pakistani anglophone fiction – cosmopolitan/national, secular/religious, female/male – can be seen as simple inversions of identities constructed in nationalist, religious, and patriarchal discourses, still relying upon the concept of identity found within the very discourses that the fiction is lauded to challenge and deconstruct. A more rigorous deconstructive reading need not necessarily lead critics to adopt a politically uncommitted approach to identity but may, on the contrary, lead them to unravel more layers of identity than the binary oppositions in which the identities are generally constructed.

In light of this discussion, we can see that critical studies of Pakistani anglophone fiction approach this fiction at two levels, the local, national level and the global, cosmopolitan level. At the local level, critical studies highlight the deconstruction of dominant identity discourses in the works of Pakistani anglophone writers. They note how fictional works challenge the hegemonic nationalist and religious discourses of identity by giving prominence to neglected and marginalised elements within Pakistani society. At the global level, critics identify in contemporary Pakistani anglophone fiction an effort to reconstruct the Pakistani Muslim identity in global, cosmopolitan terms. However, critics also attempt to redefine the concept of cosmopolitanism through their studies of Pakistani anglophone fiction. In this way, critical studies of Pakistani anglophone fiction intervene at both the national and global levels, elaborating the literary strategies of Pakistani anglophone writers through a deconstructive/reconstructive framework and contributing to the ongoing theoretical and critical debates on the questions of culture and identity in today's world.

Bibliography

Ahmed, R., Morey, P., and Yaqin, A. (eds.) (2012) *Culture, Diaspora, and Modernity in Muslim Writing*. New York: Routledge.

Barthes, R. (2003) 'The Death of the Author'. In *Modern Criticism and Theory: A Reader*. Ed. by Lodge, D. and Wood, N. 2nd edn. Delhi: Pearson Education Limited., 146–150.

Bilal, M. (2016) *Writing Pakistan: Conversations on Identity, Nationhood and Fiction*. Noida, Uttar Pradesh: HarperCollins India.

Boehmer, E. (2005) *Colonial and Postcolonial Literature: Migrant Metaphors*. 2nd edn. New York: Oxford University Press.

Brennan, T. (1997) *At Home in the World: Cosmopolitanism Now*. Cambridge, MA: Harvard University Press.

Brydon, D. (2004) 'Postcolonialism Now: Autonomy, Cosmopolitanism, and Diaspora'. *University of Toronto Quarterly* 73(2), 691–706.

Chambers, C. (2011) 'A Comparative Approach to Pakistani Fiction in English'. *Journal of Postcolonial Writing* 47(2), 122–134.

Cilano, C. (2013) *Contemporary Pakistani Fiction in English: Idea, Nation, State*. New York: Routledge.

Clements, M. (2016) *Writing Islam from a South Asian Muslim Perspective: Rushdie, Hamid, Aslam, Shamsie*. Basingstoke: Palgrave MacMillan.

Gamal, A. (2013) 'The Global and the Postcolonial in Post-Migratory Literature'. *Journal of Postcolonial Writing* 49(5), 596–608.

Gikandi, S. (2010) 'Between Roots and Routes: Cosmopolitanism and the Claims of Locality'. In *Rerouting the Postcolonial: New Directions for the New Millennium*. Ed. by Wilson, J., Sandru, C. and Welsh, S.L. New York: Routledge. 22–35.

Jalal, A. (1995) 'Conjuring Pakistan: History as Official Imagining'. *International Journal of Middle East Studies* 27, 73–89.

Jay, P. (2010) *Global Matters: The Transnational Turn in Literary Studies*. New York: Cornell University Press.

Kanwal, A. (2015) *Rethinking Identities in Contemporary Pakistani Fiction: Beyond 9/11*. Basingstoke: Palgrave Macmillan.

Malak, A. (2004) *Muslim Narratives and the Discourse of English*. New York: State University of New York Press.

Mishra, V. (2015) 'Postcolonialism 2010–2014'. *The Journal of Commonwealth Literature*, 50(3), 369–390.

Morey, P. (2011) '"The Rules of the Game Have Changed": Mohsin Hamid's *The Reluctant Fundamentalist* and Post-9/11 Fiction'. *Journal of Postcolonial Writing* 47(2), 135–146.

Said, E.W. (1983) *The World the Text and the Critic*. Cambridge, MA: Harvard University Press.

Said, E.W. (1994) *Culture and Imperialism*. London: Vintage.

Shamsie, M. (2017) *Hybrid Tapestries: The Development of Pakistani Literature in English*. Karachi: Oxford University Press.

Spencer, R. (2010) 'Cosmopolitan Criticism'. In *Rerouting the Postcolonial: New Directions for the New Millennium*. Ed. by Wilson, J., Sandru, C., and Welsh, S.L. Basingstoke: Palgrave Macmillan, 36–47.

Spivak, G.C. (1993) 'Can the Subaltern Speak?'. In *Colonial Discourse and Postcolonial Theory: A Reader*. Ed. by Chrisman, L. and Williams, P. Harlow: Pearson Education, 66–111.

Young, R. (2012) 'Postcolonial Remains'. *New Literary History* 43, 19–42.

31
ON THE WINGS OF 'POESY'
Pakistani diaspora poets and the 'Pakistani idiom'

Waseem Anwar

Hybridising a theory: the 'Pakistani (English poetic) idiom'

Whenever we talk of Pakistani art, culture, or literature, political undertones of our *Pakistaniat* or 'Pakistaniness' begin to creep in with an ever-impulsive inquisitiveness, resulting in the query: So what does it mean to be a true or real Pakistani? This investigative rootedness is also applicable to our Pakistani writers writing in English, more so to diaspora writers, but most of all to Pakistani diaspora poets whose works challenge as well as redefine 'Pakistaniness' implied through locally coined poetic but conceptual phrases. One such popular phrase is the title of the essay 'Towards a Pakistani Idiom' by our foremost Pakistani poet of English, Taufiq Rafat. We know that Rafat's notion raised concerns not only for the early Pakistani anglophone poets during the 1960s but also for many others since then. In many ways, the objective of my review of Rafat's essay is to deconstruct and hybridise our critical-poetic journey in light of colonial-postcolonial homogeneity, its 'moving poetry', which emerges from what Joshua Auerbach and Helen Zisimatos refer to in their Editors' Note to *Vallum*'s special issue *Poets from Pakistan* as 'one of the world's most dangerous countries': Pakistan (2011: 5). And then, neither to forget the conjunctive direction informed by the prepositional and positional yet purposeful 'Towards' nor to ignore the pluralising implication of the single article 'a' before 'Pakistani Idiom', the intent is to offer Rafat's notion a futuristic epistemological metaphor with unique yet universal appeal. For our purposes, therefore, I suggest inserting 'English poetic' into Rafat's seminal idea and theorising it as 'Pakistani (English poetic) idiom', making it a more interlocutory debate about *Pakistaniat* throughout this essay. I call the debate interlocutory because, in this way, it supports my argument regarding the outsider-insider or insider-outsider predicament of *Pakistaniat* and helps me to conduct our conversation in a more corroborative manner. However, some degree of overview of the global and local confluence of Pakistani-English literary history by South Asian and Pakistani critics will help us to contextualise and analyse this much-exploited term, 'Pakistani idiom', particularly with regard to its ongoing literary and poetic relevance.

The diasporic-indigenous and global-local dialectic, or what we now popularly understand as the 'glocal', is not a new phenomenon within the history of Pakistani-English poetics alongside its South Asian creative sensibility. As a historical fact, this phenomenon is also assumed to be an inevitable legacy of the *farangi* 'British Raj' period that Masood A. Raja describes in his *Constructing Pakistan*, purported to be a 'politics of difference' (2010: xix). The outcome of such a politics of difference is what the postcolonial critic Homi K. Bhabha had already recounted as 'identities of difference' (qtd. in Mansoor 2012: 16), so much so that even when one expresses oneself in a foreign language it is transformed into a universally acceptable local vernacular.[1] Today, these and many similar issues have much to do with how we like to perceive our so-called nationalistic or even selectively patriotic Pakistani identity, our *Pakistaniat* or 'Pakistaniness'. The issue of pursuing one's 'national identity in opposition to a more hybrid and ambivalent mode of thinking the nation' is again well taken care of by Raja in his article 'Exclusionary Narratives, Ambivalence, and Humanistic Studies' (2012).

Extrapolating Bhabha's theorisation of hybridity, his 'Third space of enunciation' connects to the 'transformative role of humanities' which Gayatri Spivak sees as 'the ethico-political task of the humanities' (2008: 3); Raja looks forward to an Islamic articulation of 'responsible citizenship' in Pakistan. He argues that it is through such an enunciated and articulated space that Pakistanis will learn not to 'hate, and distrust our so-called reviled others', but rather to manage and 'mobilize a narrative of love and reconciliation' (2012: 14, 20). The vivacity of a hybrid and possibly responsible and reconciling citizenship offers inclusiveness to those who are listed as separate in the name of rigid and monolithic nationalistic ideologies or agendas but who continue to pursue their global, local, or diverse Pakistani identities. Pakistani diaspora poets can be placed in similar categories of exclusive-inclusive dynamics along with so many others either labelled as minorities or segregated on grounds of their gender, religion, caste, or creed, and even somewhat humbler socioeconomic backgrounds. Given the 'form[s] of reclamation' and reconciliation regarding a pure Pakistani identity, the literary stalwart Muneeza Shamsie explores the notion of *Pakistaniat* evenly in her Introduction to *And the World Changed* by scrutinising the situation and suggesting that we need to observe diversity as a priority beyond the constraints of any monolithic or monolingual agendas (2005: vxii).

Whatever geopolitical, ideological, sociocultural, or religious factors serve as a backdrop to our obvious divide over the term *Pakistaniat* and its ever-proliferating brands, a broad understanding of 'Pakistani (English poetic) idiom' offers scope to trace the hybridised evolution of our poetic as well as our patriotic selves, our Pakistani identity beyond the rigid precincts of so-called nationalism. That Pakistan, with all its ideological underpinnings of national identities and territorial boundaries, is the focal point of most of the writers who are trying to map out *Pakistaniat* according to their understanding, interpretation, and passion is beyond question, but the nationalistic discourse in this regard remains a challenging avenue for these writers who draw our attention to the need for more diverse inclusiveness (see Afzal-Khan and Anwar 2010). In this context, Pakistani writers working in English, inside or outside Pakistan, do contribute to expanding the horizon of the Pakistani literary and poetic canvas. Based on their instinctive articulation to stay rooted in the locality of their land, yet accentuate and express themselves globally, to be cosmopolitan in spirit, poets like Rafat and Alamgir Hashmi occupy more of a 'third' space when they point out an imaginable indispensability of the Pakistani in our *Pakistaniat*. One may read Hashmi's *Pakistani Literature* (1978) or *The Worlds of Muslim Imagination* (1986) and Rafat's 'Towards a Pakistani Idiom' as conjunctive for the idea of hybridity 'of enunciation' that Raja proposes through concepts developed by critics like Bhabha and Spivak. Within this context, the term 'Pakistani', and its literary *Pakistaniat*, remains critical but salubriously open-ended, signified by what Fawzia Afzal-Khan and Waseem Anwar see as necessary, as foundational and vital, though loosely interpreted (2010: 16).

Comparing 'the best in Third World literatures in English' in his *History of Pakistani Literature in English*, Tariq Rahman also adds to the interpretative openness of literary *Pakistaniat* (1991: 290). In the same context, Sara Suleri's *The Rhetoric of English India*, its 'idioms of empire and of nations' (1992: 10) and Raja's decoding of the *farangi* ambivalence over 'politics of difference', the duality about existing/not existing in English, corroborate and help us foreground the regional specifics of *Pakistaniat* explicated by critics like Cara Cilano. In her *National Identities in Pakistan* (2010) and *Contemporary Pakistani Fiction in English* (2013), Cilano questions the notion of identity in *Pakistaniat*, given Pakistan's second partition, the breakup of its east wing for the creation of Bangladesh (the first partition being in 1947). In a way, alongside the partitioned, exilic, and diasporic imaginings of nationhood, we can see Cilano's works broadening and deepening our understanding of the terms Pakistani, Pakistaniness, and *Pakistaniat*.[2] One is thus inclined to agree with Cilano, also in light of what Shamsie points out in *And the World Changed*, vis-à-vis constraints on Pakistani monolithic and monolingual nationalistic agendas. Overall, the writers, historians, literary critics, and researchers mentioned here explore the interconnected and interlocutory uniqueness of the Pakistani literary idiom and identity within the growing context of its linguistic, cultural, political, religious, and multiple other dispersed affinities that are expanding in our global and *trans*national times. The works of these literary historians and critics also underscore what Shamsie describes in her latest work as 'hybrid Influences', influences that are bound to become part of 'Pakistani-English literature and its development [...] an almost incredible journey [...] which clearly reveals a genre which has found its sense of self' (2017: 1, 614).

Let us then go back to my hybrid interlocution inserted in Rafat's notion of the 'Pakistani (English poetic) idiom'. Far ahead of his time, and focusing on Pakistani poetry in English and its fostering of a purer spirit in idiom as well as identity, Rafat furthered Pakistani literary sensibility, making the term 'Pakistani idiom' a multidimensional symbol of poetic *Pakistaniat*. We need to understand that Rafat's description of holding on to some sort of idiom does not exclude Pakistani anglophone literature produced by diaspora Pakistanis anywhere in the world. Rafat suggests the authenticity of 'voice' to be the foremost condition for a poet becoming Pakistani beyond any reductionist nationalistic structures of exclusivity, be they geographical or political. His inclusive viewpoint on a Pakistani voice is strongly validated and detailed in Rahman's *History*, where he mentions Rafat's comment on the pre- and post-Partition Pakistani writer Ahmed Ali. Rafat explicates Ali's poetry as clearly influenced by three diverse literary traditions, English Romantic, Chinese lyric, and Urdu *ghazal*, so that the poet writes: 'Across the vast unending sky / A pigeon plies its way [...] I stand and watch it fly, / Alone' (qtd. in Rahman 1991: 153).[3] One can easily detect Ali's poetic desire to be nationalistically cosmopolitan in terms of Pakistanis who are not geopolitically bound. Further clues to the nature of an authentic Pakistani voice, its idiom and identity, are offered by the well-recognised poets Maki Kureishi, who spoke in the 1950s of 'makeshift geography' (qtd. in Rahman 1991: 160), and Zulfikar Ghose, in the 1960s, for whom 'The blood of India ran out with [his] youth' (2010: 7). Whatever else we might think, the works of such diasporic or self-alienated and self-exiled poets address the angst of multiple identity consciousness that a Pakistani writer living globally may carry. Ghose is one such multiply placed transnationalist in whose works we find intersections between his South Asian, South American, Indian, Pakistani, or other enforced or opted (dis)placements/positionalities. We see in him a more multidimensional Pakistani, one who has a broader sense of *Pakistaniat*, though generated initially through violently partitioned selves amid diverse locales of his settlement in Bombay ('The sky behind the peaks is the last of Bombay' (2010: 4)), in Sialkot ('Grandfather, if [...] Sialkot collapses, / I shall have no Mecca to turn to' (2010: 12)), and in Brazil ('Thirty-six years later [...] I walk down the Aleia das Mangueiras, the tunnel / of dark shade [...]' (2010: 94)).[4]

Examining Pakistani *trans*national identity and its multiplicity, and given the complex questions raised by Suleri regarding the 1947 Partition and then by Cilano regarding the 1971 'partitioning', geographical to generational, Shamsie dares to trace in her *A Dragonfly*

(1998) – whose title is inspired by Ghose's poem 'A Dragonfly in the Sun' (2010: 47) – the apparently 'trans-geographical' but 'deplorable tendency' of Muslim philosophies working behind Pakistani anglophone writings. These so-called Muslim philosophies, she adds, undermine 'the "Pakistani" identity of Pakistani English writers' simply because of their physical or linguistic distance from their lands of origin (Shamsie 1998: xxiii).[5] Again, in her *Leaving Home* (2001), Shamsie reviews the question of exclusion with reference to Pakistani diaspora poets: 'in Pakistan, many questioned the "Pakistani" identity of Pakistani English writers who had migrated, or had Pakistani parents and lived elsewhere' (2001: xv). One can see that throughout her multidimensional yet focused probing Shamsie excruciatingly but confidently foregrounds the 'problem of identity [that] has been […] complicated by the fact that Pakistan is an ideological state' (2001: xv). The Islamic Republic of Pakistan therefore becomes prone to complexity regarding over-ideological deliberations and over-nationalistic or over-religious propensities, which apply increasingly to marginalised, silenced, and excluded populations or groups like the subculturally or sexually segregated or the regionally, religiously, and linguistically differentiated: women, gays and lesbians, ethnic groups, diaspora writers, and many more. Whether political and religious ideologies are the source of the mentality of exclusivity of marginalised literary groups in an Islamic republic and welfare state like Pakistan is a separate matter, but that these factors add to the complicated exclusive-inclusive dynamics of Pakistani, its unique 'Pakistaniness' or *Pakistaniat*, cannot be disregarded.[6]

Given the complex intersections regarding the controversial term 'Pakistani' in 'Pakistani idiom' and Pakistani identity, and talking further about the Pakistani anglophone literary and poetic tradition, one can once again consult Rafat's mature versification in his *Arrival of the Monsoon* (1985), and in his translation of Punjabi poetry that foregrounds a modern, cross-bordered, and more cosmopolitan civilisation of love, much missed today: 'Love is a country / with its own climate' (1985: 2). While reading Rafat's love parlance in his poems, one is reminded of colloquial-metaphysical suggestiveness: 'will [morning] break on an empty bed, or a face I do not know?' (2008: 15). Again, in the poem 'Flight to London', we notice this typical colloquial-nostalgic call about his own divided self: 'Back home, we sit on the lawn, and wait' (2008: 14). Reading Rafat, then, requires sensitivity as well as sensuousness. One needs to develop a response to his 'slam' of a door as well as to his 'silence' that becomes a sign of 'affirmation' (2008: 12), because Rafat's work and its locales echo an indigenous growing in sync with a subtle but strong foreign, alienated yet 'authentic', Pakistani 'voice', the voice that Rafat approves for a poet who can be 'glocally' Pakistani. Throughout his work, Rafat's poetic culture remains universal and liberal, because like his 'deciduous love', he wants 'To see fruit ripen / By the weather's connivance' and 'to become complete' (2008: 128). His Pakistani idiomatic experimentation connects to what Rahman affirms:

> Rafat's concern with a 'Pakistani idiom' is one expression of the conflict between tradition and modernity […] Taufiq Rafat felt that […] it was better to forge an idiom which could be distinctively indigenous while reflecting contemporary and universal themes.
>
> (2013: n.p.)

The continued nervous scepticism about the 'Pakistani idiom' and its sensibility, its exclusive-inclusive dynamic that also caters to the experiences of diaspora writers writing in English, their anguish over tracing roots in their imaginary homelands, Pakistani diaspora poets offer a more multifaceted perception that keeps reifying the question of Pakistani identity as a core value for the promotion of *Pakistaniat*. With regard to *Pakistaniat* in the 'Pakistani idiom' and its diasporic-indigenous and global-local or 'glocal' growth, in his 2001 essay 'Some Recent English-Language Poetry from Pakistan', Carlo Coppola refers to seven different volumes of Pakistani anglophone poetry produced intermittently up to the golden anniversary of the country in 1997. Coppola argues that this Pakistani poetic journey presents 'a veritable embarrassment of riches' to assure 'attention [to] and appreciation' of Pakistani poets writing consciously in English (2001: 220).[7] Amid all the various phases of the ongoing Pakistani critical and poetic journey and its re/search for a 'Pakistani idiom', I analyse in the second part of this essay contemporary diaspora voices, like Waqas A. Khwaja, Moniza Alvi, Shadaab Zeest Hashmi, Zohra Zoberi, Afzal-Khan, and John Siddique, and try to trace how, one way or another, and despite all sorts of displacements, their connections to their land of origin help us review the notion of *Pakistaniat*. Although Khwaja detects an 'identity crisis' among such voices, Pakistani diaspora poetry in English today offers an element of ever-growing fluid expansion. In many ways, it foregrounds a presence that I am trying to grasp here as a fundamental part of the 'real' or true 'Pakistani (English poetic) idiom'.

Pakistani contemporary poet Ilona Yusuf's essay 'A Lively Progression: Mapping Pakistani Poetry' offers a critical-historical survey of how emerging local and contemporary diaspora poets experiment with the 'playing field of modernist and post-modernist form' to refashion 'the idea of identity' that is reliant on spatiotemporal frames beyond borders (2012: 88, 92).[8] Yusuf's poetical-political contemporaneousness in 'A Lively Progression' is concomitant with Rafat's acknowledged initiation of the 1950s in 'Towards a Pakistani Idiom', which inspired the incredible journey 'towards a more universal [and hybrid] metaphor' (Yusuf 2012: 88) and which poets and critics like Hashmi, Ghose, Suleri, Rahman, Cilano, Shamsie, Khwaja, and others investigated later and found it to be thematically 'trans-geographical'. Within the postmodernist-postcolonial myriad connotations of the prefix *trans*, as it is now all the more applicable to a historically stipulated 'Pakistani (English poetic) idiom', our choices amid its varieties of *trans*lation, *trans*literation, *trans*creation, *trans*ition, *trans*formation, or other *trans*piring forms help us synchronise the fluid diversity of Pakistani identity. Given the composite and multifarious poetics of a *trans*-Pakistani identity, one such example to refer to is Iftikhar Arif and Khwaja's *Modern Poetry of Pakistan* (2010), a complementary volume to Fakhar Zaman's *Contemporary American Poetry* (2009).

Our poetic *trans*cendence over the powerful 'wings of poesy' as represented in *Modern Poetry* makes us realise the importance of Pakistani regional rhythmical patterns that may grow and become universal. The anthology offers what Arif describes in the Preface as 'A remarkable range of poetic sentiments' (Arif and Khwaja 2010: xviii). Translations, retranslations, and transcreations in *Modern Poetry* render the Pakistani national creativity into an international co-creation, dispelling local identities as glocal fidelities beyond any imposed geopolitical rigidities. Through its cross-pollinating sentimental journey of regional works transformed into a universal tradition of transcendence of borders of nationalities, the anthology unveils multiple propositions of popular Pakistani poetics: *nazm* (controlled verse), *azad nazm* (free verse), *ghazal* (rhyming couplet), *qaafiyaa* (refraining pattern), *rubai* (Persian quatrain), *thumri* (a dance verse), *qawwali* (popular devotional verse), *sufiana kalam* (softer devotional verse), *marsiya* (martyrdom elegy), *masnavi* (epical spiritual verse), *doha* (regional couplet), *qasida* (benefactor's praise), and so on and so forth. Some of these local and regional forms, experimented with by Pakistani diaspora poets like Khwaja, Zeest Hashmi, or Afzal-Khan, who initiate the merging and mythologising of the *sufiana kalam*, *qasida*, and *ghazal* styles into their English poetic expression, open up avenues for a broad-based and sophisticated blend of multidimensionality. Do such experiments help to reduce bias against local subcultural Pakistani poetic sentiments? Does then the inclusion of local cultural/subcultural expressions and the use of bi-, tri-, trans-lingual, or transcreative discourses make the works of Pakistani diaspora writers effective 'with' as well as 'without' English? (Anwar 2014: n.p.). Many such queries are unanswered, and need to be researched, but whether the poetic ventures in *Modern Poetry* add to the polymorphous multi-dimensionality of the 'Pakistani (English poetic) idiom' and allow us to envisage how contemporary Pakistani diaspora poets urge a more hybrid yet responsible response and what Rafat, Kureshi, Ghose, Rahman, or Raja talk about as inclusive (global/glocal) and reconciling citizenship. Our critique of Pakistani anglophone poetics thus accounts for *trans*national 'glocal' poetics of diasporic writings that imagine new horizons yearning for a more homely and hybrid homeland/motherland. While many of the Pakistani diaspora poets do so, Khwaja, Alvi, Zeest Hashmi, Zoberi, Afzal-Khan, and Siddique definitely add to the kaleidoscopic multiplicity of the 'Pakistani idiom' with its growing literary precincts. Taken as a journey in continuity of 'Towards a Pakistani Idiom', their works trace the dialectics of Pakistani anglophone poetics in multiple ways, for these diverse rhymesters do theorise the dynamics of inclusiveness that I am claiming to engage for our 'Pakistani (English poetic) idiom'.

Transforming identities: some Pakistani diaspora poets

In his *No One Waits for the Train* (2007), Khwaja offers a contemplative record of multiple displacements that Amritjit Singh describes as a 'contentious legacy' and 'soulful meditation on the 1947 partition of British India'.[9] In many ways, the universal intensity of Khwaja's poems in *No One* goes beyond the original Partition, suggesting many other partitionings, displacements, and disconnects that have occurred in post-independence Pakistan. With his latest collection, *Hold Your Breath* (2017), and its 'tangible illusion', its poetic discursiveness about identity, and its 'cracking of opaqueness' (2017: 27), Khwaja's verse now spans over three decades. The range of Khwaja's sketching and symbolising between *No One* and *Hold* characterises the recurrent theme of transformed identities. Given Khwaja's own South Asian/Pakistani background, and more so his filial/familial interests in the language of his ever-expressive origination and its musicality, the *'piya torey nain'* (2017: 32–33) that takes after the classical *raga* adored by his musician uncle Khwaja Khurshid Anwar, his destinations of difference and dispersal help him compose verses that operate through fading lands of acquired belonging along with imaginable lands of assumed settlement. Call it 'diaspora' for convenience, it remains steadfast to evolve inertia in his works in terms of mobility, migration, immigration, exile, refuge, escape, nostalgia, yearning and what not! Khwaja's *Hold Your Breath* thus foregrounds the interlaced metaphoric meanderings that haunt one's glocalised sensibility, so much so that the origin and its unprecedented transformation assume an inertiatic occurrence. Overall, Khwaja's Pakistani creative impulse recreates a fair homeland for dispersed humans by playing with language, luggage, and all that such metaphors of flux may contain.

With dispersal and partitioning as a continuous trailing backdrop, the marriage and remarriage of division through difference becomes an important contact point for a 'real' as well as an 'imagined homeland' in Alvi's poems. In her work, we sense growing affinities among multiracial/multi-ethnic Pakistani groups so that identity for Alvi merges the lyrical with the epic; a fantasy that she describes as 'strange seeming' and which becomes the essence of her poetic experience within extensive imaginative possibilities for engaging feeling.[10] Alvi is conscious and confident about displacements and, therefore, asserts a comfortable position. For example, in 'I Would Like to be a Dot in a Painting by Miro' in *The Country at My Shoulder*, she contends: 'But it's fine where I am. [...] The fact that I am not a perfect circle / makes me more interesting in this world' (1993: 15).[11] Perhaps a better observer of who is or is not to be a Pakistani, and with a fascinating mobility to explore the world beyond limits of nationality by indulging in many forms of migration, Alvi declares her abode to be 'The Double City', riveting in replicas: 'I live in one city, but then it becomes another' (1996: 4). Pierced, broken, or damaged, in *Europa* (2008), Alvi finally succeeds in sailing through waters, blowing winds, and bordered lands of histories/(her) stories regarding divisions, partitions, exiles, and migrations from home or a homeland, all that she left behind long ago.

Land to motherland to home and finally to a real or imaginary homeland, the cosmopolitan spirit of Pakistani diaspora poets ventures a broadening of the 'Pakistani (English poetic) idiom' for a *trans*national poetics. Poets like Zeest Hashmi, Zoberi, Afzal-Khan, and Siddique address the issue of such convergence through their diverse experiences. Zeest Hashmi's *Baker of Tarifa* (2010) re-echoes the collectively conscious 'Cordobian' sensibility of pan-Muslim affinities through the work of local poets like Allama Mohammad Iqbal's 'The Mosque of Cordoba' and Athar Tahir's 'Andalusian Qasida'. In her venture to trace her 'Muslim Pakistaniat', Zeest Hashmi offers a sensual contemplation of a South Asian/Pakistani traveller/settler who flourishes in the lovely *ghazal*-like lyricism of luminous revelation. Zeest Hashmi's *Kohl and Chalk* (2013), textured with bilingual and multilingual dreams, and described by the poet herself in her dedication as a '*MIRROR BETWEEN BORDERS* [...] *TO SEE THE MOON LUCID*', suggests a powdery mix of cavernous grey, bracketing blacks and whites. Overall, her Eastern-Western poems in *Baker of Tarifa* and *Kohl and Chalk* fantasise the retrieval of a bygone grandeur in terms of a much-yearned-for South Asian/Pakistani identity that reciprocates with an equally desired, yet lost, Muslimhood in spaces like Spain, Turkey, or Pakistan.

As a stream of consciousness comparative to Zeest Hashmi's world of lost (Muslim) glories, Zoberi's *True Colours* is the offspring of the inner mind's universe of someone who holds their heart in their hand to make their spiritual love journey 'the greatest pilgrimage' (2012: 5). Zoberi's poetry draws on the 'Canvas of the Heart' (2012: 12) and its 'True Colours' (2012: 13) and the 'emotional landscape' of an immigrant woman blowing against the wind, to capture the true colours of 'smiling tulips' and wishful longings that finally 'embrace' (2012: 13). Self-identified as 'a Canadian-Pakistani, or a Pakistani-Canadian' in her aptly titled poem 'Hyphenated Canadian' (2012: 84), Zoberi, through her poetic flights, tries to connect back to *kamees shalwar* in her poem 'Against the Wind', 'Kalashnikov guns' in 'Afghanistan Speaks', the 'Aromas of Iram' and '*victims of the Iraq War*' in 'Car Wash Epiphany' (2012: 11, 22, 26, 33). The range of images, metaphors, similes, and symbols in Zoberi's poems address the psychology of divide through breast cancers and platonic loves (2012: 36–37). In most of her poems, Zoberi seems to be dispersed by the divinity of her diasporic being as well as by her 'psycho-neuro-endocrinologi[cal]' wisdom (2012: 74). She gathers dewdrops of (dis)connection and (un)concern to enhance a fragrance of difference that helps us unfold her glittering gift of a travelling Pakistani human insight.

With its diversity as a design for her diasporic discourse, Afzal-Khan's internationally performed and 'hip-hop influenced free verse' offers another blunt style (Afzal-Khan and Anwar 2010: 20). On the one hand, her 'Birthing Pain' reminds her of '[...] the pain / of birthing you / My poem' (2017: 89); on the other, in 'M/Other', she struggles with 'The clink-clanging of knives and forks / [...] Mindful of kitchen' and the 'madness of mothering / the Other', 'tall other' to 'embrace woman' (2017: 91–92). As a consistent though jazzy border-crosser, geographically as well as culturally and spiritually, and during her '*(Crossing into France Bastille Day, 2007)*' to compose her poem '*Flaming – Go*', Afzal-Khan notices how a 'Long neck / [...] Sinuous S / [may] Ease / her up', while in her '*Lai li la ah*', '*(En route from Lahore to New York…2010)*', the 'Arabic verse licks / [her] ears splitting / The East West / Binary [...] / Patterns [she] cannot Foretell [but are] Dedicated to some / [...] Herstory' (2017: 94–95). In general and overall, Afzal-Khan's poetic narratives, her engendered engravings in the contemporary environment, are a search for a moment of '*Looking for a Real Freak*' and '*courage to see*' (2017: 96–98) and, thus, to have 'Tea with / sex', 'Fashion / Image', 'Dress / Drugs', 'Desires […] Disrobes […] Dis / Ease' and 'Love's Foreplay' during the 'Journey' of 'Life's / Broken / Beast' (2017: 94–95). Her cross-continental journeys are like remembering the creative moments of birthing freak poems. She blends her comic-ironic and bathetically funky tone in an ingeniously experimental and adventurous nature, so that when it comes to connecting with identity, her multi-stringed poetics explores the unwrapped forbidden avenues of the sceptical Pakistani self alongside its much-debated outsider-insider dichotomy of the dispersed.

That the Pakistani diaspora poets writing in English must stay experimental, adventurous, 'bold', 'brave', and 'rebellious', yet 'pure' and 'authentic', is perhaps best illustrated through the works of Siddique – who almost, in Zulfikar Ghose and Adrian A. Husain fashion, wins laurels across borders for his love for humanity – and its sweetly savoured sensuality for all that is really forbidden. Living ahead of his time to play with the genre, Siddique's 'Six Snapshots of Partition', a prosaic-poetic narrative, describes partition as a 'thin wall made of simple materials' (2011b: 40). That the 1947 Indo-Pak Partition bloodshed could never bear purity heightens the belonging-alienating paradox in his works to 'undo' what Suleri had implied as the continued 'once-and-future' (Cilano 2009: 9) partitioning. In many ways, Siddique's latest, *Full Blood* (2011a), resonates with his *The Prize* (2005), but with differences in space, time, and distance from loved, missed, and dead ones, for its bloody search for the passionate love of the lost. In the confusion of loss and gain, 'We stand & fall in love' to kill a bird, the war-peacock and share 'bread and feast for Eid' (2005: 10). Fluttering with flowers, flames, and ever-blowing kisses, Siddique yearns for oneness in stories never told, stories of the 'Punjabi night sky' or 'the future produced by your fall' (2005: 18). In the UK, Siddique's story goes round 'The Danger and Result of Days Spent with a Narrowing Mind, Repetition, Wage Slavery and Conservatism', 'Isolated Incidents', 'Strawberries' (2005: 45, 42, 52), or the angelus he experiences. His poems in *Full Blood* and *The Prize* come forth as 'The bombs I set [to] / bloom in blood shades, / [giving] pleasure in garden' (2005: 31). Whistling amid the un-focusable darkness, Siddique furthers his themes and writes about what is mostly unspeakable, be it 'A Place of Silence', a 'Sky Burial', some 'Circumnavigations', or 'My penis and my lower belly' (2011a: 109, 107, 68–74, 56). *Full Blood* re-sounds the fulfilment of a dream dreamt in ancient times, when butterflies became 'Full Blood' to feel and live the 'Tree of Life' (2011a: 82, 75). Siddique's poems offer an 'authentic' search for the oblivious South Asian-non-South Asian and Pakistani-non-Pakistani sceptical selves drowned in the darkness of a human tropical forest filled with cutthroats, cruelties, trees, tangles, muddles, mazes. Whatever else, Siddique's brave poetic expedition and those of other diaspora poets discussed here do enable us to resist the monolithic and rigid descriptions of *Pakistaniat*. Critical discourse in their creative ventures and their 'English poetic' help us to foreground the ambivalently portrayed dialectic of our sceptical selves contained in the much clichéd phrase 'Pakistani idiom'.

Wrapping it up: so where are we now?

This short essay could not tell the tale of all the great Pakistani diaspora poets writing in English. Many old and new voices could not even be mentioned. Justice could not be done to the extensive work of the stalwarts discussed here. Close to wrapping up with reiterations, because one is also bound to be asked, On the wings of Pakistani 'poesy', where are we now?, the question of what we make of our Pakistani voices and silences, our imaginative and borderless horizons, our existing non-existences and our freer-floating homelands, motherlands, and love-lands, this essay basically underscores the outsider-insider or insider-outsider dilemma regarding our complex *Pakistaniat*. Pakistani diaspora poets, critics, and theorists have every right to abstain from the various brands of available *Pakistaniat*, including mine, while the possibilities for their 'periodizing and philosophizing' (Schwartz and Ray 2000: 5) the Pakistani literary tradition definitely add to what Paul Brians has described as: 'a colorful kaleidoscope [...] reflecting myriad [South Asian/Pakistani] realities' (2003: 6). Thus, our reading and criticism of contemporary Pakistani anglophone diaspora poets, as Ghose asserts in his *Beckett's Company*, gets 'absorbed by the reader as an experience' (2009: ix). As critical readers and citizens responsible for and reconciling with our 'Pakistani (English poetic) idiom', are we ready to accept the challenge to theorise the growing global-local interpretative viabilities of *Pakistaniat* for the future? I believe we are.

Acknowledgements: Special thanks to senior poet Athar Tahir, for his initial encouragement, and to Abdul Hameed, (former) Chairman of the Pakistan Academy of Letters (PAL), for providing relevant resources. I am grateful to the poets John Siddique and Fawzia Afzal-Khan for providing me electronically with their copyrighted materials. Thanks to Shadaab Zeest Hashmi and Zohra Zoberi for presenting their collections. I am also grateful for the access to the work of Pakistani diaspora poets offered by publication, anthologised or separately, in special issues of *South Asian Review*, *Journal of Postcolonial Writing*, *Vallum*, volumes of the Islamabad-based *Pakistani Literature* at PAL, and the Islamabad-based *Solidarity International* from PPA Publications. Thanks to Hina Saeed for posting me copies of Moniza Alvi's texts that were not available in Pakistan and to Nosheen Yousaf for helping format the chapter. This research would not have been possible without the supportive aura of many of my fellow scholar-friends at the South Asian Literary Association, including Dr Kamal D. Verma, Dr Pardhyumna S. Chauhan, and Dr Amritjit Singh.

Notes

1 Mansoor quotes Bhabha's call to go beyond a 'binary logic' (2012: 16). For Bhabha's notion of 'identities of difference', see his *The Location of Culture* (1994) and *Nation and Narration* (1990).
2 In her essay '"Freeing the Outlook of Man from its Geographical Limitations"', Cilano furthers Suleri's call for balance within Pakistan by reorienting and stabilising the 'disequilibrium' created by 'once-and-future partitions'. Cilano agrees with Suleri that post-Partition Pakistan loses its sense of land and the idea of national identity by hinging too much upon Islam and Urdu and, resultantly, constructing a monolingual Pakistani literary tradition (2009: 9).
3 On the vastness of Ali's literary profile, see also Muneeza Shamsie's biographical note (2011).
4 These references are taken from Ghose's poems 'Across India: February 1952', 'The Attack on Sialkot', and 'Returning to the Botanical Garden in Rio de Janeiro' (2010: 4–5, 11–12, 93–95). Ghose's reference to 'Plaza Pakistan' in Buenos Aires in the essay 'Brazilian Beaches, Buenos Aires and Plaza Pakistan', in *Beckett's Company*, reiterates similar ideas about how Pakistani idiom and identity and their diverse shades may get transformed amid the current global, transcultural, and transnational multiplicities: 'In Buenos Aires I remarked that while it was common for South American cities to have streets and places named after European capitals [London Palace Hotel in Montevideo ...] I was being shown the beautiful Palermo park in Buenos Aires with its associations of the Bois de Boulogne. We were driving [...] My host suddenly stopped the car and pointed to a sign that marked a clearing in front of a wooded area. The sign read: Plaza Pakistan' (Ghose 2009: 30).
5 In the article 'Islamophobia' (2013), Claire Chambers also observes that the Muslim identity has proven an increasingly useful valence for understanding Pakistani texts since a series of pivotal events between 1989 and 2005 or even after, including the Rushdie Affair, the two Gulf Wars, 9/11, 7/7, and the 'war on terror'.
6 Other critics adding dimensions to the notion about South Asian *Pakistaniat* are Chambers and Herbert (2014), Waterman (2015), Kanwal (2015), Clements (2016).

7 Coppola discusses the expanding value of Pakistani poetry in English towards world literature in English, the evolution of 'postindependence milieux' based on multiple individual *Voices* (2001: 7–9). In the same collection, Huma Ibrahim's pedagogically contextualised study of 'otherized texts', 'Transnational Migrations and the Debate of English Writing in/of Pakistan' refers to 'growing [Pakistani literary] structures of cultural cross-pollination' (2001: 35). Moving on and with some shift in emphasis, the poet-critic Waqas Khwaja's Introduction to the 2009 special issue of the *Journal of Commonwealth and Postcolonial Studies* on Pakistani literature accounts for 'sustained attempts at theorizing the heteroglossic and heteroethnic diversity of literary works of the country [Pakistan]' that have been 'conspicuously absent', resulting in an 'acute crisis of identity' (2009: 3). And then, in the same context, Afzal-Khan and Anwar highlight the theoretical-critical value of emerging Pakistani creative writing in English and offer yet another scholarly stance vis-à-vis the scope of the Pakistani literary tradition in the 2010 special issue of the *South Asian Review*. While the poetry section of this issue addresses concerns like: 'what then makes the literature Pakistani? […] What is a Pakistani [poetic] sensibility?' (2010: 17), the authors argue over the question of Pakistani and Pakistani diasporic writers exhibiting 'Pakistani skeptical selfhood' (2010: 23–28).

8 Yusuf discerns that Pakistani poets do so 'by aspiring to the universal rather than remaining confined to one place […] and time', thus imagining 'how we transcend them' (2012: 92).

9 Singh's endorsement blurb on the flap of *No One* states that Khwaja's poetry 'captures in image, narrative voice, and personal memory the terrible beauty of an innocence now lost'.

10 For details, see Encyclopedia.com (2018), where Alvi explains how the convergence of East and West is crucial for her: 'I am attracted to the strange seeming and to fantasy and find there some essence of experience'.

11 References to Alvi's poems in this chapter are from *The Country at my Shoulder* (1993), *A Bowl of Warm Air* (1996), and *Europa* (2008). However, just for information *The Split World: Poems 1990–2005* (2008) anthologises all of Alvi's previous works.

Bibliography

Afzal-Khan, F. (2017) 'Birthing Pain', 'Flaming – Go', 'La il la ah', 'Looking for a Real Freak'. In *Women: Poetry: Migration: An Anthology*. Ed. by J ortiz-Nakagawa, J. New York: Theenk Books, 89–98.

Afzal-Khan, F. and Anwar, W. (eds.) (2010) *South Asian Review*. Special Issue: *Tracing the Tradition: Embracing the Emerging* 31(3), 16–18.

Alvi, M. (1993) *The Country at My Shoulder*. Oxford: Oxford University Press.

Alvi, M. (1996) *A Bowl of Warm Air*. Oxford: Oxford University Press.

Alvi, M. (2008) *Europa*. Hexham: Bloodaxe Books.

Alvi, M. (2008) *The Split World: Poems 1990–2005*. Hexham: Bloodaxe Books.

Anwar, W. (2014) 'Transcreating the Cultural/Sub-Cultural [De]Polarization: Pakistani English Creative Writers Writing "Without" English'. Paper presented at MLA 2014 Session 795: 'South Asian Literatures – Without English' Division on Comparative Studies in 20th-Century Literature. available from <http://mla14.org/program/su> [18 July 2016].

Arif, I. and Khwaja, W. (2010) *Modern Poetry of Pakistan*. Champaign and London: Dalkey Archive Press.

Athar, K. and Siddiqui, K.K. (eds.) (2011) *Solidarity International*. Islamabad: PPA Publications.

Auerbach, J. and Zisimatos, H. (eds.) (2011) *Vallum New International Poetics* 9(1). Special Issue: *Poets from Pakistan*.

Bhabha, H.K. (1994) *The Location of Culture*. London: Routledge.

Bhabha, H.K. (ed.) (1990) *Nation and Narration*. London: Routledge.

Brians, P. (ed.) (2003) *Modern South Asian Literature in English*. London: Greenwood.

Chambers, C. (2011) 'A Comparative Approach to Pakistani Fiction in English'. *Journal of Postcolonial Writing* 47(2), 122–134.

Chambers, C. (2011) *British Muslim Fictions: Interviews with Contemporary Writers*. London: Palgrave Macmillan.

Chambers, C. (2013) '"Islamophobia": Orwellian Newspeak or Racially-inflected Hatred?'. *DAWN* [online]. Available from <www.dawn.com/news/1029946> [18 July 2016].

Chambers, C. and Herbert, C. (2015) *Imagining Muslims in South Asia and the Diaspora*. London: Routledge.

Cilano, C. (2009) '"Freeing the Outlook of Man from its Geographical Limitations": The Supraterritoriality of Pakistani English-and Urdu-Language Literatures'. *Journal of Commonwealth and Postcolonial Studies: Pakistani Literature* 16(1), 9–23.

Clements, M. (2016) *Writing Islam from a South Asian Muslim Perspective*. New York: Palgrave Macmillan.
Coppola, C. (2001) 'Some Recent English-Language Poetry from Pakistan'. In *Postindependence Voices in South Asian Writings*. Ed. by Hashmi, A. et al. Islamabad: Alhamra Printing.
Encyclopedia.com. (2018) 'Alvi, Moniza'. Contemporary Poets [online]. Available from <www.encyclopedia.com/arts/culture-magazines/alvi-moniza> [18 July 2016].
Ghose, Z. (2009) *Beckett's Company: Selected Essays*. Karachi: Oxford University Press.
Ghose, Z. (2010) *50 Poems*. Karachi: Oxford University Press.
Hashmi, S.Z. (2010) *Baker of Tarifa*. Madera, CA: Poetic Matrix Press.
Hashmi, S.Z. (2013) *Kohl and Chalk*. Madera, CA: Poetic Matrix Press.
Ibrahim, H. (2001) 'Transnational Migrations and the Debate of English Writing in/of Pakistan'. In *Post-Independence Voices in South Asian Writings*. Ed. by Hashmi, A. et al. Islamabad: Alhamra Printing, 33–48.
Kanwal, A. (2015) *Rethinking Identities in Contemporary Pakistani Fiction: Beyond 9/11*. New York: Palgrave Macmillan.
Khwaja, W. (1987) *Six Geese from a Tomb at Medum*. Lahore: Sang-e-Meel Publications.
Khwaja, W. (2007) *No One Waits for the Train*. Belgium: Alhambra Publishing.
Khwaja, W. (2009) 'Introduction'. *Journal of Commonwealth and Postcolonial Studies* 16(3), 3–8.
Khwaja, W. (2017) *Hold Your Breath*. Oxford: Onslaught.
Kureishi, M. (1997) *The Far Thing*. Karachi: Oxford University Press.
Mansoor, A. (2012) 'The Notes of a New Harp: Tracing the Evolution of Pakistani Poetry in English'. *Pakistaniaat: A Journal of Pakistan Studies* 4(1), 14–38. [online]. Available from <http://pakistaniaat.net/2012/09/pakistaniaat-print-version-of-vol-4-1-just-published/> [18 July 2016].
Rafat, T. (1985) *Arrival of the Monsoon*. Lahore: Vanguard.
Rafat, T. (2008) *Half Moon*. Lahore: Taufiq Rafat Foundation and Arslan Printers.
Rahman, T. (1991) *A History of Pakistani Literature in English*. Lahore: Vanguard.
Rahman, T. (2013) 'Taufiq Rafat' [online]. Available from <www.tariqrahman.net/literatur/Taufiq%20Rafat.htm> [18 July 2016].
Raja, M.A. (2010) *Constructing Pakistan: Foundational Texts and the Rise of Muslim National Identity: 1857–1947*. Oxford: Oxford University Press.
Raja, M.A. (2012) 'Exclusionary Narratives, Ambivalence, and Humanistic Studies'. *Journal of English Literary and Linguistic Studies* 1(1), 13–20.
Schwartz, H. and Ray, S. (eds.) (2000) *A Companion to Postcolonial Studies*. Carlton: Blackwell.
Shamsie, M. (1998) *A Dragonfly in the Sun: An Anthology of Pakistani Writing in English*. Karachi: Oxford University Press.
Shamsie, M. (2001) *Leaving Home: Towards a New Millennium*. Karachi: Oxford University Press.
Shamsie, M. (2005) *And the World Changed: Contemporary Stories by Pakistani Women*. Karachi: Oxford University Press.
Shamsie, M. (2011) 'Ahmed Ali: Centenary Year (1910–2010) – 2'. *Solidarity International* 26–27.
Shamsie, M. (2017) *Hybrid Tapestries: The Development of Pakistani Literature in English*. Oxford: Oxford University Press.
Siddique, J. (2005) *The Prize*. London: Rialto.
Siddique, J. (2011a) *Full Blood*. London: SALT.
Siddique, J. (2011b) 'Six Snapshots of Partition'. *Solidarity International* 40–43.
Spivak, G.C. (2008) *Other Asias*. Malden: Blackwell Publishers.
Suleri, S. (1992) *The Rhetoric of English India*. Chicago: The University of Chicago Press.
Waterman, D. (2015) *Where Worlds Collide: Pakistani Fiction in the New Millennium*. Karachi: Oxford University Press.
Yusuf, I. (2012) 'A Lively Progression: Mapping Pakistani Poetry'. *Vallum: New International Poetics* 9(1): 82–92.
Zaman, F. (2009) *Contemporary American Poetry: An Anthology*. Islamabad: PAL.
Zoberi, Z. (2012) *True Colours*. Canada: IOWI.

32

BRAND PAKISTAN

The case for a Pakistani anglophone literary canon

Aroosa Kanwal and Saiyma Aslam

In this culminating chapter we aim to emphasise the urgent need to canonise Pakistani anglophone literature, not only in relation to its (current) production and consumption but also in terms of its dialogical dynamics, operating in four frames of reference: the individual, the national, the regional, and the global. As Pakistani anglophone writers began to be anthologised in Commonwealth, postcolonial, and world literatures, as well as other geographically and ethnically focused collections, which gestures towards an increasing acceptance of Pakistani literature by mainstream institutions, it became important to discuss the ways in which these narratives claim a manifest or implied congruence between the development and evolution of the Pakistani literary trajectory and the development of the nation. Most importantly, acknowledgement of the existence of a national literary canon would strengthen the textual and institutional basis for Pakistani anglophone literature becoming a medium of cultural memory and a vehicle of national identificational patterns, albeit in diverse ways. It is important to emphasise here that despite being organically enmeshed within Pakistan's multilingual traditions and cultures and, at the same time, having already ushered in a stage where it is challenging the curtaining shibboleths of merely writing back to the centre, Pakistani anglophone literature is still struggling, at home, to overcome charges of being elitist and a colonial hangover. This literature, which is a product of multi-ethnic, multilingual, transnational, transcultural, and trans-local literary traditions of Pakistan, the subcontinent, and the Muslim world (and also in dialogue with other anglophone literatures from around the world), is urgently in need of being rescued from reductive misnomers. Cara Cilano recognises, in her essay 'Writing from Extreme Edges', a need to 'identify the variables that can link Pakistani English-language literary production within Pakistan's diverse array of multi-lingual literatures [and] within that subcontinent's English-language traditions' (2009: 195). While not going into the details that warranted her position, our chapter charts the terrain which anglophone literature in Pakistan has trekked over the years as a distinct literary trajectory that is enmeshed in the local and the global.

Our understanding of the Pakistani anglophone literary trajectory matches Dermot McCarthy's observation that 'The gathering of the scattered texts into a "permanent form", the selection and organization of a literary canon, and the ideological program of nation-building and identity-definition, all cohere isomorphically from the beginning in literary history' (1991: 33). In so doing, our discussion of the canonisation of the Pakistani anglophone literary tradition is significantly informed by a historical perspective that aims to reconsider past documents, including literary texts, which not only document specific ideological biases towards gender, ethnicities, religion, politics, culture, civil war, democracy, consumerism, extremism, and nuclear paroxysm, but also provide a historical and lineal contextualisation of the issues dominating today's public discourse surrounding similar issues.

Therefore, on the one hand, this chapter foregrounds the ways in which our unique literary tradition has always been in dialogue with the contemporary situation; on the other, it rebuts the discourse surrounding the Pakistani anglophone literary tradition which claims that it relies on Western discursive enclosures. We argue instead that while in dialogue with literary trends of Asian, Muslim, and subcontinental cultures and civilisations, it has morphed into a distinct Pakistani idiom. It is precisely against this backdrop that we intend to expand the capability of Pakistani anglophone writing to perform three important functions of canonisation, namely, curatorial (innovations and experiments in genre and style), normative (exemplary attitudes and wisdom), and dialogical (interaction with other literary cultures and textual fields), as we will engage with shortly. In analysing these functions, we see them as being supported by and gaining strength from other canon-making forces, such as anthologies, translations, adaptions, literary inheritances, and the increasing prominence of anglophone writers in syllabi around the world. Moreover, taking cognisance of the diverse categories (Partition fiction, post-independence narratives, post-9/11 fiction, retrospective prologues to post-9/11 fiction, chick lit, nuclear fiction, etc.) of Pakistani anglophone writing, we aim to propose how our literary legacy can 'offer a grammar promising [...] a set of models and provocations and communal identifications enabling [us] to explore new aspects of identity and give rich and contoured explanations for our choices' (Altieri 1991: 27). We cannot ignore the fact that failure to engage with the questions of value and ideals within our literary traditions would result in stasis and complacency; we are sure that as academics, we all reject this stance.

Having said this, we now lay our canon cards on the table, as it is inevitable to overlook certain questions about normative and curatorial functions of literary representations for canon constitution. Pakistani anglophone literature displays a rich kaleidoscope of works exemplifying these standards that Charles Altieri considers fundamental to the canonisation of literature. In its curatorial function, the emphasis falls on how these works exhibit a 'repertory of inventions and a challenge to our capacity to further develop a genre or style' (Altieri 1990: 33). In the normative function, the emphasis falls on studying the 'exemplary attitudes' and wisdom that works reflect. Both curatorial and normative functions address a different dimension of a literary work, and together they help to work towards a contrastive framework that Altieri calls 'cultural grammar for interpreting experience' (1983: 47).

We will now demonstrate how, in the past seventy years, Pakistani literature has expanded dramatically, epitomising normative and curatorial standards while offering what Altieri calls 'a grammar promising [...] a set of modes and provocations to communal identification enabling us to explore new aspects of identity and give rich and contoured explanations for our choices' (1991: 27). By juxtaposing the early development of Pakistani literary works with the contemporary era, we suggest how past and present literary traditions have an inherent relationship. In so doing, we propose claiming a Pakistani canon, not as the result of one or two publications or events but rather of a multitude of publications, events, and contexts interacting with authors and their works, linking both history and aesthetics in a dynamic dialogical relationship. It is precisely against this backdrop that we read our works contrapuntally, inspired by Said's *The World, the Text, the Critic* (1983), to create a distinctive (Pakistani) cultural grammar for interpreting experiences through a repertoire of inventions and developments in a genre or style.

For example, it is interesting to see how many writers of Pakistani origin, despite practising their art in the metropolis, are still attached to local cultural, historical, and generic conventions.

Hugely inspired by Taufiq Rafat's notion of the 'Pakistani idiom', Waqas Ahmad Khwaja's experimental bilingual poetry is indeed a recognisable blending of postmodern elements and the Punjabi *qissa* and *dastaan goi* traditions. The cultural delicacy of Khwaja's poetry is evident in his allusions to Baba Farid, Bulley Shah, Bhakta Kabir, and Guru Nanak. Marked by transmutations of similar rich literary traditions of the East, Shadab Zeest Hashmi's dynamic experimentation with the traditional subcontinental poetic form of the *ghazal* is a continuation of the Arabo-Persian origins of the *ghazal*s and their subcontinental fruition in the philosophical *ghazal*s of Amir Khusrau. Hashmi's writing, under the influence of the vernacular Urdu poetic tradition, is hugely informed by her readings of Allama Mohammad Iqbal, Bulley Shah, and Faiz Ahmed Faiz, masters of blending spirituality with intellect and lyricism with rhetoric. Aamer Hussein's vernacular knowledge of classical Persian and Urdu literature, especially in the Sufi tradition and the verse of Shah Abdul Latif, has enormously shaped his retellings of traditional folklore, immersed as they are in dreamlike magic and mysticism. Suhayl Saadi's narrative voice, subtly melding Scottish dialect, Urdu, English, and Punjabi, reflects different cultures and ethos that include Sufism, Jewish, Greek, and Buddhist legends, Moorish Spain, and Biblical and Quranic stories. It would not be wrong to say that Rafat's coining of the term 'Pakistani idiom' led his fellow poets to seek non-Western models to revitalise the Pakistani anglophone poetic tradition, which is a clear move away from the English canon, and to propose indigenous models and curatorial standards for the formation of a Pakistani poetic canon.

Reflecting on the rich treasure trove of Pakistani anglophone literature and its unique incarnations of craft and wisdom, we are proud to claim that Pakistani anglophone writings also strongly illustrate the normative function of our literary culture, which is not only expansive in its sweep but also dialogic in its engagement. Claire Chambers notes that:

> Pakistan's pre-Islamic civilizations (evident in the archaeological sites of Taxila, Moenjodaro, and Harappa), and its shared borders and overlapping culture with India, Afghanistan, Iran, Central Asia, and China 'has given Pakistani writers a particularly rich cultural heritage to draw on'.
>
> (2011: 122)

Absorbing and, in return, enriching its Arabo-Persian, subcontinental, and Muslim literary, philosophical, political, and cultural influences, our proposed canon presents a complex interface to engage with broader questions of identity, belonging, community, social responsibility, self-reflection, ethical challenge, and consensus, which are indispensable to an understanding of peaceful and responsible coexistence in a multicultural, multilingual world. Our writers reflect on the present against the backdrop of larger glocal geopolitical developments and centuries-old Muslim wisdom of inclusiveness and diversity, undermined in the post-9/11 era. The genesis of this debate can be found in Tariq Ali's *Islam Quintet*, written in response to a comment he heard during the 1991 Gulf War – that Muslims have no culture. Ali instead traces the tolerant, pluralistic, and intellectual side of Islamic civilisation in his five novels. Muneeza Shamsie corroborates: 'In Ali's quintet, each novel conveys illuminating insights into European and Muslim history and challenges widespread stereotypes of Islamic culture, as well as the rigid world view of Islamic extremists' (2014: 65). This excavation of the lost glories of Andalusian civilisation, particularly in response to the imperial rhetoric of the alien 'other' and the clash of civilisations, also surfaces in Imtiaz Dharker's 'Remember Andalus (Osama Bin Laden)', Zeest Hashmi's *Baker of Tarifa*, and Aamer Hussein's 'Nine Postcards from Sanlucar de Barrameda'. Similarly, the illocutionary force of the Punjabi poetry of Bulleh Shah and Qadir Yar, as exemplified in first- and second-generation poets and writers, is enormously relevant to a literary discourse that underscores the climate of fanaticism and bigotry that Zia introduced in the guise of a new (Islamic) nationalism. Nothing could provide a better foil to or a stronger rebuttal of state-sponsored repression than invoking the intertextual tradition of the centuries-old Muslim traditions of tolerance and inclusiveness, as Muneeza Shamsie aptly captures in her *Hybrid Tapestries*:

> The message of these mystics transmuted into English verse is not simply an expression of a spiritual experience, nor an attempt to merge the tradition of Pakistan's many literatures with that of English, but is also a challenge to the harsh, fanatical, highly politicized religious extremism which developed in Pakistan and other Muslim countries and communities during the last two decades of the twentieth century.
>
> (2017: 261)

Similar normative expectations are met in fictional works, too. Specifically invoking the Andalusian polymath Ibn Rushd in her epigraph – 'I believe the soul is immortal but I cannot prove it' – and occasionally referring to Aristotle, Muhammad Iqbal, al-Kindi, Ibn Sina (Avicenna) and Pascal, Uzma Aslam Khan's *The Geometry of God* contextualises the aesthetic, philosophical, ethical, and epistemological debates surrounding the discord between science and religion within the Islamic Republic of Pakistan, centred on the premise that *'there's no marriage between faith and reason. Only Adultery'* (2008: 114; emphasis original). The very title of the novel, 'The Geometry of God', gestures towards man's unique relation to God, a perfect synthesis of the physical and the spiritual. The best way to know God is through *khayal*, 'the seat of intelligence', but *zauq* (taste), a more sensual way of knowing God, is even lovelier than *khayal* because 'It's physical. Not abstract. To understand, first you need a mortal' (Aslam Khan 2008: 181). Aslam Khan draws wisdom from subcontinental, Greek, French, and Arab thinkers, philosophers, and scientists to reject any exclusivist discourse on the idea of 'pure' religion, identity, or origins. Similarly, Nadeem Aslam, in his 'mausoleum fictions', a term coined by Madeline Clements (2016: 91) for fiction such as *Maps for the Lost Lovers* (2004) and *The Wasted Vigil* (2008), draws upon Sufi mysticism, Persian, and pre-Islamic Buddhist traditions, as well as South and Central Asian aesthetic heritages. In *Maps for Lost Lovers*, 'elements from numerous legends and myths of the world have been woven' (2004 'Notes') to explain the lives of characters in Dasht-e-Tanhaii. Likewise, in *The Wasted Vigil*, Marcus' house appears as the epitome of the enduring power of art in the face of fundamentalists' resistance to arts and artefacts, especially in preserving hundreds of books nailed to the ceiling, a chest full of pictures bearing Allah's names in Arabic calligraphy but surrounded by 'images not of lovers and vines but of other living things' (Aslam 2008: 242) or a Buddha head buried under Marcus' perfume factory. In both texts, Aslam underscores the 'residual shortcoming of […] knowledge', unless supplemented by knowledge 'about history and religions, about paintings and music […] about ancient and modern events' (2008: 356). Such a normative depth replete with centuries-old wisdom, arrived at through creative engagement with other literary cultures and traditions, is not only compelling in terms of its cultural diversity and enduring commonalities with global Muslim civilisation and literature, but also reassuring in terms of our claims for canonical status.

After probing this normative cross-cultural intertextuality that echoes dialogues, it should come as no surprise that a similar literary dialogue, which provides contrastive frameworks for analysing the past, understanding the present, and predicting the future, is also manifest within individual narratives and different categories and genres of Pakistani work. These diverse categories (comprising first- and second-generation authors, and the subcategories of second-generation writings) together provide contrasting frameworks and literary critical paradigms that attest to the deep richness which our literature has already attained. One of the most productive ways to understand the strengths of Pakistani anglophone literature and culture is in terms of the perspectives and contexts that inform their diverse categories and genres; these have stemmed from a series of historical events that have given complex voice to the questions that shape any (literary) culture, from questions of individual identity and belonging to national identity formation and community identification. During the phases of the 1947 Partition and since independence, Pakistan has undergone several severe upheavals in the form of internal and external aggressions, such as the 1971 war, successive military dictatorships, the US-led Afghan *jihad*, the Talibanisation of Pakistan, wars with India, the Kashmir conflict, the war on terror, the rise of Islamic extremism and multifarious ethnic, ancestral, and sectarian crises. All these have played an enormous role in shaping Pakistani literature and literary genres. Siddharta Deb's observation remains relevant: 'The Partition has shown an uncanny ability to replicate itself through the decades, in mini-partitions, mini-massacres, and the marginalization and brutal treatment of minorities that has become the governing spirit of nationalism in South Asia' (qtd. in Kingston 2017: n.p.).

In this vein, the works by first- and second-generation writers provide compelling dialogues around important historical events, such as those in 1947 and 1971. On the events leading up to the 1947 Partition, we see a large corpus developing out of the works of first- and second-generation writers in different times and locations, adding to the 'polyphonous richness with internal divergences, with differences and tensions in evidence' (Narayan 1997: 143). Mumtaz Shah Nawaz's *The Heart Divided* (1957), Abdullah Hussein's *The Weary Generations* (1960), Ahmed Ali's *Ocean of Night* (1964), and Bapsi Sidhwa's *Cracking India* (1998) have been joined by works of second-generation writers such as Aslam Khan's *Trespassing* (2003), Khwaja's *No One Waits for the Train* (2007), Sorayya Khan's *Five Queen's Road* (2009), and Moniza Alvi's *At the Time of Partition* (2013). The importance of this rich and polyphonic legacy lies in the microhistories embedded within the historical events of 1947 and their dialogues among fictional accounts by Hindu, Muslim, and Sikh writers, whose 'unruliness' and 'leaks', as Cilano puts it, enrich, or contradict, the official history, and 'can indicate where and how the power structure that governs the archive is vulnerable' (Cilano 2010: iii). Similar questions can be raised with regard to the multiple perspectives and 'leak(s)' evoked by Pakistani and Bangladeshi writers on the 1971 war.

On the 1971 partition again, we have a rich body of works by first- and second-generation writers, such as Tariq Rahman's 'Bingo' (1975), Adam Zameenzad's *Cyrus, Cyrus* (1990), Mohsin Hamid's *Moth Smoke* (2000), Sorayya Khan's *Noor* (2006), Moni Mohsin's *The End of Innocence* (2006), Shahbano Bilgrami's *Without Dreams* (2007), Roopa Farooqi's *Half Life* (2010), Shehryar Fazli's *Invitation* (2011), and Aquila Ismail's *Of Martyrs and Marigolds* (2012). Providing a panoramic view of the angst that started with the Partition of 1947, and was aggravated in the second Partition of 1971, are works such as Mehr Nigar Masroor's *Shadows of Time* (1987), Aamer Hussein's 'Karima', and Kamila Shamsie's *Kartography* (2002). Post-independence literature is an apt reflection of the crises that continued to surge at different levels owing to internal and external sociopolitical problems affecting the nascent nation state. Ahmed Ali's *The Purple Gold Mountain* (1960), Zulfikar Ghose's *The Murder of Aziz Khan* (1967), Salman Rushdie's *Shame* (1983), Ahmed Ali's *Rats and Diplomats* (1984), and Sara Suleri's *Meatless Days* (1989) capture the post-independence challenges that vexed the country, leaving enduring reverberations that are felt to this day. These novels not only engage with the pathological violence that erupted at the time of Partition but also uncover 'those relations "outside" the "fevered sleep" of Pakistani nationalistic history that affect those who remained in or were born into Pakistan after 1971' (Cilano 2011: 1). It is interesting to note how, even in the twenty-first century, our second-generation writers are preoccupied with the catastrophic legacies of the 1947 and 1971 partitions, which underscores their 'central role in the making of Pakistani [individual and communitarian] identities in the wake of apparently irreconcilable differences that have continued to exist since 1947' (Kanwal: 2015: 21). For these significant reasons, 1947 and 1971 are important literary phases that are being continually developed by even younger writers.

The last decade experienced a boom in 'post-9/11 fiction' that emerged in response to '9/11-fiction'. Second-generation writers who are significantly writing back to the empire include Hamid, Mohammed Hanif, Ali Sethi, H.M. Naqvi, Kamila Shamsie, Maha Khan Phillips, and Feryal Ali Gauhar. Their work engages with the post-9/11 sociopolitical milieu and its repercussions for Pakistani Muslims both at home and across the diaspora. However, not all writers in the last decade have viewed 9/11 as the only marker for changed perceptions about Muslims. Efforts have also been made by Pakistani writers to trace the historical antecedents that led to the calamitous history of 9/11. Therefore, 'one more arc for the geodesic dome we build as we study the past'(Altieri 1990: 40) (in dialogic relation with the present) takes into consideration the Islamisation policies during Zia's regime and the rise of religious extremism in Pakistan, Afghanistan, and the Middle East in conjunction with the rise of Islamophobia in the West. This subgenre is labelled 'retrospective prologues to post-9/11 fiction', a term coined by Aroosa Kanwal (2015). Such literary efforts tend 'to disclose the intrinsic principles of the circle of values we inhabit' (Altieri 1990: 40), especially in the highly charged and turbulent first decade of the twenty-first century. While 'post-9/11 fiction' focuses on the impact of the September 11 terrorist attacks on the lives of Pakistanis in the diaspora and at home, and includes works such as Hamid's *The Reluctant Fundamentalist* (2007), Naqvi's *Homeboy* (2009), and Aslam's *The Wasted Vigil*, the 'retrospective prologues to post-9/11 fiction' use pre-9/11 settings in texts such as Aslam Khan's *The Geometry of God*, Kamila Shamsie's *Broken Verses* (2005) and *Kartography* (2002), and Aslam's *Season of the Rainbirds* (1993) to explore indigenous sociopolitical scenarios that, in a post-9/11 world, embroiled Pakistan in the war on terror. The two categories together provide 'a space of reevaluation' (Bromley 2000: 1) to better contextualise multifarious tensions that are local in their roots and global in their reach, or vice versa.

Recapitulating the diverse challenges that Pakistan faces today, our writers expand the canvas of their fictional worlds to provide a grand sweep of the history of 'moral dioramas [...] of unscrupulous multiplicity' (Walter Benjamin qtd. in Zevin 2005: n.p.). We call these narratives 'panoramic fiction', inspired by Walter Benjamin's panoramic literature. Panoramic fiction takes a broader perspective on the different turbulent phases in our history, such as Aslam Khan's *Trespassing* (2003), Kamila Shamsie's *Burnt Shadows* (2009) and *A God in Every Stone* (2014). Shamsie is interested in the broad sweep of history and uses the trope of archaeology as a unifying factor in *A God in Every Stone*: from ancient Persia between 485 and 515 BCE to the dissolution of the Ottoman state; from the First World War to the decline of British rule in the then Indian city of Peshawar in the 1930s. Shamsie's epic *Burnt Shadows* tells the stories of three generations marching tenaciously across Japan (1945), India (1947), Pakistan (1980), Afghanistan (1979), and America (2001). Recapitulating the mayhem and violent stories of the 1947 Partition of India and Pakistan and Pakistan's involvement in the Afghan *jihad*, both of which have had serious implications for Pakistan, the novel leads us to a 1980s Karachi plagued by sectarian violence. The final section of *Burnt Shadows* is set in Afghanistan and New York and events are framed in such a way that, through interactions between Afghan tribesmen and American mercenaries, and foreigners and the US, respectively, Shamsie reflects on post-9/11 Islamophobia in the US. Similarly, although Aslam Khan's *Trespassing* is set in the Karachi of the late 1980s and 1990s, the novel extends the debate about ethnic and sectarian crises to the wider subcontinent and the Middle East by introducing its readers to Pakistan's political, social, and religious reconfigurations during the Zia era, along with the writer's perspective on American attitudes during the Gulf War. In so doing, *Trespassing* provides a panoramic view of the expansion of Islamic practices and policies during Zia's military dictatorship by linking these to US interference in the Arab world's internal affairs during the Iran-Iraq War, and later during the First Gulf War.

In the past couple of decades, Zia's Islamic resurgence has remained popular, albeit contentious, fodder for Pakistani poets and novelists writing not only in English but also in Urdu. Given that this era is represented by many second-generation writers' fictional narratives as a turning point in the political history of Pakistan, we can identify and label these narratives as the 'legacy of Zia'. These dissident narratives of the legacy of Zia include, but are not limited to, Rushdie's *Shame* (1983), Suleri's *Meatless Days* (1989), Javaid Qazi's 'President Sahib's Blue Period' in *Unlikely Stories: Fatal Fantasies and Delusions* (1998), Aslam Khan's *Trespassing* (2003), Hanif *A Case of Exploding Mangoes* (2008), Sethi's *The Wish Maker* (2009), and Aslam Khan's *The Geometry of God* (2009). This textual corpus on the Zia regime is enormously pertinent in terms of the legislative measures and political climate that continue to implicate Pakistan, even today, in the war on terror, in human, religious minority, and women's rights debates. The measures taken by Zia under his Islamisation policy, in particular the enforcement of the Hudood ordinance and the Blasphemy Law, not only introduced religious and gender bias into Pakistani law but also had a far-reaching impact on Pakistanis abroad, bringing into the spotlight issues of racism and cultural violence. It is also important to note that honour killings, forced marriages, and women's rights gained significant public attention in the UK from the early 1980s (see Phillips 2010: 111–119; Gill and Anitha 2011). A complex concurrence of challenges afflicting Pakistan in the wake of Zia's interventions have led to tensions and differences that will likely never be reconciled. So many conflicting positions and interests have sat unevenly since then, surfacing in the tensions between Islamists, secularists, and moderates.

Just as multiple contending and conflicting positions mire Pakistan and Pakistanis in domestic and world politics, a range of genres and categories addressing these enigmas (interestingly in just as diverse a manner) have surged up in Pakistani anglophone writings – making our literature an apt register of the pulse of our changing lives and national legacies. The ghosts of the past have continued to make their presence felt in the lives of the people of Pakistan and India to this day. 'The nightmarish horrors of India's partition by the British seventy years ago on August 15, 1947, cast a long shadow into the 21st century [...] The festering wounds of hastily drawn borders remain geopolitical flashpoints that have sparked wars and terrorism' (Kingston 2017: n.p.). Most significantly, Kashmir happens to be another anomalous result of Partition, turning this region into the one such flashpoint, over which four major wars have been fought between Pakistan and India. These tense relationships and the nuclear arms race between the two countries are captured in 'nuclear fiction', such as Hamid's *Moth Smoke* (2000) and Kamila Shamsie's *Burnt Shadows*, as well as in two recent thrillers, Akbar Agha's *Juggernaut* (2015) and Munir Muhammad's *India Pakistan Nuclear War* (2016). The sociopolitical mayhem due to foreign interventions and local corruption finds expression in Karachi-based thrillers such as Hanif's *Our Lady of Alice Bhatti* (2011), Bilal Tanweer's *The Scatter Here is too Great* (2013), and Omar Shahid Hamid's *The Prisoner* (2013), *The Spinner's Tale* (2015), and *The Party Worker* (2017).

In addition to the major categories discussed above, which unequivocally gave a boost to Pakistani anglophone literature, there are numerous other genres that are exceptionally rich and vigorously engage with glocal tensions, but with nuances that are altogether different and require distinct sensibilities. For instance, comedy as a genre displays multiple variations: on the one hand, we have acerbic engagement with post-9/11 Islamophobia in Naqvi's *Homeboy*; on the other, undercutting complex geopolitical, national, and social issues, Hanif's *A Case of Exploding Mangoes* is a fine example of ebullient humour. Surprisingly impressive and notable is the chick lit genre which has blossomed over the last decade or so, gleefully captures the increasingly contentious issues of feudalism, women's agency, fundamentalism, Islamophobia, tribal customs, and forced marriages. It would not be wrong to say that:

> The light-hearted tone that is a key feature of chick lit (problematic though that term may be), is also positive in its efforts to work against the portrayal of misery and to demonstrate something light, breezy and undeniably engaged in the pursuit of happiness.
>
> (Chambers et al. 2018: n.p.)

For example, Ayisha Malik's *Sofia Khan Is Not Obliged* (2015) and its sequel *The Other Half of Happiness* (2017) engage with humorous subversions of Islamophobic stereotypes in the diaspora. Moni Mohsin's trilogy, *The Diary of a Social Butterfly* (2008), *Duty Free* (formerly *Tender Hooks*, 2011), and *The Return of the Butterfly* (2014), focuses on social chatter amidst political mayhem in contemporary Pakistan. Even 'romance fiction' comes laden with penetrating views of love, romance, and longing within the feudal structures of Pakistan, such as in Qaisra Shahraz's *The Holy Woman* (2002) and its sequel *Typhoon* (2007).

Azhar Abidi's *Passarola Rising* (2006) is highly experimental in terms of linking science and historical fiction in tracing the European past, an effort that parallels yet differs from the track taken by Tariq Ali in the *Islam Quintet*, with its emphasis on the Muslim past. Linking the private and the public in literary dialogues are autobiographies that provide important clues to local as well as global sociopolitical developments in the different phases of our national history, such as Tariq Ali's *Street Fighting Years: An Autobiography of the Sixties* (1987) and Rafia Zakaria's *The Upstairs Wife: An Intimate History of Pakistan* (2016).

Multiple sociocultural and politico-religious factors shaping the lives of women from diverse backgrounds, both at home and in the diaspora, which include but are not limited to patriarchy, misogyny, forced veiling, and wounded yet resilient subjectivities, are reflected in works such as Rukhsana Ahmad's *Song for a Sanctuary* (1993), Dharker's *Purdah* (1988), Shaila Abdullah's *Beyond the Cayenne Wall: Collection of Short Stories* (2005), Kyla Pasha's *High Noon and the Body* (2007), and Rukhsana Ahmad's *The Gatekeeper's Wife* (2014). This list of categories is by no means exhaustive, but it does indicate the vast range of genres which make up the Pakistani literary tradition and thus compel us to emphasise the canonisation of this rich and diverse literary treasure trove. What a remarkable variety we have been able to accumulate, despite the fact that our literature is still in its infancy compared to centuries-old European, British, and American traditions. What laurels we would win in the canonical inventory!

No wonder then that our writers have continued to be anthologised across the globe. While their scope and quality may vary greatly, many anthologies, collections, and literary histories include writers of Pakistani origin. For example, we find Sara Suleri, Kamila Shamsie, Bapsi Sidhwa, and Hanif Kureishi in Ato Quayson's *The Cambridge Companion to Postcolonial Novel* (2015); Rukhsana Ahmad, Tariq Ali, Nadeem Aslam, Sara Suleri, Bapsi Sidhwa, Musharraf Farooqi, Mohsin Hamid, Uzma Aslam Khan, Hanif Kureishi, Maki Kureishi, Zulfikar Ghose, Taufiq Rafat, Daud Kamal, Salman Tarik, Kaleem Omar, and Shahid Suhrawardy in Eugene Benson and L.W. Conolly's *Routledge Encyclopaedia of Post-colonial Literatures in English* (2004); Ahmed Ali, Moniza Alvi, Zulfikar Ghose, Alamgir Hashmi, Taufiq Rafat, Kaleem Omar, and

Shahid Hosain in Jahan Ramazani's *The Cambridge Companion to Postcolonial Poetry* (2017); Rukhsana Ahmad, Tariq Ali, Moniza Alvi, Nadeem Aslam, Mohsin Hamid, and Hanif Kureishi in Deirdre Osborne's *The Cambridge Companion to British Black and Asian* (2016); Mohsin Hamid, Kamila Shamsie, and Sonia Shah in Crystal Parikh and Daniel K. Yim's *The Cambridge Companion to Asian American Literature* (2015); Nadeem Aslam, Mohsin Hamid, Aslam Khan, Kamila Shamsie, Mohammed Hanif, Maha Khan Phillips, Feryal Gauhar, Sorayya Khan, and Abdullah Hussein in Janet Wilson and Chris Ringrose's *New Soundings in Postcolonial Writing: Critical and Creative Contours* (2016); Daud Kamal, Salman Tarik Kureshi, Alamgir Hashmi, and Mansoor Y. Sheikh in Peter Dent's *The Blue Wind: Poems in England from Pakistan* (1984). In addition to these foreign anthologies, our writers have appeared in anthologies compiled by Pakistani critics, such as Alamgir Hashmi's *Pakistani Literature: The Contemporary English Writers* (1987) and *The Worlds of the Muslim Imagination* (1986), Muneeza Shamsie's *A Dragonfly in the Sun: An Anthology of Pakistani Writing in English* (1997) and *Leaving Home: Towards a New Millennium: A Collection of English Prose by Pakistani Writers* (2001), Shahid Hussain's *First Voices: Six Poets from Pakistan* (1965), Yunus Said's *Pieces of Eight: Eight Poets from Pakistan* (1971) and Kaleem Omar's *Wordfall: Three Pakistani Poets* (1975). These are just a few examples of Pakistani authors' canonical itinerary. Foregrounding the prominence of Pakistani anglophone writers in the global literary market, Dent states that 'One commends these writers without reservation: they are no "backwater", but *mainstream* and affording us all valid and fruitful directions' (qtd. in Benson and Conolly 1994: 55; emphasis original). This means that as a morphing episteme, Pakistani anglophone writing has entered into pedagogical negotiations with world literatures, encouraging and promoting critical thinking among students who read canonical authors of diverse literary traditions on various university courses. William Casement's *The Great Canon Controversy: The Battle of the Books in Higher Education* (1996) usefully examines the significance of exposing students to such pedagogical negotiations that offer 'new perspectives' on and 'new ways of thinking' about questions of religious, cultural, social, gender, and national identities on the cultural battlefield. But it is important to note, as Casement does, that such 'new ideas are not preached or covertly pressured upon students; nor are they denounced. They are simply added to an already existing corpus and afforded the equal status of being deserving of consideration' (1996: 102). While Casement's idea about introducing readers to diverse perspectives is indubitably important, the notion of 'an already existing corpus' sounds generalising, especially in contemporary debates on canonisation, when literatures from around the world are being discussed primarily as part of their indigenous canon before their placement within the polymorphous richness of postcolonial, world literatures in general. We similarly view the Pakistani literary tradition as a distinct set of literary values, as well as writing with a distinct sense of a society that has to be seen for itself and that has proven its potential to echo dialogues within and across cultures and genres.

David Fishelov's dialogic approach to literature remains relevant here, according to which, great works generate dialogues with readers, writers, critics, translators, adaptors, and artists and 'a work's reputation is an institutionalized result of [...] accumulating dialogues' (2010: ix). Our preference for the term 'dialogic' is also informed by its insistence on a generous 'principle of diversity'; by focusing on Pakistani anglophone literary genres and traditions, we suggest the ways in which their '"echoes" are heterogeneously distributed' (Fishelov 2010: 47) across genre, period, and culture, both locally and globally. If, according to Fishelov, the idea of the greatness of any literary text is tied to the vagaries of its reception and dissemination across genres, which he refers to as the echoes it generates, Pakistani anglophone writing has continued to 'echo-dialogue' through adaptations and translations. This is not only a 'sign of the vitality of a literary system, but when a specific book evokes such blooming or procreation it is [also] the hallmark of its greatness' (Fishelov 2010: 24). Sidhwa's *Cracking India* (adapted as *Earth 1947*), Hamid's *The Reluctant Fundamentalist* and *Moth Smoke* (adapted as *Daira*), Hanif Kureishi's *The Buddha of Suburbia*, *My Beautiful Launderette*, and *My Son the Fanatic*, Shahraz's *The Holy Woman* (adapted as the screenplay *Dil hi tu Hai*), and Saba Imtiaz's *Karachi, You are Killing Me!* (adapted as *Noor*) are a few examples of novels adapted into films and screenplays. Despite the risk of film-makers having drastically different ideological concerns and the loss of the essence of the original, adaptations certainly have offsetting gains in terms of the size of the diversified audience and of understanding the text and its adaptation. Through diverse audience engagement, adaptations tend to reject any homogenising impulse to encourage what Fishelov describes as a 'whole range of attitudes' so that the present audience can 'adopt towards works of the past' (2010: 48). This textual re-creation and procreation tends to 'empirically test a few hypotheses about the correlation between a canonical status assigned to a work and the generation of echoes and dialogues' (Fishelov 2010: 48) over the years. Such is the case with many Pakistani novels and their adaptations.

For example, this simultaneous loss and gain in the meaning or essence of a text in the adaptation of Sidhwa's *Cracking India* into Deepa Mehta's film *Earth* is aptly captured by Rani Neutill: 'Mehta's traditional feminist perspective of representing women's subjugation obscures her ability to represent Sidhwa's novel beyond the heterosexual matrix of nationalist violence. As a result, Mehta misses the radical sites of queer and feminist resistance that Sidhwa's narrative offers' (2010: 1). Nevertheless, what needs to be emphasised here is that an adaptation is always another interpretation, in this case, of the momentous event of Partition. By juxtaposing the latter with Holocaust trauma, Mehta gives interreligious violence a global significance and reach; in other words, Mehta's adaptation recognises culturally specific as well as culturally diverse experiences of such traumas. Similarly, in adapting Hamid's monologue *The Reluctant Fundamentalist* into a political thriller, Mira Nair completely transforms Hamid's deliberate understatement and ambivalence about his protagonist's fractured identity, about his unnamed American interlocutor and the novel's structure and ending into a clear statement. As a novella, *The Reluctant Fundamentalist* was conceived so as to 'leave space for [the reader's] thoughts to echo', but its film adaptation 'collapses in a heap of wool-gathering humanism that feels warm to the touch, yet fatally hedges its political bets' (Taylor 2013: n.p.). But this is bound to happen when a text reaches a wider audience. Its dialogic dimensions also expand with the expansion of dialogic echoes. The English translation of Abdullah Hussein's short story 'Wapsi Ka Safa' ('The Journey Back') was adapted by Robert Buckler into a teleplay called 'Brothers in Trouble' for the BBC and by director Udayan Prasad as the film *Brothers in Trouble*; and together, the echoes they generated led Hussein to write a complex novel in English, *Émigré Journeys* (2000).

In addition to adaptations, when a literary work begins to circulate in translation, it demonstrates 'its openness to new sensibilities, and ensures a dynamic growth of horizons and repertoire' (Fishelov 2010: 23). We have no hesitation in claiming that Pakistani anglophone literature is not under-represented in translations, and hence is not cut 'off from the cultural capital of international recognition' (Thomsen 2017: 64). This is supported by the fact that Aslam Khan's *Trespassing* has been translated into fourteen languages in eighteen countries. Similarly, following its release in India, Aslam Khan's *The Geometry of God* was published in Spain, Italy, France, the US, the UK, and Pakistan. Hamid's three novels have been translated into more than thirty languages, ranging from Catalan to Chinese. Sidhwa's novels have been translated into Urdu and several other languages. Tehmina Durrani's *My Feudal Lord* has been translated into many languages, including an international edition co-written with William and Marilyn Hoffer. We tend to agree with Mads Rosendahl Thomsen that the 'figures that arise from translations, references and sales are not facts about the canons or an exact science, but they can be helpful in tracing changes over time and how the current interest is shaped' (2017: 56). This is indeed hugely significant in accentuating the canonisation of Pakistani anglophone literature by opening up the space required for any work to echo reverberations in other textual fields.

With reference to Pakistani anglophone writing, this is also supported by the fact that works by writers of Pakistani origin are widely taught in various disciplines across the world. Let us take a cursory look at some of the courses that have been taught in British and American universities, at different times, even reformulated in certain cases with new titles: 'Postcolonial Studies' and 'Imagining Muslims: Representations of Muslims in Britain' at the University of York, 'Fictions of Terrorism' at Durham University, 'Founding Fictions: Writing in English from Pakistan' at the University of Leeds, 'Asian Literature in English' at Michigan State University, 'Pakistani Literatures and Cultures in the South Asian Context' at Jadavpur University, India, 'Postcolonial Theory and Literary Studies' at the University of California, 'Postcolonial and the Study of English' at the University of Pennsylvania, 'Contemporary South Asian Studies' at Kennesaw State University, 'Post-9/11 Fiction' at Wilfrid Laurier University Waterloo, Ontario, 'British Muslims in Contemporary Fiction and Film' at Teesside University, UK, 'Pakistani Writing in English' at Western Illinois University, USA, 'Contemporary Pakistani Fiction in English', 'Pakistani Literature in English', and 'South Asian Fiction in English' at the International Islamic University in Islamabad. This testifies to Pakistani writers' admission into what James Atlas describes as the 'battle of the books' (1993: n.p.). Once it ascends to a sanctioned list, such as anthologies and collections, a 'work gains pedagogical value through repeated inclusion in anthologies' (Barbara Herrnstein Smith qtd. in Di Leo 2004: 91) and authors themselves become brands. On the basis of the global circulation and supranational significance of Pakistani writing in English, anglophone Pakistani writers can rightly be called the 'custodians of brand Pakistan' as they are by *Granta*'s 'How to Write about Pakistan' (n.d.: n.p.).

The literary value of Pakistani anglophone writing is also authenticated by the high visibility of Pakistani writers in the media. These authors have continued to be short-listed, long-listed, and winners of prestigious international awards, such as the Man Booker, Commonwealth, Orange, DSC Prize for South Asian Literature, Anisfield-Wolf Book Award, Windham Campbell Literature Prize, and many other international awards. No wonder then that works that achieve meritorious status and recognition through awards and prizes win over a constantly changing community of readers, which also includes academic researchers and literary critics, who are considered to be major forces in validating the canonical status of any work. Therefore, literature as a corpus or a body is created and shaped by such highly institutionalised and cultural forces.

Although it would be unfair to say that there is a dearth of literary criticism on Pakistani anglophone writing (since quite a few book-length studies, a large number of research papers, and significant numbers of anthologies and edited collections are now available tracing the trajectory of this literature's development), debates on the canonical status of any literary system as a preserver of culture can only be fuelled by literary critics. There is no denying that we have great writers and poets, we have a history of political contestation, we have a dynamic aesthetic and cultural heritage, our writers are winning acclaim and fame, and there are voices everywhere. The issue is not the absence of creative potential and a cultural reservoir, it is the absence of any critical impulse to let all the discordant chords be heard and form a unique canonical symphony. We highly regard the indispensable role that critics from outside Pakistan (such as Cara Cilano, Claire Chambers, Madeline Clements, and Rehana Ahmed) have played in the recognition of our work, signifying the many chords that enrich our literary output. Complementing the West-centric critical consciousness of our literature due to its affiliative bonds premised on 'guild consciousness, consensus, collegiality [and] professional respect', we urge more and more voices to join the scene from indigenous peoples in their filial relationship with their literature, and to be 'historical and social actors' (Said 1983: 20, 15). We urge a 'historical resituation' of our anglophone literature by 'critics who are themselves historical subjects' (Louis Montrose qtd. in Drakakis 2013: 22). This critical vacuum is chiefly responsible for the delayed efforts (such as this one) to canonise Pakistani anglophone literature. One of the best ways to strengthen the social capital required for the canonisation of Pakistani anglophone writing is to encourage our academics and research community to publish their dissertations as monographs (since many theses remain unpublished in our universities). Yet another move to strengthen this social capital is to introduce Pakistani anglophone literature as a separate discipline across all Pakistani degree-awarding institutions. We believe this vacuum can be filled by cultural idioms, competences, and dispositions, and by revitalising the critical scene with voices from within.

Bibliography

Altieri, C. (1983) 'An Idea and Ideal of a Literary Canon'. *Critical Inquiry* 10(1), 37–60.
Altieri, C. (1990) *Canons and Consequences: Reflections on the Ethical Force of Imaginative Ideals.* Evanston: Northwestern University Press.
Altieri, C. (1991) 'Canons and Differences'. In *The Hospitable Canon: Essays on Literary Play, Scholarly Choice, and Popular Pressures.* Ed. by Nemoianu, V. and Royal, R. Philadelphia: John Benjamins Publishing Company, 1–38.
Aslam, N. (2004) *Maps for Lost Lovers.* New York: Vintage.
Aslam, N. (2008) *The Wasted Vigil.* London: Faber and Faber.
Atlas, J. (1993) *Battles of the Books: The Curriculum debate in America.* New York: W.W. Norton & Co.
Benson, E. and Conolly, L.W. (eds.) (2005) *Encyclopedia of Post-Colonial Literatures in English.* 3 Vols. Oxford: Routledge.
Bromley, R. (2000) *Narratives for a New Belonging: Diasporic Cultural Fictions.* Edinburgh: Edinburgh University Press.
Casement, W. (1996) *The Great Canon Controversy: The Battle of the Books in Higher Education.* New Brunswick: Routledge.
Chambers, C. (2011) 'A Comparative Approach to Pakistani Fiction in English'. *Journal of Postcolonial Writing* 47(2), 122–134.
Chambers, C., Phillips, R., Ali, N., Hopkins, P., and Pande, R. (2018) '"Sexual misery" or "Happy British Muslims"? Contemporary Depictions of Muslim Sexualities'. *Ethnicities* 1–20.
Cilano, C. (2009) '"Writing from Extreme Edges": Pakistani English-Language Fiction'. *ARIEL* 40(2), 183–201.
Cilano, C. (2010) 'Too Soon? Pakistan and the 1971 War'. *Pakistaniaat: A Journal of Pakistan Studies* 2(3), i–x.
Cilano, C. (2011) *National Identities in Pakistan: The 1971 War in Contemporary Fiction.* London: Routledge.
Clements, M. (2016) *Writing Islam from a South Asian Muslim Perspective: Rushdie, Hamid, Aslam, Shamsie.* Basingstoke: Palgrave.
Di Leo, J.R. (ed.) (2004) *On Anthologies: Politics and Pedagogy.* Lincoln: University of Nebraska Press.
Drakakis, J. (ed.) (2013) *Shakespearean Tragedy.* New York: Routledge.
Fishelov, D. (2010) *Dialogues with/and Great Books: The Dynamics of Canon Formation.* Brighton: Sussex Academic Press.
Gill, A.I. and Anitha, S. (eds.) (2011) *Forced Marriage: Introducing a Social Justice and Human Rights Perspective.* New York: Zed Books.
Granta. (n.d.) 'How to Write about Pakistan' [online]. Available from <https://granta.com/how-to-write-about-pakistan/> [24 February 2018].
Hjartarson, P. (1995) *Making it Real: The Canonization of English Canadian Literature.* Toronto: Anansi.
Kanwal, A. (2015) *Rethinking Identities in Contemporary Pakistani Fiction: Beyond 9/11.* Basingstoke: Palgrave.
Khan, U.A. (2008) *The Geometry of God.* New Delhi: Rupa.
Kingston, J. 'The Unfinished Business of Indian Partition'. *The Japan Times* [online]. Available from <www.japantimes.co.jp/opinion/2017/08/12/commentary/unfinished-business-indian-partition/#.WyteSS2B3s0> [2 January 2018].

Lecker, R. (1993) 'A Country without a Canon?: Canadian Literatures and the Esthetic of Idealism'. *Mosaic* 26(3), 1–19.
McCarthy, D. (1991) 'Early Canadian Literary Histories and the Function of a Canon'. *Canadian Canons: Essay in Literary Value*. Ed. by Lecker, R. Toronto: University of Toronto Press, 30–45.
Narayan, U. (1997) *Dislocating Cultures: Identities, Traditions, and Third-World Feminism*. New York: Routledge.
Neutill, R. (2010) 'Bending Bodies, Borders and Desires in Bapsi Sidhwa's *Cracking India* and Deepa Mehta's *Earth*'. *South Asian Popular Culture* 8(1), 73–87.
Phillips, A. (2010) *Gender and Culture*. Cambridge: Polity.
Said, E. (1983) *The World, the Text and the Critic*. Cambridge, MA: Harvard University Press.
Shamsie, M. (2014) 'Restoring the Narration: South Asian Anglophone Literature and Al-Andalus'. In *Imagining Muslims in South Asia and the Diaspora: Secularism, Religion, Representations*. Ed. by Chambers, C. and Herbert, C. London: Routledge.
Shamsie, M. (2017) *Hybrid Tapestries: The Development of Pakistani Literature in English*. Karachi: Oxford University Press.
Taylor, E. (2013) 'Between Worlds, a "Reluctant Fundamentalist"'. New Orleans Public Radio [online]. Available from <http://wwno.org/post/between-worlds-reluctant-fundamentalist> [12 January 2018].
Thomsen, M.R. (2017) 'Changing Spaces: Canonization of Anglophone World Literature'. *Anglia* 135(1), 51–66.
Zevin, A. (2005) 'Paris: Capital of the 19th Century'. Brown University Library Centre for Digital Scholarship [online]. Available from <https://library.brown.edu/cds/paris/Zevin.html> [5 February 2018].

INDEX

7/7 109, 117, 200, 204, 250, 262, 364
9/11 23, 49–55, 59–66, 70–74, 80–91, 96–98, 106–107, 109–112, 119–120, 123, 138–147, 163–165, 168, 178, 192, 194, 200, 204, 213–214, 236, 250, 262, 364

Abdullah, Shaila 225, 229, 388
Abidi, Azhar 6, 236, 238–239, 240
Afghanistan 3, 5, 20, 36, 50–52, 63–64, 68, 71, 74, 86, 123, 131, 134, 140, 144, 153–156, 162–165, 173, 178, 310, 338, 340, 354, 376, 383, 386
Afridis 157
Afzal-Khan, Fawzia 6, 107, 108, 111, 371, 374–376
Ahmad, Jamil 143, 151–153, 339
Ahmad, Rukhsana 388–389
Ahmadis 18
Ahmed, Eqbal 22–23
Ahmed, Rehana 98–99, 210–211, 238–239, 242, 361, 391
Akbar, Agha 69, 76, 387
Akhtar, Ayad 4, 6, 58–60, 63, 65–66, 107–109, 111–112, 186, 189–190, 192–193, 195–196
Akhtar, Rizwan 297, 303–305
Al Qaeda 51, 163
Ali, Ahmed 215, 335, 372, 385, 388
Ali, Tariq 4, 23, 27, 116, 123, 335, 383, 388–389
Altieri, Charles 382, 386
Alvi, Moniza 374–378, 388–389
Anderson, Benedict 35–37, 325, 336
anti-Americanism 60, 353
anti-semitism 113
Appadurai, Arjun 285
Arab(s) 116–119, 122–123, 304, 384, 387
Arrival of the Monsoon 373
Ashraf, Saad 14–16
Aslam Khan, Uzma 134, 185, 297, 301, 336, 341–342, 365, 384–390

Aslam, Nadeem 6–7, 14, 18–20, 129, 139–141, 144, 201, 206–211, 213–216, 218–219, 236, 240–244, 246, 274–277, 279, 285–286, 288, 290–292, 336, 338, 355, 365–367, 384, 386, 388–389
assimilation 7, 133, 204, 211, 237, 239–241, 261, 289, 292

Baker of Tarifa 376, 383
Bakhtin, Mikhail 95, 97, 326, 328
Bangladesh 39–42, 44, 71, 241, 248, 265, 275, 277, 372, 385
Bano, Alia 6, 108–109, 112, 249–253, 257
BBC 98–99, 102, 132, 286, 390
Beautiful from this Angle 103
Beyond the Cayenne Wall 229, 388
Bhabha, Homi K 36–37, 49, 95, 99, 281, 285–286, 289, 291, 328, 342–343, 371
Bhutto, Benazir 174
Bhutto, Fatima 146, 151, 155–156, 174
Bhutto, Zulfiqar Ali 22–23, 156, 227–228, 306
Bihari(s) 28–29
bildungsroman 82, 103, 138, 318–320, 323, 325–329
Bilgrami, Shahbano 3, 25–26, 30, 37, 385
Bin Laden, Osama 52, 54, 111, 163, 383
binarism 362
Black Album 6, 200–201, 206–209, 211, 327, 329
blasphemy 202
Blasphemy Laws 387
Blasphemy Ordinance 128
Boehmer, Elleke 362
Book of Saladin 4, 116–118, 121
Bradford 107, 262–263, 265–266; riots 200, 204–205
Brah, Avtar 241
brand Pakistan 8, 140, 339–341, 343–345
Brennan, Timothy 118, 344
Broken Verses 5, 129–130, 133, 338, 386

Index

Brouillette, Sarah 144, 322, 336, 343–344
Buddha of Suburbia 7, 100–101, 274, 277–278, 280, 282, 298, 325–329, 384, 390
Burnt Shadows 49–51, 55, 69, 73–74, 141–143, 338, 362, 364, 386–387
burqa 164, 166–167, 254
Bush, George W. 51, 123, 163–165, 167
Butler, Judith 61, 135, 298

canon 2, 8, 229, 341, 344, 348, 350–351, 381–383, 389, 391
canonisation 8, 381–382, 388–389, 391–392
Case of Exploding Mangoes 4–5, 49, 51–54, 80, 89, 128–129, 132, 344, 349, 387–388
Casement, William 38
censorship 1, 27, 39, 91
Chambers, Claire 173, 213, 236, 261–262, 361, 363–364
Chambers, Iain 240
Charlie Hebdo 96, 185–187
China 71, 288, 298, 300, 305, 383
China-Pak Economic Corridor 300, 305
Christians 18–19, 27, 55, 113, 117–120, 189, 192–194, 264, 311, 327, 361
CIA 51–52, 54, 60
Cilano, Cara 3, 8, 23, 25–26, 28–30, 35, 38, 213–214, 337, 361–365, 372, 374, 377, 381, 385, 391
civil war 24, 26, 31–32, 43, 382
Clash of Civilisations (civilizations) 116, 118–119, 120, 123, 141, 383
Clements, Madeline 8, 338, 361–363, 365–366, 384, 391
Clinton, Bill 72, 75
Cold War 19, 51, 60, 140, 320, 323–326
colonialism 187, 188–190, 215, 298, 304, 319, 329, 348
comedy 90, 94–97, 388; family 103; Muslim-ethnic 80, 94; stand-up 94–95
Communism 20, 27, 135, 288–289, 292
conspiracy 26, 49, 51–53
Coppola, Carlo 374
cosmopolitanism 49, 55, 65, 82, 320, 341–343, 352, 360, 362, 364, 366, 368
Country at My Shoulder 375
Cracking India 15, 37, 385, 390
Crusades 116–118
cultural capital 285–292, 390
Cyrus, Cyrus 27–28, 385

deconstruction 8, 36, 360–361, 364–368
democracy 89, 90, 118, 131, 142, 156, 167, 298, 325, 382
Dhaka 22–23, 28–30, 38–39, 103
Dharker, Imtiaz 383, 388
diaspora 1–2, 4, 6–8, 32, 107–108, 113, 213, 229, 236–237, 239–240, 242, 263, 267, 274–276, 279, 282, 370–378, 386, 388

dictatorship 3, 90, 132, 387
disorientation 24, 63, 307
Disgraced 6, 58–60, 62–66, 107–108, 112, 189, 190–193
domestic violence 6, 250, 255
dramatic monologue 64, 301, 363
drone attacks/strikes 4, 77, 143–144, 156
Durrani, Tehmina 390

East is East 106, 108
East Pakistan 22–31, 36, 38–43
Egypt 118, 255–256
Empire 17, 74, 139, 188, 193, 241, 298, 309, 353, 360, 371, 386; British 241, 289; Mughal 214
End of Innocence 25–26, 213, 385
erotic 6, 185, 187, 189, 195–196, 202–203, 215, 329
Eteraz, Ali 6, 186, 189–191, 195–196
ethnocentrism 352
Exit West 6, 49, 55, 141, 185–186, 190, 197–198
extremism 1, 3, 27, 29, 158, 173, 188, 262, 337, 340, 382, 384–386

Faiz, Ahmed Faiz 128, 288, 303, 383
Fanon, Frantz 185, 189, 196, 205
farangi 370–371
Farooqi, Musharraf Ali 213
Farooqi, Roopa 3, 385
FATA 155–157
fatwa 255, 339
Fazli, Shahryar 26, 385
FBI 82, 84, 194
feminism 59, 98, 158–160, 225, 267; Postcolonial 226; Western 151–152; White 158–159
feudalism 103, 289, 388
Fishelov, David 389–390
Five Queen's Road 14, 16–17, 385
Foucault, Michel 100, 186, 286
Four Walls and Black Veils 227
forced marriages 101–102, 104, 215, 241–243, 248, 255, 262, 387–388
Forna, Aminatta 24
freedom of: expression 139, 165; movement 17, 19; speech 134–135, 186, 303
Freud, Sigmund 95, 216, 325
fundamentalism 2, 4, 8, 30, 70, 108, 127–129, 165, 217, 261, 315, 388

Gauhar, Feryal 386, 389
gaze 100, 159, 195, 228, 240, 309, 311, 322; diegetic 166; imperial 195; male 203, 206, 210; orientalising 192; orientalist 195; parodic 103–104; patriarchal 233; women's 159
gender 6, 17, 25–26, 31, 92, 108, 162, 164–165, 169, 198, 215, 227–228, 233, 237, 244, 246, 249, 267, 305, 339, 361, 364, 371, 382, 389; bias 92, 122, 387; binaries 164; chauvinism 246;

discrimination 90; diversity 8, 368; and ethnicity 36, 194; identi(ties) 180, 327; inequality 122, 246; and minority 3; norms 6, 103; perspectives 122; roles 253

gendered: agency 231, 234; body 131; history 226; identi(ties) 6, 232; ideology 234; islamophobia 236; landscape 228; nationalist consciousness 228; oppression 238; politics 233; violence 234; voices 176

Geometry of God 134, 297, 299, 301, 384, 386–387, 390

ghazal 215, 217, 372, 374, 376, 383

Ghose, Zulfikar 7, 127, 318–325, 335, 372–375, 377–378, 385, 388

Gilgit-Baltistan 352

Glasgow 274, 276, 279

global *ummah* 262, 365

globalisation 7, 58, 138, 140–142, 197, 307, 314, 335, 338–339, 344, 366

God in Every Stone 55, 151, 158, 297–300, 302–303, 386

Granta 340, 349, 353–354, 391

Greetings from Bury Park 6–7, 201, 204, 206–208, 211, 262, 287

Guantanamo 143

Gulf War(s) 3, 110, 118, 364, 383, 387

hadith 122, 255

hajj 261, 270–271

halala 242

Hamid, Mohsin 3–4, 6–7, 30, 49, 53–55, 58–62, 64, 66, 68–71, 75–77, 129, 139–142, 144, 185–190, 194, 196–197, 213–219, 236, 307, 309–316, 336, 338–339, 344, 349, 353, 362–363, 365–367, 385–390

Hamoodur Rahman Commission 23

harem 97, 121–122, 195

Hashmi, Alamgir 1, 371, 388–389

He Named me Malala 172, 176, 178, 180

Heart Divided 336, 385

hedonism 200, 202, 208, 325

heterosexual 226, 232, 390

hierarchy 132, 190, 232, 242, 298, 349

hijab 98–100, 166, 253

Hold Your Breath 375

Holy Woman 225, 230–234, 388, 390

Home Boy 4, 80, 82–83, 86–87, 89–91, 112

homosexual 53, 87–88, 109

honour killing 101, 155, 209, 213, 215, 241, 243, 245, 255, 274, 387

Hosain, Shahid 389

How to Get Filthy Rich in Rising Asia 7, 49, 54, 307, 312

humour 4, 53, 80–92, 94–95, 97–104, 202, 329; benign 4, 81–82, 84, 91; dark 140; ebullient 82, 388; hybrid 81; ironic 89; irreverent 97; malign 81–83; punch-down 81, 91; push back 82, 84; Rabelaisian 87

human rights 1–5, 74, 123, 127, 129–130, 133–135, 138–147, 246

Huntington, Samuel P 116, 118–120, 123

Hussein, Aamer 3, 28–29, 227, 339, 367, 383, 385

Hussein, Abdullah 385, 389–390

Hutcheon, Linda 120

Hybrid Tapestries 23, 335, 384

hybridity 44, 54, 60, 229, 278, 281, 336, 362, 371

hypersexual 160

I am Malala 145–146, 162, 172–177, 179–180

Ice-Candy Man 24

idealism 83, 132, 243, 315, 328

Identity: crisis 4, 35, 82, 140, 236, 254, 265, 277, 282, 309, 365, 374; cultural 35, 151, 158, 280, 338, 361; diasporic 275; formation 4, 37, 59, 275, 280, 282, 385; Muslim 8, 22, 29, 174, 194, 200, 261, 267, 271, 335–336, 339, 344, 361, 364, 366–368; national 8, 14, 16, 35–37, 228, 265, 274, 325, 337, 351, 360, 362–364, 371; Pakistani 15, 35–36, 44, 64, 129, 134, 141, 206, 253, 342, 361–362, 364, 366–367, 371–374, 376; politics of 131, 134, 285, 325, 338, 361; religious 17, 241, 267, 368; tribal 151–152, 158–161

Imaginary Homelands 280, 373

Imtiaz, Saba 103, 390

In the Name of Honour 145

In Other Rooms, Other Wonders 144–145

India 2, 4, 13, 15–17, 20, 22–23, 26–27, 30–31, 36, 50, 60, 68, 70–72, 77, 88, 143, 154, 157, 214, 216, 227, 275, 278, 288, 298, 300, 303, 319–320, 337, 341, 353, 372, 383, 385–387, 390–391

India Pakistan Nuclear War 69, 73, 76–77, 387

Indus Valley civilisation 300, 302

Invitation 26, 385

Iqbal, Allama Mohammad 376, 383

Iran 92, 144, 166, 249, 353, 383, 387

Iran-Iraq War 387

Iraq 110, 163, 249, 376, 387

Islam Quintet 383, 388

Islamism 159, 196, 262, 267

Islamisation 3, 14, 127, 129, 131, 134, 147, 173, 214, 228, 301, 386–387

Islamophobia 3, 55, 80–82, 94–95, 97, 100, 109–111, 135, 196, 209–210, 236, 267, 386, 388

Islamophobic : attitudes 4; discourse 97; jokes 99; stereotypes 388, 236; verbal abuse 4

Ismail, Aquila 3, 29, 385

Jalal, Ayesha 15–16, 22–23, 35, 68, 361

Jalib, Habib 128

jihad 3, 51, 70, 76, 101, 385–386

jihadist 173, 188, 267, 353, 355

jilbab 98

Jinnah, Muhammad Ali 3, 13–14, 19, 23, 71

jirga 144

Juggernaut 69, 73, 75–77, 287

Kamal, Daud 388–389
Kanwal, Aroosa 8, 132, 173, 240, 361–363, 365, 386
Karachi 20, 22, 26, 28–29, 31, 42, 44, 50, 55, 73, 76, 94, 96–97, 103, 143, 145, 155–156, 158, 229, 230, 263, 288, 314, 316, 324, 336, 386–387, 390
Kartography 3, 25, 31, 42–44, 50, 229, 338, 385–386
Kashmir, 13, 36, 70, 77, 157, 352–354, 385, 387
Khan, Ayub 285, 288
Khan, Ghaffar 158–159
Khan, Liaquat Ali 17
Khan, Nusrat Fateh Ali 207, 217, 276
Khan, Sahabzada Yaqub 22
Khan, Sorayya 3, 14, 16–18, 24–26, 37–39, 40, 42, 385, 389
Khan, Wali 22
Khan, Yahya 22
Khwaja, Waqas Ahmad 335, 374–375, 383, 385
Kohl and Chalk 376
Kumstlerroman 326, 328
Kureishi, Hanif 6–7, 100–101, 110, 112, 200–208, 236, 240, 263, 274, 277–281, 318, 325–327, 329, 388–390
Kureishi, Maki 372, 388

Lahore 16–17, 27, 30, 53–54, 64, 75–76, 187, 189, 213–214, 216–218, 237, 303–306, 301, 336, 338, 344, 349, 376
Leila in the Wilderness 181
life writing(s) 1, 7, 145, 261–262, 267, 271–272
Love in Headscarf 98, 102–103, 264, 269

madrasa(s) 263, 266
magic realism 40, 128, 319–325, 356
Mai, Mukhtar (Mukhtaran) 5, 145, 162, 168–169, 365
Making of Mr Hai's Daughter: Becoming British 7, 262, 268, 285
Malak, Amin 364
Malik, Ayisha 4, 94, 388
Mamdani, Mahmood 365
Manchester 264
Maps for Lost Lovers 6, 7, 201, 206–211, 213–217, 219, 236, 240, 274–277, 282, 285, 338, 384
Marcuse, Herbert 325–328
marginalisation 30, 129, 155
Martyrs and Marigolds 29, 385
masculinist: history 6; ideologies 6, 185; melancholia 186; postcolonialism 6
Masoor, Mehr Nigar 29–31, 385
McCarthy, Dermot 381
Meatless Days 27, 385, 387
Mecca 261, 269, 271
media 7, 23, 28, 38, 51, 60, 62, 65, 98, 103–104, 112–113, 116, 118–121, 123, 139, 144–145, 156–157, 172–173, 175, 177, 186, 200, 225, 248, 257, 261, 276, 286, 299, 327, 335, 337, 339, 391
Mehta, Deepa 390

melancholia 6, 186, 191
Memory of Love 24
memoir(s) 5, 27, 29, 98, 102, 138, 145–147, 162–163, 168, 172–180, 201, 204–207, 261–262, 264, 266, 268–269, 285, 287
Mernissi, Fatima 111, 250
metropolitan: audiences 8, 348, 351–353, 357; cultures 348, 357; habitus 357; market 8, 343, 348–350; readers 8, 173, 348, 354–355
Middle East 118, 174, 386–387
Midnight's Children 31, 87, 118, 351
migrancy 362, 364
migration 3, 7, 14–16
mimicry 60, 278, 285, 342
Mir-Hosseini, Ziba 254–255
misogyny 90, 190–192, 195, 388
mobility 7, 13–15, 19, 108, 285, 289–290, 301, 327, 329, 336, 375
modernism 7, 215, 318–323, 325
Modood, Tariq 285–286, 365
Mohammad, Munir 69, 76, 387
Mohammed, Hanif 3–5, 49, 80, 128, 236, 349, 367, 386–389
Mohsin, Moni 25–26, 213, 385
Moore, Lindsey 215
Morey, Peter 8, 64, 66, 119, 123, 200, 361, 363–365
Moth Smoke 30, 53–54, 69–70, 75–76, 213–217, 219
Mueenuddin, Daniyal 2, 140, 144, 145, 336, 339, 344, 349
muhajir 31
mujahideen 51, 60, 144
Mukti Bahini 24, 30–31
mullah 132, 179
multiculturalism 7, 204, 239, 289, 291–292, 325
Murder of Aziz Khan 127, 320, 385
Musharraf, Pervez 23
muslimness 186
My Feudal Lord 390
My Son the Fanatic 201, 390

Naqvi, H. M. 4, 80, 112, 386, 388
narrative perspective 307–310, 314, 316
narrative structure 310
National Identities in Pakistan 23, 372
nationalism 28–29, 55, 74, 110, 127, 134, 234, 272, 311, 365, 384
nationhood 14, 337, 348, 372
Native Believer 6, 189–191, 195
nazm 374
Nehru, Jawahar Lal 17
neo-colonial 60
Night of Power 262, 267
niqab 98, 166
No One Waits for the Train 375, 385
nomadism 153–154, 159, 281
nomadology 151, 275, 280
North Waziristan 155–157

nuclear: age 69, 75; bomb 69, 73–74, 76; club 68, 77; detonation 69, 73; explosion 73, 217; fiction 73, 382, 387; *jihad* 76; *jihadis* 70, 77; novel 4, 69–71; power 71; question 69–70; tests 31, 71–72, 75–76, 214, 303; thrillers 69, 76–78; war 69, 73, 76–78, 387; weapons 68–72, 75, 142

Of Martyrs and Marigolds 29, 385
Omar, Kalim 388–389
orientalism 116, 155, 163
otherness 3, 31, 188, 196, 198, 276, 340, 343, 344, 368
Our Lady of Alice Bhatti 55, 144, 387

Pakistani idiom 1, 8, 370–377, 382–383
Pakistaniat 8, 370–374, 376–378
Pakistaniness 1, 370–373
Parachinar 157
Parsee 237–238, 245
Partition 2–4, 14–15, 17–18, 24, 28–29, 31–32, 36–37, 40, 50, 69, 71, 74, 89, 127, 143, 155, 319–320, 325, 336, 372, 375, 377, 382, 385–387, 390
Pasha, Kamran 4, 116, 123
Pashtun 144, 152, 154–160, 172–175, 300
Pashtunwali 144
Passarola Rising 388
pastiche 234, 322
pastoral 154–155, 266
pastoralism 154
patriarchy 25, 145, 165, 209–210, 225, 233, 242, 255, 351, 357, 388
performativity of faith 194
Peshawar 158, 298, 300, 386
Phillips, Maha Khan 103, 386, 389
phoenix 5, 162–163, 168–170
pluralism 127, 142, 164
Postmaster 14, 15
postmemory generation 3, 37–38, 40, 43
postmodernism 120, 215
post-postcolonial 7, 297–299, 305, 307
progressivist 151–152, 158–159, 160
propaganda 19, 23, 24, 175, 205, 212
Psychoraag 7, 274
psychosexual 189
Punjabi 14, 26, 28, 30, 32–33, 55, 206, 265, 276, 337, 373, 377, 383

qaafiyaa 374, 376
qawwali 207, 373
The Qur'an 89, 127–128, 192, 194, 231–232, 254–255, 267–268

racism 4, 42–44, 63, 84, 95–97, 109–110, 209, 250, 329, 387
Rafat, Taufiq 370–375, 383, 388
Rahman, Sheikh Mujibur 22–23

realism 5, 7, 127–128, 193, 214–216, 219, 319–325
refugee(s) 15–16, 31, 83, 197, 249, 323
Reluctant Fundamentalist 6–7, 49, 54–55, 58–61, 66, 68, 141, 187–190, 194, 307, 309–311, 370–375, 383, 388
Riaz, Fehmida 225, 227–228, 234
Rohina, Malik 107
romance 5–6, 86, 103, 151, 215, 219, 225–231, 233–34, 388
Roy, Arundhati 78, 341
Rubai 374
Rushdie Affair 262
Rushdie, Salman 35, 49, 91, 97, 118, 128, 280, 321, 335, 351, 385, 387

Said, Edward 116, 155, 163, 318, 355, 360
Said, Yunus 389
Salih, Tayeb 185, 186
Satanic Verses 97, 200, 201
Saudi Arabia 2, 134, 298, 355
Scatter Here is Too Great 7, 307, 312, 314
Season of Migration 6, 185–190, 195–197
Season of the Rainbirds 14, 18, 338, 386
sectarianism 4
Sethi, Ali 386–387
sex 6, 70, 75, 92, 101, 104, 130, 191, 197, 200–203, 205–207, 211, 216, 218, 237, 243, 245, 251–253, 377
sexuality 6, 108, 159, 160, 201, 204, 207, 210, 214, 216, 218, 225, 233, 238, 244–245, 248, 250–253, 255, 280, 326
Shades 108–109, 112, 251–253
Shadow of the Swords 4, 116, 120, 123
Shadows of Time 29, 31, 385
Shah, Bina 339
Shah, Sonia 389
Shah Nawaz, Mumtaz 385
Shahraz, Qaisra 6, 225, 229, 234, 236, 341–342, 388, 390
Shame 35, 91, 128, 129, 351, 385, 387
Shamsie, Kamila 3, 5, 6, 37, 42, 49, 69, 129, 140, 151, 173, 185, 214, 225, 236, 297, 336, 343–344, 362, 385–386
Shamsie, Muneeza 3, 20, 127, 237, 335, 339, 371, 383, 384, 389
Sharia Law 89, 127, 134–135, 144
Sialkot 372
Siddique, John 374, 377–378
Sidhwa, Bapsi 6, 15, 24, 37, 185, 228, 236, 336, 385, 388, 390
silence 5, 24, 26, 28, 38, 42–43, 65, 128–135, 179, 228, 231, 268, 303, 373, 377
Sindhi 44, 231, 233, 337
Singh, Khushwant 15, 24
Sofia Khan is Not Obliged 94, 96–98, 102, 388
Soviet Union 20, 236
Soviet-Afghan war 60, 143

Soviets 52, 134
space(s) 3, 6–7, 14–16, 18, 40, 100, 133, 143, 151, 159–160, 175–176, 179, 186, 192–194, 217–218, 228–230, 233–234, 236, 240–243, 245, 261–272, 274–282, 289, 291, 299–300, 302, 305, 324, 336, 349, 357, 363, 371, 377, 386, 391; aesthetic 53; cultural 276–277; of diaspora 7, 274–276, 282, 287–288; domestic 18, 102, 240, 269, 271; female 159; of female subjectivity 6; fictional 215–216; geographical 18, 40, 322; identity and 7, 26, 274; Islamic 7, 261, 264, 266, 268–269, 271–272; liminal 36, 236, 278; lived 3, 14–15; matrimonial 6, 236; migratory 229; and mobility 7, 19; Muslim 270; nomadic 153; personal 277; political 234; postcolonial 274; private 18, 41, 262; public 160, 228, 265, 268, 324; religious 7, 262, 267–269, 272; sacred 271; social 7, 160, 215, 239, 262; smooth 151–153, 156–157, 160; third 81, 281, 365, 371; transnational 230; of worship 261
spatial 4, 13–14, 16–17, 19, 49, 64, 155, 230, 262, 265, 267, 269, 275–278, 280–282, 291, 300, 355, 357
Spivak, Gayatri 98, 130, 289, 292, 367, 371
stereotypes 2, 4, 54, 61, 81, 95–99, 101, 116, 121, 127, 160, 175, 187, 192–193, 236, 239, 252, 281, 351, 353–356, 366, 383, 388
Story of a Widow 213
subaltern 5, 7, 118, 129–132, 135, 145, 188, 286, 291, 367
subalternity 298, 302
subcontinent 13, 17, 36, 50, 71–73, 75, 139, 158, 201, 207, 214–215, 303, 305, 381, 387
subjectivity: female 6, 175; human 298–299, 304, 365; Islamic 98; Muslim 6, 213, 262; Pakistani 308; worldly 213
Sufi: aesthetics 201, 207; literature 208; music 207; mysticism 384; perspective 206; poetry 217; *qawwalis* 207; *qissa* 207, 209; saints 208; shrines 355; singer 276; tradition 383
Sufiana kalam 207
Sufism 207, 210–211, 383
Suhayl, Saadi 7, 274, 383
Suhrawardy, Shahid 388
Suleri, Sara 3, 27, 371–372, 374, 385, 387–388
Suxavat tribe 320, 322–323
symbolic capital 290, 292
Syria 2, 118, 120, 255

talaq 209, 242
Taliban 86, 107, 144, 157, 162, 165, 169, 172, 173, 176–179
Tanweer, Bilal 7, 307, 339, 387
Tarik, Salman 388–389
terrorism 1, 3–4, 51, 73, 82, 84–85, 116, 142–143, 165, 214, 272, 337, 339, 344, 351, 387, 391
terrorist(s) 54, 60–61, 66, 82, 85–86, 95, 107, 110–111, 144, 156, 164–165, 173, 196, 312, 314, 340, 353, 361, 363, 386
thumri 374
Train to Pakistan 15
transnationalism 143, 153, 362, 366
Trespassing 341, 385–387, 390
Triple Mirror of the Self 319–325
Twilight 6, 236–223, 245
Typhoon 341, 388

ummah 128, 131, 262, 266, 269, 365
uncanny 25, 82, 323, 385
unveiled 63, 107
Upstairs Wife: An Intimate History of Pakistan 388

Wandering Falcon 143, 151–153, 339–340
war on terror 3, 5, 51, 54, 60, 73, 75, 110, 123, 138–146, 155, 157–158, 164–165, 167, 173, 175–176, 180, 267, 298, 306, 310, 338–339, 344, 363–364, 385–387
Wasted Vigil 141, 338, 384, 386
We are a Muslim, Please 7, 262, 267
West Pakistan 3, 13, 22–23, 29–32, 37–38, 40–42
Without Dreams 25–26, 37, 385
World Trade Centre 110, 309, 339
writing back 5, 141, 172, 175–176, 180, 344, 381, 386

xenophobia 236, 238, 241

Yaqin, Amina 61–62, 119, 123, 200, 288, 361
Yaqub-Khan, Sahabzada 22
Yousafzai, Malala 5, 145, 162–163, 166, 168–169, 172–180
Yusuf, Ilona 297, 302–303, 305, 374

Zameenzad, Adam 27–28, 385
Zeest Hashmi, Shadaab 374–376, 383
Zia-ul-Haq 51, 52, 86–87, 127, 216, 228
Zoberi, Zohra 374–376

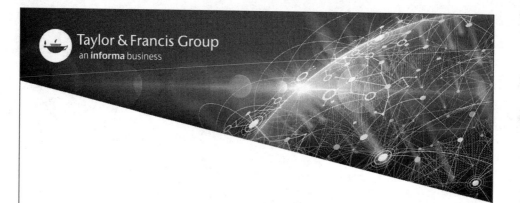